Sleep Mechanisms and Functions

in humans and animals — an evolutionary perspective

The Comparative Psychology of Animals and Humans

Series Editor: Professor W. Sluckin, University of Leicester

The comparative perspective — viewing animals and human beings side by side — is best suited to a range of topics within psychology. The nature/nurture issue has traditionally been considered in this way, and more narrowly circumscribed areas of study, such as conditioning, have for a long time been investigated in animals as well as in humans. In more recent times, developments in the related fields of ethology and sociobiology have focused attention on the comparative approach to selected psychological topics.

The aim of this series is to produce books dealing in a comparative manner with a variety of topics. The multiple authorship of each book ensures a thorough and in-depth coverage of the topic, while at the same time great care is taken that the chapters cohere according to an overall structure provided by the book's editor. Each volume is under the separate editorship of a specialist in the given field. All the books review and evaluate research in the respective fields, and give an up-to-date summary of the present state of knowledge.

Sluckin	Fear in animals and man
Colman	Cooperation and Competition in humans and animals
Archer & Birke	Exploration in animals and humans
Mayes	Memory in animals and humans
Mayes	Sleep Mechanisms and Functions in humans and animals

Sleep Mechanisms and Functions

in humans and animals — an evolutionary perspective

Edited by

Andrew Mayes

Department of Psychology
Manchester University

VNR (UK) Van Nostrand Reinhold (UK) Co. Ltd.

Published by Van Nostrand Reinhold (UK) Co. Ltd.
Molly Millars Lane, Wokingham, Berkshire, England

Library of Congress Cataloging in Publication Data

Main entry under title:

Sleep mechanisms and functions in humans and animals.

(The comparative psychology of animals and humans)
Includes index.
1. Sleep—Physiological aspects—Addresses, essays, lectures. 2. Evolution—Addresses, essays, lectures. 3. Sleep—Psychological aspects—Addresses, essays, lectures. I. Mayes, Andrew Richard. II. Series.
[DNLM: 1. Sleep. WL 108 S631]
QP425.S676 1983 156′.4 83-6935
ISBN 0-442-30540-0

Printed in Great Britain at the University Press, Cambridge

Preface

The chapters in this book provide a comprehensive view of our knowledge about sleep. This knowledge is changing and developing very rapidly, partly because of the dramatic increase in sleep research which has been continuous since the 1950s. This increase has been associated with, and probably stimulated by, the introduction of new techniques and approaches. Techniques, which have been refined in the past few years, include single unit recording from identified neurons in behaving animals and the spectral analysis of EEG, aided by relatively cheap computer technology. New approaches have included attempts to analyse sleep in different mammalian species and see how sleep parameters relate to constitutional and ecological factors, and to study sleep as a periodic activity which interacts with other periodic processes. Knowledge derived from these new techniques and approaches has sometimes upset confidence in strongly supported hypotheses. For example, many hypotheses of the 1960s and 1970s about the nature of slow-wave and active sleep mechanisms now seem untenable, and researchers now assert restorative theories about sleep's function in a much more qualified fashion as a result of the influence of ethological ideas. As the functions of sleep are adaptations to evolutionary pressures, several chapters in this book lay stress on comparisons of sleep in species facing different environmental pressures. It is hoped that the identified relationship of sleep processes to environmental factors will illuminate their possible functions and, to a lesser extent, their mechanisms.

To convey an impression of this rapidly changing picture, there are chapters on rhythmical aspects of sleep, on sleep phylogeny (with a complete bibliography of sleep studies on all animal groups), sleep ontogeny, sleep mechanisms (both physiological and biochemical), sleep functions, dreaming, and the final chapter, briefly considers research arising from the recent taxonomy of sleep disorders. In the introductory chapter, Bernie Webb sets the scene with a brief history of modern sleep research which focuses on the major discoveries such as the distinction between active and quiet sleep. He then outlines theories of sleep functions which have guided contemporary research. The theories are divided into two groups: restorative and behavioural. Webb indicates their differences and then points out that as sleep is complex, it may have both restorative and behavioural functions.

This last theme of Webb's is taken up by several contributors to the book and developed by them. In his chapter on sleep as a biological rhythm, Ken Hume argues that whereas active sleep (or REM) follows a circadian periodicity, amounts of slow wave sleep are determined by length of previous wakefulness. Both he and Webb refer to Borbély's theory that the sleep–wake system is controlled by a combination of a circadian oscillator and a self-regulatory process. Alex Borbély develops this theory in the context of biochemical mechanisms, in his chapter on pharmacological approaches to sleep. The same theme is also returned to by Jim Horne in his detailed discussion of the possible functions of sleep. His distinction between obligatory and facultative forms of sleep fits well with Borbély's theory, as obligatory sleep is controlled by a self-regulatory process whereas facultative sleep is more influenced by circadian factors. Finally, Ray Meddis in his chapter on sleep's evolution, shows that quiet sleep (slow wave sleep) and active sleep times in mammals are only weakly associated, which suggests that they are determined by unrelated influences. Whether these two aspects of sleep serve different functions remains to be proved however.

The ontogeny of sleep provides a window on sleep mechanisms and functions as these emerge gradually and slowly disintegrate. This is one of the areas which has benefited by the use of more sophisticated recording and analysing techniques. Ronald Harper, Zehava Frostig and David Taube review the rapid changes in sleep patterns which occur in the first sixth months of full-term infants. They also describe how developmental abnormalities in these indices may be related to disorders such as the sudden infant death syndrome. Harold Zepelin then gives a careful account of how sleep changes across the life span and initially assesses what these changes reveal about sleep mechanisms and functions.

Three chapters review recent advances in our understanding of the mechanisms which control sleep. Mircea Steriade describes his exciting work which relates activity in midbrain reticular formation neurons to wakefulness and active sleep. This is a case where modern techniques have confirmed and extended earlier beliefs, which had been neglected until recently. In contrast, Steriade casts doubt on the popular view that there are active, sleep-producing mechanisms in the brain stem, when he concludes that we have returned to something like Bremer's classical deafferentation concept of slow wave sleep generation. Jerome Siegel reviews lesion and recording studies of active sleep control and shows how the two approaches complement each other. His work with colleagues, using single unit recording from moving animals, has itself shown that previous research, purporting to find cells which specifically increased their firing rates in active sleep, was overly simple. Most such cells also increase their firing when there is movement in the waking state — they are probably high-level motor control neurons. In his chapter on sleep pharmacology, Alex Borbély considers the effects of benzodiazepines, antidepressants and serotonin depletion on sleep and the search of endogenous sleep substances, before relating such work to his two-process model.

In his chapter on dreaming, David Foulkes develops a very interesting argument about whether animals other than humans dream. His sceptical conclusion is reached after assessing the available 'suggestive' data on animals and the cognitive requirements of dreaming in intact adults. The argument is also developed in relation to his own recent research on the ontogeny of dreaming in children, which seems to indicate that non-human animals lack the cognitive equipment to dream in the fully human sense. Andrew Mayes briefly highlights some of the main themes of the book in his final chapter, and outlines the recent taxonomy of sleep disorders. Work, associated with this taxonomy, is discussed by Hume, Harper, Frostig and Taube, Zepelin and Borbély, as well as in the final chapter.

Sleep functions are still matters for speculation. Sleep mechanisms have not yet been fully elucidated and the course of sleep evolution is highly controversial. Readers must hold these fundamental uncertainties constantly in mind. This book depicts a stage of knowledge which is nevertheless an exciting one in resolving these important uncertainties.

Contents

CHAPTER 1

Theories in Modern Sleep Research

Wilse B. Webb

This introductory chapter is about theories of sleep. It may seem a bit odd to begin a book with theories, but Immanuel Kant stated a most reasonable dictum many years ago: 'Concepts without factual content are empty . . . data without concepts are blind. By their union only can knowledge be produced'.

This book will present, in detail, the selected observations on contemporary sleep research. These have been generated by the individual interests and the decisions of researchers. These, in turn, have arisen from a wide variety of training backgrounds and have been modulated by technological developments, the availability of funds and choice determinants (Webb, 1961).

The concern of this chapter, however, is with the conceptual schema or theories about sleep. Since one of the prime purposes and uses of theories is that of coordinating and explaining data, it is to be hoped that this approach may lend perspective to or serve as an overview of the chapters that follow.

In order that these schema should not be totally abstract and 'empty' the first section is a skeletal outline of the prominent features of the development of sleep research. The final section explores the theories which have arisen to coordinate these emerging data.

1.1 Contemporary Sleep Research

Attempts to comprehend the nature and role of sleep have an ancient and honourable history. Aristotle wrote on sleep and dreams in his *De Natura*. The Hippocratic writings included the manifestations of sleep and their implications.

Early systematic research, however, essentially parallels the development of life science research which began to emerge in the 1800s. Table 1.1 provides estimates of the number of papers published annually on sleep. These were derived from the comprehensive references in Pieron's *Le Problème Psychologique du Sommiel* (1913), Kleitman's revision of his 1939 *Sleep and Wakefulness* (1963) and publications of the Brain Research Institute which has annually published yearly annual bibliographies of sleep research since 1968 (Brain Research Institute, 1968–1980), as well as a bibliography covering the years 1963–1967 (Rechtschaffen & Eakins, 1968). It is clear from this table that there was a slow steady growth in sleep research papers up to 1950 which may parallel the general growth in scientific literature. However, it is also clear that an emergent and highly active programme of contemporary sleep research began in the 1950s and 1960s, and it has shown a remarkable accelerated growth.

The recency of the contemporary research era permits some understanding

Table 1.1 Yearly Averages of Cited References

Pieron	Kleitman	Brain Information Service
*1801 - 1820 = 0.5	*1921 - 1930 = 44	*1963 - 1967 = 450
1821 - 1840 = 1	1931 - 1940 = 95	1968 - 1972 = 648
1841 - 1860 = 4	1941 - 1950 = 72	1972 - 1977 = 1418
1881 - 1910 = 21	1951 - 1960 = 180	1978 - 1980 = 1892

* Note different yearly groupings.

of the dynamics. From the 1920s there was a period of rapidly accelerating research on the functions of the central nervous system by cutting pathways, removing sections and electrically stimulating parts of the brain. For sleep research, a climax was reached in 1949 when the Italian researcher, Moruzzi, working with Magoun in the United States, demonstrated the role of the reticular activating system at the base of the brain in the maintenance of attention and activity. It seemed that the 'waking centre' had been found.

Earlier a critical development had occurred. While exploring the uses and characteristics of the electroencephalographic (EEG) measures of the ever-changing electrical potential of the brain, clear and specific changes associated with sleep were noted in the late 1930s by several investigators. A coding of these changes was published by Loomis, Hobart and Harvey in the *Journal of Experimental Psychology* in 1937. Not only could sleep be seen to be a highly active and dynamic process, but also it could now be measured continuously and objectively.

The seminal paper of the modern sleep research period can be specifically cited. While further exploring the meaning of the EEG measures, Nathaniel Kleitman and his student, Eugene Aserinsky, reported on the spontaneous and intermittent appearance of an 'activated' EEG pattern resembling wakefulness associated with rapid eye movements (REM). Their paper, 'Regularly occurring periods of eye motility and concomitant phenomena during sleep', was published in *Science* in 1953. One of the 'concomitant phenomena' was dream recall! They had quickly established that awakening from this period resulted in a high probability of dream recall (20 of 27 occasions) and a low probability of dream recall on awakening at other times (4 of 23 occasions).

The discovery was surrounded by good fortune. Kleitman was certainly an appropriate midwife. He was fully prepared by a lifetime of devotion to sleep research. He had published his first paper on sleep in 1923 and published his landmark book *Sleep and Wakefulness* in 1939. Most critically he was joined by a young colleague at Chicago — William Dement. Dement was quick to see the importance of the REM period of sleep and in rapid succession he examined REM periods in schizophrenics in 1955, with Kleitman described a new coding schema to include REM sleep in 1957, and reported on the presence of activated sleep in the cat in 1958. By 1960 he had conducted REM sleep deprivation experiments with humans.

Meanwhile an intensive exploration of the neurophysiology of REM sleep had begun. Moruzzi had returned from Magoun's laboratory to Pisa and had begun a series of publications about the reticular activating system. Reports on a 'paradoxical' sleep in cats, characterized by an activated central nervous state during sleep, and its correlative relations to the reticular area of the brain were soon forthcoming from Moruzzi's laboratory in the early 1960s. Michael Jouvet, a French neurologist, had also studied with Magoun in California. He returned to Lyons in 1956 and began work on habituation of responses in the brain to test Pavlov's theories about the role of the cortex in learning. He did this by studying chronically decorticated cats. During long-term recording he noticed a strange phenomenon. Even without a cortex the cats were showing an alternative pattern of activity in the brain! Recording normal cats, it was seen that there was indeed, within sleep, a period of high cortical activity with a loss of muscle tonus and eye movements. It was evident that there was an activated sleep very different from the rest of sleep and the mechanism 'had to be triggered by a structure located in the lower brain stem'. This led to an elegant series of experiments in the late 1950s and early 1960s which precisely located structures in the pontine reticular formation which controlled REM sleep.

Research on the nature of the cognitive content of dreams and the implications of its association with the REM state were accelerated. Between 1955 and 1956 there were at least 18 studies reporting on the differential character of recall from REM and non-REM sleep. By 1966 Foulkes had published his book, *The Psychology of Sleep*, which was focused on the REM–dream relationship. Human and animal REM deprivation experiments became widespread. The presence and character of REM or activated sleep in neonates and an increasing range of species were measured.

By the mid-1960s the research area had become a lively one. An association with an annual meeting had been formed (the Association for the Psychophysiological Study of Sleep). Books had begun to appear, e.g. Oswald's *Sleep and Dreaming* (1962), Kleitman's revised *Sleep and Wakefulness* (1963), *Sleep and Altered States of Consciousness* (1965), *Sleep Mechanisms* (1965).

As were the earlier pioneers in sleep research, the participants in the area were drawn from a wide range of primary disciplines: neuroscientists, pediatricians, psychiatrists, pharmacologists, engineers, animal behaviourists, physiologists and psychologists. The multi-disciplinary presence reflected the wide range of interests and skills directed towards the comprehension of sleep.

Table 1.2 summarizes the extended nature of sleep research and some of its dynamics. Three years have been selected from the Annual Bibliography of world-wide sleep research published by the Brain Research Institute. The categories used are those coded in this bibliography. Clearly the range of research interests are broad; from single nerve cell firings to dream content, from endocrinology to sleep deprivation effects, from biochemistry correlates to sleep disorders, from pharmacology to biological rhythms.

Significant shifts in interest can be seen between 1968 and 1977 which are affirmed by a continuation of this trend between 1977 and 1980. The year 1968 was perhaps the peak of laboratory-centered research and much of that research focused on the search for the neurophysiological bases for REM sleep and for behavioural correlates of REM deprivation. Both of these areas showed sharp declines between 1968 and 1977 and continue to decline in relative emphasis. (It should be noted that due to the rise in absolute numbers of publications from 542 in 1968 to 1904 in 1977 that there has, in fact, been a slight rise in the absolute number of articles (142 vs. 150) in the neurophysiological area.) On the other hand there has been a significant rise in the clinical area (personality,

Table 1.2

Subject matter	1968	1977	1980	Advances and declines
Neurophysiology	26	14	8	– 12
Physiology	5	5	6	
Biochemistry*		4	5	
Pharmacology*	(17)***	13	12	+ 4
Endocrinology*		4	5	
Infancy & ageing	3	7	8	+ 4
Animal sleep	2	2	2	
Dream content	3	4	4	
Personality, patholody & disorders of sleep	22	26	27	+ 4
Sleep deprivation	7	3	2	– 4
Instrumentation	1	3	3	
Biological rhythms*		6	6	
Less than 3% each (books and reviews, hypnosis and altered states, electrosleep, behaviour correlates, external stimuli, etc.)				

* Not differentiated in 1968.
*** Three categories combined in 1968.

pathology and disorders) and in the areas of biochemistry, pharmacology, endocrinology and infancy and ageing. Finally, the coding of articles under the category of Biological Rhythms is a significant development.

The meaning of these shifts cannot be certainly ascertained. Midst one's own time perspective it is hard to come by the meaning of great battles. An historic moment is usually understood, not by the participants of that time, but in elegant retrospective and global interpretations of historians. Do we attribute the decline in neurophysiological research to a waning of funds, or, as Jouvet suggests, the grand discoveries have been made and we approach the more wearisome and less attractive research of 'backing and filling'? Has the driving force behind REM research faded before unproven relevance or our failures of ingenuity? Does increased emphasis on clinical problems and the blossoming of Sleep Clinics reflect an increased body of applicable knowledge, pressures of rising public interest or economic sensibility? Is the conception of sleep as a biorhythm a meaningful schema, a passing precept or a response to practical problems of shift work, jet lag, cyclical sleep disturbances and the sleep/waking interface? Indeed, is the present scene and its variations more than another transition of interests towards an unknown end?

If uncertainty lies in understanding a current time, even greater uncertainty lies in prescience about the future. However, a few guesses seem reasonable. The need to know about and to use information about sleep has become an irrevocable part of the future. Chronic and acute sleep disturbances are pervasive. More than 70 million dollars are spent on prescription sedatives each year. Any one night millions and millions will struggle with their sleep. The Edison world of 24 hours of potential light has ripped away sleep's cocoon of darkness and cut sleep loose to float in a world of shiftwork and continuous entertainment. Airplanes toss sleep across time zones. Sleep, stubbornly defending its existence, needs all the help it can get.

Research has been and is building a solid foundation of facts. The neurophysiological mapping approaches completion and the assault on the biochemical secrets continue apace. Disorders of sleep — disturbances of sleep's fundamental mechanisms, such as seen in narcolepsy — are now viewed more clearly and more certainly. New relations between sleep and other life-systems have become more apparent, as seen in apneas — respiratory disturbances in sleep. Sleep's place in time and its relations to its surround are being described. The deviations and variations are better known. The search for the magical control by drugs is intensive. The topography, landscape and laws of the dark kingdom become more apparent. Whether we will become better citizens thereof increasingly becomes a choice to be made.

And the dreams? Nearly 80 years ago Freud wrote, rather fretfully, as he began to interpret the dream: 'the scientific theories of dreams leave no room for any problem of interpreting them, since in their view a dream is not a mental act at all, but a somatic process signalizing its occurrence by indication registered in the mental apparatus.' The discovery of the conjunctive relation of the somatic signal — REM — and the presence of the cognitive state of dreaming joined signal and significance inextricably. This cannot help but bring us closer to finally deciphering the measuring of that rich mysterious and intricate domain.

What may not be apparent in this brief overview of sleep research is that it has been almost fiercely empirical. This was noted in 1963 'sleep research has been almost exclusively atheoretical in its general approach and has been diligently devoted to the collection of empirical facts. No one can object to gathering in empirical data [but] data gathering in absence of theory or concepts may result in a mound of facts which often miss ultimate causes and effects or indeed may even bury them (Webb, 1968)'.

Oversimplified, the field has devoted itself primarily to descriptions of what happened to electrophysiological defined sleep as a function of variations in the central nervous system resulting from surgical, chemical and biochemical interventions, ageing, species variations, physical disorders, time schedules; the description of the concomitants of sleep such as threshold changes, dreams, and physiological measures; the consequences of sleep loss and stage deprivations.

This should be neither surprising nor humiliating. In the earlier cited source, it was noted that 'there is good reason for this state of affairs'. In the first place sleep research emerged piecemeal for many disparate interests and disciplines and still reflects this. It has never been a central concept within any one discipline. Further, sleep research is indeed young and its facts are only beginning to emerge. There is in research the alternative caveat. 'Theorizing without sound data is an equally futile exercise' (Webb, 1968).

However, explanatory constructs did begin to emerge. Since the data base was almost exclusively focused on the REM state throughout the 1960s it is not surprising that these constructs were attempts to explain or conceptualize these phenomena. We will briefly review these before turning to our primary concern — the more general theories about sleep.

1.2 Theories of Dream

We confine ourselves to those models emerging in the 1960s in response to the experimental data associated with REM sleep. In general there were four such models: psychodynamic, homeostatic, memory and learning processing, and restoration.

The psychodynamic models were essentially extensions of the Freudian concept of a 'drive discharge' model in which dreaming permitted a discharge or release of instinctual drive held in check by the preconsciousness. This appears to be the concept underlying Dement's early experimentations which 'Blocked' (deprived) the subject of REM (dreams) with the resultant appearance of personality disturbances and enhanced drive levels in deprived subjects. This concept was elaborately discussed by Fisher (1965).

The homeostatic model was introduced by Ephron and Carrington (1966). This conceived of sleep as a sharply reduced level of cortical functioning which must be 'offset' by cortical excitation associated with REM sleep. Roffwarg, Muzio and Dement (1966) 'explained' the large amount of REM sleep in neonates (over 50%) as a necessary endogenous stimulation for the development of the cortex in the long-sleeping and sensorily deprived infant.

Three variants of this endogenous stimulation model were posed. Snyder (1967), basing his observations on lower animals, proposed a 'sentinel' role of REM as it periodically activated the animal to monitor the environment during the period of reduced vigilance of sleep. Berger (1969) proposed a REM function in maintaining binocular vision efficiency. Hawkins (1966) suggested that REM periodic events were needed to pattern regularly recathexis (combining the psychodynamic and biological stimulation theories).

The earliest learning memory models were 'computer analogy' models (Evans & Newman, 1965; Gaader, 1966; Dewan, 1970). These proposed various 'programmings', 'consolidations', 'reprogramming' and 'clearing' processes during REM sleep.

The later learning 'theories' could be conceived of as 'miniature theories' developed to account for the complex and often conflicting experimental studies of learning and retention. The most consistent of these has been that of Greenberg and Pearlman who have suggested a selective role of dealing with the integration of 'new' and 'unprepared' material within the personality of the person (1978). A detailed review of the studies of REM and memory functions may be found in Fishbein and Gutwein (1977).

Finally, there is the restoration concept, i.e. during REM sleep daytime 'wear and tear' is endogenously 'repaired'. Morruzzi (1966) presents an elaborate discussion of such a proposition relative to the neurons or synapases which are associated with 'learning and conditioning'. Hartmann (1973), drawing together a wide range of data, concludes that 'D-sleep (REM) could function in the restoration concept perhaps by means of synaptic rebuilding, using macromolecules previously synthesized of the catecholamine-dependent systems which play a role in psychological mechanisms including attention, secondary processes and guidance during waking' (p. 150).

We shall now turn to theories about sleep. A significant lunge forward relative to coordinative theories about sleep occurred with the publication of Hartmann's *The Functions of Sleep* (1973). While his book was primarily concerned with the role of D-sleep (REM), he unequivocally hypothesized the role of sleep as being a 'restorative' one. In his book he points out that 'In sleep research, as in other areas of scientific inquiry, *why* is often the first question asked and the last question answered, or left unanswered' (p. 3). As we shall see some efforts are being made to amend this gloomy state.

1.3 Theories of Sleep

Kleitman, in *Sleep and Wakefulness* (1963), points to Pieron's division of sleep theories into 'partial' and 'complete' theories. Complete theories are those which attempt to 'account for the existence of the sleep-wakefulness cycle itself, for the necessity of sleep'. Partial theories are those which explain 'not why but how one falls to sleep (and) are often content to elucidate the mechanism of change from wakefulness to sleep' (p. 341). Kleitman further notes that, 'Complete theories usually also account for the partial theory'.

Partial theories are not at issue. The search for the mechanism — or 'how' — of sleep should and will continue along various dimensions, e.g. neurochemistry, neurophysiological, developmental, temporal. This data will coordinate circumscribed areas in various languages and be responsive and changing relative to new findings. Our concern is with the 'complete theories' — those schema whose intent has been to explain the presence or the 'why' of sleep.

An earlier review (Webb, 1979) divided the extant theories of sleep somewhat arbitrarily into five groupings:

Restorative theories: Sleep is a period of recovery or restoration of physiological, neurological and/or psychological state (Aristotle, Shakespeare, Hartmann, Oswald).

Protective theories: Sleep protects the organism from excessive wear and tear of the waking state (Claparède, Coriat, Pavlov).

Energy conservation: Sleep serves to conserve or reduce energy expenditure (Rechtschaffen, Berger).

Ethological theories: Sleep is an adaptive behavioural response (Allison, Meddis, Webb).

Instinctive theories: Sleep is an elicited instinctive response (Moruzzi, Meddis, Webb, McGinty).

Within the review (and even more so retrospectively) it was apparent that these groupings were not independent positions. Indeed, in the bare outline presented above one would readily consider the 'energy conservation' concept as a variation or specification of the 'protective' theories and the 'instinctive' theories as a particular form of 'ethological' theories. Indeed, broadly interpreted, both a 'restorative' theoretical position and an 'ethological' position could be said to serve a 'protective' function. Further, within each category, individual theorists escape the designated boundaries, e.g. Pavlov: protective–restorative; Moruzzi: instinctive–partially restorative (neurological not physiological); Allison: energy conservation–ethological; Webb (early) ethological–instinctive.

As noted in that review, we are not without 'theories' at this point. 'Rather than finding ourselves midst a whirl of incoordinate data points without thoughts of their meaning, we are faced with a variety of entangled organizing presumptions about the underlying purposes of sleep. . . . In the face of these dissonances there is certainly a tendency to say "Enough of this idle speculation. Let us return to collecting our facts" ' (p. 28).

We find good grounds for rejecting this position. First it is difficult to believe that this ubiquitous and time-consuming event does not have a purpose. The challenge alone is worth the search. Moreover, it is a 'first question asked'. Stated some 300 years ago by Samuel Johnson: 'No searcher has yet found either the efficient or final cause . . . or what benefits the animal receives from this alternative suspension of its active powers.' Few laymen in their inquiries about sleep fail to include the ultimate question: Why do we sleep? If the sleep researcher does not seek that answer, who is to do so? More critically, whatever the answer — tentative, implicit, correct or incorrect — it contains great power. A theory or conceptualization is a belief and for all men, laymen and scientists alike, beliefs direct behaviour. For the scientist in particular, such beliefs structure his language and communication, provide ideas to pursue and direct his attention toward particular 'causes' and 'effects'.

Although our earlier brief outline of the existing theories of the function of sleep was not encouraging, a further examination indicates the presence of two significantly different approaches to explicating the purpose of sleep. The resultant conceptualizations, while converging in many aspects, continue to have relevant and different constructs. These can be labelled the 'restorative' theories and the 'behavioural' theories.

1.4 Restorative Theories

The restorative theories of sleep can be generally characterized as follows:

Wakefulness (and its associated activities) results in (causes) an internal state which is antithetical to continued wakefulness; sleep results in (causes) the modification of that state (is restorative).

The particular theories differ in the specificity and the designation of the internal state. Specificity ranges from 'getting tired and becoming refreshed' to detailed analyses of cellular energy charges or peptide levels. To capture the flavour of these theories let us consider a few of them.

Certainly one of the oldest is that of Aristotle. He states that 'if (sense perception) continues beyond its appointed time limit . . . it will lose its power, and will do its work no longer'. 'Sleep . . . is a state of powerlessness arising from excess of waking . . . and rising of necessity . . . for the sake of conservation'. He further specifically states 'that the nutrient part does its work better when the animal is asleep than when it is awake. Nutrition and growth are then especially promoted'.

The blossoming life science research of the late 1800s brought forth a number of 'theories' about sleep, most of which were implicitly 'restorative'. These were described elsewhere (Webb, 1975): 'The period extending from 1870 to the 1920s was marked by increasing information about physiology and neurology, and typically these finding became combined into 'grand theories'. These theories took two general forms: 'humoral' theories, in which some toxic substance resulted in the dysfunction of the central nervous system, and 'inhibitory' theories in which the central nervous system (or parts thereof) ceased to function. These 'action' theories of sleep stand in opposition to 'passive' theories which would later attribute sleep to an absence of stimulation. There was a remarkably uniform pattern to the emergence of sleep theories during this period. A new set of findings would be developed about a physiological system and within a few years these findings would serve as an explanatory basis for sleep. For example, as information about the vascular system became available, theories of cerebral anaemia or congestion were put forth as the likely causes of sleep. The most prominent of these theories was that of Mosso in the 1870s.

Information about nerve cells provoked the initial inhibition theories of sleep. These ranged from general theories generated by Darwinian influences and Brown-Sequard's hypothesis, in the late 1880s, that sleep was an inhibitory reflex, to the more specific dendritic theory of Lengendre in the early 1900s that the dendrites retracted in sleep, resulting in reduced functioning. The general increase in information about the central nervous system, combined with his own clinical observations, led Mauthner in 1890 to posit one of the first sleep-centre theories, placing it in the periventricular grey and suggesting a break in the conducting pathways to and from the cerebral cortex.

New data about and interest in haemotology, and in particular oxygen and CO_2 characteristics of the blood, led to a plethora of humoral theories of sleep. Kleitman in *Sleep and Wakefulness* (1963) reviews the humoral theories of sleep, and cites 18 substances which have been suggested as triggers for the sleep process over the years. A new theory seemed to emerge with each new discovery of the biochemical process (p. 341)'.

In the context of this chapter these were not 'grand theories' but 'partial' theories in search of the sleep mechanism. Indeed, Hess (1965), in speaking of the purpose of sleep at a symposium on sleep mechanism in 1964, felt impelled to comment: 'It might be feared that my paper would be purely theoretical and thus superfluous, as giving facts can only advance our understanding . . . [However] it is an illusion to suppose that simple facts have by themselves the power to constitute a theory. It is only the inference based upon them that will advance our viewpoints' (pp. 3–4).

In spite of Hess's wise words the early trends described have been the dominant approach into the present. The empirical explorations of the central nervous system's proximal role in sleep onset continued apace and the increasing emphasis on biochemical approaches here seen a resurgence of 'humoral' 'theories'.

Several authors, however, have explicitly espoused a 'restorative' position. Hess (*op.cit.*) in 'coordinating' his findings and others, concluded that 'Like hunger and thirst, physical and mental fatigue automatically made itself felt. This is the subjective signal that the performance of the individual is no longer up to the external demands made on it . . . With the onset of fatigue a reestablishment of equilibrium is introduced . . . and the explanation can be no other than restorative processes . . . sleep is the expression of a predominance of a trophopic component of the automatic system . . . A question that still remains unanswered is by what means restitution of tissues occurs . . . Oxidative mechanisms can probably be excluded, since they are already regulated during the active phase and immediately afterwards . . . One is led more strongly to consider the compensation of defects in the structural organization, either at the cell membranes or conditions within the cell.' (pp.5–6).

The most recent and extensive statements of the restorative position have been that of Hartmann (1973), Adams and Oswald (1977) and Adams (1980).

While both suggest independent functions of REM sleep, both view a primary sleep function to be 'a time for restoration and repair of the body and the brain'. Specifically stated: 'It appears that the rest/activity cycle of simple organisms and the sleeping/waking rhythm of higher animals induce concomitant fluctuations in cellular work and, hence, in the cellular energy change. As a consequence metabolic balance alters so that degradative processes are inevitably favored during activity' (Adams & Oswald).

1.5 Behavioural Theories

The behavioural theories of sleep ascribe the purpose of sleep as a mode of behavioural adaptation to the environment. They may be generally characterized as follows: sleep is a behavioural state of diminished responsivity. The amount, period lengths, and placement of sleep are species specific endogenously determined tendencies. The purpose of these episodes is to adapt effectively the organism for survival in its particular ecological niche.

We noted that the restorative position has had a long history and, as noted by Hess, has tended to be an atheoretical search for the 'cause-to-be-reversed'. Contrawise the behavioural theories have been more recent*, more speculative, less specific, and more oriented towards distal (evolutionary) causes rather than proximal ones. As such they have enjoyed less attention and, perhaps, suffered less.

A behaviourally derived approach to variations in sleep was stated by Allison & Van Twyer (1970). While the major thrust of this paper was concerned with the evolutionary emergence of 'paradoxical' or 'activated' sleep (REM sleep in animals), they suggested that sleep characteristics may be determined by predator–prey relationships and by the security of the sleep environment. (They also suggested that the function of slow wave sleep was energy conservation.)

Meddis (1975, 1977), specifically rejecting a restorative position, proposed 'that sleep, in conjunction with a sleep instinct and circadian influences, acts to implement a behavioral strategem which is carefully tailored to promote survival' (1975, p. 676). In *Sleep Instinct* (1977) Meddis writes: 'the time spent sleeping by a given species of mammals depends mainly upon the amount of time available for sleep. Across species, at least, the sleeping time appears to expand to fill up an animal's spare time. By spare time it is meant time which is not needed for other essential activities or which, for other reasons, cannot be used for these activities. In this way time can be classified as spare if an animal has already completed all the jobs necessary for survival or if it is too dangerous to carry them out even though they are outstanding needs' (pp. 23–24). As for the purposes of sleep he states: 'The benefits depend, of course, upon the species. For some the conservation of energy is most valuable, for others the

*Recency here excludes such quasi-behavioural theories as that of Pavlov's protective-inhibition theory (clearly derived from behavioural observations) or Claparède's 'biological theory' (1905) that we sleep to prevent exhaustion or the overall psychological notion of 'tiredness' and 'recovery' since all are propaedeutic schema to recovery hypotheses.

protection from predation is paramount, whilst for others the cardinal benefit comes from the timing element which helps them anticipate dramatic changes in the environment'. (pp. 28). He summarizes his position by stating relative to sleep 'enforcement': 'First, it influences an animal to withdraw to safety of a sleep site where it adopts an energy conserving posture. Second, it uses some internal clock arrangement to ensure this withdrawal will occur at a time that is most valuable. Third, by altering the consciousness of the animal, it produces a state of unawareness which helps to keep the animal in its sleep site until the appropriate time for venturing forth again' (p. 28).

Since 1971 I have espoused a similar theory (Webb, 1971, 1974, 1975). (Meddis in his Preface (1977) notes: 'Latterly, I have found that I am not alone. Bernie Webb, a respected elder statesman [sic] of the sleep research world, has independently drawn conclusions which match my own'.) Its two basic postulates were: 'periods of non responding are necessary for survival and sleep serves as a necessary condition to aid in maintaining these periods of non responding' (1975, p. 13). This was described as 'an evolutionary theory in that it assumes that sleep evolved as an adaptive process for survival of each species in its ecological niche'. Functionally, sleep was viewed 'as an inherent, unlearned response system, adaptively developed and species-specific which is released in the nervous system by appropriate internal and external zeitgebers (time cues)' (1974 p. 1026).

There has been a single essential change in my schema. In my earlier papers, I described 'instinctive behaviour' as the primary mediational condition. Sleep was 'released' by internal and/or external cues and 'This release controls or directs the behavior of the organism to adaptive ends. Like all instincts, the more developed the species the more flexible the relationship of the behavior to the environmental events' (1974, p. 1096).

I currently prefer to consider sleep to be a manifestation of a biological rhythm system. In such a system the 'cues' for sleep and waking are endogenous, time-determined state variables which reoccur at approximately fixed sidereal time intervals. The zeitgebers signal the initiation of and sustain the maintenance of the complex behaviour sequences associated with the sleep and the waking state.

My preference for the biological rhythm construct is predicated upon two primary considerations. In its classical form instincts are viewed and studied as stereotypic responses to external 'releasor' stimuli, (cf. Tinberger, 1969). While internal states may serve as modulators or determinants of threshold, the emphasis is on the particular external stimulus. For example, a recent text states: 'Instincts can be considered species-specific behavior emerging in reasonably complete form the first time an animal of a certain age and motivational state encounters a particular stimulus' (Alcock, 1975, p. 66). The most cursory consideration of the appearance of sleep or waking in almost every mammal reveals no such 'tight' relationship of sleep to particular stimuli.

Contrawise the biological rhythm research area, which has shared a common time of development with sleep research, has emphasized an endogenous cue system. In its research of a remarkable array of states and behaviours it has developed methodologies and concepts which have remarkable utility and potential transfer to the phenomenon of sleep (Enright, 1960; Webb, 1982).

1.6 Comparison of Theories

We have now the outlines of two concepts of sleep. On one hand we have a theory which explicates a certain purpose for sleep — that of a restorative state — and oriented inwardly toward the search for that changing state. On the other hand, we have a theory with a more amorphously stated purpose — behavioural adaptation — and oriented towards a comprehension of behaviour and environmental interactions.

Are we to view these as irreconcilable and opposing theories in which the establishment of one abrogates the other? Certainly this position has been taken. Hess has stated relative to the reparative position: 'The more differentiated an organism, the more it depends on conscious elaboration of, and appropriate reaction to, signals from the outside world. During sleep these cognitions are depressed and the individual is left defenseless. The fact that all highly organized creatures accept this risk for a considerable part of their life suggests that sleep must have a vital function. We consider it a reparative process which obviously cannot take place in the higher creatures while they are active' (1954, p. 117). Equally adamant is the position stated by Meddis: 'I have tried to rid the sleep concept of its century old associations with the need for rest and recovery. In my opinion there is no necessary connection between the two. The belief that there is a connection is probably one of the heaviest anchors currently slowing our progress toward more useful theories of the nature and function of sleep' (1977, p. 126).

We may take a more neutral approach conceiving of each position as independent enterprises. 'My postulates are orthogonal to these [restorative] notions and would be neither enhanced nor modified by the presence of restorative functions of any type or in any species' (Webb, 1975, p. 16). I suspect a restorative theorist would be equally inclined to accept evidence of behaviour–environment coordinates.

However, a more useful approach at this time would be to take neither an all-or-none approach nor a neutral one. Rather let us briefly examine areas of probable agreement and disagreement.

First let us consider salient points where the positions need not be considered incompatible. The behavioural models tend to emphasize their 'innate' (generally meaning unlearned), 'inherent' (generally implying genetically transmitted), 'adaptive' (translated, in the context, to mean 'having survival values'), and species-specific. There is no apparent reason that such terms could not be appropriately applied to a 'restorative' system. Indeed, it is difficult to conceive of a restorative system that would not be so described.

The behavioural model proponents also typically refer to themselves as 'evolutionary'. The implication here is that the particular system evolved across the species history as a functional survival system relative to its pressures. Again it would seem unnecessary and unlikely that a restorative theorist would demur.

A primary tenet of the restorative theories is that the determinant of sleep onset and termination is an endogenous state change. The behavioural theories, however, particularly in the biological systemic formulation of them, finds no quarrel with the generalized precept. Both would accept the assumption that such states could be modulated, delayed, interfered with by exogenously cued demands.

Reflecting their emphasis on the phenomonal manifestations of sleep, the adaptive theorists have emphasized the systematic and repetitive time aspects of sleep. They, as a result, have increasingly embraced the tenets and concepts of chronobiology which is a system concerned with such events. However, it should be noted that the restorative position, by utilizing a homeostatic or feed-back loop system with appropriate assumptions, can be modelled into an orderly, repetitive timed system. In the simplest terms, human sleep could hypothetically reflect a system which requires approximately one-half a recovery period time relative to expenditure time (8 hours 'recovery' for 16 hours of wakefulness 'expenditure').

How then do these positions differ? Are there differences which make a difference? At this stage the answer appear to be Yes.

The restorative position is a unifactor reversal theory. A particular state changes and sleep is a period during which there is a reversal of that state. The experimental design in such a model would then dictate a search for State X which was high (or low) during waking and was conversely low (or high) in sleep. The refinement of such a finding would then be to determine the time course of the state change and, in turn, determine the effective independent variables related to the state change.

The behavioural model (we are here assuming a biological rhythm model) does not assume a continuous state change across either sleep or waking. Rather a state change is assumed at the onset and termination of the two periods. The resultant experimental paradigms are those used classically in the area of chronobiology which serve to define the presence and stability of endogenous, time-determined biological events: time-free environments, phase-change designs involving displacements in the presumed time sequence and altered time sequences (see Webb, 1982). Hence, refinements and extensions of these designs involve studies of synchronies and dysynchronies of various rhythm and re-entrainment times.

The most fundamental resultant difference between these models is the role of implications ascribed to the sleep behaviour of the organism. In a 'hard core' restorative model, the behaviour of sleep is merely a condition for the occurrence of the state reversals. Furthermore, its onset and termination time is a direct function of the level of the state variables and thus the time of occurrence will be predicted by that level. In contrast the role and implication of sleep behaviours in the behavioural model are ecologically defined, i.e. based upon the organism–environmental relationship. For example, changes of predator–predatee relations, foraging needs, reduction of environmental stresses, energy expenditure reduction. As such, sleep may serve a range of functions. Indeed, restorative states may be adjunctively included. Moreover, the prediction of the timing of the event is to be based upon the observation of behaviour and its repetitive character rather than on the measurement of a state variable.

There is an odd paradox here. The restorative position, with a firm and functional teleological purpose — restitution — is driven past a predictive theory into a search for mechanisms. In contrast, the less certain teleogical behaviour theory, with its 'adaptive' purpose, searches for predictions of temporal aspects of sleep with a more casual regard for 'how' these events are determined. It is strongly possible that divergent approaches may emerge with the findings which will meld into a 'complete' theory of sleep.

An alternative approach is to combine these theories. Before closing,

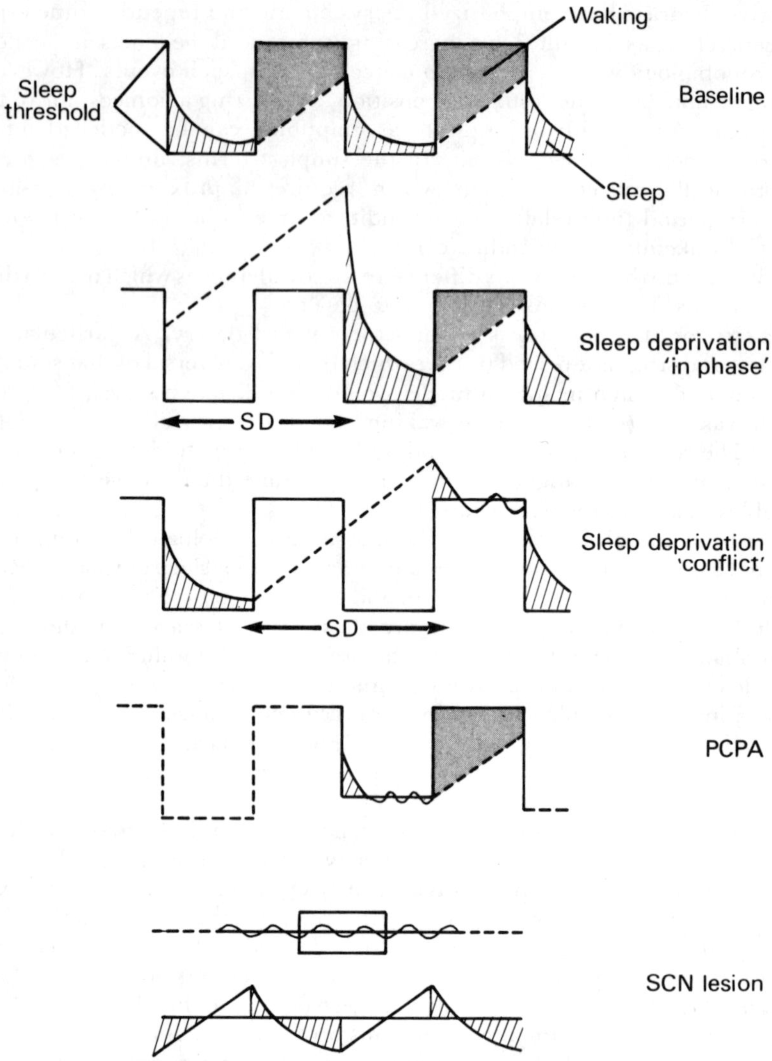

Fig. 1.1 Reproduced from A. A. Borbély (1981) in F. Obal and G. Genedeau (Eds.), *Environmental Physiology*, Vol. 18, Pergamon Press, by permission.

reference should be made to the developing position taken by Borbély and his associates (Borbély, 1981; Borbély *et al.*, 1981). This model is illustrated in Fig. 1.1. Quoting: 'In the model illustrated . . . the sleep-wake is shown as a combination of a clock triggered and a self-regulated process. A circadian oscillator is assumed to determine two levels of sleep threshold; a high level in the waking-phase and a low level in the sleep-phase. The self-regulated process is represented by a regulatory variable whose level increases as a function of sleep time. The propensity for sleep or waking is assumed to depend on the level of this variable relative to the sleep threshold (hatched areas). During the usual sleep-wake cycle, sleep propensity is highest at the beginning of the daily sleep phase, and gradually declines with the progression of sleep' (Borbély, 1981). Borbély has begun elegantly to test the predictions of this model utilizing biological rhythm research designs coupled with a measure of sleep (Stage 4 'density') as an inferential measure of sleep 'need' and recovery.

1.7 Conclusion

It has not been the intent of this review of sleep theories to marshal data and choose between the conceptual positions. Rather, as initially stated, the hope has been to lend perspective to the panorama of the mass of emerging data about sleep and to indicate the heuristic and conceptual aspect of these schema about these data.

It should not matter that the schema are incomplete nor, at points, incompatible. This is the nature of science as it gropingly attempts better to describe the facts of nature presented to it in even greater detail. The incompleteness and points of incompatibility are important parts of future sleep research. Indeed, aspects of the book that follow are steps in current clarifications.

And from all the systems certain common notions about sleep can be drawn which are useful in beginning to comprehend its fundament. It is a highly complex but highly organized biological event comprised of a coordinate system extending from the biochemical and cellular level of the central nervous system through the physiological systems and extending into behaviour. It is an inherent and unlearned system and, as such, displays typical species-specific, developmental aspects and intraspecies individual differences. These characteristics and its very ubiquity lend themselves to interpreting sleep as having evolved across time in an adaptive form.

Though simply stated, these are, in fact, strong and directive constructs — coordinate and organized systems, unlearned, inherent, adaptive, evolved. Yet, on the whole and, with thought, I believe they fit the extant data and, at least, the implicit assumptions of the research field.

The chapters following will do much to elucidate the Aristotelian formal, material and efficient causes of sleep. We must await time, technology, diligence and, perhaps, fancy to sort out more certain answers among our present theories to yield Aristotle's fourth level of causation — the final cause or its teleological purpose. Only then will we have the answer to the problem posed by Samuel Johnson more than 300 years ago.

'Sleep is a state in which a great part of every life is passed . . . Yet of this change, so frequent, so great, so general, and so necessary, no searcher has yet found the efficient or final cause; or can tell by what power the mind and body are thus chained down in irons, stable stupefication; or what benefits the animal receives from this alternate suspension of its active powers.' (*The Idler*, 25 November 1758).

References

ADAMS, K. (1980). Sleep as a restorative process and a theory to explain why. In: MCCONNELL, BOER RONIJN, VAN DE POLL and CORNER (Eds.), *Adaptive Capabilities*

of the Nervous System, Progress in Brain Research, Vol. 53, Elsevier/North-Holland Biomedical, pp. 289–305.
ADAMS, K. and OSWALD, I. (1977). Sleep is for tissue restoration. *J. Royal College of Physicians*, **11**, 376–388.
ALCOCK, J. (1977). *Animal Behavior: An Evolutionary Approach*, Sunderland, Massachusetts: Sinauer Associates.
ALLISON, T. and VAN TWYVER, H. (1970). The evolution of sleep. *Natural History*, **79**, 56–65.
BERGER, R. (1969). Ocularmotor control: a possible function of REM sleep. *Psychological Review*, **76**, 144–164.
BORBÉLY, A. A. (1981). The sleep process: circadian and homeostatic aspects. In: F. OBAL and G. GENEDEAU (Eds.), *Environmental Physiology*, Vol. 18, Oxford: Pergamon Press.
BORBÉLY, A. A., TOBLER, I. and GROOS, G. (1981). Sleep homeostasis and the circadian sleep-wake rhythm. Symposium 'New Perspectives in Sleep Research' (February 1981, Santa Monica, CA) Spectrum Publications.
DEWAN, E. M. (1970). The programing (P) hypothesis for REM sleep. In: E. HARTMANN (Ed.), *Sleep and Dreaming*, Boston: Little, Brown, pp. 295–307.
ENRIGHT, J. T. (1980). *The Timing of Sleep and Wakefulness*, New York: Springer-Verlag.
EPHRON, H. S. and CARRINGTON, P. (1966). Rapid eye movement sleep and cortical homeostasis. *Psychological Review*, **73**, 500–526.
EVANS, C. R. and NEWMAN, E. A. (1964). Dreaming: An analogy for computers. *New Scientist*, **419**, 577–579.
FISHBEIN, W. and GUTWEIN, B. (1977). Paradoxical sleep and memory storage processes. *Behavioral Biology*, **19**, 425–464.
FISHER, C. (1965). Psychoanalytic implications of recent research on sleep and dreams. *J. Amer. Psychoanalytic Association*, **13**, 197–303.
GAARDER, K. (1966). A conceptual model of sleep. *Arch. Gen. Psychiatr.*, **14**, 253–260.
GREENBERG, R. and PEARLMAN, C. (1974). Cutting the REM nerve: an approach to the adaptive role of REM sleep. *Perspectives in Biology and Medicine*, Summer, 1974, 513–521.
HARTMANN E. (1973). *The Functions of Sleep*. New Haven, Conn: Yale University Press.
HAWKINS, D. R. (1966). A review of psychoanalytic dream theory of psychophysiologic sleep research. *Brit. J. Med. Psychol*, **39**, 85.
KLEITMAN, N. (1963). *Sleep and Wakefulness*, Chicago: University of Chicago Press.
MEDDIS, R. (1975). On the function of sleep. *Animal Behavior*, **23**, 676–691.
MEDDIS, R. (1977). *The Sleep Instinct*, London: Routledge & Kegan Paul.
MORUZZI, G. (1966). The functional significance of sleep with particular regard to the brain mechanisms underlying consciousness. In: J. C. ECCLES (Ed.), *Brain and Conscious experience*, New York: Springer.
PIERON, H. (1913). *Le Problème Physiologique du Sommeil*, Paris: Masson.
RECHTSCHAFFEN, A. and EAKIN, D. (1967). *Sleep and Dream Research, A Bibliography*, Los Angeles: Brain Research Institute, Publication **0701**.
ROFFWARG, H., MUZIO, J. and DEMENT, W. (1966). Ontogenetic development of the human sleep-dream cycle. *Science*, **152**, 604–619.
SNYDER, F. (1967). In quest of dreaming. In: H. A. WITKIN and H. B. LEWIS (Eds.), *Experimental Studies of Dreaming*, New York: Random House.
TINBERGEN, N. (1969). *The Study of Instinct*, New York: Oxford Press.
WEBB, W. B. (1961). The choice of the problem. *Amer. Psychol*, **16**, 223–227.
WEBB, W. B. (1968). *Sleep: An Experimental Approach*, New York: Macmillan.
WEBB, W. B. (1971). Sleep as a biorhythm. In: W. P. COLQUHOUN (Ed.), *Biological Rhythms and Human Performance*, London: Academic Press.
WEBB, W. B. (Ed.) (1973). *Sleep: An Active Process*. Glenview, Ill.: Scott, Foresman.
WEBB, W. B. (1974). Sleep as an adaptive response. *Percept. Mot. Skills*, **38**, 1023–1027.

WEBB, W. B. (1974). The adaptive functions of sleep patterns. In: P. LEVIN and W. P. KOELLA (Eds.), *Sleep 1974*, Basel: Karger, pp. 13–19.

WEBB, W. B. (1974). The rhythms of sleep and waking. In: L. SCHEVING and F. HALBERG (Eds.), *Chronobiology*, Tokyo: Igakushoin, pp. 481–486.

WEBB, W. B. *Sleep: The Gentle Tyrant*, Englewood Cliffs, NJ: Prentice-Hall.

WEBB, W. B. (1979). Theories of sleep functions and some clinical implications. In: R. DRUCKER-COLIN, M. SHKUROVICH, and M. B. STERMAN (Eds.), *The Functions of Sleep*, New York: Academic Press, pp. 19–36.

WEBB, W. B. (1982). Biological rhythms and sleep. In: W. B. WEBB (Ed.), *Biological Rhythms, Sleep and Performance*, London: Wiley.

CHAPTER 2

The Rhythmical Nature of Sleep

Kenneth I. Hume

2.1 Introduction

An organism's activity depends to a large extent upon its environment. Life on earth is responsive to the daily oscillation in many major environmental variables produced by this planet's rotation about its poles. One obvious effect of this rotation is the alternation of day and night and associated with this is a regular alternation between behavioural activity and relative quiescence throughout the animal kingdom. In humans, as in most other animals studied, the relatively quiescent phase of this biological rhythm is usually associated with sleep. Such rhythms with a periodicity of about 24 h were described as circadian by Halberg (1969).

Observations along the phylogenetic scale, although incomplete, suggest that sleep and circadian rhythms have a long evolutionary history. The 24 h periodicity in environmental variables associated with the alternation of day and night must have been one of the major influences that presumably helped shape the physiology and behaviour of human beings' ancestors as they evolved the capacity to live on the land.

In temperate climates most adult humans adopt a similar daily pattern where the major sleep period is generally confined to the nocturnal phase of the nychthemeron and wakefulness is usually associated with the diurnal phase (Kleitman, 1963). In the rat and other nocturnally active animals, the position of sleep and wakefulness is reversed. Thus, although different species can be active at different times of day they still demonstrate an obvious circadian rhythm of sleep and wakefulness.

The recording of activity patterns has been a central theme in the study of circadian rhythms (see Aschoff, 1981, for reviews). However, sleep has usually been treated as a unitary process and recorded simply as the opposite of wakefulness. In this way the rhythmical pattern of sleep and wakefulness was recorded but there was usually no information gathered on the nature of sleep.

The early study of sleep was restricted by the lack of a useful measure of the phenomenon. The early researcher relied upon simple and indirect measures such as body movements, duration, arousal thresholds and subjective reports of sleep experience. All of these were inadequate to describe fully the process of sleep. A suitable measure was not forthcoming until the EEG provided an objective measure of brain activity.

The EEG as a tool to investigate sleep became firmly established in the late 1930s (Loomis *et al.*, 1937). The next great impetus to sleep research was when Aserinsky and Kleitman (1953) noticed that sleeping subjects had two kinds of eye movement, slow and rapid. The discovery of dramatic changes in the physiology of the sleeper accompanying these bouts of rapid eye movement lead to formulations (reviewed by Dement and Mitler, 1974) of a dichotomy of sleep into two distinct states, REM (rapid eye movement) and NREM (non-REM) sleep. Thereafter sleep could no longer be regarded as a single state that varied along a continuum in depth (Dement & Wolpert, 1958). The method of polygraphic sleep recording where the EEG, EOG and EMG are recorded simultaneously has allowed substantial progress in sleep research over the last two decades, clearly demonstrating that sleep is not a unitary process.

This polygraphic method of dividing sleep into sleep stages according to electrophysiological criteria has been refined the most for the human. The clarity of description of human sleep is due in part to the general acceptance by most sleep laboratories of the Rechtschaffen & Kales manual (1968). The division of a sleep episode into sleep stages has allowed a detailed picture of the temporal organization of sleep, what is frequently called its infrastructure.

Therefore, consideration of the rhythmical nature of sleep involves two aspects, the pattern of sleep and wakefulness as well as sleep's infrastructure of sleep stages. However, as other authors have noted (Webb, 1971), in the large number of studies into circadian rhythms conducted in the last 30 years (e.g. Aschoff, 1960; Halberg, 1969; Conroy & Mills, 1970; Wever, 1979) sleep has usually been treated as a unitary process and a time when useful measures are more difficult to obtain. Studies investigating the relationship of the temporal infrastructure of sleep to circadian rhythms have been rare. This chapter will be concerned with the temporal and rhythmical aspects of the infrastructure of sleep, both in the context of the normal and abnormal patterns of sleep and wakefulness.

Also, the chapter will be mainly concerned with sleep in young adult humans as man is the species in which we have the largest body of knowledge of the infrastructure of sleep and this is where the majority of work in this area has been directed over the last couple of decades.

This chapter continues with a broad outline of the general principles and methods of rhythm research to allow a fuller appreciation, for those readers unfamiliar with rhythm research, of the experimental designs and rationales encountered later; fuller accounts can be obtained elsewhere (Aschoff, 1981; Minors & Waterhouse, 1981). Next, there is a discussion of the relationship between sleep and rhythm research followed by a consideration of the rhythmical aspects of nocturnal sleep in humans. The main body of the chapter will be concerned with the infrastructure of sleep during abnormal sleep/activity schedules which have provided for a greater understanding of the rhythmical nature of sleep. Some consideration is then given to the ways that the sleep–wakefulness rhythm can affect other rhythms, e.g. temperature and hormone secretion. A brief account of pathologies and mechanisms associated with the sleep–wakefulness rhythm follows, before a final discussion of the functional implications of rhythms in sleep.

2.2 Principles and Methods of Rhythm Research

An organism's activity depends to a large extent upon its environment. However, major environmental variables are not constant but vary rhythmically with a period of 24 h due to the earth's rotation, e.g. the variation in light intensity associated with the alternation of day and night. Therefore organisms on the earth are subjected to continual daily oscillations in their environment and this has determined behavioural patterns of activity, rest and sleep.

If an organism demonstrates a 24 h rhythm in one of its variables, it is possible that this is simply a reflection of some rhythmical variation in one of the environmental variables to which it was exposed. The body rhythm would then be described as being under *exogenous* control. Evidence for such a case would be obtained if on removal of the organism from the environmental variable the body rhythm ceases. On the other hand, if the observed rhythm continued in the absence of any rhythmical environmental influence this suggests that it is the result of some internal oscillator or clock which is responsible for the overt rhythm. Under these circumstances the controlling influence would be *endogenous*.

Much effort has centred on identifying which of the many observed rhythms are endogenous and a large number of rhythms in physiological variables have been clearly demonstrated and well documented to be of endogenous origin (Minors & Waterhouse, 1981; Aschoff, 1981).

When a rhythm is endogenous and therefore driven by some internal oscillator the rhythmical environmental influences still play an important role in keeping the internal clock in step with the environment. The rhythmical environmental influences which provide the organism with cues to the solar time are known as *zeitgeber* or time-givers. The process by which zeitgeber synchronize the internal oscillators to maintain an exact 24 h periodicity in the usual nychthemeral environment is called *entrainment*.

It is worthwhile to consider briefly the general methods employed within biological rhythm research in order to clarify the rationales and procedures which will be encountered later in this chapter.

The conditions which have to be satisfied for a rhythm to be considered endogenous have been outlined previously, e.g. Conroy and Mills (1970). There are two main approaches which involve observing the response of the rhythm to (1) constant conditions, i.e. without zeitgebers, and (2) a shift in the phase or period of the external zeitgeber.

The major method for studying rhythms has involved observing if they continue in an environment where all rhythmic influences likely to affect them have been removed. This method involves temporal isolation under constant conditions where any potential zeitgeber such as temperature, noise and humidity are kept constant. It is not usually possible, nor deemed necessary by most researchers, to remove all the subtle geophysical rhythms e.g. γ rays. Although it has not been established that animals can detect such variables, nevertheless a small minority of authors, e.g. Brown (1976) consider that such geophysical time cues are important determinants of circadian rhythms.

There are two natural locations where environmental conditions can be relatively constant; down deep caves and at the north and south poles. Such locations have produced valuable information particularly in the early days of rhythm research (Conroy & Mills, 1970) but these places are not readily accessible and are inhospitable which must put strain on the subjects and the data-gathering systems. Therefore, a number of isolation units have been constructed for the purpose of allowing subjects to live in an environment where they do not receive any natural or other indications of the solar time (Elliott *et al.*, 1972; Aschoff, 1965; Weitzman *et al.*, 1979; Webb & Agnew, 1974).

The implicit assumption in such 'time-free' environments is that the internal oscillators are allowed to 'free-run' at a more natural frequency. This natural frequency does not correspond with the exact 24 h period observed in the presence of external zeitgeber, i.e. under entrained conditions. This condition where the endogenous rhythms continue at a frequency different from the exact 24 h rhythms of the environment is known as *external desynchronization*. In humans it is a common finding that the period of free-running rhythms is increased by about 1 h from that recorded in a normal nychthemeral environment (e.g. Wever, 1979) while some species adopt periods slightly less than 24 h (Aschoff, 1981). Research into the rest/activity patterns of free-running animals have shown that the period lengths are species specific, genetically influenced and remain constant from months to years (Pittendrigh & Daan, 1976).

If variables continue to oscillate with the same period in the absence of external zeitgeber this can indicate a possible causal nexus. In this way free-running experiments have provided valuable information of the relationships between rhythms and helped towards elucidating the mechanisms associated with the internal circadian oscillators. Further consideration will be given to these topics in the free-running section which follows.

Free-running rhythms are usually different from the exact 24 h period of the environmental variables in nychthemeral conditions but frequently are very similar to the new rhythmical pattern of habits, particularly the sleep–wakefulness rhythm. For example, the temperature and sleep–wakefulness rhythms are frequently closely associated at the start of a free-running experiment. However, in some individuals, as the free-running experiment progresses these rhythms of temperature and sleep–wakefulness become dissociated and the two rhythms adopt distinct periods. This condition is referred to as *internal desynchronization*. On the other hand, if different rhythms in the same individual change their mutual phase relationship this is known as *internal dissociation*.

The second main approach to establish the endogeneity of a rhythm involves the response of the rhythm to a sudden shift in the phase or period of the environmental rhythms.

Shifts of phase are experienced by air travellers after transmeridian flights on arrival in the new time zone where initially their internal clocks are still set to the time zone from which they departed. Another applied case in which phase shifts of the pattern of sleep and activity can be incurred is with shift workers, particularly night workers (see later for further discussion).

If a bodily rhythm adjusts immediately to the new phase setting of the environmental rhythms, there is little case for attributing the rhythm to an internal oscillator. On the other hand, if there is a delay before the rhythm is again back in synchrony with the rhythms of the environment, there is clear evidence for an internal oscillator which requires a suitable duration to become re-set to the new phase of the environmental periodicities. The evidence for endogeneity would be further improved if once it has become entrained to the new phase setting it does not immediately revert to its former phase when the original phase of the environmental periodicities is restored. This can be used as an investigative tool, as the rates at which the various rhythms adapt to the new phase setting can give indications of possible causal relationships (Conroy & Mills, 1970).

The response of rhythms to changes in the period of the zeitgeber is a less used experimental technique than free-running or phase-shifts and of more theoretical than practical interest. When a different period is imposed for the rhythms of habits and environment, an endogenous rhythm would initially retain an approximately 24 h period. If it did become entrained to the new period it would not revert immediately to its former period when the original rhythm of habits and environment are restored. Organisms can adjust in time to any new phase setting of the environmental periodicities. This is clearly not the case with new periods, there are limits, the *range of entrainment* outside of which an endogenous circadian rhythm cannot be entrained by zeitgeber.

2.3 Sleep and Rhythm Research

An obvious question to arise from the above consideration of the principles and methods employed in rhythm research is — What has been gained by the application of these techniques to our understanding of the rhythmical nature of sleep?

Unfortunately, there are a number of difficulties that arise in the study of the rhythmical nature of sleep as compared to more easily described and measured phenomena such as body temperature. Other authors have commented on some of these difficulties (Conroy & Mills, 1970; Minors & Waterhouse, 1980).

Sleep and wakefulness are alternating states of the organism, unlike other physiological variables, e.g. temperature, which is a continuous variable that can be sampled throughout the 24 h, allowing a clear description of the rhythm in body temperature. To overcome this limitation one can look for continuous variables that are related to the sleep–wakefulness rhythm that can be measured over the 24 h. These can be objective, e.g. locomotor activity, or subjective, e.g. sleepiness/fatigue scales, but the precise relationship of these measures to sleep or any putative sleep–wakefulness oscillator is unknown.

In addition, the occurrence of sleep is not determined exclusively by a putative endogenous oscillator, whether the subject is under temporal isolation in an isolation chamber or in the world outside. An individual 'decides to' then 'attempts to' sleep which may or may not be forthcoming. The decision to attempt to sleep depends on the level of interest in what one is doing or what is happening in the environment and how much sleep one intuitively feels from experience one 'needs' for their scheduled activity on the following day. Also, the need-one-feels to sleep depends on the previous sleep–wakefulness pattern, in particular how much sleep was obtained during the previous bedrest and how long ago that was. (This will be considered in more depth in a later section on sleep duration.) One's previous activity during wakefulness also determines the need-one-feels to sleep. For example, after unusually large amounts of physical exertion one feels 'shattered' and welcomes the opportunity to sleep. How one's sleep is altered by such activity is a more contentious issue; see Horne (1981) for a review.

When one is trying to sleep, it may not be achieved, even with an otherwise normal healthy individual, due to temporary anxiety associated with an unresolved problem which can delay the onset and shorten the duration of sleep.

In spite of these difficulties, considerable information has been gathered over the last 30 years (e.g. Wever, 1979) on the nature of the sleep–wakefulness rhythm, particularly from free-running experiments, which is discussed in a later section. However, this information relates mainly to the pattern of sleep and wakefulness, the details of the infrastructure of the sleep phase, e.g. time taken to fall asleep and the sleep stage profile have been largely ignored.

Interest and research effort into biological rhythms and sleep developed at about the same time yet surprisingly, for two closely related areas, little cross-fertilization seems to have occurred. There were some exceptions, notably Kleitman (1939 and revised in 1963) in the only early reference work entitled 'Sleep and Wakefulness' does emphasize strongly both the infrastructure of sleep and its periodic nature.

One major cause of this mutual lack of understanding between the two related fields of study has been ascribed to the sleep researchers' early pre-occupation with the psycho-physiology of dreaming (Hobson, 1969). Another possible cause of the lack of intercourse between sleep and biological rhythm research, which is more long-lasting, is the large amount of specialized terminology which is peculiar to these two specialisms. They both rely heavily upon jargon for brevity and ease of communication within the specialisms but, similar to all jargon, it tends to obscure the subject matter to the uninitiated. Both the Chronobiologic Glossary (Halberg & Katinas, 1973) which runs to 32 pages, and the Rechtschaffen and Kales (1968) manual of standardized terminology, techniques and scoring system for sleep stages of human subjects, can be 'heavy going' for those readers without good reason to understand fully the nuances of these two specialisms. The extent to which confusion can occur just within the sleep literature is illustrated in a review by Freemon (1972) where 25 different labels for REM sleep and NREM sleep are listed, some of which are still in use today.

There have been some recent attempts (Czeisler *et al.*, 1980) to provide a standardized terminology to help to integrate biological rhythm and sleep research. One simple example of the confusion that can exist between the two specialisms can be found in studies where the bedrest–activity cycle is altered and periods are designated for sleep with the lights out and the subject in bed, which the unwary rhythm researcher may record as sleep. However, one can only be sure that the subject is asleep if suitable electrophysiological recordings are taken. A similar problem can result if sleep occurs during designated wakefulness periods unless suitable monitoring precautions are taken. This type of problem has been highlighted in mice (Mitler *et al.*, 1977) when sleep has been recorded in addition to wheel-running activity rhythms. Sleep occured during the active as well as the inactive phases of the wheel-running rhythm and on occasions there were poorly defined sleep rhythms on days when the wheel-running activity rhythm remained very distinct.

2.4 Rhythmical Aspects of Nocturnal Sleep

Before consideration of the rhythmical aspects of nocturnal sleep in the adult human it is fitting to consider briefly what developmental changes have occurred in the pattern of sleep and wakefulness. Developmental aspects of human sleep are covered in more depth in a later chapter.

2.4.1 *Development*

A circadian organization of sleep and wakefulness is not usually present at birth. However, rhythmical behaviour is usually evident, e.g. the human infant exhibits a 50–60 min ultradian rhythm of rest and activity (Aserinsky & Kleitman, 1955) with naps taken throughout the nychthemeron. However, within a few weeks there appears an unequal distribution of sleep between day-time and night with slightly more sleep during the latter (Hellbrügge, 1960). At birth the neonate spends about 16 h of each 24 h asleep (Kleitman & Engelmann, 1953).

As the child develops, the amount of sleep during night naps increases while the total duration of sleep per 24 h decreases. Maturation is paralleled by an increased ability to remain awake longer and to sleep 'continuously' at night (Kleitman, 1963). Development continues with a progressive decrease in the total sleep per 24 h until, for the young adult, sleep is nocturnally placed, lasts in general for 7 to 8 h, and occurs once every 24 h.

The length of time each species spends asleep each day varies considerably, e.g. the bat is asleep for about 20 h while the elephant sleeps only 4 h. Similar to humans, the majority of the species can be characterized by sleeping at a particular time of day (Aschoff, 1981).

The ability to concentrate sleep in the night, as development continues, occurs whether the infant is hospitalized, with the added environmental encouragement to sleep at night, or whether the child is allowed an on-demand schedule (Kleitman & Engelmann, 1953). This sleep–wakefulness rhythm appears to develop spontaneously with the long sleep taken during the night if the child develops in an environment which is exposed to day and night. However, if the child is kept in continuous light with on-demand feeding, although the circadian rhythm develops, the sleep does not necessarily correspond to the night-time (Martin-du-Pan, 1970). This establishment of a circadian sleep–wakefulness rhythm, out of phase with the world outside, provides good evidence that this rhythm is not imposed by some environmental factor and points to the natural development of this rhythm by the infant (Mills, 1975). Further evidence for the innate predisposition for this circadian rhythmical behaviour has come from a study by Valatz & Bugat (1974) who has shown that families of mice kept under constant environmental conditions of lighting, temperature, and so on, showed clear circadian rhythms even after six generations had passed.

Polygraphic sleep recordings from infants are different from those in the adult, therefore the adult criteria (Rechtschaffen & Kales, 1968) cannot be applied strictly, to the extent that a separate manual has been developed for infants (Anders *et al.*, 1971). This presents a serious difficulty for the consideration of the development of the infrastructure of sleep. Nevertheless, in parallel with the considerable changes in the sleep–wakefulness pattern there are equally substantial changes in the infrastructure which mainly concern REM.

A most striking discovery was that the neonate spends about one-third of each 24 h, which represents one-half of its sleep time, in active REM sleep, the precursor of stage REM sleep in the adult (Roffwarg *et al.*, 1966). This high level diminishes progressively to approximately 30% of the sleep at about 4 years and reaches adult values of 20–25% soon after the age of 10 (Williams *et al.*, 1974). There is some evidence for a circadian variation in the tendency for REM to occur in the infant with the least REM recorded in the afternoon (Sostek *et al.*, 1976). The REM–NREM rhythm is clearly evident at birth with a period of 50–60 min which increases to reach adult values of approximately 100 min between the ages of about 5 and 10 years (Williams *et al.*, 1974).

2.4.2 REM–NREM Cycle

One of the clearest impressions to remain with a sleep researcher after spending his first night recording the continuous electrical activity from the scalp of a sleeping person is the rhythmical nature in which the sleep stages unfold across the night. The regular cyclic appearance of REM and NREM sleep, with a period of about 90 min, was a striking characteristic reported by Dement & Kleitman (1957). This basic cycling within sleep has been amply corroborated by numerous authors (e.g. Kales *et al.*, 1967; Hartmann, 1968; Globus, 1970; Brezinova, 1974) and is present in other animals although the cycle length varies considerably between species (Zepelin & Rechtschaffen, 1974).

There is at present considerable controversy over whether or not this basic oscillation, which manifests itself during sleep as the REM–NREM cycle, continues to operate with the same periodicity into the waking hours. Kleitman (1963) on the basis of the REM–NREM cycle was the first to propose such an ultradian (period less than 21 h) oscillation in certain neurophysiological functions, which continues through sleep and waking. He described this as the Basic Rest Activity Cycle (BRAC). It has been proposed that this BRAC is responsible for the ultradian rhythms that have been detected during wakefulness in a number of variables (reviewed by Kripke, 1974) including oral activity (Friedman & Fisher, 1968; Oswald *et al.*, 1970), psychomotor performance (Globus *et al.*, 1971), fantasy (Kripke & Sonnenschein, 1973), waking gastric activity (Hiatt *et al.*, 1975) resting heart-rate (Orr *et al.*, 1972) and eye movements (Othmer *et al.*, 1969; Aserinsky, 1973).

This view is not held by others (Lewis, 1974; Brezinova, 1974; Moses *et al.*, 1975; Brezinova *et al.*, 1975) who consider that the REM–NREM cycle is a manifestation of a sleep dependent oscillation, which terminates on awakening and starts again at the next sleep onset. One of the main arguments against the REM–NREM cycle being a sleep independent oscillation, is that the cycle length is sensitive to factors within sleep, e.g. the amounts of SWS (slow wave sleep, Stages 3 plus 4) and the amounts of wakefulness that occur within the cycle (Brezinova, 1974; Brezinova *et al.*, 1975).

Other authors (Moses *et al.*, 1975; Moses *et al.*, 1978; Johnston, 1980) have compared the REM–NREM cycle length in nocturnal sleep and in grossly abnormal bedrest–activity schedules, e.g. 60 min bedrest followed by 160 min activity maintained for 40 h. If the oscillator responsible for the appearance of REM is sleep independent as is envisaged in the BRAC hypothesis then REM should occur at approximately equidistant time intervals throughout the sleep obtained on the altered bedrest–activity schedules independent of the amount of sleep or wakefulness between subsequent REM periods. On the other hand, if this oscillator is sleep dependent then REM onset should be related to the amount of sleep, not just the time elapsed, since the last REM episode. The results of these experiments favour a sleep dependent oscillator governing the appearance of REM, i.e. intervening wakefulness lengthens the REM–NREM cycle. However, Johnston (1980) also states that there may well be more than one oscillatory system responsible for rhythms seen during sleep and wakefulness.

In opposition to the sleep dependent model, Shultz *et al.* (1980) favour a periodically driven process which incorporates the concept of a clock or oscillator of higher precision than the overt REM–NREM cycle. This delivers triggers for REM sleep appearances at intervals throughout the day and night, as envisaged in a BRAC model. This author's results reveal that the length of one cycle depends on the length of the preceding cycle such that a long cycle length will be followed by a short cycle and vice versa. This shows a tendency to correct for the previous cycle length, evoking the idea of a controlling influence (a clock) beyond the sleep process *per se* which would be necessary for the BRAC model to operate.

In addition, an intriguing observation was made from longitudinal studies (Shultz *et al.*, 1975) of a gradual forward shift (5–10 min) in REM sleep onset time (apart from the first REM episode which was determined by sleep onset) from night to night. This indicated that the length of the REM–NREM cycle was not a sub-multiple of 24 h but drifted in a regular fashion from night to night. This would suggest that the mechanism responsible for the REM–NREM cycle is not under the control of an exact 24 h oscillator but rather an independent free-running oscillator that has a period slightly longer than an exact sub-multiple of 24 h. This lends support to the concept of a REM–NREM cycle which is controlled by a sleep independent, periodically driven process.

The results obtained by Carskadon & Dement (1975, 1980) using 90 min 'days' where 30 min bedrest was followed by 60 min of activity, neither supported nor rejected the sleep independent nor the sleep dependent theories of REM oscillators. For these authors other factors have to be taken into consideration and for them the most striking results in the timing of REM sleep on the 90 min 'day' was the recurrence of REM sleep on alternative bedrest episodes. On 56% of occasions REM sleep occurred on alternate bedrests while on only 8% of occasions did REM sleep occur on consecutive bedrest. Also, there appeared to be a mutually exclusive relationship between REM sleep and SWS in the sleep episodes during the times of greatest sleep tendency.

The answer to some of the unresolved questions posed by the above work may lie with a number of trigger and clock mechanisms normally acting in unison which is lost when grossly abnormal ultradian sleep–wakefulness patterns, such as those above, are employed. Any model would have to explain the large variability observed in the REM–NREM cycle. This variation in the cycle length is present both within and between subjects (Williams *et al.*, 1974).

The usual REM–NREM cycle length quoted for a night's sleep is the mean of about 4 cycles. However, there is clear evidence that within a night there is a clear difference with the serial order of the REM–NREM cycles, both in their length and the duration of the component sleep stages. The first and last cycle lengths are on average shorter than those in the middle of the night (Brezinova, 1974; Hume, 1978; Feinberg & Floyd, 1979).

A rare piece of evidence for the suggestion by Globus (1970) that the period of the REM–NREM cycle is modulated by a circadian component was presented by Taub & Berger (1973). They found that as sleep commenced progressively later from 20.00 to 04.00 the average period of the REM–NREM cycle significantly decreased. However, this finding has not been corroborated by other workers who have studied sleep at various times across the nychthemeron. The situation is further confused by the finding of an ultradian rhythm with a period of about 15 min in eye movements within REM sleep (Lavie, 1979).

Therefore, a number of key issues are still unresolved; whether the REM–NREM cycle is controlled by an oscillator that operates during both sleep and wakefulness, if ultradian rhythms in other variables are coupled to this oscillator and if this ultradian oscillator is linked to circadian oscillators such as the one which controls the rhythm of sleep and wakefulness.

2.4.3 Nocturnal Distribution of SWS and REM

The first NREM episode of the night contains a large proportion of SWS then successive NREM episodes contain progressively less. By the end of the night, SWS is not common and when present, appears only in small amounts, mainly as Stage 3. Detailed analysis of EEG delta activity, the principal component for defining SWS, has shown a distribution across the night which is fitted well by a damped sinusoidal rhythm with a period of about 100 min (Lubin *et al.*, 1973).

There is a progressive increase in the durations of the REM episodes as the night's sleep proceeds (Dement & Kleitman, 1957; Verdone, 1968) and consequently a shortening of the interval between REM episodes (Williams *et al.*, 1974).

This predominant occurrence of REM sleep in the latter part of the night while SWS appears predominantly early on in sleep (Dement & Kleitman, 1957; Williams *et al.*, 1974; Webb & Agnew, 1969) is a striking temporal characteristic of the sleep structure of nocturnal sleep.

Two studies have demonstrated the stability of this differential distribution: more intense arousal efforts were required to eliminate Stage 4 sleep from the first third of the night compared to later portions of the night. The opposite was found for REM, which was more difficult to displace from the last third of sleep (Williams *et al.*, 1967). An attempt to force Stage 4 sleep to occur during the last third of sleep and REM to occur during the first third was only partially successful (Agnew & Webb, 1968).

A similar differential distribution has been reported in the monkey (Crowley *et al.*, 1972). The rat shows a predominance of SWS at the beginning of the daily rest phase, and REM shows a slight increase over the rest plane (Borbély, 1980).

2.5 Sleep during Abnormal Bedrest–Activity Schedules

The normal bedrest–activity pattern, in which the 24 h are divided into about 16 h of activity followed by a nocturnally placed sleep episode, can be altered by varying the duration of sleep episodes, the number of sleep episodes, the temporal position of the sleep episodes, or any combination of these variables. Abnormal bedrest–activity patterns can also result when the 24 h cycle length is shortened or lengthened, e.g. to 21 h and 27 h 'days', whereby the ratio of bedrest to activity is maintained but the actual length of bedrest and activity is altered as is the solar time of the sleep episodes which shifts continually.

2.5.1 Bedrest Duration

Reducing the duration of bedrest, sleep deprivation, has been used extensively and has become a vital part of sleep research. The amount of sleep has been decreased in three ways: total sleep deprivation; partial sleep deprivation; selective sleep stage deprivation in which a particular stage is prevented from continuing by arousal and which, although not a wholesale sleep deprivation, is a fractional deprivation of the normal sleep process. The result of sleep deprivation can be summarized as follows. (See review by Horne (1978 & *ibid.*) for further details.)

Studies involving a reduction in the amount of sleep from that usually obtained during the normal sleep–wakefulness pattern suggest important roles for SWS and REM sleep. Selective sleep stage deprivations suggest a 'need' for SWS and REM sleep in that the 'debt' incurred is partially repaid on recovery nights (Dement, 1960; Agnew *et al.*, 1964). In response to total sleep deprivation and the concomitant prolonged wakefulness there is a compensatory increase in TST (total sleep time) and SWS which takes precedence over REM sleep on recovery night (Berger & Oswald, 1962). When either SWS or REM sleep is increased in recovery from deprivation it is usually at the expense of Stage 2 sleep (Freemon, 1972). Response to partial sleep deprivation emphasizes the priority of SWS over other sleep stages; SWS suffers the least decrease in its duration yet is increased on recovery nights, while REM sleep was reduced and remained low showing no compensation until after SWS on recovery nights (Webb & Agnew, 1974; Johnson & Macleod, 1973). Studies with individuals who habitually sleep for short durations give similar conclusions to studies using experimental restriction of sleep duration (Hartmann, 1973).

It is worthwhile to reflect that owing to the dichotomy of life between sleep and wakefulness the sleep-deprived person not only has lost sleep but also has gained wakefulness and lost the normal overt rhythm of sleep and wakefulness. Most early researchers only considered the loss of sleep as the reason for any observed changes in the physiology or psychology of the sleep-deprived yet wakefulness-satiated person.

There is an interesting interaction between total sleep deprivation and circadian rhythms. Froberg *et al.* (1972) studied the effect of 75 h without sleep on fatigue and performance at a target task in a group of soldiers. There was a general increase in the reported fatigue and a decrease in performance as the duration of wakefulness increased. However, superimposed upon these trends were clear circadian rhythms with fatigue and performance worse at the time of the habitual nocturnal sleep episode and both improved during the daytime.

Extending nocturnal sleep (Verdone, 1968; Phoebus *et al.*, 1970; Feinberg *et al.*, 1980) revealed a positive linear relationship between sleep duration and REM sleep, up to about 9 h, and maintenance of the differential distribution, where SWS predominates early while REM sleep is maximal later in the sleep episode. The extra morning sleep (after habitual rising time) was similar in composition to the last few hours of a normal night's sleep i.e. mainly Stage 2 and REM sleep. A further important finding was that a large 'overdose' of REM sleep on one night did not decrease REM sleep on the subsequent night.

When subjects were confined to bed for 54 h (Aserinsky, 1973) a large amount of the time in bed was spent asleep (on average 32 h, with a wide range between individuals 23–40 h) and clear circadian rhythmicity was obtained with sleep concentrated in the nocturnal phase and the time of maximum appearance of NREM and REM sleep was different, 21.00 to 03.00 and 03.00 to 09.00 respectively. Similar results were obtained from subjects who spent 24 h in bed (Nakagawa, 1980). The striking result here was despite initial instructions to keep their eyes open and remain awake during the daytime (with daylight in the laboratory), the young healthy subjects reported an uncontrollable desire to fall asleep and they slept for 30–60% of the daytime in addition to nocturnal sleep. In the present author's experience of putting subjects to bed at all hours on various regimens, even 2 h naps within busy daytime schedules, sleep is usually easily achieved.

2.5.2 · Nocturnal Bedrest plus Naps

A nap after lunch or dinner is to many people an enjoyable flirtation with sleep. Such naps taken in addition to the habitual nocturnal slumber constitute another way of obtaining extra sleep each 24 h and a common feature of the sleep–wakefulness pattern in the very young as with the very old, and is a major cultural tradition in some tropical countries.

Maron *et al.* (1964) investigated reports and personal experience of 'full blown dreams' occurring at sleep onset, especially during daytime naps. Subjects were instructed to maintain their normal bedrest–activity cycle before the study and were split into two groups. One group attempted to nap during the early afternoon and the other during the evening. Comparison between the two groups revealed that REM sleep latency was shorter, and the amount of time spent in REM sleep was longer in the afternoon, whereas the amount of time in SWS was longer in the evening. This was the first clear demonstration that the nature of sleep obtained at two times within the daytime was different indicating a possible circadian variation in the infrastructure of sleep. The authors concluded prophetically:

> . . . apparently at different points in the diurnal cycle, there is a different potential for having REM periods during sleep . . .

and they postulated a 'REM period potential curve' which was suggested to be inversely related to the known temperature rhythm (Kleitman, 1963). Later studies involving morning, afternoon and evening naps (Webb *et al.*, 1966; Webb & Agnew, 1967; Karachan *et al.*, 1970) supported the suggestions that the potential for REM sleep depended upon the time of day and the direct relationship between Stage 4 and the duration of preceding wakefulness (Webb & Agnew, 1971).

From the early to mid-1970s it was becoming clearer, that temporal factors are major determinants of the sleep stage pattern. In particular SWS was preserved in preference to the other stages of sleep and maintained its early position within sleep whatever the time of day that sleep was taken. Also, the amount of SWS seemed to be directly dependent on the length of wakefulness before the sleep episode. However, this relationship did not hold completely, when a number of nights' sleep were missed the amount of SWS in the recovery sleep did not compensate fully for the 'lost' SWS that would have normally accrued, had sleep occurred as usual.

REM sleep appeared to be different, it did not seem to be related to the duration of preceding wakefulness but it was related to the length of sleep and the time of day. The study of daytime naps hinted at an underlying potential for REM sleep to be maximal in the early morning with a progressive decrease as the nap occurred later in the day. However, problems existed with this early work in that the durations of prior wakefulness were uncontrolled and the naps occurred in addition to the habitual sleep, thus producing extra sleep per 24 h.

In order to demonstrate unambiguously any circadian aspects of sleep stages, sleep needed to be studied at various times of the day without interference from variations in duration of prior wakefulness or excessive or reduced sleep per 24 h, and preferably in such a manner that adaptation to the new schedule of sleep and wakefulness did not occur.

These considerations present a minefield of problems for the researcher trying to design experiments to resolve whether sleep stages have a rhythmical component that oscillates with a circadian period. Sleep has to be sampled as frequently as possible over the 24 h, yet sleep being a discontinuous state presents far more difficulty to sample than a continuous variable such as body temperature which can be recorded relatively easily at all hours regardless of whether the subject is asleep or awake. In addition, when sleep is taken at abnormal times this automatically changes the duration of preceding wakefulness which can cause an alteration of the sleep stage pattern at the start of the altered sleep–wakefulness regimen which could lcad to sleep deprivation or satiation with possible rebound phenomena in later sleep episodes. The final cause for concern is that while investigating the circadian pattern the experimental regimen may work to upset that system with the possibility of adapting to that altered regimen.

2.5.3 Habitual Bedrest Split

There have been two major approaches to circumvent the above problems. One involved splitting the usual 8 h of bedrest into two 4 h episodes (Webb & Agnew, 1971; Hume & Mills, 1977). The other involved a more radical departure from the normal circadian pattern of sleep and wakefulness in which ultradian 'days' of 3 h 40 min (Moses *et al.*, 1975), 3 h (Weitzman *et al.*, 1974) and 90 min (Carskadon & Dement, 1975) were employed where the bedrest to activity ratio was maintained at about its usual value.

In these ultradian bedrest–activity cycles, sleep episodes were scheduled at frequent intervals throughout the 24 h, the duration of wakefulness before the bedrests was constant and the cycle lengths were so far removed from the circadian range that entrainment of any putative endogenous circadian oscillators to these ultradian periods seemed highly unlikely. The main problem that was encountered with these extreme departures from the normal sleep–wakefulness pattern was sleep deprivation, e.g. the subjects slept on average for 56% of the time allowed, compared to 90% in the control periods. This was reflected by increased TST, SWS and a small increase in REM sleep during the early part of a post-experimental recovery week (Weitzman *et al.*, 1974).

However, there were some interesting results that were consistent between the three studies. The most striking results from the 3 h 'day' (Weitzman *et al.*, 1974) was the clear circadian pattern of the amount of sleep obtained in the 1 h when it was allowed. The four 1 h sleep periods commencing at 03.00, 06.00, 09.00 and 12.00 accounted for 70% of the sleep with roughly equal and maximum sleep obtained at 06.00 and 09.00. The distribution of REM sleep throughout the 24 h was even more restricted, almost no REM sleep occurring in the 1 h sleep periods commencing at 21.00 and 24.00, while 75% of the REM sleep occurred during the 06.00, 09.00 and 12.00 periods. Sleep Stages 1 and 2 closely followed the distribution of TST, while SWS was more evenly distributed with less tendency towards circadian rhythmicity. The SWS was the least affected by the ultradian condition and was maintained at 75% of its control amount. Similar results were found in the other two ultradian studies except the time of peak sleep and REM sleep were slightly delayed (09.00 to 12.30 and 07.00 to 14.00 respectively) on the 90 min 'day' (Carskadon & Dement, 1975).

Another intriguing result was the high incidence of 'sleep onset REM periods' (SOREMPs) where REM sleep appears within 10 min of sleep onset. This is far earlier than usual when REM sleep follows the major episode of SWS and takes about 80–90 min to appear after sleep onset (Williams *et al.*, 1974). In the Moses *et al.* (1975) study, with bedrests of 1 h commencing every 220 min, two-thirds of the REM episodes were described as SOREMPs and on the 20 occasions when both SWS and REM sleep occurred in a nap, only twice was REM sleep preceded by SWS. A similar result was obtained on the 90 min 'day' (Carskadon & Dement, 1975), here REM sleep appeared on average before SWS.

These ultradian studies provided strong evidence for a circadian rhythm in the ability to sleep and in the distribution of REM sleep over the 24 h, but the high degree of sleep deprivation suffered by the subjects casts some doubt on the findings. However, the demonstration of circadian rhythmicity on such imposed ultradian regimens, which one might expect to erode the circadian system along with sleep deprivation and its accompanying stress, attests to the resilience and endogeneity of such rhythms.

The other main approach for elucidating the circadian organisation of sleep stages involved splitting the 8 h of bedrest into two 4 h episodes. This was first employed by Webb & Agnew (1971) then later refined and extended by Hume & Mills (1977). The rationale behind the split-sleep design is that one 4 h bedrest (anchor bedrest) is positioned at the habitual retiring time, e.g. 24.00 to 04.00, while the second 4 h bedrest (drift bedrest) can be positioned at various times during the remainder of the 24 h. Continuation of this split-sleep regimen, while varying the position of the 'drift bedrest', for a number of days yields a set of 'anchor sleeps' with various preceding wakefulness values, and a set of 'drift sleeps' at various times of day with the same set of preceding wakefulness values. This design allows a powerful comparison between the effects of the duration of preceding wakefulness and the time of day on sleep. Maintaining one bedrest at the habitual time of retiring should serve to anchor the circadian system under study, while having only one abnormally placed bedrest per 24 h does not present such a strain to that system as one might expect from the ultradian studies previously mentioned.

The results showed that the amount of REM sleep followed a clear circadian rhythm. This was rigorously defined (Hume & Mills, 1977) by means of cosinor analysis providing a maximum at 10.26. The amount of SWS was largely dependent upon the duration of prior wakefulness (from 2 to 16 h in steps of 2 h). Also, REM sleep showed a weak but significant negative correlation with the duration of preceding wakefulness. This is most likely due to the strong positive association of SWS which usually takes precedence over other stages of sleep, reducing the time available in the 4 h bedrest–sleep episode for REM sleep to occur.

Therefore as a result of extending nocturnal sleep, napping, and in particular, the ultradian and split-sleep studies outlined above, the appearance of REM sleep depends in part on a circadian rhythm. On a normal nychthemeral existence the circadian rhythm is maximal during the morning and declines to a minimum during the evening. On the other hand SWS is little affected by the time of day and far more dependent on the duration of wakefulness before the sleep episode. This association holds well for periods of wakefulness up to 16 h but for longer durations the relationship is not as strong. It is surprising how unresponsive SWS is to the type of activity undertaken during the preceding wakefulness, e.g. there is considerable controversy (Horne, 1981) as to whether exercise affects the amount of SWS, and when a significant rise is reported it is usually a minor response occurring after considerable exercise (e.g. Buguet *et al.*, 1980).

2.5.4 Free-Running

Free-running has been a fruitful line of enquiry in circadian rhythm research. The subject lives in an environment for long periods of time where information to the time of day is excluded. (See Section 2.2 on Principles and Methods of Rhythm Research.) This is in complete contrast to the studies considered above in which the infrastructure of sleep was obtained from subjects who were following as closely as possible an habitual nychthemeral existence. There the experiments were routinely carried out under entrained conditions with the subjects in full knowledge of the time of day and the unusual hour of some bedrests. In addition, little attempt was usually made to remove zeitgeber except to remove light and noise during unusually placed bedrests.

Free-running human subjects usually increase the period of their 24 h sleep–wakefulness cycle by about 1 h (Mills, 1964; Wever, 1979). However, the pattern of sleep and wakefulness does not always present a clear picture; there can be considerable variability between individuals. In general, as the duration of the free-running experiment increases so does the variability of the sleep-wakefulness rhythm with periods of up to about 50 h common. Also, there is considerable variability in the length of sleeps in the longer free-run experiments (Czeisler, 1978). The various types of anomalies have been described in detail elsewhere (Minors & Waterhouse, 1981).

There are very few studies concerned with free-running subjects in which sleep has been polygraphically recorded. Webb & Agnew (1974) gave half of their subjects a heavy exercise schedule for the two weeks of a free-running experiment. All subjects showed a sleep–wakefulness rhythm greater than 24 h (mean 25.3 h) with no difference in period extension between the exercised and the non-exercised group. The overall amount of sleep increased in the time-cue-free environment and exercise increased the variability in the distribution of sleep and wakefulness. However, the relative amount and distribution of sleep stages did not differ between control, exercised and non-exercised free-running conditions.

Chouvet *et al.* (1974) published results from three male subjects who spent 5–6 months in deep caves. All subjects showed some degree of circabidian rhythm (34 h of wakefulness/14 h of sleep). One subject adapted completely to this new rhythm and maintained it for longer than two months. Approximately half of the sleep was polygraphically recorded.

Some of the results puzzled the authors, e.g. the length of the sleep episodes were not correlated with the duration of prior wakefulness. One might predict intuitively that a long wakefulness episode would be followed by a long compensatory sleep. Some authors (Aschoff *et al.*, 1971; Dirlich *et al.*, 1977) have suggested an oscillatory model which proposes an inverse relationship between the length of sleep and the duration of prior wakefulness. In essence they suggest that sleep onset is determined by some oscillating function falling below some threshold level and subsequent awakening would occur when the function rises above the threshold. In this manner, if the sleep onset is delayed, awakening would not be similarly delayed but would still occur at the same time, i.e. determined by the rising oscillatory function reaching the threshold. The net effect of this is that the longer an individual remains awake the shorter the subsequent sleep. Although this is an interesting suggestion which fits some data (Aschoff *et al.*, 1971), such a model does not always account for observed sleep-wakefulness patterns (Czeisler, 1978).

Another puzzling result obtained by Chouvet *et al.* (1974) was that latencies were shorter with frequent sleep onset REM periods in two subjects unable to maintain a circabidian rhythm, while the subject with a well-adapted rhythm had the usual delay before REM sleep appeared.

An exciting and major contribution to this area of research, which helps to explain the French authors' results, was made by Czeisler (1978) in a team lead by Elliott Weitzman. They recorded sleep and other physiological variables from subjects who were allowed to live by self-selected routines for long periods (up to 189 days) in their isolation facility. One group of subjects presented the 'classical picture' where their free-running rhythms remained internally synchronized with approximately identical periods of about 25 h. On the other hand the remainder of the subjects had a number of very long sleep–wakefulness cycles (up to 50 h) while they maintained a normal ratio of sleep to total time (about 0.30) and near 24 h rhythms in body temperature. This uncoupling of rhythms which are normally linked in close temporal order has been referred to as 'internal desynchronization' (Wever, 1979). Similar patterns of very long sleep–wakefulness cycles interspersed with cycle lengths in the circadian range have been reported from other laboratories, where subjects have been allowed to free-run for long periods (Aschoff, 1965; Wever, 1979; Mills *et al.*, 1974; and Chouvet *et al.*, 1974). However, these wide variations in sleep duration had been described previously as random and irregular.

It was not the length of prior wakefulness (provided they were awake for longer than 14 h) that was controlling the length of these self-selected sleeps. Czeisler *et al.* (1980) revealed an important relationship between the phase of the body temperature rhythm and the nature of sleep. They noticed that short sleep episodes usually began just at or after the mid trough of the temperature cycle and then the average sleep length was 7.8 h (similar to the internally synchronized subjects) and they tended to wake at the end of the rising phase of body temperature. However, when the subjects selected their bedtime at about the circadian temperature cycle maximum, then sleep length averaged 14.4 h, i.e. wake times occurred on the next 'up slope' of the temperature curve.

In this way the duration of the sleep episodes was highly correlated with the circadian phase of the body temperature rhythm at sleep onset and not with the length of prior wakefulness. Not only did the organization of sleep and wakefulness depend in part on the phase of the temperature cycle, but also the infrastructure of sleep stages varied with this rhythm. In particular there was a clear and close relationship between the rhythms in REM sleep propensity and body temperature, a relationship which had first been hinted at in nap studies (Maron *et al.*, 1964) and ultradian bedrest–activity cycles (Moses *et al.*, 1977). The first 50 min of REM sleep were accumulated on average 2 h earlier when sleep began just after the temperature minimum (Czeisler *et al.*, 1980). In addition SOREMPs reliably occurred when subjects chose to go to bed just after the temperature cycle trough (and the early REMPs were longer). In contrast to the substantial shift in REM sleep distribution the total amount of REM sleep and its percentage of the sleep periods remained constant in the entrained and free-running condition.

Similar findings have been reported from Germany (Zulley, 1980) where free-running subjects had more REM sleep at the beginning of sleep episodes in which the temperature minimum occurs earlier as compared with episodes in which the temperature minimum occurs later. This was due to reduced time before the first REM sleep episode and its longer duration. The author suggests that the first as opposed to subsequent REM sleep episodes may be particularly influenced by circadian parameters associated with the temperature rhythm.

On the other hand, SWS maintained its early position in the sleep episode for both the entrained and free-running conditions while its percentage of the total sleep time did increase to a small extent from the entrained (27.8%) to the free-running (29.8%) condition (Weitzman *et al.*, 1980). An interesting finding for the long sleep episodes was the reappearance of SWS after 12–18 h of sleep. There were occasional awake sequences but these were not long enough to explain the reappearance of SWS. On this basis, Weitzman *et al.* (1980) suggest that SWS may be related to the length of elapsed time since the last appearance of SWS, not the duration of prior wakefulness. Unfortunately, there does not appear to be any detailed analysis where the amounts of SWS are compared with the length of prior wakefulness.

Further validation of the important relationship between sleep, REM and the phase of the temperature circadian rhythm was sought (Czeisler *et al.*, 1980) by reanalysing earlier data (Weitzman *et al.*, 1974) from an imposed ultradian bedrest–activity schedule with a cycle length of 3 h. The results were in full agreement with the free-running data, with subjects finding great difficulty in sleeping (and with virtually no REM) at the peak of their temperature cycle whilst most sleep was obtained at the nadir of the cycle which was the time of maximum appearance of REM.

2.5.5 *Phase Alterations*

In adults, apart from the usual small variation in the temporal position of sleep within the 24 h, there are two common cases of large deviations from the usual pattern of sleep and wakefulness. These occur with night shift working and rapid change of time zones as experienced by air travellers, who fly significant distances eastward or westward.

Phase alterations of the bedrest–activity cycle have been employed in numerous studies concerned with the circadian rhythmicity of physiological measures and psychological performance (Kleitman, 1963; Conroy & Mills, 1970; Colquhoun, 1971; Minors & Waterhouse, 1981). The adaptability of rhythms to new phase settings has been gauged in order to determine if they are of endogenous or exogenous origin (see earlier section).

Much research has centred on identifying which of the many observed rhythms are endogenous and what relationships exist between endogenous rhythms. This is necessary to uncover any causal nexus which may exist between them and understand the oscillating and controlling influences on the observed rhythms. In most phase shift studies sleep was treated as a unitary process and it was not customary to include polygraphic recording of sleep (Webb, 1971).

There were clear indications from early survey work (Wyatt & Marriott, 1953; Dirken, 1966; Tune, 1969) that a good proportion of night workers were dissatisfied with their lot. They frequently complained about a loss of sleep, being fatigued and the associated disruption of their social life. Workers on rotating shifts (morning, evening and night) reported that the night shift led to disturbed sleep, tiredness and restrictions on their social life in 52%, 80% and 77% respectively of those questioned (Wedderburn, 1978). This area is difficult to review because of the large number of different shift systems that are employed. See the review by Rutenfranz *et al.*, (1977) for details of some of the possible shift systems.

The first major study of night workers in which daytime sleep was polygraphically recorded was carried out by Kripke, Cook & Lewis (1971). The authors experienced great difficulty in getting subjects to report for recording sessions, even though the subjects had initially been selected as the most stable and regular sleepers of the night workers. Sleep-logs filled in by the subjects showed that the bedrest–activity patterns were very variable with all subjects reverting to night sleep on their 'off-duty' periods. These problems appear to have been common in most studies carried out on shift workers. The sleep patterns were generally similar to matched controls from other sleep laboratories. However, subsequent studies have found clear differences of the infrastructure of day sleep in night workers.

Alterations in quantity and distribution of sleep stages in nurses working night shifts and sleeping by day, were observed by Bryden and Holdstock (1973). The amount of SWS decreased in the day-sleep condition. Differences in REM sleep were confined to its distributions within the sleep period, where it occurred sooner with appreciably more REM sleep in the first third and less in the last third of the diurnal sleep, compared with nocturnal sleep. However, these nurses frequently napped during their work period (this would explain the reduced amount of SWS recorded during the day) and reverted to normal social patterns, with sleep at night, on their 'off-duty' periods.

The French authors Foret and Lantin (1972) showed that even workers who had worked shifts for two years exhibited extremely irregular bedrest–activity patterns. There were no significant differences in the amounts of SWS and REM sleep between nocturnal and diurnal sleep. But, as with the findings of Bryden and Holdstock (1973) the distribution of REM sleep was affected, with more REM sleep during the early REM–NREM cycles of day-sleep. As with all the recorded day-sleep of the night workers the duration of sleep was reduced by about 1.5 h. In order to reduce an accumulating sleep deficit these authors argue (Foret & Benoit, 1978) in favour of a rapid rotating shift system which would allow earlier recovery from shortened diurnal sleep. Webb & Agnew (1978) studied a simulated rapidly rotating shift system in which the subjects were allowed ad lib sleep when not scheduled for a shift. They found the subjects slept as late as possible prior to the morning shift, went to bed shortly after the night shift and slept midway between shift on the afternoon shift even though this involved retiring much later than normal, e.g. 03.00. This could be explained if the subjects free-ran during the experiment with a period greater than 24 h and sleep onset times becoming progressively later when the schedule allowed. Unlike the sleep–wakefulness pattern the infrastructure was not markedly changed.

Recently, Dahlgren (1981) showed that permanent night workers (more than 3 years' experience) exhibited a better adjustment of the body temperature rhythm to night work and day sleep and had fewer disturbances to their sleep stage pattern than workers on rotating shifts. A close relationship between the degree of adjustment of temperature and REM sleep was observed which agrees with Czeisler *et al.* (1980), but there was some indication that the temperature and REM rhythms were not completely coupled.

Experimental simulated phase alterations of the bedrest–activity cycle have been employed in a few studies primarily interested in sleep (e.g. Weitzman *et al.*, 1970; Webb *et al.*, 1971; Knauth & Rutenfranz, 1972; Taub & Berger, 1973; Hume, 1980).

The first 'phase reversal' of the bedrest–activity cycle in which sleep was polygraphically recorded was reported by Weitzman *et al.* (1970). The subjects were scheduled for a 180° (12 h) phase reversal of their bedrest–activity cycle. Webb *et al.* (1971) in a similar study used a 9 h phase delay. Both studies involved the initial loss of a night's sleep and in both these experiments little attempt was made to control the environment during the wakefulness portion of the regimens. Hence the subjects were aware of the real time, and the abnormality of their routine, by a multitude of environmental time cues, a situation similar to that experienced by shift workers.

The results from the two studies showed similar alterations in the sleep patterns. The most striking change in the displaced sleep was a clear shift of REM sleep towards the early part of the sleep episode, with a concomitant decrease in the last 2 h when waking frequently occurred. This early preponderance of REM sleep was brought about, in part, by a decreased REM latency but the basic REM–NREM cycle length was preserved. SWS suffered little change and appeared to shift immediately with the phase change, retaining its former position, predominantly in the first half of the sleep period.

Knauth and Rutenfranz (1972) reasoned that with sleep in the daytime the general level of noise is increased compared with at night. Sleep was recorded during nocturnal and diurnal bedrest sessions with and without noise added to the sleeper's environment. The results showed that the distribution of REM sleep was markedly affected in the daytime sleep with a shift towards the beginning of the sleep period. Noise caused a shorter duration of sleep, a reduction of Stage 4 and REM sleep and an increase in the number of stage changes during both daytime and nocturnal sleep. This indicates that differences between diurnal and nocturnal sleep infrastructure cannot be explained simply on the basis of disruption of sleep, similar to that caused by noise. Recently these authors (Knauth *et al.*, 1980) after reviewing evidence conclude that the 'qualitative sleep disturbance' of shift workers might be due to noise rather than time of day effects, while the duration of sleep seems to be dependent on the time of day.

Taub and Berger (1973) investigated the effect of shifting the position of sleep both earlier (retiring at 20.00 and 22.00) and later (retiring at 02.00 and 04.00) compared to the habitual position (24.00 to 08.00). The results as summarized by the authors were:

> . . . As sleep commenced progressively later from 20.00 to 04.00: Stage 4 significantly increased, but predominated during the first third of sleep in all conditions; REM also increased significantly and the length of the REM cycle significantly decreased. Compared to habitual sleep, REM latency was significantly reduced with retiring at 04.00.

The authors appreciated that the relative effects of sleep period displacement, and the length of prior wakefulness, could not be directly assessed as both factors varied concomitantly. However, they considered that these results, together with previous findings (e.g. Webb *et al.*, 1971), indicated a circadian rhythm of REM sleep, whereas the propensity for stage 4 sleep was determined primarily by prior length of time awake.

This approach has been extended recently by Akerstedt and Gillberg (1981). For one day each week, sleep was displaced, in steps of 4 h, to a total of seven times of day. While awaiting for the scheduled sleep on the experimental day the subjects were isolated from external time cues and the sleep was then allowed to terminate spontaneously. Despite the confusing variation in prior wakefulness, most sleep occurred after bedtimes at 19.00 and 23.00, while the least was after bedtimes at 07.00 and 11.00. The tendency to awake coincided with the peak time of least tiredness and clustered around noon. A time of day when the authors considered a barrier existed to further sleep because with increased accumulation of wakefulness, as sleep was delayed from its usual time (23.00) to 11.00, sleep length decreased. This fits the model of Aschoff *et al.* (1971) in which awakening is determined by a circadian sleep–wake function rising to a threshold level irrespective of the length of prior wakefulness or sleep.

These results agree with the idea of REM sleep being controlled in part by endogenous circadian factors while the amount and distribution of SWS is mainly dependent on exogenous factors, i.e. the duration of preceding wakefulness.

The early phase shift studies (Weitzman *et al.*, 1970; Webb *et al.*, 1971) were not aimed primarily at the rate of adaptation of the sleep stage profile to the new phase of the bedrest–activity cycle. However, in the Weitzman *et al.* (1970) study there were some signs of adaptation in the second week following the new regimen. Hume (1980) investigated the time course of adaptation of the sleep stage pattern to both an 8 h phase advance and delay of the bedrest–activity cycle. Such an 8 h phase advance in the nychthemeral rhythm of environment is experienced by anyone who flies eastward across 8 time zones and an 8 h phase delay occurs with a westward flight of the same magnitude.

Sleep was recorded in an isolation unit, described by Elliott *et al.* (1972), in which the natural cues to the time of day were absent. The subjects were warned of the phase shifts during the previous day and after the 'shift' (alteration of the clocks) they continued to follow their usual routine in which bedrest was scheduled from 23.30 to 07.30, by the clock inside the isolation unit.

The results showed that the mean amount of REM sleep was significantly increased after the westward shift, with sleep between 07.30 and 15.30 (GMT), while there was significantly less REM sleep after the eastward shift with sleep at 15.30 to 23.30 (GMT). This would be predicted if REM sleep followed a circadian rhythm that was not shifted or only partially shifted in phase, since REM sleep has previously been shown to follow a circadian rhythm, with maximum propensity for REM sleep in the morning (Hume & Mills, 1977). Unlike the difference in the amount of REM sleep in response to the eastward and westward phase-shifts, there was a similar significant change in the distribution of REM sleep across the sleep episode for both directions of shift with REM sleep becoming far more prominent in the first and less prominent in the last third.

Similar to other experiments with abnormal sleep–wakefulness patterns the mean amount of SWS was not significantly affected as a result of the phase-shifts. It occupied a similar position within sleep before and after the shifts maintaining a clear predominance in the first third of sleep episodes commencing at 23.30, 07.30 and 15.30 (GMT).

On arrival in a new time-zone after air travel, the traveller encounters a host of external 24 h rhythms of environment and society which are out of step with one's internal rhythms which are still in phase with the rhythms of the home time-zone. The collective subjective feelings of 'out-of-sorts' associated with this period of adjustment during which the internal rhythms synchronize with the external rhythms of environment and habit is commonly termed 'jet-lag'.

There are additional factors besides this loss of synchrony between the body and environment rhythms which determine one's well-being after a long flight: (1) fatigue and stress of flying, (2) excitement and apprehension associated with the purpose of the flight, e.g. holiday or tightly scheduled business trip, (3) non-rhythmical aspects of the unfamiliar environment, e.g. diet, climate, social customs, accommodation. All of these could lead to disturbed nights with early awakening. The effect on sleep of real time-zone changes incurred on trans-Atlantic flights was investigated by Evans *et al.* (1972). Early morning awakening was a frequent complaint of these time-zone travellers, particularly with older subjects. But there were no changes in the distribution of REM sleep. However, Endo *et al.* (1978) studied trans-Pacific air travellers and found a decrease in the amount of REM sleep after an initial 7 h eastward shift and an increase in REM sleep together with a change in its distribution after the return westward shift. These results are similar to those obtained in other 'field' studies (Moiseeva *et al.*, 1976; Klein *et al.*, 1976) and the laboratory-based studies of Hume (1980).

The extent of the alterations in the sleep stage pattern, and the time course of adaptation following a phase-shift, varied between individuals (Weitzman *et al.*, 1972; Hume, 1980). Similar results have been obtained for other circadian rhythms, where the effect of real and simulated time zone shifts have been investigated (Elliott *et al.*, 1972).

There was variation in the rate of adaptation of the sleep infrastructure between subjects in the laboratory study (Hume, 1980) but this was generally accomplished within a week for the westward shift. This finding was reinforced by a similar initial response to a second identical phase-shift which occurred one week after the first. Adaptation was not as clear after an eastward shift and a further identical shift a week later gave indication that adaptation had not been fully achieved. This has been observed after real flights, e.g. Klein *et al.*, (1976), where in response to an 8 h time zone transition it took on average 6.5 days for re-entrainment after an eastward flight and on average 5.1 days for a westward flight. The different rate of adjustment of various circadian rhythms to shifted zeitgeber depending upon the direction of the shift has been described as the 'Asymmetry effect' (Aschoff, 1978). This more rapid adaptation to an 8 h phase delay would agree with the numerous demonstrations that the free-running period in humans is slightly greater than 24 h, as adaptation would be expected sooner with a phase delay than a phase advance. In the former case there would be fewer intervening days before the free-running period (about 25 h) had 'caught up with' the new phasing. If this explanation is valid it would be predicted that animals whose free-running rhythms are less than 24 h would behave in the opposite manner and adapt more rapidly to phase advance (eastward shift) than phase delay (westward shift) of the zeitgeber. This has been observed (Aschoff *et al.*, 1975).

Besides the direction of shift the conditions surrounding the phase shift are very important factors affecting the rate of adaptation. Shift workers are subjected to a multitude of cues informing the subjects that they are living on an abnormal routine. Complete adaptation to diurnal sleep was not achieved by French railway workers, some of whom had worked rotating shifts for two years (Foret & Benoit, 1974). This suggests that naps and off-duty nocturnal sleep keep the REM sleep rhythm fixed with a high propensity for REM sleep in the morning.

In the isolation unit (Hume, 1980) there were no cues informing the subjects that they were living on an abnormal routine. Neither were there strong stimuli suggesting and encouraging the new routine, nor any change in the environmental variables. Only the clock inside the unit was altered and they had instructions to live according to clock time.

The situation is obviously different for air travellers experiencing a new time-zone. They are in receipt of strong stimuli suggesting and encouraging adaptation to the new phase position. Subjects who had to stay in their hotel rooms after a 6 h time-zone transition (Klein & Wegmann, 1974), took longer for re-entrainment of their circadian rhythms than subjects who were allowed to go out of doors, thereby experiencing more environmental cues to the new phasing.

It would be worthwhile to investigate the relative importance of the environmental cues which increase the rate at which an individual's sleep adapts to a new phase position, and which environmental stimuli, at what levels of stimulation, cause disruption of sleep and delay in adaptation. Which zeitgeber are most important for entraining the human sleep–wakefulness and other circadian rhythms has not been resolved finally. The most important periodic stimuli which synchronize rhythms in other animals including non-human primates is the light dark cycle (Pittendrigh, 1960; Moore-Ede *et al.*, 1976a). So potent and lawful is the entraining capacity of the light–dark cycle that Aschoff has been able to draw up a general rule of its effect on the free-running periods of certain species, i.e. with increasing intensity of illumination light/diurnal active animals decrease their free-running period while dark/ nocturnal active animals increase their free-running period. However, this rule does not hold when applied to humans and other primates.

Wever (1969) after experiments in an isolation unit, concluded that light–dark cycles were not capable of entraining human circadian rhythms.

However, certain flaws have been pointed out (e.g. Czeisler, 1981b) in the experimental detail of these experiments. In particular, the additional lighting, e.g. bedside lamps, that were available to the subjects in the isolation facility. Czeisler *et al.* (1981b) attempted to untangle and reassess the evidence for the importance of five major factors in entrainment; light–dark cycles, knowledge of time, meal-times, social contacts and bedrest–activity schedules, and presented new evidence which suggests that light–dark cycles alone are capable of entraining human circadian rhythms.

Knowledge of the time on its own does not seem to be an important influence as a subject living alone in a cave could not maintain a 24-h existence despite having a watch (Mills, 1964). Aschoff (1971) and Wever (1979) consider social cues in particular the timing of meals, work, rest, bedrest onset and termination to be the most important factors for entrainment. This view is based on observations such as the majority of subjects in group free-running experiments remain synchronized with each other at a period greater than 24 h suggesting that social interaction must be strong enough to entrain their circadian system to a common free-running period.

A constant difficulty in this area is how to untangle the effects of social cues, e.g. experimenters asking someone to go to bed, from the effects of the schedule, i.e. if they go to bed when asked. Regularity of the behavioural scheduling rather than social cues was considered to be the most important factor by Webb & Agnew (1974) who found a rigid schedule of bedrest sufficient for entrainment. They observed that circadian rhythms could be strictly entrained to a 24-h day if the wake time was rigidly controlled, but a bell was sounded at the same time in the morning as the room lights were turned on. Therefore the relative effects of lighting and wake time are difficult to determine.

It is feasible that entrainment is due to summation of various zeitgeber influences. Minors & Waterhouse (1981) after an exhaustive discussion of the evidence conclude that more than one zeitgeber is made use of and the relative important of zeitgeber will vary for different individuals under different circumstances.

2.5.6 Period Alterations

An alteration in the period of the sleep–wakefulness rhythm presents a more complex situation than an alteration in the phase of the rhythm. A phase shift changes the timing of the sleep period whereas a period alteration involves three variables, duration of prior wakefulness, length of time asleep and time of day of the sleep period, each of which can influence sleep. Despite study of numerous physiological measures (Conroy & Mills, 1970) no polygraphic recordings of sleep were obtained in investigations involving a change of the sleep–wakefulness period until the mid-1970s.

It has been found that there are marked inter-individual differences in the ability to adapt to abnormal periods of the bedrest–activity rhythm when imposed 'artificially'. In particular it has been consistently difficult to entrain successfully 12 h or 48 h temperature rhythms, while some success has been recoded with periods nearer 24 h, e.g. 22 or 27 h (Kleitman, 1963).

A systematic alteration of 'day' length with sleep recordings and bedrest–activity periods near to 24 h was reported by Webb & Agnew (1975). 'Days' of 30 h, 18 h, 12 h and 9 h were employed, with a constant ratio of bedrest to activity of 1:2. The results showed all the modified bedrest–activity schedules resulted in reduced sleep duration with an increase of Stage 1 sleep and a decrease of Stage 2 sleep with little sign of adaptation.

The effect of lengthening and shortening the habitual 24 h period by 3 h to 27 and 21 h, where sleep commences respectively 3 h later or earlier on successive days, was studied in an isolation unit by Hume (1978). These are periods within the circadian range (20–28 h) and similar to those used by rhythm researchers who have reported (Kleitman, 1963; Lewis & Lobban, 1956) some success in the entrainment of rhythms, mainly temperature, to the new period.

In general the subjects reported little difficulty in sleeping and staying awake at the scheduled times while living on 27 and 21 h days in an isolation unit (Hume, 1978). The subjects were informed at the start of the experiment that the clocks may not indicate solar time, but not how such a discrepancy might occur. After a few days some felt that there was 'something amiss' but none deduced that the frequency of the electrical supply to the clocks in the isolation unit had been changed, so the clocks registered 24 h in either 27 or 21 h of solar time. The most popular suggestion was the clocks were altered while they were asleep.

However, sleep was clearly disturbed, with significant increases in the amount of wakefulness, movement and Stage 1 sleep during the sleep episodes for both these lengthened and shortened days. Predictably, the duration of sleep was increased on the 27 h day with 9 h available for sleep, and decreased on the 21 h day with only 7 h for sleep. In full agreement with the direct relationship between the length of sleep and the amount of REM sleep (Verdone, 1968), there was more REM sleep in the longer sleep episode with the 27 h day and less in the 21 h day than was obtained on the control 24 h days. Likewise, the relationship between the duration of preceding wakefulness and the amount of SWS was upheld, with more SWS after 18 h and less after 14 h than was obtained after the habitual 16 h of activity. Similar to other abnormal sleep–wakefulness schedules, alteration of the external zeitgeber period had no significant effect on the length of the REM–NREM cycle.

In general there are three types of results from experiments involving artificial day lengths (Minors & Waterhouse, 1981): (1) a rhythm shows no sign of adaptation to the altered daylength and retains a period of about 24 h which would be free-running and provides evidence for an endogenous nature, (2) the rhythm takes up a period equal to the artificially imposed daylength and this indicates its exogenous origin, or (3) the most common result where there are signs of two periodic influences present due to the interaction of endogenous and exogenous factors attributable to a free-running rhythm with a period of about 24 h and the other equal to the artificial daylength.

Analysis on a daily basis (Hume, 1978) revealed few signs of adaptation of the infrastrucure of sleep to the new cycle lengths of the external zeitgeber. Near 24 h rhythms were still apparent, resulting in 'daily' variations in the amount of sleep and REM sleep. Both were at a minimum in the late afternoon to evening and maximal in the morning by solar time.

The continuation of these near 24 h rhythms were more apparent for the 21 h than the 27 h days. This would be predicted if, in the absence of 24 h zeitgebers, these endogenous rhythms 'free-ran' and a period longer than 24 h would be expected. This happened with the temperature rhythm, which had periods of about 24.3 h for the 21 h days (Mills *et al.*, 1977). Therefore the longer free-running period would be better matched with a 27 h than to a shortened 21 h day.

The maximum amount of REM sleep was observed slightly later with regards to solar time during the first and second weeks of 21 h days; this indicates the extent of maladaptation to the zeitgeber period. The minutes of REM sleep during each 7 h sleep episode, when plotted against the mid-point of the bedrest on solar time, were well fitted by a cosine curve with an acrophase (projected time of maximum) at 10.55 (Hume & Mills, 1977). The data points did not allow precise definition of the period and could just as well be fitted by a cosine of period slightly over 24 h as by one of 24 h.

2.6 Sleep–Wakefulness, Temperature and Hormonal Rhythms, Pathology and Mechanisms

So far, the rhythmical aspects of sleep and sleep stages have been considered without any consideration of how the pattern of sleep and wakefulness can affect other circadian rhythms. Variables which possess endogenous rhythmicity are responsive to behavioural events such as exercise, bedrest or eating meals. These 'masking effects' (Aschoff *et al.*, 1975) or 'evoked responses' (Czeisler, 1978) are normally superimposed upon the endogenous rhythm when an individual follows a normal nychthemeral existence. Sleep and wakefulness exert a major direct effect on many rhythms.

2.6.1 Temperature

A circadian rhythm of body temperature was one of the first to be recognized (Conroy & Mills, 1970) and is possibly the most widely recorded variable in humans because of its comparative ease of measurement. Its close association with sleep duration and the REM sleep potential rhythm (Czeisler *et al.*, 1980) make it particularly relevant here. It is generally found that on an entrained nychthemeral existence the body temperature reaches its peak in the evening, about 20.00, and falls rapidly at sleep onset and then more gradually to reach a minimum at about 05.00. It rises sharply at about the time of awakening and then more gradually through the day.

The marked temperature drop during the first few hours of sleep is observed whatever the time of day of sleeping. This temperature drop associated with sleep is superimposed upon the endogenous temperature rhythm. Interestingly, the size of this sleep-induced drop in temperature is itself dependent on the time of day, such that the drop is less during the daytime than at the habitual time of sleeping (Mills *et al.*, 1978). A similar time of day effect is found for the temperature elevation due to exercise (Crockford & Davies, 1969). The situation is further complicated by the inactivation of the thermo-regulatory process during REM sleep (see review by Parmeggiani, 1980). The extent to which such masking effects are to be considered nuisance factors which obscure the true endogenous rhythm or are important effects of entraining zeitgeber is not yet clear. There is some evidence that sleep can act as a zeitgeber (Minors & Waterhouse, 1981). It was observed by these authors that when subjects lived on imposed irregular schedules of sleep and wakefulness their rhythms free-ran. However, when one 4 h portion of sleep (anchor sleep) was routinely taken at a fixed time of day, i.e. similar to the first half of an habitual night's sleep, it stabilized the rhythms to a 24 h pattern. These authors emphasize that it is unresolved what aspects of sleep, e.g. posture, inactivity or sleep stages, are responsible for the masking or zeitgeber influences. See Minors & Waterhouse (1981) for further discussion.

In free-running subjects, temperature and other rhythms can remain internally synchronized but the phase relationship between the bedrest–activity cycle and the temperature rhythm often changes with the temperature minimum occuring at about sleep onset as opposed to the last half of sleep (Wever, 1979; Czeisler *et al.*, 1980). Some subjects show internal desynchronization where the periods for temperature and sleep-wakefulness become distinct with consequently no consistent phase relationship between them. In this situation the temperature rhythm tends to be more regular and nearer 24 h than the sleep–wakefulness rhythm. Therefore, although these rhythms are usually closely linked and affect each other, there is a strong case for their separate control via two independent oscillators.

2.6.2 Hormones

The relationships between sleep, sleep stages and hormonal rhythms has received considerable attention and provides some good examples of the possible interaction between these rhythmical processes. Sleep is a major determinant of the 24 h pattern of hormone secretion. It has a variable but important influence upon the overt phasing of the rhythms of human growth hormone (HGH), thyroid stimulating hormone (TSH), luteinizing hormone, testosterone and prolactin and has masking effects upon their waveforms (Parker *et al.*, 1980). Detailed consideration of the circadian rhythms of hormones is given elsewhere (Parker *et al.*, 1980).

Clearer resolution of relationships between hormones, sleep and sleep stages has been achieved as a result of the development of techniques which allow for more sensitive assay methods, e.g. radio immuno assays and procedures which enable more frequent plasma samples during both sleep and wakefulness (Hellman, *et al.*, 1970; Weitzman, 1976) as opposed to methods which relied upon urinary measurements of derived metabolic products. This is particularly important when inferences about the relationship between sleep stages and endocrine secretions are to be drawn, as one is a composite measure of electrophysiological activity associated with the CNS which is scored in 30 s epochs while endocrine secretion is subject to delay before CNS control mechanisms are reflected in hormonal level changes in blood. Because of these different processes the relationships between them cannot be precise. HGH and cortisol are good examples to illustrate the types of possible relationships between the rhythms of sleep and hormones.

HGH is secreted in an episodic manner (Weitzman, 1976) with short periods of secretion (1–2 h) then long intervals with no detectable HGH. The major secretory period is associated with the first few hours of sleep (Daly & Evans, 1974; Parker *et al.*, 1980). In addition, there are other smaller peaks of secretion later in the day which may be related to the times of feeding (Parker *et al.*, 1980). For further discussion of factors which cause secretion of HGH see the review by Quabbe (1977).

The close association between the major HGH release and sleep has held under various experimental procedures, which include: delay or advance of the sleep episode (Takahashi *et al.*, 1968; Honda *et al.*, 1969), reversal of the sleep–wakefulness cycle (Sassin *et al.*, 1969) ultradian (3 h) sleep–wakefulness regimen (Weitzman *et al.*, 1974) and free-running experiments (Weitzman *et al.*, 1979) where subjects showed internal dissociation of the sleep–wakefulness and temperature rhythms. These studies show a strong relationship between sleep and HGH with no indication that HGH is controlled by an independent endogenous circadian oscillator. Is this sleep-related secretion associated with a particular stage of sleep?

SWS is implicated for this association as it occurs predominantly in the first few hours of sleep and retains this position within sleep regardless of the time of day of sleep. Sassin *et al.* (1969) showed a clear tendency for HGH to be released during SWS under a habitual regimen of sleep and wakefulness and this association was retained and immediately adjusted to a 12 h shift (phase reversal) of the sleep–wakefulness rhythm. Therefore, HGH secretion similar to SWS does not display the characteristics of an endogenous circadian rhythm as it adapts immediately to a change in the timing of sleep within the 24 h with no residual secretion at the habitual time of maximal secretion.

The relationship between SWS and HGH is not precise, secretion occurs after sleep onset but prior to epochs which are scored as either Stage 3 or Stage 4 (i.e. SWS). This was clearly demonstrated in studies by Karacan *et al.* (1971) and Sassin *et al.* (1969) who employed the technique of SWS deprivation and were only partially successful in achieving the suppression of HGH as some was secreted before SWS had occurred. However, the secretion may be related to EEG delta activity which is maximal during SWS.

The scoring criteria provide clear but arbitrary delineation between an epoch score for Stage 3 and Stage 2 (which usually precedes Stage 3) based on the percentage of EEG delta activity; less than 20% for Stage 2 while more scores Stage 3. A detailed investigation (Pawel *et al.*, 1972) of the relationship between EEG delta activity and HGH levels in which the sleep recordings were scored in 10 s epochs (as opposed to the more usual duration of 20 or 30 s) and blood samples were taken every 4 min (compared with the usual interval of about 20 min) showed that EEG delta activity consistently occurred before the rise in plasma HGH. From the little data available, it seems that the amount of HGH released is not directly related to the duration of SWS, rather the EEG delta activity acts as a trigger for HGH release.

Cortisol, similar to HGH, has a consistent 24 h pattern of secretion under nychthemeral conditions (Daly & Evans, 1974; Parker *et al.*, 1980) and is released in an episodic manner (Weitzman, 1976). Plasma levels are lowest during the hours immediately preceding and just after bedtime, then rise during sleep to the main secretory phase during the last 2 hours of sleep and first hours of wakefulness, thereafter they decline across the daytime when the episodes of secretion are intermittent until secretion is again at a minimum at bedtime.

Given the similarity between this distribution and the REM potential rhythm (Hume & Mills, 1977) this stage of sleep was considered a likely contender for possessing a close relationship with cortisol secretion. However, there is clear evidence that cortisol rhythm is independent of sleep stages and the sleep–wakefulness rhythm. Sleep is not necessary to observe a normal pattern of cortisol secretion (Nichols & Tyler, 1967); following air travel across numerous time-zones there was dissociation between the cortisol and sleep–wakefulness rhythms which took days before the original temporal relationship was regained (Flink & Doe, 1959; Conroy & Hall, 1969) and such a temporal relationship was not re-established up to 3 weeks after a phase reversal of the sleep–wakefulness cycle (Weitzman *et al.*, 1968, 1970). Therefore unlike the close association between HGH and SWS, the cortisol and REM rhythms can be completely dissociated by rescheduling sleep and wakefulness.

A change in the endogenous pattern of cortisol secretion was reported for some subjects under free-running conditions (Weitzman *et al.*, 1979). There was a phase advance (6–8 h, relative to sleep onset) and the average rate of increases after the minimum was much more gradual but the maximum levels were still at about the end of the sleep episode. In addition to this endogenous component a clear inhibition of cortisol secretion was observed for the first 2–3 h following sleep onset. Further evidence for such an effect comes from a thorough investigation of endocrine rhythms in young adult men under nychthemeral conditions (Parker *et al.*, 1980) where the minimum occurs early in sleep with a clear reduction in variance of the rhythm at this point compared to the rest of the day which is suggestive of a sleep-related inhibition of cortisol secretion.

Two components were present in the cortisol secretion pattern in subjects living on a 3 h 'day' (Weitzman, 1974). Besides the marked endogenous circadian components there was some ultradian component presumably resulting from the sleep or bed-rest related inhibition of cortisol. This result was quite different from that of HGH which showed an ultradian period of 3 h with no circadian component. Therefore, apart from the main endogenous secretory rhythm, sleep does seem to affect the secretory pattern of cortisol. Again it is not known for sure what component of the sleep process is responsible for this inhibition of cortisol secretion at sleep onset.

2.6.3 Pathology

The mechanisms that control the sleep–wakefulness cycle and allow entrainment to a precise 24 h rhythm, can function abnormally, similar to all physiological systems. Sleep and rhythm pathologies are just beginning to receive systematic classification and study. See Weitzman (1981) and the Association of Sleep Disorders Centers' — Diagnostic Classification of Sleep and Arousal Disorders (1979) for full detailed accounts.

There are reports of individuals exposed to normal nychthemeral environments who have great difficulty in keeping in step with the rest of society. Some experience great difficulty in retiring and rising at regular times from day to day and similar to normal subjects isolated in time-free environments they go to bed and wake up progressively later each day, producing sleep–wakefulness periods greater than 24 h.

Miles *et al.* (1977) reported a case of a hyper-nychthemeral rhythm in a man blind from birth who showed a persistent 25 h rhythm in sleep–wakefulness and plasma cortisol. Such desynchronization seems to be more common in blind than sighted individuals (Miles *et al.*, 1977). One can readily appreciate that blindness and the consequent removal of a major zeitgeber makes blind individuals more prone to lose 24 h entrainment.

However, similar cases have been reported in normally sighted individuals

(Elliott *et al.*, 1970; Kokkoris *et al.*, 1978; Weber *et al.*, 1980) who report less difficulty in maintaining a sleep–wakefulness period greater than 24 h than a rigid 24 h schedule. There is some evidence that these individuals can maintain a normal 24 h period when the socializing pressures are increased and this has lead some authors (Weber *et al.*, 1980) to emphasize the importance of social zeitgeber for normal 24 h entrainment.

Another condition in the category of Disorders of Sleep–wakefulness Schedule is the delayed sleep phase syndrome. This involves a delay of sleep onset and difficulty in morning awakening. This differs from the non-24 h sleep–wakefulness syndrome in that there is no progressive shift of the sleep and awake times rather the phase of the sleep–wakefulness rhythm is delayed by a set number of hours. There has been some success at resetting the phase of the sleep–wakefulness cycle in such individuals via chronotherapy (Czeisler *et al.*, 1981a) as opposed to the traditional remedy for all types of insomnia — drug therapy. These authors postulated that these individuals could not phase advance their sleep–wakefulness rhythm to a normal phasing. Therefore, they were placed on a 27 h sleep–wakefulness regimen which involves a phase delay of 3 h per day, this was maintained for about 6 days until the subjects were now sleeping at normal times. The procedure was successful in shifting the sleep times from about 05.00–13.00 to 00.30–08.00 and subsequently all subjects reported a lasting resolution of their problem. However, the problem may reappear later if the subjects do not adhere to a strict bed-rest time, e.g. following a late party.

Another example of modifying the circadian rhythm in order to effect relief from illness is seen with phase advance of the sleep–wakefulness cycle which can act as an antidepressant (Wehr *et al.*, 1979). These authors and others noticed the similarity between depressed patients' sleep and normal subjects whose circadian rhythms of temperature and REM sleep are phase advanced, i.e. REM sleep occurs earlier in the sleep episode. Therefore, a phase advance of the sleep–wakefulness cycle of depressed patients was tried to compensate for the abnormal timing and to realign these rhythms. A 6 h phase advance of the sleep–wakefulness cycle was effective in clearing the depression in a manic-depressive woman but the relief was only temporary and similar in duration to the desynchronization with jet lag. However, this represents an interesting departure from the traditional drug therapy and indicates that abnormal sleep patterns in some types of depression are due to abnormal internal phase relationships of circadian rhythms.

2.6.4 *Mechanisms*

Some brief consideration follows of the control mechanisms that have been identified to account for rhythmicity in sleep. Reviews of the neurophysiological and neurochemical substrates of sleep and arousal mechanisms are to be found elsewhere (see chapters by Steriade, Siegel and Borbély). However, all putative sleep mechanisms should incorporate the circadian and ultradian timing systems into their final models.

In the 1970s the importance of the suprachiasmatic nucleus (SCN) of the hypothalamus in non-human primates and other mammals as a clock or oscillator for their circadian timing system became clear. See Rusak & Zucker (1979) and Moore (1979) for reviews. The retino-hypothalmic tract (RHT), originating in the retina, innervates the SCN and accounts for the powerful phase control which the light–dark cycle exerts on circadian rhythms in these species (Moore, 1979). Lesions of the SCN in the squirrel monkey eliminates circadian rhythmicity in activity, feeding and drinking but not temperature (Fuller *et al.*, 1981). This indicates that the SCN is just one of the key pacemakers in what must be a multi-oscillator system.

In humans the same structure cannot be identified as rigorously but a small cluster of loosely packed neurones in the supra-chiasmatic region which may be homologous to the SCN in other primates has been reported (Lydic *et al.*, 1980). Existence of RHT in humans cannot be shown for ethical reasons but mathematical modelling of the human circadian system (Kronauer *et al.*, 1982) provides further support for a circadian pacemaker in humans homologous to the SCN in other primates which drives rest–activity cycles and is directly coupled to zeitgeber inputs such as the light–dark cycle.

Therefore, it is envisaged that the SCN provides a time base which exerts a major influence that either sets the time when sleep is possible, thus allowing the sleep regulatory mechanism to put the animal to sleep during its inactive period, or keeps the animal awake during its active period.

2.7 Review and Functional Implications

Sleep is an inherently rhythmical process in which the endogenous sleep–wakefulness rhythm is the most obvious. The free-running paradigm reveals the organization of sleep and wakefulness, particularly the most likely time for sleep onset and its duration, is determined partly by the phase of the temperature rhythm. However, the position is far from clear as there is a body of evidence for two separate oscillators controlling sleep–wakefulness and temperature rhythms (Aschoff, 1981; Wever, 1979; Moore-Ede *et al.*, 1976). The relative importance of the various zeitgeber which entrain human circadian rhythms is unresolved.

The appearance of REM sleep depends on two endogenous cyclical phenomena, one circadian and the other the ultradian REM–NREM rhythm. There is conflicting evidence and divided opinion whether the ultradian oscillator continues to operate and influence other processes into the waking hours as envisaged by Kleitman (1963). This oscillator has been extremely resistant to experimental manipulation and therefore has proved very difficult to study. Only Borbély (1975) has reported entrainment of the REM–NREM cycle length in the rat by external time cues — short periodic light–dark cycles. There is very little evidence for circadian modulation of the REM–NREM cycle length despite various abnormal bedrest–activity schedules in humans.

There is overwhelming evidence that the potential for REM sleep follows a circadian rhythm, with a maximum in the morning at about the time of getting up and a minimum in the evening, under entrained conditions. This is closely coupled to the phase of the body temperature rhythm such that REM sleep propensity is greatest a couple of hours after the trough of the temperature rhythm and lowest a few hours after the temperature maximum. These rhythms can become dissociated from the sleep–wakefulness rhythm, i.e. internal desynchronization during free-running. The concept of an endogenous circadian rhythm in the potential for REM sleep implies that the oscillator responsible for the timing of REM sleep or, a process which REM sleep reflects, is sleep independent. This does not preclude sleep from having a major influence on this process and by definition REM sleep occurs only during sleep. A stark reminder that rhythmical aspects are not the only determinants of REM sleep is that REM sleep deprivation is followed by a compensatory REM sleep rebound indicating that a certain amount of REM sleep must be maintained across sleep episodes, although the deprivation threshold for REM sleep compensation is higher than that for SWS. The circadianly rhythmical properties of REM sleep contrast markedly with SWS which is primarily dependent on the length of preceding wakefulness, irrespective of the time of day of sleep.

Does knowledge of the rhythmical nature of sleep help us decide between the suggested functions of sleep? There are two main approaches to the function of sleep, as discussed fully in the first chapter, restorative and behavioural.

The restorative school views sleep as a time for recovery in which various neurochemical and neurophysiological systems operate to reverse the effects of wakefulness. Therefore, this model could easily incorporate a rhythm dimension where the sleep–wakefulness rhythm is viewed as reflecting a restoration –depletion rhythm.

It is quite plausible to expect, similar to all other physiological processes, a time of day when restorative processes are most efficient and this for humans has been considered to be at night when we are asleep. Common sense would suggest the system has evolved to withstand a certain duration of depletion and take subsequently a relatively fixed duration for recovery.

The strong association between the duration of wakefulness before sleep and the amount of SWS together with SWS's association with the release of HGH fit nicely into a restorative model. However, there have been questions raised about the association between HGH and tissue repair (see chapter by Horne). Furthermore, as a result of evolution it would be expected that this rhythm becomes coupled with the environmental variables which favour survival, with rest and activity at the most appropriate time. This point crosses the artificial divide between restorative and behavioural theories.

The behavioural/ethological approach is constructed around a circadian timing dimension in that sleep is viewed as a response to the environmental periodicities which would make activity less beneficial than enforced immobility with the consequent energy conservation. Therefore, sleep–wakefulness cycle is seen as reflecting an inactivity–activity rhythm which increases the safety of the animal and its chances of survival.

This seems perfectly plausible for sub-human species for whom environmental variables are critically important but this argument is much less strong for humans. Man has learnt progressively to control and manipulate his environment to his advantage ever since, for example, he clothed himself and was able to harness fire. In parallel with technological developments for environmental control the need to sleep has not apparently diminished even today and is still one of the most potent influences on the organization of our lives. This would suggest that for humans sleep must serve some other function than just keeping us out of harm's way.

This is one of the conclusions arrived at by Horne (*ibid.*) after a review of the evidence he puts forward a model which incorporates aspects of the two positions. He suggests that there is some sleep that we need (obligatory sleep) normally in the first part of the night and composed mainly of SWS and about half of our nightly REM sleep. This obligatory sleep allows restitution for the brain, particularly the cerebrum. The remainder of our nightly sleep (optional sleep) mainly Stage 2 and REM, is taken as the result of a sleep drive but we can do without it and is merely a way of keeping us occupied during darkness.

There seem to the present author to be strong parallels between Horne's position and the more mechanistic models of Borbély and co-workers (1980 & *ibid.*). The Borbély model of sleep regulation involves two separate processes: A sleep-dependent, self-regulated process (S) whose level increases during wakefulness, decreases in sleep and has characteristics similar to SWS in particular its close association to duration of prior wakefulness. The other process (C) is largely sleep independent and reflects mainly the circadian rhythm of sleep propensity which in humans is maximal in the early morning and minimum in the late afternoon and is a rigidly programmed rhythm controlled by a circadian oscillator. Sleep propensity or sleep intensity is the sum of S and C.

The sleep-dependent process (S) could be viewed as the function associated with obligatory sleep which is composed of mainly SWS and allows restitution after depletion during wakefulness. The sleep-independent, circadian rhythm process (C) fits nicely into the concept of optional sleep with the idea of a phylogenetic precursor of sleep which humans can do without. REM sleep is more awkward to accommodate in either model but as there is a need for a certain amount of REM sleep this obligatory minimum can be included within the sleep-dependent process S while the strong circadian aspect of REM sleep could be generated as part of process C.

It is encouraging to see such converging lines of explanation which include an important role for the rhythmical nature of sleep and REM sleep. However, there are many problems still to be resolved.

References

AGNEW, H. W. jun and WEBB, W. B. (1968). The displacement of Stages 4 and REM sleep within a full night of sleep. *Psychophysiology*, **5**, 142–148.

AGNEW, H. W. jun., WEBB, W. B. and WILLIAMS, R. L. (1964). The effects of Stage 4 sleep deprivation. *Electroencephalog. Clin. Neurophysiol.*, **17**, 68–70.

AKERSTEDT, T. and GILLBERG, M. (1981). The circadian variation of experimentally displaced sleep. *Sleep*, **4(2)**, 159–169.

ANDERS, T., EMDE, R. and PARMELEE, A. (1971). (Eds.) A Manual of standardized techniques and criteria for scoring of states of sleep and wakefulness in newborn infants. UCLA Brain Information Service, NINDS Neurological Information Network.

ASCHOFF, J., GERECKE, U., KURECK, A. *et al.* (1971). Interdependent parameters of circadian activity rhythms in birds and man. In: M. MENAKER (Ed.), *Biochronometry*, Washington, DC: National Academy of Sciences, 3–27.

ASCHOFF, J. (1960). Exogenous and endogenous components in circadian rhythms. Cold Spr. Harb. Symp. Quant. Biol., **25**, 11–28.

ASCHOFF, J. (1965). Circadian rhythms in man. *Science*, **148**, 1427–1432.

ASCHOFF, J. (1978). Features of circadian rhythms relevant for the design of shift schedules. *Ergonomics*, **21**, 739–754.

ASCHOFF, J. (1981) *Handbook of Behavioural Neurobiology, Vol. 4, Biological Rhythms*. New York: Plenum.

ASCHOFF, J., HOFFMANN, K., POHL, H. *et al.* (1975). Re-entrainment of circadian rhythms after phase shifts of the zeitgehr. *Chronobiologia*, **2**, 23–78.

ASERINSKY, E. (1973). Relationship of REM density to the prior accumulation of sleep and wakefulness. *Psychophysiology*, **10(6)**, 545–558.

ASERINSKY, E. and KLEITMAN, N. (1953). Regularly occurring periods of eye motility and concomitant phenomena during sleep. *Science*, **118**, 273.

ASERINSKY, E. and KLEITMAN, N. (1955a). A motility cycle in sleeping infants as manifested by ocular and gross bodily activity. *J. Appl. Physiol.*, **8**, 11–18.

ASSOCIATION OF SLEEP DISORDERS CENTERS. (1979). Diagnostic Classification of Sleep and Arousal Disorders, 1st ed, prepared by the Sleep Disorders Classification Committee. H. P. ROFFWARG, Chairman, *Sleep*, **2**, 1–137.

BERGER, R. J. and OSWALD, I. (1962). Effects of sleep deprivation on behaviour, subsequent sleep and dreaming. *J. of Mental Science*, **108**, 457–465.

BORBÉLY, A. A., HUSTON, J. P. and WASER, P. G. (1975). Control of sleep states in the rat by short light-dark cycles. *Brain Research*, **75**, 89–101.

BORBÉLY, A. A. (1980). Effect of light and circadian rhythm on the occurrence of REM sleep in the rat. *Sleep*, **2(3)**, 289–299.

BREZINOVA, V. (1974). Sleep cycle content and sleep cycle duration. *Electroencephalog. Clin. Neurophysiol.*, **36**, 275–283.

BREZINOVA, V., BECK, U. and OSWALD, I. (1975). Sleep cycle duration and timing of REM periods in interrupted night sleep. *Intern. J. of Chronobiol.*, **3**, 81–87.

BROWN, F. A. (1976). Evidence for external timing of biological clocks. In: J. D. PALMER, (Ed.) *An Introduction to Biological Rhythms*. New York: Plenum.

BRYDEN, G. & HOLDSTOCK, T. L. (1973). Effect of night duty on sleep patterns of nurses. *Psychophysiol.*, **10(1)**, 36–42.

BUGUET, A., ROUSSEL, B., ANGUS, R. *et al.* (1980). Human sleep and adrenal individual reactions to exercise. *Electroencephallog. Clin. Neurophysiol.*, **49**, 515–523.

CARSKADON, M. A. and DEMENT, W. C. (1975). Sleep studies on a 90-minute day. *Electroencephalog. Clin. Neurophysiol.*, **39**, 145–155.

CARSKADON, M. A. and DEMENT, W. C. (1980). Distribution of REM sleep on a 90-minute sleep-wake schedule. *Sleep*, **2(3)**, 309–319.

CHOUVET, G., MOURET, J., COINDET, J., SIFFRE, M. and JOUVET, M. (1974). Periodicite bicircadienne du cycle veille-sommeil dans des conditions hors du temps. Etude polygraphique. *Electroencephalog. Clin. Neurophysiol.*, **37**, 367–380.

COLQUHOUN, W. P. (1971). (Ed.) *Biological rhythms and human performance,* New York: Academic Press.

CONROY, R. T. W. L. and HALL, M. D. (1969). Adrenal cortical function and body temperature rhythms after a transatlantic flight. *Journal of Physiology* (London), **200**, 123.

CONROY, R. T. W. L. and MILLS, J. N. (1970). *Human Circadian Rhythms*. London: Churchill.

CROCKFORD, G. W. and DAVIES, C. T. (1969). Circadian variations in responses to sub-maximal exercise on a bicycle ergometer. *Journal of Physiology* (London), **201**, 94P–95P.

CROWLEY, T. J., KRIPKE, D. F., HALBERG, F., PEGRAM, G. V. and SCHILDKRAUT, J. J. (1972). Circadian rhythms of Macca mulatta: sleep, EEG, body and eye movement, and temperature. *Primates*, **13(2)**, 149–168.

CZEISLER, C. A. (1978). Human circadian physiology: internal organisation of temperature, sleep-wake and neuro-endocrine rhythms monitored in an environment free of time cues. PhD thesis, Stanford University.

CZEISLER, C. A., BORBÉLY, A., HUME, K. I., *et al.* (1980). *Sleep,* **2(3)**, 287–288.

CZEISLER, C. A., RICHARDSON, G. S., COLEMAN, R. M. *et al.* (1981a). Chronotherapy: resetting the circadian clocks of patients with delayed sleep phase insomnia. *Sleep*, **4(1)**, 1–21.

CZEISLER, C. A., RICHARDSON, G. S., ZIMMERMAN, J. C. *et al.* (1981b). Entrainment of human circadian rhythms by light-dark cycles: A reassessment. *Photochemistry and Photobiology*, **34**, 239–247.

CZEISLER, C. A., WEITZMAN, E. D., MOORE-EDE, M. C. *et al.* (1980) Human sleep: its duration and organization depend on its circadian phase. *Science*, **210**, 1264–1267.

DAHLGREN, K. (1981). Adjustment of circadian rhythms and EEG sleep functions to day and night sleep among permanent night workers and rotating shift workers. *Psychophysiology*, **18(4)**, 381–391.

DALY, J. R. and EVANS, J. I. (1974). Daily rhythms of steroid and associated pituitary hormones in man and their relationship to sleep. *Advances in Steroid Biochemistry and Pharmacology*, **4**, 273–283.

DEMENT, W. C. (1960). The effect of dream deprivation. *Science*, **131**, 1705–7; **132**, 1420–2;

DEMENT, W. C. and KLEITMAN, N. (1957). Cyclic variations in EEG during sleep and their relation to eye movements, body motility and dreaming. *Electroencephalog. Clin. Neurophysiol.*, **9**, 673–690.

DEMENT, W. and MITLER, M. (1974). An introduction to sleep. In: O. PETRE-QUADENS and J. SCHLAG (Eds.) *Basic Sleep Mechanisms*, New York: Academic Press, pp. 271–296.

DEMENT, W. C. and WOLPERT, E. (1958). The relation of eye movements, body motility and external stimuli to dream content. *J. Exp. Psychol.*, **55**, 543–553.

DIRKEN, J. M. (1966). Industrial shift work; decrease in well-being and specific effects. *Ergonomics*, **9**, 115–124.

DIRLICH, G., ZULLEY, J. and SCHULZ, H. (1977). The temporal pattern of the REM sleep rhythm. Proceedings: Twelfth International Conference, International Society for Chronobiology. Milan, Italy: 11 Ponte, pp. 483–493.

ELLIOTT, A. L., MILLS, J. N., MINORS, D. S. and WATERHOUSE, J. M. (1972). The effect of real and simulated time-zone shifts upon circadian rhythms of body temperature, plasma 11-hydroxycorticosteroids, and renal excretion in human subjects. *J. Physiol.*, **221**, 227–257.

ELLIOTT, A. L., MILLS, J. N. and WATERHOUSE, J. M. (1970). A man with too long a day. *J. Physiol.*, **212**, 30–31P.

ENDO, S., YAMAMOTO, T. and SASAKI, M. (1978). Effects of time-zone changes on sleep west–east flight and east–west flight. *Jikeikai Med. J.*, **25**, 249–268.

EVANS, J. I., CHRISTIE, G. A., LEWIS, S. A., DALY, J. and MOORE ROBINSON, M. (1972). Sleep and Time-Zone Changes. *Arch. Neurol.*, **26**, 36–48.

FEINBERG, I. and FLOYD, T. C. (1979). Systematic trends across the night in human sleep cycles. *Psychophysiology*, **16**, 283–291.

FEINBERG, I., FEIN, G. and FLOYD, T. C. (1980). EEG patterns during and following extended sleep in young adults. *Electroencephalog. Clin. Neurophysiol.*, **50**, 467–476.

FLINK, E. B. and DOE, R. P. (1959). Effect of sudden time displacement by air travel on synchronization of adrenal function. *Proceedings of the Society of Experimental Biology and Medicine*, **100**, 498–501.

FORET, J. and BENOIT, O. (1974). Structure du sommeil chez des travailleurs a horaires alternants. *Electroencephalog. Clin. Neurophysiol.*, **37**, 337–344.

FORET, J. and BENOIT, O. (1978). Étude du sommeil de travailleurs à horaires alternants: adaptation et récupération dans le cas de rotation rapide de poste (3–4 jours). *Eur. J. Appl. Physiol.*, **38**, 71–82.

FORET, J. and LANTIN, G. (1972). The sleep of train drivers: an example of the effects of irregular work schedules on sleep. In: COLQUHOUN, W. P. (Ed.) *Aspects of human efficiency*, pp. 273–283.

FREEMON, F. R. (1972). *Sleep Research: A Critical Review.* Springfield, Ill: Charles C. Thomas.

FRIEDMAN, S. and FISHER, C. (1968). On the presence of rhythmic diurnal, oral instinctive drive in man: a preliminary report. *J. Amer. Psychonal. Assoc.*, **15**, 317-323.

Froberg, J., Karlsson, C. G., Levi, L. *et al.* (1972). Circadian variation in perform ance, psychological ratings, catecholamine excretion and diuresis during prolonged sleep deprivation. *Int. J. Psychobiol.*, **2**, 23–36.

Fuller, C. A., Lydic, R., Sulzman, F. M. *et al.* (1981). Circadian rhythm of body temperature persists after suprachiasmatic lesions in the squirrel monkey. *American Physiological Soc.*, R385–391.

Globus, G. G. (1970). Rhythmic functions during sleep. *Int. Psychiat. Clin.*, **7**, 15–21.

Globus, G. G., Drury, R. L., Phoebus, E. C. and Board, R. (1971). Ultradian rhythms in human performance. *Percept. Mot. Skills*, **33**, 1171–1174.

Halberg, F. (1969). Chronobiology. *Ann. Rev. Physiol.*, **31**, 675–725.

Halberg, F. and Katinas, G. S. (1973). Chronobiologic glossary. *Int. J. Chronobiol.*, **1**, 31–63.

Hartman, E. L. (1968). The 90-minute sleep dream cycle. *Arch. Gen. Psychiat.*, **18**, 280–286.

Hartmann, E. L. (1973). *The functions of sleep*. New Haven, Conn: Yale University Press.

Hellbrügge, T. (1960). The development of circadian rhythms in infants. *Cold Spr. Harb. Symp. Quant. Biol.*, **25**, 311–323.

Hellman, L., Nakada, F., Curti, J., Weitzman, E. D., Kream, J., Roffwarg, H., Ellman, S., Fukushima, D. K. and Gallagher, T. F. (1970). Cortisol is secreted episodically in normal man. *Journal of Clinical Endocrinology and Metabolism*, **30**, 411–422.

Hiatt, J. F. and Kripke, D. F. (1975). Ultradian rhythms in waking gastric activity. *Psychosomatic Medicine*, **37(4)**, 320–325.

Hobson, A. (1969). Sleep and biorhythmicity. *Science*, **165** (3896), 932–933.

Honda, Y., Takahashi, K., Takahashi, S., Azumi, K., Irie, M., Sakuma, M., Tsushima, T. and Shizume, K. (1969). Growth hormone secretion during nocturnal sleep in normal subjects *Journal of Clinical Endocrinology and Metabolism*, **29**, 20–29.

Horne, J. A. (1978). A review of the biological effects of total sleep deprivation in man. *Biological Psychology*, **7**, 55–102.

Horne, J. A. (1981). The effects of exercise upon sleep: a critical review. *Biological Psychology*, **12**, 241–290.

Hume, K. I. (1978). Some electrophysiological studies of sleep from subjects on varying sleep-wakefulness schedules. PhD thesis, University of Manchester.

Hume, K. I. and Mills, J. N. (1977). Rhythms of REM and Slow-Wave Sleep in subjects living on Abnormal Time Schedules. *Waking and Sleeping*, **1(3)**, 291–296.

Hume, K. I. (1980). Sleep adaptation after phase shifts of the sleep-wakefulness rhythm in man. *Sleep*, **2(4)**, 417–435.

Johnson, L. C. (1980). The REM cycle is a sleep-dependent rhythm. *Sleep*, **2(3)**, 299–307.

Johnson, L. C. and Macleod, W. L. (1973). Sleep and awake behaviour during gradual sleep reduction. *Percept. Motor Skills*, **36**, 87–91.

Kales, A., Jacobson, A., Kales, J. D., Kun, T. and Weissbuch, R. (1967). All night EEG sleep measurements in young adults. *Psychonom. Sci.*, **7**, 67–68.

Karacan, I., Finley, W. W., Williams, R. L. and Hursch, C. J. (1970). Changes in Stage 1-REM and Stage 4 sleep during naps. *Biological Psychiatry*, **2**, 261–265.

Karacan, I., Rosenbloom, A. L., Williams, R. L., Finley, W. W. and Hursch, C. (1971). Slow wave sleep deprivation in relation to plasma growth hormone concentration. *Behavioral Neuropsychiatry*, **2**, 11–14.

Klein, K. E. and Wegmann, H. M. (1974). The resynchronization of human circadian rhythms after transmeridian flights as a result of flight direction and mode of activity. In: L. E. Scheving, F. Halberg, and J. E. Pauly, (Eds.), *Chronobiology*, Tokyo: Igaku Shoin, pp. 564–570.

Klein, K. E., Wegman, H. M., Athananenas, G., Hohlweck, H. and

KUKLINSKI, P. (1976). Air operations and circadian performance rhythms. *Aviation, Space & Environmental Med.*, **47(3)**, 221–230.

KLEITMAN, N. (1963). *Sleep and Wakefulness*, 2nd edn, Chicago: University of Chicago Press.

KLEITMAN, N. and ENGELMANN, T. G. (1953). Sleep characteristics of infants. *J. Appl. Physiol.*, **6**, 269–282.

KNAUTH, P. and RUTENFRANZ, J. (1972). Investigations of the problems of sleep in connection with experimental shiftwork. *Int. Arch. Arbeitsmed.,* **30**, 1–22.

KNAUTH, P., RUTENFRANZ, J., SCHULZ, *et al.* (1980). Experimental shift work studies of permanent nights and rapidly rotating shift systems. *Int. Arch. Occup. Environ. Hlth.*, **46**, 111–125.

KOKKORIS, C. P., WEITZMAN, E. D., POLLAK, C. P., SPIELMAN, A. J., CZEISLER, C. A. and BRADLOW, H. (1978). Long-term ambulatory monitoring in subject with a hypernychthemeral sleep-wake cycle disturbance. *Sleep*, **1**, 177–190.

KRIPKE, D. F. (1974). Ultradian rhythms in sleep and wakefulness. In: E. D. WEITZMAN (Ed.), *Advances in Sleep Research*, Vol. 1, Spectrum Pubs, New York: Wiley.

KRIPKE, D. F., COOK, B and LEWIS, O. F. (1971). Sleep of night workers: EEG recordings. *Psychophysiology*, **7(3)**, 377–384.

KRIPKE, D. F. and SONNENSCHEIN, D. (1973). A 90-minute daydream cycle. Paper read to the Association for the Psychophysiological Study of Sleep, San Diego, May 1973.

KRONAUER, R. E., CZEISLER, C. A., PILATO, S. F. *et al.* (1982). Mathematical model of the human circadian system with two interacting oscillators. *Am. J. Physiol*, **242**(11), R_3–R_{17}.

LAVIE, P. (1979). Rapid eye movements in REM sleep-more evidence for a periodic organisation. *Electroencephal. Clin. Neurophysiol.*, **46**, 683–688.

LEWIS, P. R. and LOBBAN, M. C. (1956). Patterns of electrolyte excretion in human subjects during a prolonged period of life on a 22-hour day. *J. Physiol.*, **133**, 670–680.

LEWIS, S. A. (1974). The paradoxical sleep cycle revisited. In: L. E. SHEVING, F. HALBERG and J. E. PAULY (Eds.), *Chronobiology*, Tokyo: Igaku Shoin, pp. 487–490.

LOOMIS, A. L., HARVEY, E. N. and HOBART, G. A. (1937). Cerebral states during sleep as studied by human brain potentials. *J. Exp. Psychol.*, **21**, 127–144.

LUBIN, A., NUTE, C., NAITOH, P. and MARTIN, W. B. (1973). EEG delta activity during sleep as a damped ultradian rhythm. *Psychophysiology*, **10**, 27–35.

LYDIC, R., SCHOENE, W. C., CZEISLER, C. A. *et al.* (1980). Supra chiasmatic region of the human hypothalamus: homolog to the private circadian pacemaker? *Sleep*, **2**, 355–362.

MARON, L., RECHTSCHAFFEN, A. and WOLPERT, E. A. (1964). Sleep cycle during napping. *Arch. of Gen. Psychiatry*, **11**, 503–508.

MARTIN-DU-PAN, R. (1970). Le role du rhythme circadien dans l'alimentation du nourrisson. *La Femme et l'Enf.*, **4**, 23–30.

MILES, L. E. M., RAYNAL, D. M. and WILSON, M. A. (1977). Blind man living in normal society has circadian rhythms of 24.9 hours. *Science*, **198**, 421–423.

MILLS, J. N. (1964). Circadian rhythms during and after 3 months in solitude underground. *J. Physiol.* (London), **174**, 217–231.

MILLS, J. N. (1975). Circadian rhythms in infancy. *Chronobiologia*, **11(4)**, 363–371.

MILLS, J. N., MINORS, D. S., and WATERHOUSE, J. M. (1977). The physiological rhythms of subjects living on a day of abnormal length. *Journal of Physiology*, **268**, 803–826.

MILLS, J. N., MINORS, D. S., and WATERHOUSE, J. M. (1974). The circadian rhythms of human subjects without timepieces or indication of the alternation of day and night. *Journal of Physiology (London)*, **240**, 567–594.

MILLS, J. N., MINORS, D. S. and WATERHOUSE, J. M. (1978). The effect of sleep upon human circadian rhythms. *Chronobiologia*, **5**, 14–27.

MINORS, D. S. and WATERHOUSE, J. M. (1981). *Circadian rhythms and the human*, Bristol: Wright.

MITLER, M. M., LUND, R., SOKOLOVE, P. G., PITTENDRIGH, C. S. and DEMENT, W. C. (1977). Sleep activity rhythms in mice. *Brain Research*, **131**, 129–145.

MOISEEVA, N. J., BOGOLOVSKY, M. M., SIMONOV, M. Y. and TONKOVA, N. V. (1976). Characteristics of the circadian sleep rhythm in relation to environmental factors associated with the rotation of the earth and to biological macrorhythms in man. *J. Interdiscipl. Cycle. Res.*, **7**, 15–24.

MOORE-EDE, M. C., KASS, C. A. and HERD, J. A. (1976a). Transient circadian internal desynchronization after light-dark phase shift in monkeys. *American Journal of Physiology*, **232(1)**, R31–R37.

MOORE-EDE, M. C., SCHMELZER, W. S., KASS, D. A. and HERD, J. A. (1976b). Internal organization of the circadian timing system in multicellular animals. *Federation Proceedings*, **35(12)**: 2326–2332.

MOORE, R. Y. (1979). The anatomy of central neural mechanisms regulating endocrine rhythms. In: D. T. KREIGER (Ed.) *Endocrine Rhythms*. New York: Raven Press.

MOSES, J., NAITOH, P. and JOHNSON, L. C. (1978). The REM cycle in altered sleep wake schedules. *Psychophysiology*, **15**, 569–575.

MOSES, J. M., HORD, D. J., LUBIN, A., JOHNSTON, L. C. and NAITOH, P. (1975) Dynamics of nap sleep during a 40 h period. *Electroencephalog. Clin. Neurophysiol.*, **39**, 627–633.

NAKAGAWA, Y. (1980). Continuous observation of EEG patterns at night and in daytime of normal subjects under restrained conditions. 1. Quiescent state when lying down. *Electroencephalog. Clin. Neurophysiol.*, **49**, 534–537.

NICHOLS, C. T. and TYLER, F. H. (1967). Diurnal variation in adrenal cortical function. *Annual Review of Medicine*, **18**, 313–324.

ORR, W. C., HOFFMAN, H. J. and FRAZIER, T. W. (1972). A 90-minute heart rate biorhythm: complex demodulation and period analysis. Paper read at APSS Lake Minewaska, New York.

OSWALD, I., MERRINGTON, J. and LEWIS, H. (1970). Cyclic 'on demand' oral intake by adults. *Nature*, **225**, 959–960.

OTHMER, E., HAYDEN, M. P. and SEGELBAUM, R. (1969). Encephalic cycles during sleep and wakefulness in humans: a 24 hr pattern. *Science*, **164**, 447–449.

PARMEGGIANI, P. L. (1980). Temperature regulation during sleep: A study in homeostosis. In: J. OREM and C. D. BARNES, (Eds.) *Physiology in sleep*. New York: Academic Press, pp. 98–145.

PARKER, D. C., ROSSMAN, L. G., KRIPKE, D. F. *et al.* (1980). Endocrine rhythms across sleep-wake cycles in normal young men under basal state conditions. In: J. OREM and C. D. BARNES, (Eds.) *Physiology in sleep* New York: Academic Press, pp. 146–180.

PAWEL, M. A., SASSIN, J. F. and WEITZMAN, E. D., (1972). The temporal relation between HGH release and sleep stage changes at nocturnal sleep onset in man. *Life Sciences*, **11**, 587–593.

PHOEBUS, E., TAUB, J. M., GLOBUS, G. G. and DRURY, R. (1970). Sleep stage characteristics of extended sleep in normal subjects. *Percept. Mot. Skills*, **71**, 526.

PITTENDRIGH, C. S. (1960). Circadian rhythms and the circadian organization of living systems. *Cold Spring Harbor Symposium on Quantitative Biology*, **25**, 159–184.

PITTENDRIGH, C. S. and DAAN, S. (1976). The stability and lability of spontaneous frequency. *Journal of Comparative Physiology*, **106**, 223–252.

QUABBE, H. J. (1977). Chronobiology of growth hormone secretion. *Chronobiologica*, **4**, 217–246.

RECHTSCHAFFEN, A. and KALES, A. (1968). (Eds.), A Manual of standardized terminology, techniques and scoring system for sleep stages of human subjects. Bethesda, MD, National Inst. of Health Publication **204**.

ROFFWARG, H. P., MUZIO, J. N. and DEMENT, W. C. (1966). Ontogenetic development of the human sleep-dream cycle. *Science*, **152**, 604–619.
RUTENFRANZ, J., COLQUHOUN, W. P., KNAUTH, P. *et al.* (1977). Biomedical and psychosocial aspects of shift work: a review. *Scand. J. Work Environ. Hlth.*, **3**, 165–182.
RUSAK, B. and ZUCKER, I. (1979). Neural regulation of circadian rhythms. *Physiol. Rev.*, **59**, 449–526.
SASSIN, J. F., PARKER, D. C., MACE, J. W., GOTTIN, R. W., JOHNSON, L. C. and ROSSMAN, L. G. (1969). Human growth hormone release: relation to slow wave sleep and sleep-waking cycles. *Science*, **165**, 513–515.
SCHULZ, H., DIRLICH, G., BALTESKONIS, S. and ZULLEY, J. (1980). The REM-NREM sleep cycle: renewal process or periodically driven process. *Sleep*, **2(3)**, 319–329.
SCHULZ, H., DIRLICH, G. and ZULLEY, J. (1975). Phase shift in the REM sleep rhythm. *Pflugers Arch. ges Physiol.*, **358**, 203–214.
SOSTEK, A. M., ANDERS, T. F. and SOSTEK, A. J. (1976). Diurnal rhythms in 2 and 8 week old infants: sleep-waking state organization as a function of age and stress. *Psychosom. Med.* **38**, 250–256.
TAKAHASHI, Y., KIPNIS, D. and DAUGHADAY, W. (1968). Growth hormone secretion during sleep. *Journal of Clinical Investigation*, **47**, 2079–2090.
TAUB, J. M. and BERGER, R. J. (1973). Sleep stage patterns associated with acute shifts in the sleep-wakefulness cycle. *Electroencephalog. Clin. Neurophysiol.*, **35**, 613–619.
TUNE, G. S. (1969). Sleep and wakefulness in a group of shift workers. *Brit. J. Industr. Med.*, **26**, 54–58.
VALATX, J. L. and BUGAT, R. (1974). Facteurs genetiques dans le determenisme du cycle veille-sommeil chez la souris. *Brain Res.*, **69**, 315–330.
VERDONE, P. (1968). Sleep satiation: extended sleep in normal subjects. *Electroencephalog. Clin. Neurophysiol.*, **24**, 417–423.
WEBB, W. B. (1971). Sleep behaviour as a biorhythm. In: W. P. COLQUHOUN. (Ed.) *Biological rhythms and human performance.* New York: Academic Press.
WEBB, W. B. and AGNEW, H. W. Jun. (1967). Sleep cycling within 24 hr periods. *J. Expt. Psychol.*, **74**, 158–160.
WEBB, W. B. and AGNEW, H. W. Jun. (1969). In: L. E. ABT and B. F. RIESS (Eds.) *Progress in Clinical Psychology*, Vol. 8, Dreams and Dreaming pp. 2–27, New York: Grune & Strattton.
WEBB, W. B. and AGNEW, H. W. Jun. (1971). Variables associated with split period sleep regimes. *Aerospace Med.*, **42(8)**, 847–850.
WEBB, W. B. and AGNEW, H. W. Jun. (1971). Stage 4 sleep: influence of time course variables. *Science*, **174**, 1354–1356.
WEBB, W. B. and AGNEW, H. W. Jun. (1974). Regularity in the control of the free-running sleep wakefulness rhythm. *Aerospace Med.*, **45**, 701–704.
WEBB, W. B. and AGNEW, H. W. Jun. (1978). Effects of rapidly rotating shifts on sleep patterns and sleep structure. *Aviat. Space Environ. Med.*, **49(2)**, 384–389.
WEBB, W. B. and AGNEW, H. W. Jun. (1974). Sleep and waking in a time-free environment. *Aerospace Med.*, **45**, 617–622.
WEBB, W. B. and AGNEW, H. W. Jun. (1975). Sleep efficiency for sleep-cycles of varied lengths. *Psychophysiol.*, **12**, 637–641.
WEBB, W. B., and AGNEW, H. W. Jun. and STERNTHAL, H. (1966). Sleep during the early morning. *Psychon. Scie.*, **6**, 277–278.
WEBB, W. B., AGNEW, H. W. Jun. and WILLIAMS, R. L. (1971). Effect on sleep of a sleep period time displacement. *Aerospace Med.*, **42(2)**, 132–155.
WEBBER, A. L., CARY, M. S., CONNOR, N. *et al.* (1980). Human non-24 hr sleep-wake cycles in an everyday environment. *Sleep*, **2(3)**, 347–354.
WEDDERBURN, A. A. I. (1978). Some suggestions for increasing the usefulness of psychological and sociological studies of shift work. *Ergonomics*, **21**, 827–833.

WEHR, T. A., WIRTZ-JUSTICE, A., GOODWIN, F. K. *et al.* (1979). Phase advance of the circadian sleep-wake cycle as an anti-depressant. *Science*, **206**, 710–713.

WEITZMAN, E. D., (1976). Circadian rhythms and episodic hormone secretion in man. *Annual Review of Medicine*, **27**, 225–243.

WEITZMAN, E. D., CZEISLER, C. A. and MOORE-EDE, M. C. (1979). Biological rhythms of man living in isolation from time cues. In: *Sleep, Wakefulness and Circadian Rhythms*, AGARD Lecture Series **105**, AGARD, Chapter 7.

WEITZMAN, E. D., CZEISLER, C. A., ZIMMERMAN, J. C. *et al.* (1980). Timing of REM and Stages 3 + 4 sleep during temporal isolation in man. *Sleep*, **2(4)**, 391–409.

WEITZMAN, E. D., GOLDMACHER, D., KRIPKE, D., MACGREGOR, P., KREAM, J. and HELLMAN, L. (1968). Effect on sleep stage pattern and certain neuroendocrine rhythms. *Trans. Am. Neurol. Ass.*, **93**, 153–157.

WEITZMAN, E. D., KRIPKE, D. F., GOLDMACHER, D., MACGREGOR, P. and NOGEIRE, C. (1970). Acute reversal of the sleep-waking cycle in man. *Arch. Neurol.*, **22**, 483–489.

WEITZMAN, E. D., NOGEIRE, C., PERLOW, M., FUKUSHIMA, D., SASSIN, J., MACGREGOR, P., GALLAGHER, T. F., and HELLMAN, L. (1974). Effects of a prolonged 3 hr sleep-wake cycle on sleep stages, plasma cortisol growth hormone and body temperature in man. *J. of Clin. Endocrinol & Metab.*, **38(6)**, 1018–1030.

WEITZMAN, E. D. (1981). Sleep and its disorders. *Ann. Rev. Neurol.*, **4**, 381–417.

WEVER, R. (1979). *The Circadian System of Man. Results of experiments under Temporal Isolation*, Berlin: Springer Verlag.

WILLIAMS, R. L., AGNEW, H. W. Jun. and WEBB, W. B. (1967). Effects of prolonged Stage 4 and REM deprivation. *USAF School of Aerospace Med.* Report SAM-TR-66-59.

WILLIAMS, R., KARACAN, I. and HURSCH, C. (1974). *Electroencephalography (EEG) of human sleep: clinical application.* New York: John Wiley.

WYATT, S. and MARRIOTT, R. (1953). Night work and shift changes. *Brit. J. Industr. Med.*, **10**, 164–172.

ZEPELIN, H. and RECHTSCAFFEN, A. (1974). Mammalian sleep, longevity and energy metabolism. *Brain Behaviour Evolution*, **10**, 425–470.

ZULLEY, J. (1980). Distribution of REM sleep in entrained 24 hour and free-running sleep-wake cycles. *Sleep*, **2(4)**, 377–391.

CHAPTER 3

The Evolution of Sleep

Ray Meddis

3.1 Introduction

Evolution is a type of modern myth, a delicate blend of fact and conjecture, which seeks to make sense of the present in terms of an epic story of things past. Like the myths of other societies — each fervently believed in their day to be true — our modern tale of the evolution of species stretches back through unimaginable time and features terrible and often unlikely beasts experiencing strange metamorphoses in everchanging and unfamiliar landscapes. For Titans we substitute Tyrannosaurs; for the forces of good and evil we substitute the impersonal principle of the survival of the fittest.

These accounts are theories which are not true or false in any simple sense but more or less satisfactory as frameworks for organizing what we know about the world around us now. Darwin's theory of the evolution of species was stimulated by the diversity of living things and the challenge of a number of fossils which indicated a past quite different from the present. Sleep studies are quite untroubled by any fossil record and it seems unlikely that it ever will be. But it is troubled by an astonishing diversity of sleep patterns among extant species and some account is needed to make sense of these. For example, sleep in cattle is recognizably similar to sleep in a chimpanzee; but there are many differences. Cattle sleep only half as much as chimps. They spend much time in a special state called drowsiness which chimps enjoy hardly at all. Quiet sleep in the chimp is characterized by two quite distinct phases which contrast with a single more or less uniform pattern in cattle. While both intermittently emit the electrical brain signal known as spindles (12 Hz EEG activity) during sleep, only the chimp emits K-complexes (isolated high voltage slow waves). The chimp is often difficult to wake while cattle start at the slightest stimulus. The list continues and many other lists of differences exist for other pairs of species. A theory of the evolution of sleep is one way of attempting to make sense of the variety of sleep patterns in modern animal species.

It might seem a simple matter to link sleep patterns with the constitutional requirements of a species or the demands of its ecological niche. Unfortunately, it is not as simple as linking the shape of a bird's beak to the kind of job it is best suited for. In the case of the beak, we already have a rough idea that its function is to gain access to food and to process it in some way before delivering it to the alimentary canal. The function of sleep, however, is still shrouded in mystery. While there is no shortage of theories on the topic, it is fair to say that none has emerged so far which has won universal approval. Rechtschaffen (1979), in a recent discussion of the methodological difficulties facing theorists in this area, is very pessimistic. It seems difficult to find a theory which will embrace all of the known facts and he suggests 'that theories of sleep function should be offered more modestly until they are supported by evidence from several research strategies'. The absence of a clear idea of the function served by sleep is a serious handicap to any attempt to unravel the tangle of evidence bearing upon the matter of sleep's evolution.

It is possible that sleep serves not one but a multitude of purposes and that many of the theories already proposed are, in fact, simultaneously applicable. Sleep *may* be a necessary period of rest and recuperation when certain essential repair or maintenance processes are accelerated. It *may* be simply a time for minimizing physiological stresses when energy can be conserved and tissue damage minimized. It *may* be a time for consolidating the effects of new experiences and integrating them with old learning. It *may* be a period of enforced immobilization which minimizes predatory threat or contact with a hostile environment. It may even be all of these. The last two decades of sleep research have witnessed an increase rather than a reduction in the number of hypotheses. The most important development to note is the loosening of the stranglehold of the time-honoured view that the primary and essential function of sleep is detoxification. We now have a wide range of possible functions, each of which may apply to a different degree in different species.

The second major impediment to the smooth progress of developing evolutionary theories of sleep is the paucity of data. While we have enough evidence to show that sleep varies enormously in quantity and quality, at least among mammals, this evidence is based on a relatively small number of species studied in university laboratories. In fact we have very little data concerning the sleep of animals in their natural habitat. The data may be available somewhere but it is not easily accessible. Naturalists appear to regard sleep as an unimportant phenomenon even though most mammalian species spend more than half of their life in this state. Most accounts either do not mention sleep at all or, at best, do so only incidentally. As a result, our most detailed information comes from electrophysiological studies of sleep carried out in the laboratory. To sleep in a recording chamber with electrodes implanted deep in the brain is to sleep in a most unnatural setting. However, with few exceptions, this is the data which we are dependent upon to begin our explorations of the evolution of sleep.

A summary of this data is given in Table 3.3. Estimates of various aspects of the sleep of 65 mammalian species are given along with measures of some constitutional and ecological variables. The table is based mainly on a compilation by Zepelin & Rechtschaffen (1974) and amendments by Allison & Cicchetti (1976) who also give detailed accounts of how the data were arrived at. There are many problems with such compilations; for example, the sample of species is not random and the estimates are only as good as the research reports which supplied them. Nevertheless, they supply a useful first approximation which succeeding generations can refine or remodel.

A third major problem facing theories of the evolution of sleep comes from the recency of much of our knowledge of the internal structure of sleep. So much has been discovered in such a short time that the new facts remain only partly digested and we are left with the certain knowledge that many important, and possibly crucial, facts are still awaiting discovery. For example, before 1950, few people even suspected the fact that mammalian sleep was made up of two dramatically different states, active sleep (AS, also known as paradoxical sleep, rapid eye movement sleep and dreaming sleep) and quiet sleep (QS, also known as slow wave sleep and orthodox sleep). Since the pioneering work of Aserinsky & Kleitman (1953) and Jouvet (1961), research into AS has produced surprise after surprise including the exceptionally high response thresholds to external stimuli, its association with dream reports in humans, the simultaneous occurrence of penile erections, the discovery that AS appears before QS in the foetus and is preponderant in sleep in the first few weeks, irregularities in autonomic functioning (e.g. heart rate and respiration fluctuations) and, more recently, evidence that thermo-regulatory mechanisms — so vital to birds and mammals — may operate abnormally if at all during AS. Who knows what new properties are waiting to be discovered?

Our conceptualization of QS has also become more complex during this period. Four classifications are needed (Stages 1–4) to describe normal variations in human QS. Cats seem to require only two which are called deep quiet sleep (DQS) and light quiet sleep (LQS). Many other mammals, however, show a rather uniform picture which can be summarized as a single state (QS). In what follows, we shall ignore the differences of pattern and stick to the general term QS even though these differences cry out for an explanation in terms of their evolution and function. We are almost wholly ignorant on this point.

There is also the phenomenon of drowsiness which is particularly prominent in cats, dogs, hedgehogs, foxes and cattle. The state is characterized by a 'sleepy' appearance, relaxation and its own EEG pattern but shows very low response thresholds. Should we class this as sleeping or waking? Table 3.1 does not include figures for drowsiness in the QS total but this is necessarily an arbitrary decision. Any future analysis of the concept of sleep will need to grasp this nettle.

We are, therefore, faced in our search for a theory of the evolution of sleep with a complete lack of any fossil record, no generally accepted theory of the function of sleep, a very short supply of somewhat imperfect data and a rapidly shifting conception of the nature of sleep and its properties. Few sane men would tackle the problem with any hope of success. At the very least, we must expect Rechtschaffen's plea for modesty to apply as much to the proffering of evolutionary scenarios as it clearly does to issues of function. Nevertheless, questions of the origin of sleep and the influences affecting the radiation of sleep patterns through evolutionary history, press themselves upon us and we must make a start however inadequate. To this end, I shall begin with a review of a number of issues currently under discussion, followed by a statistical analysis of the data in Table 3.3 in the manner pioneered by Hartmann (1968), Zepelin & Rechtschaffen (1974) and Allison & Cicchetti (1976).

3.2 Evolutionary Origin of Sleep

In the absence of any fossil record of sleep patterns, we are very dependent upon the 'common ancestor' model of evolution in our search for the origin of sleep. The argument runs thus: if two species both display sleep phenomena then *either* (1) a common ancestor also displayed a similar phenomenon *or* (2) the sleep pattern in question evolved separately in the two species. In the latter case, a common ancestor may or may not have been 'pre-adapted' to facilitate the evolution of the phenomenon in its descendants. Typically, we disregard the second possibility in the interests of parsimony. For example, there are many similarities between the sleep of humans and chimpanzees which make us feel that we inherited similar mechanisms from our common ancestor. It seems inconceivable that we would independently evolve such similar mechanisms. We are, however, unable to check the fossil record as we could if the argument concerned, say, the position of eyes in the head. The way forward, therefore, seems to involve drawing up a list of all extant species which show sleep patterns and then, with reference to a standard phylogenetic tree, find the most recent common ancestor of all of these species. This common ancestor will then help pinpoint the earliest certain date of the presence of sleep phenomena in the evolution of life.

I have already attempted the exercise (Meddis, 1975, 1977 Chapter 2) with a rather surprising result. From a perusal of the literature, I satisfied myself that sleep was present in at least some species of all the various vertebrate phyla (mammals, birds, reptiles, amphibia and fish) and also among some invertebrates (e.g. molluscs, insects). It began to look as if the search would never end — after all, even flowers sometimes close up at night — so I stopped with the limp conclusion that 'sleep was of great evolutionary age'. I was certainly a long way from finding a youngest, common, sleeping ancestor!

The biggest problem facing the investigator in this area is the difficulty of defining sleep. Despite many interesting differences — of which more later — sleep among mammals is fairly consistent, both behaviourally and electrophysiologically. Most mammals retire to a safe place, assume a posture which is not very tiring to maintain and close their eyes. EEG records of the same animals are typically dominated by the high amplitude slow waves (1–3 Hz) and intermittent spindle activity (12–16 Hz) of QS alternating with shorter periods of the low amplitude high (but variable) frequency activity of AS. Birds show a directly analogous pattern. However, when we arrive at reptiles we find a sharp discontinuity in that their sleeping EEG shows no universally agreed resemblance with either AS or QS in birds and mammals. We are therefore obliged to rely upon behavioural criteria which are difficult to formulate. As a first approximation we can say that sleep is a period of immobility with raised response thresholds in a species-typical posture and a species-typical site and with a circadian organization. The definition is unsatisfactory on various counts, however. First, we can always find examples of sleep which do not fit these criteria such as the soldier asleep standing up on sentry duty or animals which show very low response thresholds during sleep. Secondly, the definition lies dangerously close to alert resting. Thirdly, the definition is so loose as to risk embracing the sleeping flower! It seems likely that the concept of 'sleep' will not stand up to the rigours of too general a usage.

The second problem is that too loose a definition of sleep makes us vulnerable to the error of falsely rejecting the possibility that mechanisms producing sleep-type behaviour may have evolved independently in some species. For example, hibernation is a very common phenomenon in the animal kingdom but it takes on many different forms in different species and phyla. It seems that the frequency of occurrence of hibernation phenomena is a function of the frequency with which environmental pressures oblige animals to cease trading until such times as business can recommence. This may be for only a few days during a food shortage, for a whole season of intense heat or cold or for many years of drought. We do not need to evoke a common ancestor to explain the widespread occurrence of the hibernation strategem. Indeed the enormous variety in the detailed mechanisms of hibernation would soon contradict this. We do not have as much detailed comparative data on sleep as we do on hibernation but we must consider the possibility that they are analogous in this respect; that sleep patterns may evolve independently in response to similar constitutional or ecological pressures.

In the case of sleep, we can recognize the environmental pressures which might promote its independent appearance in many different species. The daily fluctuations in light intensity bring with them a host of changes which challenge the adaptive ability of every animal; changes in temperature, in the availability and accessibility of food sources and in the danger from predators. Scheduling activity so as to optimize the chances of survival will inevitably involve circadian fluctuations in mobility and conspicuousness. It also seems reasonable that varieties of 'unconsciousness' or manifestations of raised response thresholds should emerge as mechanisms for enforcing periods of inactivity in animals which are otherwise easily provoked into action by stimulation. The ubiquity of sleep-type phenomena may therefore represent little more than a reflection of the need of animals to adapt to fluctuations in environmental conditions.

Clearly, we cannot rule out the possibility that sleep has been invented many times among animals in general. However, the similarity of the manifestations of sleep among all mammals so far studied makes the idea of parallel evolution highly unlikely within this particular class. What seems more likely is that the sleep patterns in mammals represent a series of refinements of a common mechanism handed down from a very early mammalian common ancestor. Moreover, the existence of very similar sleep patterns among birds and mammals argues very strongly that both have adapted a common inheritance to their own needs. Unfortunately, the argument cannot be easily sustained because no reptile has been found to show electrophysiological sleep patterns which closely resemble those of birds and mammals. Birds and some modern reptiles who do not show mammalian/avian sleep patterns are thought to have a common ancestor more recent than their common ancestor with mammals (see Fig. 3.1). Therefore, we have to face the possibility that parallel evolution is the best explanation of the similarity between sleep in birds and mammals. We shall review this question in more detail in the following section.

3.3 Evolution of Active and Quiet Sleep States

The cyclic alternation of QS and AS in the sleep of mammals presents us with very special problems on two fronts. First, it is proving very difficult to uncover the function of this alternation; that is, it remains unclear as to why the process of natural selection should have favoured this pattern. Secondly, a considerably mystery surrounds the parallel evolution of the same pattern in both mammals and birds. If we knew what function was being served by the AS/QS alternation, the answer to the parallel evolution problem would probably be easier to find. However, we do not know its function for sure and, while we shall be guided by theories of possible functions, the bulk of our analysis must mainly involve similarities among the sleep patterns of living species.

Both birds and mammals are believed to have evolved independently from reptilian stock (Fig. 3.1). Both birds and mammals show a QS/AS alternation during sleep but no modern reptile studied so far shows a similar sleep pattern. How, then, can we explain the similarity between birds and mammals? There are a number of possible answers. First, it might be that the distant reptilian

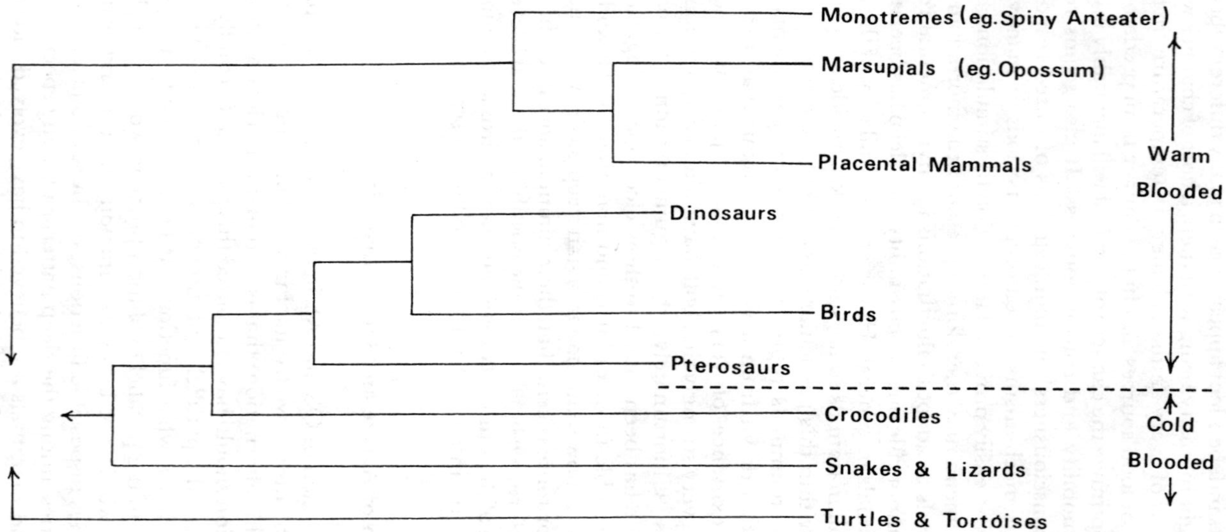

Fig. 3.1 Phylogenetic tree for mammals, birds and reptiles (see, for example, Desmonds, 1977, Appendix 1).

stock (which is ancestral to modern birds, mammals *and* reptiles) did show a QS/AS alternation during sleep but modern reptiles have acquired a new style of sleeping. Sleep in modern amphibia, however, (see bibliography) shows a great similarity to sleep in modern reptiles. Since modern amphibia are our only window on the sleep of the ancient extinct amphibia from which reptiles were derived, it begins to look as if avian and mammalian sleep constitute a departure from their reptilian heritage.

An alternative explanation is that the new style of sleep evolved independently in birds and mammals, possibly in response to a common need such as homeothermy. An important piece of evidence in favour of this view is the finding of an absence of a QS/AS cycle in the echidna (or spiny anteater), a primitive egg-laying mammal (Allison *et al.*, 1972). Specifically, the echidna shows QS but no AS. It can be seen from Fig. 3.1 that the absence of the QS/AS cycle in monotremes forms the basis of an argument that the reptilian ancestors of mammals did not show the cycle either. This is because the monotremes formed their own separate line of evolution very early in the emergence of mammals.

Since the AS/QS cycle is not to be found in either modern reptiles or monotremes, it seems reasonable to conclude that this sleep pattern has emerged independently in birds and mammals. Since the echidna's sleep is unambiguously QS, we might also conclude that QS is the original kind of sleep and that AS is an evolutionary novelty. Allison *et al.* (1972) have suggested that its absence in the echidna may be linked to the fact that it lays eggs, but, since birds also lay eggs, the matter remains unresolved.

The twin postulates of (1) the independent evolution of the QS/AS alternation pattern of sleep and (2) the phylogenetic primacy of QS are central to the traditional and still dominant view of the evolution of sleep. Its main supporters have been the French school led by Jouvet and two American groups led by Allison and Rechtschaffen, although they differ in some details. Hermann *et al.* (1964), when reporting an investigation of sleep in the tortoise which did not appear to have any AS, expressed the matter succinctly when concluding that reptiles stand 'at the point on the evolutionary ladder where AS disappears'. However, this position has not gone unchallenged. Berger and his colleagues are hostile to the idea of a reptilian origin of QS (Berger, 1975) and, more recently, they have hardened on the idea that AS is, in fact, phylogenetically older than QS (Walker & Berger, 1980). My own preference (Meddis 1977, 1979), when reviewing this material, has been for the idea that QS is an evolutionary novelty and that AS is vestigial and potentially maladaptive in birds and mammals. The issue remains controversial, of course, but the discussion which follows will emphasize reasons for not accepting the traditional view.

3.4 The Similarity of Avian and Mammalian Sleep

The astonishing similarity of the complex sleep of birds and mammals makes it difficult to accept the theory of parallel evolution. Table 3.1 is an attempt to summarize the results of most of the available literature on the electrophysiological study of sleep in birds. All avian species, studied so far, reveal two clearly different kinds of sleep which can easily be identified with mammalian QS and

Table 3.1 Summary of Results of some Major Studies of the Characteristics of Avian Sleep

See text for explanation, and bibliography for references. HVSW = high voltage slow waves; REMS = rapid eye movements; EMG = electromyogram; ✓ = present; × = not present; — = not commented on.

	QS		AS								
Species	HVSW	Spindles	Epoch length(s)	REMS	EMG drop	Irregular EKG	Raised thresholds	Follows QS only	Hippocampal theta	% of TST	Author
Starling	✓	×	16	✓	✓	—	—	✓	—	2–6	Tymicz *et al.* 1975
Falcon, Hawk	?	×	3–15	✓	—	—	✓	✓	—	7–10	Rojas-Ramirez *et al.* 1970
Pigeon	✓	×	9	✓	?	✓	✓	—	×	7	Van Twyver *et al.* 1972
	✓	×	11	✓	?	—	✓	—	—	7	Berger *et al.* 1972
	✓	—	few	✓	✓	—	—	—	—	—	Tradardi 1966
Owl	✓	×	9	×	rarely	✓	—	✓	×	3	Susic *et al.* 1973
Burrowing owl	✓	×	11	×	×	—	—	✓	×	5	Berger *et al.* 1972
Chickens	✓	×	1–8	✓	✓	✓	—	✓	×	0.5–16	Summary of 7 studies*
Chaffinch	✓	—	27	?	×	—	—	✓	—	7.14	Tymicz 1975

* Hen/chicken studies used were: Karmanova *et al.*, 1971; Klein *et al.*, 1963; Hishikawa *et al.*, 1969 Ookawa, 1972; Schelhuber *et al.*, 1974; Sugihata *et al.*, 1973.

AS. QS is characterized by high voltage slow waves (HVSW) in the EEG while AS has many of the features of mammalian AS such as desynchronized, low voltage EEG, irregular heart rate, raised response thresholds and rapid eye movements (REM) — except the owls whose eyes do not move during waking either. Neck muscle tonus (EMG) reduction is often but not always reported, although most authors remark that the birds' heads did droop during AS. Most conspicuous, however, is the alternation of QS and AS throughout the sleep period; AS always follows QS and never follows waking. These two features are strongly reminiscent of the mammalian pattern.

On the debit side, we may note some differences. Spindles (10–14 Hz bursts of EEG activity), which are very characteristic of mammalian QS are never reported in birds. Similarly, hippocampal theta (steady synchronous electrical rhythm, 6–9 Hz) is reported absent in avian AS. In birds, AS epochs are considerably shorter (3–15 s duration) and occupy a smaller proportion (2–10%) of total sleep time than is common for mammals.

Striking as these differences undoubtedly are, they do little to minimize the impressiveness of the similarities. Spindles, it should be noted, are also absent from the QS of the monotreme, echidna (Allison *et al.*, 1972) which counts as a mammal from most points of view. Moreover, mammalian AS epochs do vary enormously in length from species to species. We do not know, for certain, why this is but small mammals do tend to have much shorter epochs. The birds studied so far are indeed small with high basal metabolic rates by the standards of most mammals. This goes part of the way to explaining the shortness of their AS epochs, although, it must be admitted, it is not a complete explanation.

On balance, the parallels seem too strong to admit of an explanation in terms of convergent evolution. Unfortunately, it is equally difficult to see how a common origin can be found. The fossil record is generally interpreted to show a close affiliation between birds and crocodiles and also a (less close) affiliation between mammals and turtles (chelonia). Since neither crocodiles nor turtles have electrophysiological sleep patterns anything like those of birds or mammals, an explanation of the sleep parallels in terms of common ancestors seems to be ruled out. It is true that recent research (see Desmond, 1977, for a palatable review) has shown that homeothermy may have been more common in reptiles such as dinosaurs and pterosaurs than hitherto believed. Nevertheless, I know of no suggestion of a direct link between the evolution of homeothermy in mammals and that in birds. The only remaining possibility is that the stem reptiles ancestral to birds, mammals, turtles and crocodiles must have been pre-adapted to develop this kind of sleep pattern under certain conditions (such as homeothermy). Although difficult to defend in detail, this suggestion merits further analysis and investigation.

3.5 The Reptilian Heritage

Although modern reptiles are different from the extinct stem reptiles which are ancestral to all higher vertebrates, they supply the only available clues to our reptilian sleep heritage and therefore deserve close scrutiny. Fortunately, we now have a number of electrophysiological studies of sleep in reptiles. Table 3.2 summarizes the results of the bulk of these investigations. The most certain conclusion from all investigators is that the avian/mammalian pattern of QS/AS alternation is not present in any order of reptiles. What similarities then, if any, can we find between our sleep and reptilian quiescence?

All but one study report an absence of high voltage slow waves (HVSW) during the behavioural immobility, presumed to be sleep, in reptiles. The only exception to this rule is a report on young crocodiles (Warner *et al.*, 1977) living in a colony. The authors of this report imply that the failure of other investigators to observe HVSW may result from abnormal conditions of alertness in the animals caused by the stress of isolation and the recording procedures. The weight of evidence does seem to be against them, but their suggestion remains a tantalizing possibility. However, their results do show that it is physiologically possible for crocodiles to show HVSW. This undermines any suggestion that the absence of HVSW in reptiles is due to 'the absence of appropriate physiological substrates' (Flanigan *et al.*, 1973).

Almost all investigations show a low voltage desynchronized EEG during quiescence, distinguished only from the waking EEG by a modest slowing of the dominant frequencies. In mammals and birds we identify AS mainly in terms of quiescence accompanied by a desynchronized EEG. Can we not, therefore, equate reptilian sleep with avian and mammalian AS? Normally, we look for reduced tone in the major neck muscles to confirm that this is, in fact, AS and not waking. Muscle tone in the neck muscles in reptiles is indeed low during sleep or even altogether absent. AS is also characterized by phasic events such as eye movements or twitching of paws, which are less often reported in reptiles. About half of the studies do indicate some such events although typically widely spaced throughout the sleeping periods. With so many indications in favour of a diagnosis of AS why are investigators so reluctant to accept it?

Part of the problem may be historical. QS was known first to researchers while AS discovered relatively recently. It is not surprising therefore that QS might come to be known as 'orthodox' sleep while the new, and surprising AS might attract the name 'paradoxical' sleep (see e.g. Oswald, 1974, p. 97). Our natural assumption is that reptilian sleep is 'orthodox'. We then go on to wonder if 'paradoxical' sleep is present *as well*. As a result, most investigators have been looking for periods of AS interrupting QS. The majority have been reluctant to invest the occasional appearance of eye movements with the status of 'paradoxical sleep'. What has rarely been considered seriously, is the possibility that the *whole* of the sleep period in reptiles may be analogous to AS in mammals and birds. After all, mammalian and avian AS is generally considered to consist of a continuous or 'tonic' set of features such as desynchronized EEG and isoelectric EMG which are interrupted at intervals by phasic events such as eye movements and other muscle twitches (Grosser & Siegel, 1971). Normal reptilian sleep may, therefore, correspond to the 'tonic' aspect of mammalian AS. Their eye movements and twitches would then be the phasic events.

Currently the major objection to the acceptance of this idea is based on the observations of spikes or sharp waves in the EEG and electrocorticogram of some reptiles (see Table 3.2). One school of thought (e.g. Flanigan *et al.*, 1973; Hartse, 1980) believes that these spikes are analogous to similar spikes observed in the ventral hippocampus of cats during QS. If this view can be substantiated then it would constitute a strong piece of evidence in favour of a QS interpretation of reptilian sleep. But why are reptilian spikes not identified with the well-known PGO waves which, in mammals, 'can be recorded from the reticular

Table 3.2 Summary of Sleep Features in Major Studies of Sleep in Reptiles

See text for explanation. Failure to observe sleep is reported in the sea turtle, *Caretta caretta* (Susic, 1972), *Alligator mississipiensis* (Van Twyver, 1973). See bibliography for references. HVSW = high voltage slow waves.

Species	EEG change in sleep: HVSW	EEG change in sleep: Lower frequency	EEG change in sleep: amplitude	EEG change in sleep: Sharp waves/spikes in sleep	Eye movements in sleep: Present	Eye movements in sleep: Duration	Authors
Lizards							
Iguana							Huntley *et al.*, 1977
dipsosaurus dorsalis	×	✓	reduced	✓	✓	—	Huntely *et al.*, 1980
ctenosaura pectinata	×	✓	reduced	during waking	✓	1–3 min	Tauber *et al.*, 1968
ctenosaura pectinata } *iguana iguana* }	×	✓	reduced	✓	×	—	Flanigan, 1973
iguana iguana	×	✓	same	✓	×	—	Peyrethan *et al.*, 1969
Chameleon							
chameleo jacksoni } *chameleo melleri* }	×	✓	same	✓	✓	1–7 min	Tauber *et al.*, 1966
Crocodiles							
Caiman latirostris	×	✓	same	—	✓	1 min	Peyrethan *et al.*, 1969
Caiman sclerops	×	✓	slight increase	—	×	—	Rechtschaffen *et al.*, 1968
Caiman sclerops	×	✓	same	✓	✓	4–7 s	Flanigan *et al.*, 1973
Caiman sclerops (juvenile)	✓	✓	increase	×	—	—	Warner *et al.*, 1977
Snakes							
python saebe	×	✓	increase	✓	×	—	Peyrethan *et al.*, 1969
Turtles							
Testudo marginata	possibly	✓	increase	×	×	—	Hermann *et al.*, 1964
Testudo denticulata	×	same	same	✓	×	—	Walker *et al.*, 1973
Terrapene carolina	×	✓	lower	✓	×	—	Flanigan, 1974b
Emys orbicularis	×	✓	same	—	(15% of animals 15 s)		Vasilescu, 1970
Geochelone carbonaria	×	×	same	✓	×	—	Flanigan, 1974a

formation of the pons, from the lateral geniculate and from the occipital cortex' (Jouvet, 1969)? These PGO waves are associated with REMs and, in the waking animal, can be recorded during visual attention. Apparently analogous monophasic spikes have been observed in the optic tectum of chickens with a close relation to eye movements. These spikes are not observed during QS but do occur in AS in association with REMs (Sugihara & Gotoh, 1973). Flanigan *et al.* (1973), in their study of the crocodile, indicate that cortical spiking was accompanied by spikes in the optic tectum which were, in turn, synchronous with 'spikes recorded from electrodes implanted in extra-ocular muscles'. Despite the parallels with avian tectal spiking Flanigan *et al.* (1973) and Hartse (1980) prefer to interpret the observations in terms of QS on pharmacological grounds; the spikes responded to two drugs — MAO inhibitors and reserpine — in a manner which was contrary to expectations based on studies of mammalian PGO spikes but consistent with expectations based on studies of spike potentials found in the ventral hippocampus of cats.

The matter is clearly very technical and one hesitates to argue with the specialists. However, not all the specialists are in agreement on the matter; Walker and Berger (1980) disagree. They do not feel that the spiking issue constitutes strong enough evidence to undermine their view that 'perhaps . . . [AS] is a vestige of a reptilian poikilothermic state of waking inactivity'. The term 'waking' here reflects their conviction that reptilian quiescence should not be equated with sleep at all! This view is based on a failure to observe response threshold changes during quiescence in the tortoise (Walker *et al.*, 1973). In this, they agree with Van Twyver's (1973) conclusions following studies in the American alligator but disagree with Flanigan's (1973) demonstration of reduced reactivity during quiescence (but not necessarily spiking periods) in the crocodile. Whether or not the name 'sleep' ought to be applied to this condition, we should note that some scientists claim it as a precursor of AS and others of QS.

3.6 AS and Homeothermy

Indirect evidence in favour of a reptilian origin for AS comes from some intriguing research findings which suggest that various mechanisms used to regulate body temperature in mammals (e.g. panting, sweating, nasolabial secretions in cattle, peripheral blood flow changes, shivering and non-shivering thermogenesis) are not mobilized during AS in response to thermal stress (see e.g. Parmeggiani, 1977; Walker *et al.*, 1977; Toutain *et al.*, 1972). It appears that a mammal would be vulnerable during AS periods if these periods were to last for a long time in extremes of environmental temperature; an animal's only defence in such conditions is to reduce greatly the amount of time spent in AS (Parmeggiani, 1977). These thermoregulatory responses do function normally, however, in QS. Since poikilothermia is a characteristic of reptiles, it seems possible that poikilothermia in mammalian AS may reflect a parallel between AS and reptilian quiescence (Walker & Berger 1980; Meddis 1977, 1979).

The matter goes beyond there, however. In a series of studies (reviewed in Walker & Berger, 1980) it has been shown that states of torpor or hibernation in mammals and birds are associated with large reductions in the proportion of sleep time devoted to AS. As the body temperature is lowered, so AS is reduced in amount. For example, in the ground squirrel, AS is rarely observed at body temperatures below 27 °C while QS may be present almost all of the time. Similarly, in the ring-necked dove, no AS is observed below body temperatures of 30 °C. Presumably, AS is suppressed during torpor or entrance to hibernation because thermoregulatory mechanisms are required continuously both to prevent too precipitious a fall in body temperature and to effect a gradual return to normal at the end of torpor. It is interesting in this connection to note that the echidna, a non-therian mammal which shows no AS, normally maintains a normal body temperature of 30 °C, which is much lower than that of therian mammals. This does suggest a possible starting point in the search for a solution to the riddle of the absence of AS in the echidna.

Such data offer strong support to the early intuition of investigators that the emergence of the AS/QS pattern in birds and mammals was linked with homeothermy in some way (e.g. Allison *et al.*, 1972). It is clear that the poikilothermia of AS is not a practical proposition for homeothermic animals. An obvious function for QS is to provide for long periods of immobility while regulating body temperature appropriately. What then is the function of AS? Walker and Berger (1980) and Horne (1977) have suggested that AS contributes to energy conservation through a reduced metabolism relative to QS. While the evidence on this point is still limited, it is reasonable to presume that any failure to mobilize expensive thermogenesis must constitute an energy saving in environments below body temperature.

My own preference in this matter (Meddis 1977, 1979) has been to view AS as vestigial in homeotherms and as having no function. If AS is, indeed, a poikilothermic condition, having its roots in reptilian quiescence, then it would appear to be a lethal heritage which needs to be suppressed. In fact, AS typically occupies less than 20% of mammalian sleep and appears for only brief periods — epochs measured in seconds in birds and minutes in mammals. Later it will be argued that the length of an AS epoch is closely linked to the thermal vulnerability of an animal. Thus, small animals, whose body temperature might fall very quickly in a poikilothermic condition, experience very short AS epochs.

3.7 AS and Ontogeny

In foetal mammals and neonates, AS occupies a much larger proportion of the animals total sleep time (Jouvet *et al.*, 1961; Roffwarg *et al.*, 1966). In most mammalian species studied so far, AS is the first kind of sleep to be seen; QS develops later and comes slowly to occupy a greater and greater proportion of total sleep. Berger (1975) has made a strong case for a coincidence in the timing of the appearance of AS and of the maturation of the young animal's ability to maintain a constant temperature in a cold environment. It is, as if, AS can be tolerated in large amounts only when an animal is not required to thermoregulate (e.g. in utero). When neonates take on themselves the responsibility of maintaining their own body temperature, then AS declines in prominence and QS begins to dominate its sleep.

The coincidence of the maturation of thermoregulatory abilities and the emergence of QS is an invitation to speculate that the ontogenetic sequence is reflecting the phylogenetic sequence. This would be consistent with the view proposed here that AS is phylogenetically ancient and that the evolution of QS was a necessary accompaniment of the evolution of homeothermy. The notion that ontogeny recapitulates phyologeny has had a long and chequered history (Gould, 1977) and it would be foolish to base a theory on this oracular principle alone. However, I have argued elsewhere (Meddis, 1979) that the principle holds good for the ontogenetic–phylogenetic parallels in the emergence of electrophysiological indicators (e.g. K-complexes, the division of QS into light and deep stages and sleep spindles) and may hold equally well for AS.

However, the ontogeny data are subject to an alternative explanation. It could be that AS is a foetal adaptation, a state which serves an important function in the maturation of the foetus (Roffwarg, 1966). If this is the case, then thermoregulatory capacity would be irrelevant, since the foetus does not need to thermoregulate, anyhow. It would also explain why AS comes to occupy an extremely small proportion of the 24 h period in adult mammals. Roffwarg *et al.* (1966) have suggested that the activated character of AS might be instrumental in promoting rapid maturation of the developing nervous system.

AS as a foetal adaptation is a strong theory but it is not clear, as with much evolutionary speculation, how it can be tested. For example, no one has ever shown that AS really does stimulate neural growth. We must simply wait for more pieces of the jigsaw to become available. Certainly we have enough material to stimulate hypothesis, but not enough to decide between hypotheses which seem to be flatly contradictory. It is clear that sleep characterized by an AS/QS cycle is restricted to birds and mammals (marsupial and placental). The parallel evolution of this pattern is most likely linked either to some aspect of homeothermy or the special needs of their developing foetuses. Both states may have evolved independently but evidence has been presented here in favour of a common reptilian origin of AS. However, there remain well-informed schools of thought which continue to prefer a common reptilian origin for QS. While I am happy to join battle in favour of one side, it is clear that neither theory is currently guaranteed ultimate acceptance.

Recent research by Warner and Huggins (1977) and Meglasson and Huggins (1979) does provide us with yet another possibility. Almost alone among investigators, they have found high voltage slow waves in the EEG of resting juvenile crocodiles. At the very least, this suggests that modern reptiles may yet supply evidence for the view that the ancient stem reptiles were 'pre-adapted' for the development of QS as we know it in birds and mammals. This sleep with slow waves was found *in addition* to the quiescence with spiking reported by Flanigan *et al.* (1973) in their adult crocodiles. Spiking disappeared during sleep with slow waves. It is therefore possible that 'quiescence with spikes' maps onto AS in homeotherms while 'sleep with slow waves' maps onto QS. It is intriguing to note that 'sleep with slow waves' has been reported only in relatively high environmental temperatures (29–38 °C) which means that the body temperatures of the crocodiles would be relatively close to those of homeotherms. It is too early to speculate in any detail on this point but the persistent pointers to a link between QS and raised body temperature cannot be ignored.

A possible function of high voltage cortical slow waves may be to reduce response thresholds. If this is so, slow waves would serve little purpose at low body temperatures when the animal is inactive in any case.

3.8 Evaluation of Specific Sleep Adaptations in Mammals

I have dwelt at some length on the evolution of AS and QS states but it is only one of many topics on which a whole new research industry could be based. Among mammals alone we can identify a number of adaptations of their sleep patterns which invite explanations in terms of the ecological or constitutional pressures which have influenced their evolution. For example, the AS/QS cycle may be an almost universal feature of mammalian sleep but the organization of cycles into sleep periods is subject to differences between species. In some species (e.g. higher primates) the cycles are joined into a single continuous episode while in others (e.g. cats and rats) a polyphasic pattern is observed with a number of distinct sleep episodes per day each composed of one or more cycles. Large herbivores (e.g. horses, cattle, sheep) on the other hand, have such disturbed sleep that the cycles are often difficult to discern. The total sleep time (TST) per 24 h is also highly variable. Table 3.3 shows a range of 17.1 h from 2.6 h (roe deer) to 19.9 h (little brown bat). It is likely that these variations represent adaptations to various ecological niches but the detailed process of linking manifest selection pressures to varieties of sleep pattern has only just begun.

Quiet sleep is often treated as a single homogenous state under the title slow wave sleep even though in some species — especially the higher primates — the major proportion of QS displays no slow waves at all. This has led to the distinction of light quiet sleep (LQS) with few, if any, slow waves and deep quiet sleep (DQS) with a predominance of slow waves. The distinction is particularly useful in cats but the classification is refined even further in the higher primates to include four stages of discriminable sleep patterns. Whereas the rat shows only a simple version of QS, in humans QS is a medley of different patterns. The reason for this development has attracted very little speculation but may be linked to the benefits of reduced response thresholds in LQS.

The function served by slow waves in the EEG of a sleeping mammal is also open to speculation. The absence of slow waves in AS shows that they are not a *necessary* condition of sleep. Furthermore, research has shown that animals can display slow waves while awake (Vanderwolf, 1975, for review) which shows that slow waves are also not a *sufficient* condition of sleep. In addition to slow waves we find further mysteries in the intermittent spindles (bursts of 12 Hz activity) and K-complexes (isolated high voltage slow waves). Whereas slow waves are present during QS in both birds and mammals, spindles are found only in mammals except possibly in the echidna, the most 'primitive' of mammals. K-complexes, however, are found only in higher primates. This evolutionary puzzler is discussed at greater length elsewhere (Meddis, 1979) but I know of no strong theory to explain the evidence.

Drowsiness is yet another phenomenon which is present in different amounts in different species. Ungulates, carnivores and some insectivores are known to spend hours of each day in the state of drowsiness. At these times, animals are inactive, uninterested in their surroundings and demonstrate occasional spindles in the EEG recording. Nevertheless, investigators are reluctant to classify it as sleep because the animals typically show low response thresholds. If we accept Walker *et al.*'s (1980) call to include hibernation at one extreme of the QS depth continuum, we might also want to add drowsiness to the other end. Ruckebusch's (1972) studies of drowsiness in farm animals clearly support the idea of a continuity between drowsiness and QS. To extend our idea of QS so far into wakefulness at one end and torpor at the other will inevitably impose a great strain on our concept of sleep as a simple unitary phenomenon but the problems of sleep description will have to be faced sooner or later. For our purpose, however, drowsiness raises the issue of why some species have so much of it while others — such as humans — have so little. Immobility *with vigilance* may be better suited to some species than others but I know of no pattern which offers the basis of a general explanation.

3.9 Statistical Analysis of Comparative Sleep Data

Solutions to the puzzles described above clearly require a multi-disciplinary approach. The physiologist, ecologist, palaeontologist and sleep researcher must pool their resources and share their different perspectives if we are to make much progress. The analyses described below give a flavour of the kind of results which can emerge from such an enterprise. These involve the accumulation of a database containing estimates of sleep parameters for various mammalian species along with measures of constitutional variables and aspects of their ecology. Using these data, we can calculate correlation coefficients between the variables and try to decide what is associated with what. Below I shall briefly describe the achievements of a number of researchers who have used this technique (Hartman, 1968; Zepelin & Rechtschaffen, 1970, 1973; Daillaire *et al.*, 1974; Allison & Cicchetti, 1976; Lorant, 1976), discuss a number of issues raised by their work and finally attempt a reanalysis of the available data in the light of these issues.

The database to be used in my analysis is given in Table 3.3. Although many additions and changes have been made the original compilation is the considerable achievement of Zepelin and Rechtschaffen whose thorough account of the origin of many of the values in the table must be studied carefully by any serious student of this topic. Allison and Cicchetti (1976) extended the list of species, made a few detailed changes in the light of research since the original compilation and added the estimates of 'predatory danger', 'sleep exposure' and 'overall danger'. I have added some more data points from the recent literature and have dropped the incomplete entries for Kangaroo, Giraffe, Marmot and Okapi. I have not attempted to improve or add to any of Allison and Cichetti's 'ecological' data points except for some estimates which appeared recently (Allison *et al.*, 1977). Although the echidna is reported to have no AS, I have entered this in the table as an unknown value to side-step certain statistical problems. I am grateful to Truett Allison for supplying his unpublished database and for discussing his statistical procedures with me. My own database and the computer program used to analyse it are available from me as a line printer listing or an ASCII punched paper tape. I am conscious of many shortcomings in the data and the analysis procedure and I invite potential critics to adjust either to suit their taste and reanalyse the data.

3.9.1 Statistical Notes

The basic technique used by all authors in this group is the Pearson product moment correlation coefficient. This estimates the 'goodness of fit' of a straight

Table 3.3 Sleep Parameters, Constitutional Variables and Ecological Measures for 65 Species

The data are taken from Zepelin and Rechtschaffen (1974), incorporate changes and new data in Allison and Cicchetti (1976) and include some new recently published figures. TST = total sleep time; QST = quiet sleep time; AST = active sleep time; Cycle = AS/QS cycle length; LFS = life span; BMR = basal metabolic rate; BDW = body weight; BRW = brain weight; GP = gestation period; PI = predation index; SE = sleep exposure; OD = overall danger; ADV = brain advancement at birth.

Order / *Family* / Species	QST (h)	TST (h)	AST (h)	Cycle (min)	LFS (yrs)	BMR ($0_2/cm_3/g/h$)	BDW (kg)	BRW (g)	GP (days)	PI	SE	OD	ADV
Monotremata													
Tachyglossidae													
Echidna	8.6	8.6	—	—	50	0.22	3	25	—	2	2	2	—
Marsupialia													
Didelphidae													
N. Amer. opossum	19.4	13.8	5.6	22.5	5	0.52	1.7	6.3	12	2	1	1	—
Water opossum	19.4	12.8	6.6	—	3	—	3.5	3.9	14	2	1	1	—
Phalangeridae													
Phalanger	13.7	11.9	1.8	—	13	—	1.62	11.4	17	2	1	2	—
Insectivora													
Tenrecidae													
Tenrec	13.3	11.0	2.3	—	4.5	—	0.9	2.6	60	2	1	2	—
Erinaceidae													
Europ. hedgehog	10.7	6.6	4.1	17.0	6	0.75	0.785	3.5	42	2	2	2	0.089
Desert hedgehog	10.3	7.6	2.7	—	—	—	0.55	2.4	—	2	1	2	—

Order / *Family* / Species	QST (h)	TST (h)	AST (h)	Cycle (min)	LFS (yrs)	BMR $(0_2/cm_3/g/h)$	BDW (kg)	BRW (g)	GP (days)	PI	SE	OD	ADV
Talpidae													
E. Amer. mole	8.4	6.3	2.1	10.4	3.5	1.9	0.075	1.2	42	1	1	1	—
Star-nosed mole	10.3	8.1	2.2	7.4	3.5	—	0.060	1	—	3	1	2	—
Soricidae													
L. Short tailed shrew	9.1	7.7	1.4	8.8	2.6	8.5	0.005	0.14	21	5	2	4	—
G. Short tailed shrew	14.9	12.6	2.3	7.6	2.7	3.4	0.019	0.29	20	4	3	3	—
Musk shrew	12.8	10.8	2.0	11.0	2	1.8	0.048	0.33	30	4	2	3	—
Chiroptera													
Vespertilionidae													
Little brown bat	19.9	17.9	2.0	12.0	24	2.89	0.01	0.25	50	1	1	1	—
Big brown bat	19.7	15.8	3.9	7.5	19	0.7	0.023	0.3	35	1	1	1	—
Primates													
Tupaiidae													
Tree shrew	15.8	13.2	2.6	13.9	2.3	—	0.104	2.5	46	3	2	2	0.168
Lorisidae													
Slow loris	11.0	—	—	—	12.7	—	1.4	12.5	90	2	2	2	0.312
Galago	10.7	9.5	1.2	33.0	10.4	—	0.2	5	120	2	2	2	—
Cebidae													
Owl monkey	17.0	15.2	1.8	—	12	0.51	0.48	15.5	140	2	2	2	—
Cebinae													
Squirrel monkey	9.9	—	—	—	20	0.83	0.61	20	—	—	—	—	—
Cercopithecidae													
Vervet	10.3	9.7	0.6	—	24	—	4.2	58	210	4	3	4	—
Patas monkey	10.9	10.0	0.9	—	20.2	—	10	115	170	4	4	4	—

Order / *Family* / Species	QST (h)	TST (h)	AST (h)	Cycle (min)	LFS (yrs)	BMR (0_2/cm_3/g/h)	BDW (kg)	BRW (g)	GP (days)	PI	SE	OD	ADV
Rhesus monkey	9.6	8.4	1.2	44.5	29	0.43	6.8	179	164	2	3	2	0.586
Baboon	9.8	9.1	0.7	40.0	27	0.3	10.5	179.5	180	4	4	4	0.296
Pongidae													
Chimpanzee	9.7	8.3	1.4	90.0	50	0.25	52.2	440	230	1	1	1	0.376
Gorilla	12.0	—	—	—	39.3	—	207	406	252	1	4	1	0.559
Hominidae													
Man	8.0	6.1	1.9	95.8	100	0.22	62	1320	267	1	1	1	0.258
Edentata													
Dasypodidae													
Giant armadillo	18.1	12.0	6.1	—	7	—	60	81	—	1	1	1	—
Nine-banded armadillo	17.4	14.3	3.1	22.8	6.5	0.25	3.5	10.8	120	2	1	1	0.292
Lagomorphia													
Leporidae													
Rabbit	8.4	7.5	0.9	29.0	18	0.42	2.5	12.1	31	5	5	5	0.134
Rodentia													
Aplodontiidae													
Mountain beaver	11.2	8.4	2.8	—	—	—	1.35	8.1	45	3	1	3	—
Sciuridae													
Ground squirrel	13.8	10.4	3.4	12.5	9	0.87	0.101	4	28	5	1	3	—
Arctic ground squirrel	16.5	—	—	—	—	0.59	0.92	5.7	25	5	2	3	—
Cliff chipmunk	14.9	—	—	—	—	—	0.067	—	—	3	1	2	—
Eastern chipmunk	16.3	—	—	—	8	1.25	0.122	1.97	31	3	1	2	—
Cricetidae													
Golden hamster	14.4	11.0	3.4	11.6	3.9	0.93	0.12	1	16	3	1	2	0.054

Order / *Family* / Species	QST (h)	TST (h)	AST (h)	Cycle (min)	LFS (yrs)	BMR (0_2/cm_3/g/h)	BDW (kg)	BRW (g)	GP (days)	PI	SE	OD	ADV
Giant pouched rat	8.3	6.3	2.0	—	4.5	—	1	6.6	42	3	1	3	—
Cotton rat	11.3	10.1	1.2	—	3	1.1	0.148	1.18	27	3	3	3	0.432
Spalacidae													
Mole rat	10.6	8.2	2.4	—	—	0.77	0.122	3.0	30	2	1	1	—
Muridae													
Rat	13.2	10.6	2.6	8.5	4.7	0.86	0.28	1.9	21	3	1	3	0.118
Mouse	13.2	11.9	1.3	12.3	3.2	1.49	0.023	0.4	19	4	1	3	0.200
Gerbil	15.3	13.6	1.7	18.6	—	—	0.065	1.04	21	—	—	—	0.138
Cavidae													
Guinea Pig	8.2	7.4	0.8	12.1	7.6	0.74	1.04	5.5	68	5	3	4	0.589
Chinchillidae													
Chinchilla	12.5	11.0	1.5	6.5	7	—	0.42	6.4	112	5	4	4	0.387
Carnivora													
Canidae													
Dog	8.6	6.16	2.5	20.0	20	0.36	14.0	70	63	1	1	1	0.097
Grey wolf	13.0	—	—	—	16.2	0.32	36.33	119	63	1	1	1	—
Red fox	9.8	7.4	2.4	20.7	9.8	0.43	4.23	50.4	52	1	1	1	—
Arctic fox	12.5	—	—	—	14	0.52	3.38	44.5	60	1	1	1	—
Procyonidae													
Raccoon	12.5	—	—	—	13.7	0.39	4.29	39.2	63	2	2	2	—
Felidae													
Cat	12.4	9.0	3.4	20.0	28	0.44	3.3	25.6	63	1	2	1	0.197
Jaguar	10.8	—	—	—	22.4	—	100	157	100	1	1	1	—
Viveridae													
Genet	6.1	4.8	1.3	—	34	—	1.4	17.5	—	1	2	1	—

Order / *Family* / Species	QST (h)	TST (h)	AST (h)	Cycle (min)	LFS (yrs)	BMR ($0_2/cm_3/g/h$)	BDW (kg)	BRW (g)	GP (days)	PI	SE	OD	ADV
Phocidae													
Grey seal	6.2	4.7	1.5	—	41	—	85	325	310	1	3	1	—
Hyracoidea													
Grey rock hyrax	6.6	5.7	0.9	—	7	—	0.75	12.27	225	2	2	2	—
Rock hyrax	5.4	4.9	0.5	—	6	—	3.6	21	225	3	2	3	—
Tree hyrax	5.4	4.9	0.5	—	7.5	—	2	12.3	200	3	1	3	—
Proboscidea													
Elephantidae													
Asian elephant*	3.9	2.1	1.8	124.0	69	0.07	2547	4603	624	3	5	4	—
African elephant*	3.3	—	—	—	38.6	—	6654	5712	645	3	5	3	0.368
Perissodactyla													
Equidae													
Horse*	2.9	2.1	0.8	15.5	46	0.15	521	655	336	5	5	5	0.517
Donkey*	3.1	—	—	—	40	0.2	187	419	365	5	5	5	—
Tapiridae													
Brazilian tapir*	6.2	5.2	1.0	54.0	30.4	—	160	169	392	4	5	4	—
Artiodactyla													
Cervidae													
Roe deer*	2.6	—	—	—	17	—	14.8	98.2	150	5	5	5	—
Bovidae													
Goat*	3.8	3.3	0.5	19.2	20	0.19	27.7	115	148	5	5	5	0.577
Sheep*	3.8	3.2	0.6	16.5	20	0.24	55.5	175	151	5	5	5	0.416
Cow*	3.9	3.2	0.7	16.0	30	0.13	600	423	281	5	5	5	0.436
Suidae													
Pig	8.4	6.5	1.9	—	27	0.12	192	180	115	4	4	4	0.167

* Animals classified as 'grazers' (see text).

line function relating two variables. Its most easily understood expression is in the form of the square of the correlation coefficient which represents the proportion of common or shared variance between two variables; the greater the shared variance, the more accurately we can predict one variable from a knowledge of the other. We compute the percentage shared variance (%SV) thus

$$\%SV = 100\, r^2$$

where r is the correlation coefficient. Although r is normally used in reports of this kind, it is considerably less transparent in this context and it has no advantages whatsoever over %SV. Just as we conventionally affix a minus sign to r to indicate an inverse function, we apply the same convention to %SV. For example, if AS time is correlated −0.59 with gestation period, we say

$$\%SV = 100\, x - |0.59^2| = -34.8\%$$

which means that 34.8% of the variance of AS time is predictable using an inverse function from a knowledge of gestation time, i.e. the longer the gestation time the less the AS time. This also implies, of course, that 65.2% of the variance remains 'unexplained'.

The technique of *partial correlation* can be used to assess the value of a third variable in explaining some or all of this unexplained or residual variance (%SVR). Using this technique we will find that 'overall danger' has a partial correlation (after removal of gestation period effects) of −0.69 with AS time. This means that approximately 48% of the residual variance is 'explained' by 'overall danger'. Since the residual variance constituted only 65.2% of the original variance to be explained, our third variable (overall danger) adds only 48% of 65.2% which is 31% of the original variance.

We may now compute the total shared variance (%SVT) explained by both gestation time and overall danger by simply adding the two shared variance estimates:

$$\%SVT = 34.8\% + 31\% = 65.8\%$$

This procedure is more commonly known as the technique of *multiple correlation*. For our purposes, we need merely note that 65.8% of the variance of the AS time of a species is predictable from a knowledge of its gestation period and Allison's estimate of the 'overall danger' to which it is typically exposed. For a more traditional account of correlation, partial correlation and multiple correlation see Guilford (1965, Chapter 16).

These statistical procedures are purely descriptive and refer only to the collection of values in the database. Since our sample of species is not in any sense random, we cannot conjure up any statistical justification for treating our results as typical of the complete population of mammalian species. Accordingly tests of 'statistical significance' are of limited value and I have abandoned Zepelin and Rechtschaffen's (1974) approach in this respect. Nevertheless, for presentation purposes only I have omitted %SV values of less than 10% from the shared variance matrices (Tables 3.4 and 3.5) on the grounds that they must be of little interest. This corresponds to a significance test rejection level for correlations below 0.32. (Note that $r = 0.31$ is the critical value at the 5% significance level for sample sizes of 30. This means that all values appearing in Tables 3.4 and 3.5 would have been significant using Zepelin and Rechtschaffen's method.) The results of our calculations, therefore, merely summarize the strength of the relationships observed between variables over the limited collection of species available to us in Table 3.3.

Because our techniques can cope with only linear relationships between variables, it is often necessary to transform the scales on which variables are measured, in order to obtain the best straight-line fit. Our variables show the strongest correlations when subjected to a logarithmic transformation. Therefore, all variables were transformed in this way except Allison's ecological variables and the binary 'grazing' variable. *Unless otherwise stated, all future references to variables are to be understood as referring to logarithmic transforms of these variables.* For example, a large negative %SV between metabolic rate and AS/QS cycle length implies an inverse linear function relating *log* metabolic rate to *log* cycle length.

Table 3.3 is not complete and we need to take care over the matter of missing data. The %SV values in Table 3.4 and 3.5 are based on all pairs of scores for which data are available on both variables. As a result, the sample size (*N*) for each %SV value will vary somewhat but never fall below 30. Table 3.3 can be used to find *N* for any pair of variables. Partial and multiple correlation values must likewise be based only on complete triplets of scores. Details are given in the text whenever this situation arises.

3.9.2 Previous Studies

Hartmann (1968) wrote the first short chapter when he reported, using data from six mammalian species (mouse, rat, rabbit, cat, man and elephant), a perfect rank order inverse correlation between the 'QS/AS cycle' length of a species and its characteristic metabolic rate. Thus, a mouse (which has an extremely high metabolic rate) is found to have a very short AS/QS cycle length — less than 5 min — while the elephant (with a low metabolic rate) was found by visual observation (Hartmann *et al.*, 1967) to have a very long cycle. Unfortunately, it was not clear from this article that metabolic rate was, in fact, the key variable. Both brain weight and body weight — among other variables — are known to be strongly correlated with metabolic rate. It remained possible that these may be even more closely related to cycle length. The matter was taken up in later investigations.

At about the same time Zepelin and Rechtschaffen (1970, 1974) took an interest in the relationship between daily sleep quotas and longevity which became apparent as increasing amounts of data became available. They were aware, of course, that life span (LFS) was also linked to that cluster of constitutional variables including basal metabolic rate (BMR), body weight (BDW), brain weight (BRW) and gestation period (GP). The result of their labours was a very comprehensive correlational study of all of these variables with a number of estimates of sleep parameters including total sleep time per day (TST), total quiet sleep time (QST), total active sleep time (AST), percentage of TST spent in active sleep (AS%) and AS/QS cycle length (CYCLE). Altogether 53 mammalian species were used in their database which is meticulously described in their paper (Zepelin & Rechtschaffen, 1974).

It is difficult and, in some respects, unfair to summarize briefly the results of such a detailed and carefully argued presentation but we can inspect some of the main conclusions. To begin with cycle length, we find that Hartmann's finding for 6 species remains valid for the 24 species for which cycle length estimates were then available. In fact large %SVs (around 72%) were found for all of the constitutional variables. Since the data were relatively sparse, Zepelin and Rechtschaffen were reluctant to select a best predictor but eventually nominated brain weight after inspection of a variety of partial correlation results. For 22 species brain weight has 85%SV with cycle length which is remarkably high in view of the uncertainty of the individual measures of each species' brain weight and cycle length.

The superiority of brain weight over metabolic rate seems surprising since it is much easier to think of the AS/QS cycle as just another physiological process controlled by the general pacemaker (BMR) which seems to influence most bodily process rates. However, brain size has been implicated in the control of other process rates by Sacher (1974) who showed that the rate of growth of body tissue in the foetus is limited by the rate of growth of nervous tissue. Presumably, this protects the all-important brain by not allowing other organs to grow rapidly at the brain's expense. Such an approach allows us to link cycle length and brain size through the idea of the thermoregulatory threat during AS described above. Since large brains heat up and cool down relatively slowly they are less threatened by short periods of loss of thermoregulatory control. It follows that small animals with small brains are more vulnerable. If the purpose of the AS/QS cycle is to break up AS into a number of tolerable episodes, then we might expect small animals to have shorter cycles since these involve shorter AS episodes. Both brain weight and body weight show strong correlations with cycle length, but the superior brain weight correlation presumably results from the fact that brain temperature is more crucial to survival than body temperature.

A new variable was introduced to the database in the form of a simple estimate of the active sleep episode length (ASE):

$$\text{ASE} = \text{CYCLE} \times \text{AS\%} / 100$$

This estimate assumes that each cycle is composed wholly of sleep (i.e. no waking) and that only one AS episode occurs per cycle. Although neither of these two assumptions necessarily holds, ASE serves as an easily computed first approximation which allows us to explore a possibility. My expectation was that brain weight would show a stronger relationship with ASE than cycle length.

Zepelin and Rechtschaffen's results were qualified by an almost simultaneous publication by Dallaire and Ruckebusch (1974) which claimed that published correlations between metabolic rate and cycle length had been exaggerated. Their own graphs based on 22 species showed a more impressive relationship between cycle length and encephalization, where encephalization refers to the extra development of neural tissue over and above what is predictable from body size alone — human beings and the primates, for example, show a high degree of encephalization. Lorant (1976) using correlation methods confirmed their finding. Taking these two studies together and examining their data in detail we can see that the problem has its origins in differences in the species included in the database. The French investigators reject Hartmann's data on the elephant but include data of their own (not available to Zepelin and Rechtschaffen) showing relatively short cycles for goats, ponies and cattle. The point here is that these species have relatively great bodyweight (low metabolic rate) but little encephalization.

So far the problem remains unresolved. In the analysis below, we shall include an encephalization variable (ENC) which is calculated from the other variables thus:

$$ENC = BRW / (0.12\ BDW^{0.667})$$

where BRW is measured in grams and BDW in kilograms. This procedure follows that adopted by Lorant (1976) and others (see e.g. Russell, 1979). A high value of ENC indicates a relatively large brain for the body size of that species.

We shall compute two shared variance matrices; one including and one excluding large herbivores, since this group contains all of the controversial species (Tables 3.4 and 3.5). If cycle length is closely linked with encephalization we might reasonably expect the relationship to hold even when the controversial species are excluded.

Zepelin and Rechtschaffen also found usefully large correlations between TST and constitutional variables. Their result implies that small animals sleep more than large animals. Since small animals have higher metabolic rates (i.e. a higher rate of energy expenditure per gram of body tissue), it also follows that longer sleep is associated with higher rates of energy expenditure. This finding is used by Horne (1977) and Walker *et al.* (1980) to support their view that sleep may serve the purpose of minimizing energy expenditure. However, the results again showed that *brain weight* was a better predictor of TST than either body weight or metabolic rate. Nevertheless, Zepelin and Rechtschaffen were reluctant to conclude firmly in favour of any necessary relationship between TST and constitutional variables because the results were not reliable within subgroups of species. For example, positive correlations were found between metabolic rate and TST among marsupials, primates, perissodactyls and carnivores while negative correlations were found among insectivores and artiodactyls.

We can see in Fig. 3.2 that large herbivores display very much less sleep than the other species. This may simply be explained in terms of the vulnerable nature of the habitat of large herbivores. Sleep may expose them to predators and therefore needs to be reduced to tolerably low levels. If we were to remove them from the graph, the remaining points do not appear to indicate any linear relationship between metabolic rate and total sleep time. To explore this possibility further, I included a new binary variable (GRZ) into the database which scored 1 for grazing animals and 0 for non-grazing animals. I also analysed the results twice with and without the grazers.

The pattern of Zepelin and Rechtschaffen's results for QST was broadly the same as TST which is not surprising since QST occupies 80–90% of TST. AST was, however, largely independent of QST having only 34% SV. Its main correlation was with gestation period (41% SV). The authors were, however, disappointed in their ability to predict AST from constitutional variables. They contrasted AS with QS which in many additional respects appear to be very different kinds of sleep. They did not comment on the correlation between AS and gestation time. AS% was uncorrelated with any of the constitutional variables in their study.

In their discussion, Zepelin and Rechtschaffen sympathetically consider a proposal by Allison and Van Twyver (1970) that 'the status of a species as predator or prey and the security of a species' sleeping arrangements are decisive factors with respect to sleep time'. After informally reflecting on a

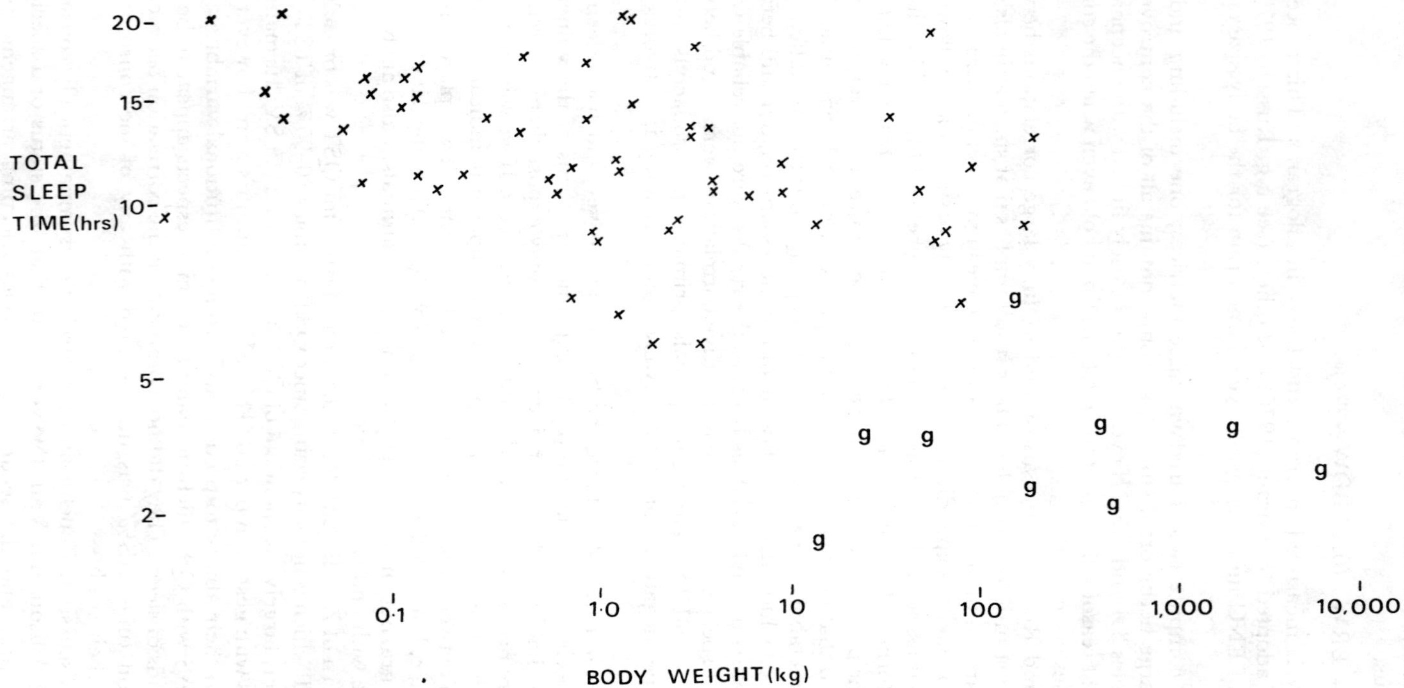

Fig. 3.2 Plot of log bodyweight (kg) against log total sleep time (h) for various mammalian species. Original data given in Table 3.3. Grazing animals are shown as 'g', while non-grazing animals are shown as 'x'.

number of species which appear to contradict this thesis, they conclude that 'none of these factors seems to possess explanatory power comparable to that of energy metabolism'. In their original study, Allison and Van Twyver had found that 'good sleepers' (species who slept more than 8 h per day) typically either were predators or chose to sleep in very secure sleep sites. In either case the animals had little to fear while asleep. 'Poor sleepers' by contrast were typically prey species who slept in exposed places. To defend his position Allison, with Cicchetti, set out to reanalyse Zepelin and Rechtschaffen's data with a view to correlating ecological as well as constitutional variables with estimates of AS and QS amounts for a range of species.

Allison and Cicchetti (1976) added three new variables (all five-point scales) to characterize 'predation', 'sleep exposure' and 'overall danger'. On all three scales a low score indicated minimum threat. The predation index (PI) indicated the authors' assessment of the extent to which a species was preyed upon in its natural habitat. The sleep exposure (SE) scale reflected the degree of protection offered by the typical sleep site of a species. The overall danger (OD) scale provided a general estimate of predatory danger which took both of the preceding scales into account. Some other variables were dropped, however: these were TST, AS%, CYCLE length and BMR. They added a small number of species and supplied some missing constitutional data points. They then discarded all species for whom complete data were not available leaving 39 species. They used correlation, partial correlation and multiple correlation techniques. In addition, they factor analysed their correlation matrix.

Their ecological variables were all interestingly correlated with sleep parameters. Overall danger had −47%SV with AST and sleep exposure had −34%SV with QST — to quote the best two predictors. Among the constitutional variables, gestation period had −42%SV with AST and body weight had 51%SV with QST. It was clear that AS and QS were multiply determined. To find the best joint predictors of the sleep variables, Allison and Cicchetti partialled out the strongest single predictor (body weight for QST and overall danger for AST) and then looked for the variable with the highest shared variance with the residuals. These turned out to be overall danger for QST and gestation time for AST. A best fit equation predicting QST from a combination of body weight and overall danger accounted for 58% of the variance of QST. A second best fit equation predicting AST from a combination of overall danger and gestation time accounted for 66% of the variance of AST. The results clearly support Allison and Van Twyver's (1970) hypothesis that predatory danger is an important influence on sleep patterns in mammals.

Allison and Cicchetti were moved to speculate about the significance of the inclusion of gestation period in the predictive equation for AST. One possible explanation offered was that species with prey status may have longer gestation times than would be predicted from their body weights. In this way gestation period would, in part at least, be yet another reflection of predatory danger. This explanation was not supported by useful correlation between gestation period and predatory danger so the possibility was rejected in favour of an alternative which implied that animals with shorter gestation periods need more AS (in the foetus at least) to hasten the development of the foetal nervous system. To clarify the picture I decided to include an additional measure of gestational delay (DELAY) in the database. This was simply the ratio of a species' typical gestational period to that which would have been predicted on the basis of the adult brain weight of the species:

$$\text{DELAY} = \text{GP} / (27.4\ \text{BRW}^{0.365}).$$

This formula was derived from an expression in Sacher (1974).

Since the first draft of this paper, Zepelin (1980) has shown that approximately 50% of the variance of AST can be predicted from neonatal brain weight (expressed as a percentage of adult brain weight). Animals born relatively mature (precocial) have more developed brains at birth compared with those born in a more immature, helpless condition (altricial). Advancement (ADV) is the ratio of neonatal brain weight to adult brain weight. Zepelin showed that this measure of advancement was highly correlated with an independent 'four-point altricial-precocial rating with more points for quicker maturation'. He argues that his result explains Allison and Cicchetti's finding of an association between AST and overall danger since precocity is generally considered to be a defence strategem against vulnerability. To evaluate this point, 25 estimates of brain advancement at birth (ADV) were taken from Sacher and Staffeldt (1974) and included in the data base.

In view of the interesting correlations between the ecological variables and both AST and QST, it is unfortunate that Allison and Cicchetti did not include TST in their computations. Similarly the omission of AS% is greatly to be regretted. It is relevant to our study of the evolution of AS to know whether danger affects the total amount of AS per day or whether it works indirectly by allowing TST to be set by other factors while influencing only the proportion of time spent in AS. If it is the raised thresholds of AS which makes it maladaptive in the face of danger, then we might well expect danger to be more strongly correlated with AS% than AST. Alternatively, the correlation may be even stronger with AS episode length (ASE, described above), since the longer the AS episode, the longer before an animal will become aware of any present danger. In our more complete analysis below we shall be able to tackle all of these points.

3.9.3 Results

Table 3.4 shows the percent shared variance matrix for all of the data given in Table 3.3 ($N = 65$). Values less than 10% have been omitted; to convert to correlation coefficients simply divide by 100 and take the square root. Where this matrix overlaps with those of Zepelin and Rechtschaffen (1974) and Allison and Cicchetti (1976) the results are broadly similar. The main exception is the reduced strength of the relationship between cycle length and brain weight (as well as the other 'size' variables). This must be due to the inclusion of new data on farm animals from the French researchers Ruckebusch and Dallaire. Table 3.5 shows the result of a second analysis which excludes all grazing animals. In this table, the association between total sleep time (as well as quiet sleep time) and the 'size' variables is considerably weakened. Cycle length and brain weight, however, show a greater proportion of shared variance. We shall now look at the variables individually.

Total sleep time (TST). Table 3.4 shows a slightly weakened relationship between TST and its best predictor, body weight (– 37%SV), compared to Zepelin and

Rechtschaffen's best predictor which was brain weight (– 50%SV). This must be due to the inclusion of new species. However, in this analysis at least, danger variables were better predictors of TST, as we might have expected from Allison and Cicchetti's separate correlations between danger and both QST and AST. Our best danger predictor of TST was sleep exposure with – 48% shared variance. Both constitutional and ecological variables were beaten into second place, however, by the simple binary variable which indicated whether or not we were dealing with grazing animals. Grazing had – 62% shared variance with TST. Since grazing showed considerably more shared variance with TST than body weight we cannot explain the effect of grazing on TST in terms of the obvious weight differences between grazers and non-grazers.

The simplest explanation of our result is that TST is reduced in grazing animals as a result of the peculiar pressures on such animals. Since grazing animals are typically heavier than non-grazers this produces the appearance of an association between weight and TST which is misleading. We can check this suggestion in Table 3.5 which looks at the variables within the non-grazer group. Here, no obvious relationship can be detected between TST and *either* size variables (body weight, brain weight, metabolic rate) or danger variables (predatory index, sleep exposure or overall danger). Note that the large reduction in size of the correlation cannot be explained in terms of the reduction in sample size since large herbivores constitute only a small proportion of the total group. Small correlations exist for gestation period but, as we shall see below, these are considerably weakened when the marsupial species (with their abnormally short gestational periods) are withdrawn from the database. *We may, therefore, conclude that a grazing life-style is accompanied by reduced daily sleep quotas. We must also conclude that among non-grazing animals (Table 3.5) there exists little correlation, if any, between TST and any of the size or danger variables included in this study.*

Quiet sleep time (QST). QST shows the same pattern of results as for TST which is not surprising since it occupies 80–90% of TST. It is interesting to note that QST shows only a very weak association (19%SV) with active sleep time (AST) among non-grazing animals. This supports the idea that AST and QST are determined by unrelated influences.

Active sleep time (AST). The best predictor of AST in Table 3.4 is neonatal brain advancement (ADV) with – 53%SV. Overall danger (OD) is only second best with – 44%SV. This appears to support Zepelin's (1980) contention that ADV is a *prior* explanation, that is, the AST/ADV correlation explains the AST/OD correlation. However, the matter is not so simple. To begin, there is no correlation between OD and ADV in Table 3.4 (< 10%SV). This implies that, contrary to Zepelin's (and Allison and Cicchetti's) assumption, precocity cannot be taken as a simple indicator of vulnerability to predation. Moreover, ADV is negatively correlated with DELAY. This implies that long gestation periods are not necessarily associated with brain advancement at birth. These apparent contradictions warrant further analysis.

One complication is that the correlations between AST and the ecological variables are based on a much larger sample (N = 51) than those involving ADV (N = 22). In a supplementary analysis I used only the 25 species for

Table 3.4 Percent Shared Variance Matrix for all Species in Table 3.3

Variables and the shared variance concept are defined in the text.

	TST	QST	AST	AS%	CYCLE	ASE	LFS	BMR	BDW	BRW	ENC	GP	DEL	PI	SE	OD	GRZ	ADV
TST	100																	
QST	94	100																
AST	50	28	100															
AS%			48	100														
CYCLE	– 12	– 14			100													
ASE	– 13	– 23		31	78	100												
LFS	– 22	– 22	– 11		52	41	100											
BMR	32	35			– 46	– 46	– 58	100										
BDW	– 37	– 45			49	52	52	– 87	100									
BRW	– 33	– 42	– 13		60	57	65	– 81	81	100								
ENC	– 11		– 15		48	33	43	– 21	16	40	100							
GP	– 49	– 42	– 37		44	32	54	– 59	59	67	36	100						
DELAY			20	20		10						– 22	100					
PI	– 16		– 26	– 13		– 15								100				
SE	– 48	– 35	– 38				20	– 24	33	26		36		37	100			
OD	– 36	– 22	– 44	– 14										85	59	100		
GRZ	– 62	– 52	– 16				17	– 30	36	27		31		22	56	39	100	
ADV	– 25	– 22	– 53	– 14			12		19	21	10	38	– 27		28		21	100

Table 3.5 Percent Shared Variance Matrix for Non-grazing Species in Table 3.1

Variables and the shared variance concept are defined in the text.

TST	100																
QST	89	100															
AST	46	19	100														
AS%			69	100													
CYCLE	− 14	− 12			100												
ASE	− 10	− 21		20	72	100											
LFS					55	38	100										
BMR					− 56	− 54	− 49	100									
BDW	− 10	− 17			65	63	41	− 82	100								
BRW	− 10	− 19			72	63	58	− 73	73	100							
ENC	− 13		− 18		56	38	47	− 23	17	48	100						
GP	− 32	− 24	− 35	− 13	46	23	42	− 41	39	53	44	100					
DELAY			25	24		24		− 20				− 25	100				
PI			− 14	− 21	− 15	− 35	− 17	10	− 13	− 10				100			
SE			− 27	− 25								12		21	100		
OD			− 32	− 34		− 28								83	37	100	
ADV			− 37	− 29						12	12	32	− 29		13		100
	TST	QST	AST	AS%	CYCLE	ASE	LFS	BMR	BDW	BRW	ENC	GP	DEL	PI	SE	OD	ADV

whom ADV scores were available; 24 of these had ratings for PI, SE and OD. On this occasion the best predictor of AST was not ADV but overall danger (– 61%SV). The increase in %SV for OD from – 44 to – 61 illustrates how influential sampling effects can be. This does not mean that OD is a prior explanation since we have already established that OD and ADV are not correlated. We might, therefore, be dealing with two largely independent influences on AST. The results of a partial correlation analysis are given in Table 3.6. When variance explained by OD is removed, ADV accounts for the bulk of the residual variance (– 69%SVR). By combining OD and ADV using multiple correlation (Table 3.6) we can explain 88% of the variance of AST which is gratifyingly high. As new estimates for ADV become available it will become possible to assess the robustness of this result. A reduction in the %SVT is highly likely but even if it stays as high as 70% it will still be a credit to the insights of Allison, Cicchetti, Zepelin and Rechtschaffen.

Table 3.6 Results of Various Calculations Involving Regression of AST on Seven Candidate Predictors

Predictor =	GP	DELAY	PI	SE	OD	GRZ	ADV
Simple shared variance using all available data ($N \leq 65$)							
%SV	– 37	20	– 26	– 38	– 44	– 16	– 53
Simple shared variance using only data for species with ADV estimate ($N \leq 25$)							
%SV	– 20	<10	– 50	– 59	– 61	– 41	– 53
Residual shared variance after partialling out OD ($N \leq 25$)							
%SVR	– 37	<10	<10	– 16		– 12	– 69
Residual shared variance after partialling out ADV ($N \leq 25$)							
%SVR	<10	– 14	– 16	– 43	– 75	– 26	
Total shared variance when OD is added to a second variable ($N \leq 25$)							
%SVT	76	62	64	68		66	88
Total shared variance when ADV is added to a second variable ($N \leq 25$)							
%SVT	53	60	82	73	88	65	

The results indicate a two-process model whereby AS is suppressed by both vulnerability to predation and by early maturation of the nervous system, where these two effects are possibly independent. The effect of danger in suppressing AST is probably a necessary consequence of the raised response thresholds during this type of sleep. It seems logical that a survival advantage will accrue to vulnerable species if they spend less time in AS. The brain advancement at birth finding is open to two interpretations. First, we might surmise that a high ADV score reflects a species' need to be very mature at birth and that this need is met by delaying birth until the foetus is mature. This explanation is contradicted by the low (even negative) relationship between DELAY and ADV variables. Alternatively, we might interpret a low ADV score as reflecting a sustained period of growth of nervous tissue *after birth*. This latter effect is generally recognized to be a neotenous feature (Gould, 1977). Neoteny is a process whereby some foetal and infant characteristics develop more slowly and persist into adulthood. In our case, neoteny may result in the persistence of infantile sleep patterns in adult sleep.

It is probably unwise to speculate concerning the function of increasing AST in this way since it may simply be a passive consequence of a neotenous strategem which can confer a very wide range of benefits on a species in certain kinds of environment (Gould, 1977). The neoteny hypothesis does not predict any strong relationship between ADV and QST since QST does not change as dramatically in ontogeny as AST once it has reached its maximum value around birth. Zepelin (1980) has made the interesting suggestion that the relatively small amount of AS in birds may be explained by the fact that they are 'relatively mature at birth'.

Active sleep percent (AS%). Correlations between AS% and other variables were conspicuous by their absence. Extensive analysis involving multiple and partial correlation techniques also failed to reveal any patterns. This result is wholly consistent with all previous reports. When taken together with the lawfulness of absolute amounts of AS per 24 h, it begins to look as if AS% is not a measure of any biological importance. One view is that total sleep time is determined by constitutional and ecological variables with the proportions of AS and QS being secondarily determined by separate factors. The data do not support this view. The poor correlation between QST and AST (28%SV) suggests that they vary independently and are subject to different influences. That this association is further reduced in Table 3.5 (19%SV), when only non-grazing animals are used, reinforces this conclusion.

QS/AS cycle time (CYCLE). Constitutional variables show strong correlations with CYCLE; the best predictor being brain weight (BRW) with 60%SV (*N* = 33, Table 3.4). This is considerably weaker than the 85%SV reported by Zepelin and Rechtschaffen. Dallaire and Ruckebusch's (1974) and Lorant's (1976) postulated relationship with encephalization (ENC) fared less well but still creditably at 48%SV. It was suggested above that the differences in the results of the French and American investigators might have been due to their different selection of species. Since these differences were concentrated among grazing animals, it was decided to repeat the analysis using the 27 non-grazing animals for whom CYCLE data were available. This resulted in a substantial increase in correlation for both brain weight (72%SV) and encephalization (56%SV) — see Table 3.5. In Fig. 3.5, we can see that species are arranged fairly neatly along the regression line, including the two 'grazers', elephant and tapir. However, goat, sheep, horse and cow all show very short cycles for their brain weight. Since the data for all four species originate from Ruckebusch's laboratory (see Lorant, 1976, for data), it is possible that we are simply dealing with differences in scoring techniques or laboratory conditions. Until independent assessments are available, it is pointless to speculate on these exceptions.

In both Tables 3.4 and 3.5, basal metabolic rate (BMR) shows a less substan-

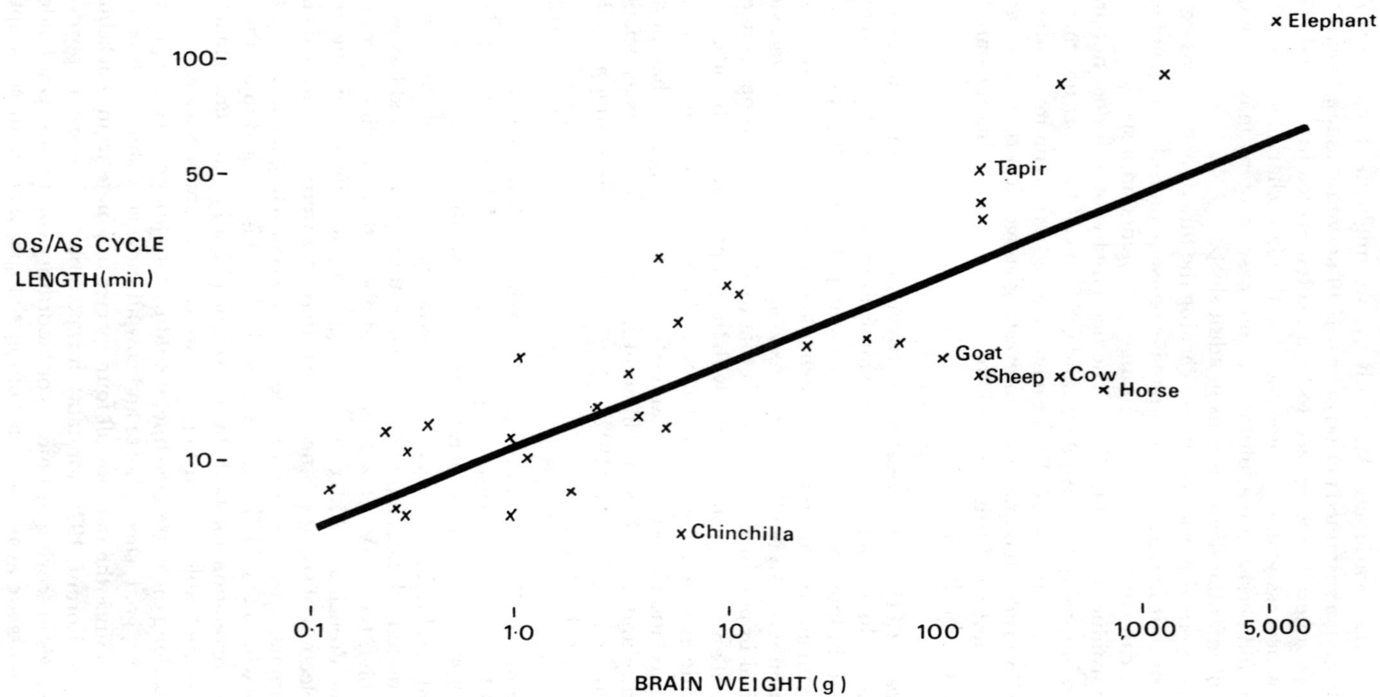

Fig. 3.3 Plot of log brain weight (g) against log QS/AS cycle length (min) for various mammalian species. Original data given in Table 3.3. Certain species of particular interest (see text) have been named.

tial association with CYCLE (– 46%SV and – 56%SV) than brain weight. In this respect, Hartmann's (1968) metabolic hypothesis seems increasingly less likely and Zepelin and Rechtschaffen's finding in favour of brain weight has survived the addition of new species to the database. The significance of the relationship, however, remains in doubt. We may argue that species with small brains in some way need to experience frequent periods of AS. This would be consistent with Horne's (1977) and Walker and Berger's (1980) view that AS is a time of low energy expenditure. Since smaller animals expend energy at a faster rate than larger animals, they may need AS more often. Alternatively, we might contemplate the other possibility that AS is a time of thermoregulatory threat (Meddis, 1979) because of the absence of homeostatic response to variations in body temperature. Since body temperature fluctuates more rapidly in smaller species and since the brain is the organ most easily damaged by thermal irregularities, it may be that rapid cycling with short AS periods is a better strategem for small-brained species than slow cycling with prolonged AS periods. If this latter hypothesis is true, then it may be more profitable to examine the length of the AS epoch than the cycle itself.

Active sleep episode length (ASE). It can be seen from Tables 3.4 and 3.5 that ASE has roughly comparable correlations with brain weight, if slightly smaller, than those for CYCLE. Smaller correlations with predatory index (PI) and overall danger (OD) are also present, being strongest for the non-grazing animals. These negative correlations imply that more vulnerable species have shorter ASEs. This is consistent with the observation that response thresholds are highest during AS. Using only species for whom ASE values are computable, multiple correlations were computed using BRW in combination with the three ecological variables (PI, SE and OD). For these species, the %SVT were 72, 68 and 72 respectively. For non-grazing species ($N = 27$), they were 74, 75 and 76. In both cases, the ecological variables added more than 10%SV to an already strong relationship between ASE and BRW.

These results provide support for the idea that ASE is maladaptive in mammals by virtue of raised response thresholds and thermoregulatory threat. As a consequence active sleep episodes are kept short in adult mammals. This effect is intensified in mammals with smaller (and therefore thermally more vulnerable) brains and in species exposed to predatory danger. The mechanism by which this shortening of ASE is achieved appears to involve shortening the AS/QS cycle in proportion with brain weight and, more directly, by further reducing the length of the ASE in proportion to predatory threat. Since the ASE values were computed from CYCLE and AS%, these conclusions must remain tentative until the relationships can be confirmed using actual measurements of active sleep episodes.

Gestation. Table 3.5 shows a negative correlation between gestation period and TST (– 32%SV) and QST (– 24%SV). This cannot be explained in terms of gestational delay since this variable shows no sizeable correlation with either TST or QS. Even so, the correlation is inflated by the presence of the marsupials which have abnormally short gestation times while the two species of oppossum have very long TSTs. Removing all three marsupial species brings the correlations down to – 24%SV for TST and – 18%SV for QST which are too small to warrant further consideration. Nor may we hypothesize that marsupials as a group are long sleepers since the phalanger weighs in at only 13.7 h sleep per day which is close enough to the average for non-grazing animals. In the absence of marsupials, gestation period shows poor correlations with AST (−28%SV) and AS% (<10%SV). A good correlation between gestation and cycle length (48% SV) does not survive partialling by brain weight (<10%SVR). *In general, gestation period* (per se) *does not appear to be useful as an explanatory variable for any aspect of sleep.*

The measure of *gestational delay* was particularly disappointing. No substantial correlation was found between this and any of the sleep variables. This piece of negative information is useful, however, in that it eliminates yet another possibility from our list.

3.9.4 Summary of Results

Statistical analysis of correlates of mammalian sleep parameters over the last two decades have made a number of advances. It seems that the amount of active sleep in adults can be explained in terms of exposure to predatory threat and degree of neoteny characterizing a species. On the one hand, species exposed to predatory danger have reduced active sleep amounts while, on the other hand, species whose major growth of nervous tissue occurs after birth have increased active sleep amounts as adults. The length of individual epochs of active sleep is shorter for species of smaller size and for species exposed to greater predatory threat. This result is consistent with the hypothesis that AS is maladaptive in mammals by virtue of the inactivity of thermoregulatory mechanisms and the raising of behavioural response thresholds which are observed at these times. The former would be a greater threat for smaller animals and the latter would be a greater threat for species more preyed upon than preying.

Quiet sleep has not yielded up many of its secrets, however, and its correlates remain a mystery. Whereas it was previously believed that quiet sleep could be predicted from the size of a species, this appears to be a statistical artifact. Grazing animals have typically reduced sleeping times. Since they are also typically larger than the other species for which we have available data, this creates the false impression of a relationship between size and quiet sleep time. Among non-grazing animals, no such relationship is observed. Furthermore, quiet sleep amounts appear to be unrelated to active sleep amounts and determined by different factors. Since quiet sleep makes up the bulk of total sleep, it is equally true to say that we still know of no systematic determinants of total sleep time beyond the simple assertion that herbivores typically sleep much less than other species.

3.10 Conclusions

Any discussion of the evolution of sleep patterns must have an evanescent quality. We are speculating about events which took place long ago and which left no trace except in the distorted mirror of the genetic heritage of modern species. Nor can we even be sure of the appropriateness of a genetic explanation of the similarities among sleep patterns in animals currently available for study. Such similarities may arise through parallel (or convergent) evolution, shaped merely by similarities in environmental or constitutional pressures. But the effort of seeking an evolutionary theory is still worthwhile. The search necessarily focuses our attention on broader issues such as the function of sleep, the relationship between sleep-control mechanisms and constitution, the interaction between the pattern of sleep and environmental pressures and the complementarity of sleep and waking behaviour. Things went smoothly as long as sleep research continued to stumble on new phenomena (EEG slow waves, spindles, K-complexes and spikes; active sleep with its autonomic variability, rapid eye movements, postural relaxation, penile erections; variations in amounts of sleep among species; exotic sleep disorders such as narcolepsy and sleep apnea; etc., etc.). No doubt, we shall continue to discover new and surprising facts about sleep but sooner or later we must try to make sense of this jumble of data. Arguments about the evolution and function of sleep provide a necessary forum for clarifying the issues, testing general theories and inspiring well-directed research projects. So far, the theories remain a poor match for the data, but the richness of the data is such that powerful theories do seem to be just around the corner.

Acknowledgement

I would like to acknowledge many helpful discussions on this topic with my colleagues Jim Horne, Nick Norgan and Phil Peters and to thank Ralph Berger for his comments on the final draft.

Note by Harold Zepelin

Dr Meddis has graciously allowed this comment. Despite valuable insights, he has, in my opinion, reached some unjustified conclusions. Demonstration of sleep's relationship with body weight and metabolic rate requires a wide range of values. This indicates the existence of only a moderately strong relationship, but it does not mean that previous findings are 'statistical artifacts'. Dr Meddis's designation of 'grazing' species is arbitrary and allows him to test for this relationship in variance-deprived subsamples. Why not include as grazers the gorilla, rabbit, mountain beaver, chipmunk, giant pouched rat, guinea pig, chinchilla, and rock hyrax — all strictly herbivorous? (It might be argued that some are grazers, others browsers, but this is hairsplitting.) In a subsample constituted of these species together with Dr Meddis's 'grazers' the correlation of log body weight and log TST in his data is -0.75 ($p < 0.0001$); in the remainder of the sample it is -0.31 ($p < 0.05$). Hardly artifacts! Dr Meddis's position on tests of significance allows him to brush aside meaningful correlations (e.g. -0.32 for TST and body weight in his 'non-grazers'; $p < 0.05$), but his view is dogmatic and incorrect in practice. His judgement of sleep-related danger may also be biased because the PI, SE, and OD ratings were not generated, as they should be, by persons with no stake in the ongoing controversy.

Rejoinder to Harold Zepelin's Comments by Ray Meddis

I am grateful to Dr Zepelin for his careful attention to my article and his efforts in reworking some of the correlations. I certainly agree that the ratings of PI, SE and OS should, ideally, have been made by an independent authority. That is not to say that I (or, I presume, Dr Zepelin) question the integrity of the suppliers of *all* of these figures — Drs Allison and Cichetti — but dispassionate observers are more likely to meet the strict criteria of scientific analysis. It is not clear, however, that Allison and Cichetti are so inaccurate in their ratings that a new set would greatly affect the correlations in such a large sample. Despite requests, I have never succeeded in inducing a suitably qualified scientist to take on the task of rating the animals but, like Dr Zepelin, I would be very encouraged to have a new and possibly extended set of ratings for the purpose of reanalysis.

Of course, I am quite unable to agree with him that my definition of 'grazing' animals is arbitrary. The term is used in the article to describe a group of animals which have a great deal in common in terms of their ecology. Put a gorilla, rat and guinea pig in among an elephant, horse, donkey, deer, goat, sheep, cow and pig and even a seven-year-old would find the odd men out. I accept the argument — possibly implied — that a common herbivorous diet may rule out diet as an explanation of the short sleep of grazing animals, thus making exposure to predation a more likely candidate. It does nothing, however, to shore up the case in favour of a weight or metabolic determinant of total sleep time. Among non-grazers — even by Dr Zepelin's revised criteria — the correlation between these two variables is only 0.31 (or 10% explained variance) despite a body weight range from 0.005 g to 207 kg and a total sleep range of 5.4 to 19.9 h. By any standards this is a paltry correlation and no basis whatsoever for a scientific theory and it is unworthy to resort to the concept of 'statistical significance' to keep it alive. At 0.31, the correlation coefficient would only just make the generous $p = 0.05$ level of significance even if the animals were a random sample from the mammalian order. Since the sample is very non-random, statistics would require a very much higher correlation than this to qualify as significant. In which case the correlation is seen to be significant neither in the statistical sense nor in terms of common parlance. On this point my position remains that the correlation is low enough to be considered an artifact, that it is not meaningful and that, as a consequence, it should be set aside.

References

ALLISON, T. and CICCHETTI, D. V. (1976). Sleep in mammals: ecological and constitutional correlates. *Science*, **194**, 732–734.

ALLISON, T. and VAN TWYVER, H. B. (1970). The evolution of sleep. *Nat. Hist.*, **79**, 56–65.

ALLISON, T., VAN TWYVER, H. B. and GOFF, W. R. (1972). Electrophysiological studies of the echidna, *Tachyglossus Aculeatus*. *Arch. Ital. Biol.*, **110**, 145–184.

ALLISON, T., GERBER, S. D., BREEDLOVE, S. M. and DRYDEN, G. L. (1977). A behavioural and polygraphic study of sleep in the shrews *Suncus murinus*, *Blarina brevicauda* and *Cryptotis parva*. *Behav. Biol.*, **20**, 354–366.

ASERINSKY, E. and KLEITMAN, N. (1953). Regularly occurring periods of eye motility and concomitant phenomena during sleep. *Science*, **118**, 273–274.
BERGER, R. J. (1975). Bioenergetic functions of sleep. *Fed. Proc.*, **34**, 97–102.
DALLAIRE, A., TOUTAIN, P. L. and RUCKEBUSCH, Y. (1974). Sur la périodicité du sommeil paradoxal: faits et hypothèses. *Physiol. Behav.*, **13**, 395–400.
DESMOND, A. J. (1977). *The Hot-Blooded Dinosaurs*, London: Futura.
FLANIGAN, W. F. jun., WILCOX, R. H. and RECHTSCHAFFEN, A. (1973). The EEG and behavioural continuum of the crocodilian *Caimon sclerops*. *Electroenceph. Clin. Neurophysiol.*, **34**, 521–538.
GOULD, S. J. (1977). *Ontogeny and Phylogeny*. Cambridge, Mass: Harvard University Press.
GROSSER, G. S. and SIEGEL, A. W. (1971). Emergence of a tonic-phasic model for sleep and dreaming. *Psychol. Bull.*, **75**, 60–72.
GUILFORD, J. P. (1965). *Fundamental statistics in psychology and education*, New York: McGraw Hill.
HARTMANN, E. (1968). The 90-minute sleep-dream cycle. *Archs. Gen. Psychiat.*, **18**, 280–286.
HARTMANN, E., BERNSTEIN, J. and WILSON, D. (1967). Sleep and dreaming in the elephant. Paper presented at the 7th annual meeting of the Association for the Psychophysiological Study of Sleep, Santa Monica.
HARTSE, K. M. (1980). The limbic spike: an electrophysiological correlate of sleep in mammals and reptiles. *Sleep Research*, **9**, 30.
HELLER, H. C., WALKER, J. N., FLORANT, G. L., GLOTZBACH, S. F. and BERGER, R. J. (1978). Sleep and hibernation: electrophysiological and thermoregulatory homologies. In: L. WANG and J. W. HUDSON, (Eds.), *Strategies in cold: Natural thermogenesis and torpidity*, New York: Academic Press.
HORNE, J. A. (1977). Factors relating to energy conservation during sleep in mammals. *Physiol. Psychol.*, **5**, 403–408.
JOUVET, M. (1961). Telencephalic and rhombencephalic sleep in the cat, pp. 188–208. In: G. E. W. WOLSTENHOLME and M. O'CONNOR, (Eds.), *The Nature of Sleep*. Boston, Mass: Little, Brown.
JOUVET, M. (1967). Neurophysiology of the states of sleep. *Physiol. Rev.*, **47**, 117–177.
JOUVET, M. (1969). Biogenic amines and the states of sleep. *Science*, **163**, 32–41.
LORANT, J. (1976). *Etude phylogenetique des états de sommeil*. Thèse Docteur-Vétérinaire. L'Université Paul Sabatier, Toulouse, France.
MEDDIS, R. (1975). On the function of sleep. *Animal Behaviour*, **23**, 676–691.
MEDDIS, R. (1977). *The Sleep Instinct*, London: Routledge & Kegan Paul.
MEDDIS, R. (1979). The evolution and function of sleep. In: D. A. OAKLEY, and H. C. PLOTKIN, (Eds.), *Brain, Behaviour and Evolution*, London: Methuen.
MEGLASSON, M. D. and HUGGINS, S. E. (1979). Sleep in a crocodilian *Caimon sclerops*. *Comp. Biochem. Physiol.*, **63A**, 561–567.
OSWALD, I. (1974). *Sleep*, Harmondsworth: Penguin.
PARMEGGIANI, P. L. (1977). Interaction between sleep and thermoregulation. *Waking and Sleeping*, **1**, 123–132.
RECHTSCHAFFEN, A. (1979). The function of sleep: methodological issues. In: R. DRUCKER-COLIN, M. SHKUROVICH and M. B. STERMAN, (Eds.), *The functions of sleep*, London: Academic Press.
ROFFWARG, H., MUZIO, J. and DEMENT, W. (1966). Ontogenetic development of human sleep-dream cycle. *Science*, **152**, 604–618.
RUCKEBUSCH, Y. (1972). The relevance of drowsiness in the circadian cycle of farm animals. *Animal Behaviour*, **20**, 637–643.
RUSSELL, I. S. (1979). Brain size and intelligence: a comparative review. In: D. A. OAKLEY and H. C. PLOTKIN, (Eds.), *Brain, Behaviour and Evolution*, London: Methuen.

SACHER, G. A. and STAFFELDT, E. F. (1974). Relation of gestational time to brain weight for placental mammals. *American Naturalist*, **108**, 593–615.
TOUTAIN, P. and RUCKEBUSCH, Y. (1972). Secretions nasolabiales au cours du sommeil paradoxal chez les bovins. *C. R. Acad. Sc.* (Paris), **274**, 2519–2522.
SUGIHARA, K. and GOTOH, J. (1973). Depth electroencephalograms of chickens in wakefulness and sleep. *Jap. J. Physiol.*, **23**, 371–379.
VANDERWOLF, C. H. (1975). Neocortical and hippocampal activation in relation to behaviour. *J. Comp. and Physiol. Psychol.*, **88**, 300–323.
VAN TWYVER, H. and ALLISON, T. (1973). Polygraphic studies of the American Alligator. *Sleep Research*, **2**, 87.
WALKER, J. M. and BERGER, R. J. (1980). Sleep as an adaptation for energy conservation functionally and physiologically related to hibernation and shallow torpor. *Prog. Brain Res.*, **53**, 255–278.
WALKER, J. M., GLOTZBACH, S. F., BERGER, R. J. and HELLER, H. C. (1977). Sleep and hibernation in ground squirrels (Citellus spp.): electrophysiological observations. *Am. J. Physiol.*, **233**, R213–R221.
WARNER, B. F. and HUGGINS, S. E. (1978). An EEG study of sleep in young caimans in a colony. *Comp. Biochem. Physiol.*, **59A**, 139–144.
ZEPELIN, H. and RECHTSCHAFFEN, A. (1974). Mammalian sleep, longevity and energy metabolism. *Brain, Behav. and Evol.*, **10**, 425–470.
ZEPELIN, H. and RECHTSCHAFFEN, A. (1970). Mammalian sleep and longevity. *Psychophysiology*, **7**, 306.
ZEPELIN, H., (1980). REM sleep and the altricial-precocial dimension. *Sleep Research*, **9**, 114.

Bibliography of Animal Sleep Studies

Primates

ADAMS, P. M. and BARRATT, E. S. (1974). Nocturnal sleep in squirrel monkeys. *Electroenceph. Clin. Neurophysiol.*, **36**, 201–204.
ADEY, W. R., KADO, R. T. and RHODES, J. M. (1963). Sleep, cortical and subcortical recordings in the chimpanzee. *Electroenceph. Clin. Neurophysiol.*, **28**, 368–373.
BALZAMO, E., BRADLEY, R. J. and RHODES, J. M. (1972). Sleep ontongeny in the chimpanzee: from two months to forty-one months. *Electroenceph. Clin. Neurophysiol.*, **33**, 47–60.
BALZAMO, E. (1972). Organisation du sommeil nocturne au cours de l'ontogenese chez le chimpanze age de 42 mois. *Rev. E.E.G. Neurophysiol.*, **2**, 379–394.
BALZAMO, E., BRADLEY, R. J., BRADLEY, D. M., PEGRAM, G. V. and RHODES, J. M. (1972). Sleep ontogeny in the chimpanzee: from birth to two months. *Electroenceph. Clin. Neurophysiol.*, **33**, 41–46.
BALZAMO, E., BRADLEY, R. J., PEGRAM, G. V. and BERT, J. (1973). Etude des états de vigilance du Babouin. *Papio papio* adulte realizee par telemetric en milieu africain. *C. r. Soc. Biol.* (Paris), **167**, 70.
BERGER, R. J. and WALKER, J. M. (1972a). A polygraphic study of sleep in the tree shrew (*Tupaia glis*). *Brain, Beh. and Evol.*, **5**, 54–69.
BERT, J. (1971). Adaptation du sommeil aux conditions experimentales d'enregistrement chez deux Cercopithecinae (*Papio papio et Macaca radiata*). *Medical Primatology*, (Proc. 3rd Conf. exp. Med. Surg. Primates), pp. 49–53. Basel: Karger.
BERT, J. (1970). Sleep in primates: a review of various results. *Medical Primatology (Proc. 2nd Conf. exp. Med. Surg. Primates*, New York: 1969), pp. 308–315. Basel: Karger, 1971.
BERT, J. and COLLOMB, H. (1966). L'electroencephalogramme du sommeil nocturne chez le babouin; etude par telemetrie. *J. Physiol.* (Paris), **52**, 258–301.

BERT, J., COLLOMB, H. and MARTINO, A. (1967). L'electroencephalogamme de sommeil d'un pro-simien; sa place dans l'organisation du sommeil chez les primates. *Electroenceph. Clin. Neurophysiol.*, **23**, 342–350.

BERT, J., KRIPKE, D. F. and RHODES, J. (1970). Electroencephalogram of the mature chimpanzee - 24 hr. recordings. *Electroenceph. Clin. Neurophysiol.*, **28**, 368–373.

BERT, J., PEGRAM, V., RHODES, J. M., BALZAMO, E. and NAQUET, R. (1970). A comparative sleep study of two Cercopithecinae. *Electroenceph. Clin. Neurophysiol.*, 28, 32–40.

BERT, J., PEGRAM, V. and BALZAMO, E. (1972). Comparison du sommeil de deux macaques (*Macaca radiata* et *Macaca mulatta*). *Folia. Primatol. (Basel)*, **17**, 202–208.

BERT, J. (1973). Similitudes et differences du sommeil chez deux babouins, *Papio hamadryas* et *Papio papio*. *Electroenceph. Clin. Neurophysiol.*, **35**, 209–212.

FREEMON, F. R., MCNEW, J. J. and ADEY, W. R. (1971). Chimpanzee sleep stages. *Electroenceph. Clin. Neurophysiol.*, **31**, 485–489.

FREEMON, F. R. and MCNEW, J. J. (1973). Comparison of chimpanzee and human sleep. *Sleep Res.*, **2**, 85.

KRIPKE, D. F., REITE, M. L., PEGRAM, G. V., STEPHENS, L. M. and LEWIS, O. F. (1968). Nocturnal sleep in rhesus monkeys. *Electroenceph. Clin. Neurophysiol.*, **24**, 582–586.

MCNEW, J. J., HOWE, R. C. and ADEY, W. R. (1971). The sleep cycle and subcortical-cortical EEG relations in the unrestrained chimpanzee. *Electroenceph. Clin. Neurophysiol.*, **30**, 489–503.

MEIER, A. and BERGER, R. (1965). Development of sleep and wakefulness in the infant rhesus monkey. *Expl. Neurol.*, **12**, 257–277.

PEGRAM, V. (1972). Comparison of field versus laboratory sleep in the baboon (*Papio papio*), developmental sleep patterns in the young (Ed.), baboon, and comparison of sleep for old world primates. In: M. H. CHASE (Eds.), *The Sleeping Brain*, pp. 33–36 (Brain Information Service — Brain Research Institute, Los Angeles).

PERACHIO, A. A. (1969). Sleep in New World Monkeys. *Psychophysiol.*, **6**, 227.

PERACHIO, A. A. (1970). Sleep in the nocturnal primate (*Aotus trivirgatus*) *Proc. 3rd Int. Congr. Primatol.*, **2**, 54–60.

REITE, M. L., RHODES, J. M., KAVAN, E. and ADEY, W. R. (1965). Normal sleep patterns in macaque monkeys. *Arch. Neurol.*, (Chicago), **12**, 133–144.

RISS, D. and GOODALL, J. (1976). Sleeping behaviour and associations in a group of captive chimpanzees. *Folia Primatol.*, **25**, 1–11.

SCHALLER, G. B. (1963). *The Year of the Gorilla*, pp. 140–149. Chicago: University of Chicago Press.

TENAZA, R., ROSS, B. A., TANTICHAROENYUOS, P. and BERKSON, G. (1969). Individual behaviour and activity rhythms of captive slow lorises (*Nycticebus coucang*). *Anim. Behav.*, **17**, 664–669.

VUILLON-CACCUITTOLO, G., BALZAMO, E., PETTER, J. J. and BERT, J. (1976). Sleep-wakefulness cycle studied by telemetry in a lemur, *Lemur macaca fulvus*. *Rev. EEG. Neurophysiol. Clin.*, **6**, 34–36.

WEITZMAN, E. D., KRIPKE, D. F., POLLACK, C. and DOMINGUEZ, J. (1965). Cyclic activity in sleep of *Macaca mulatta*. *Arch. Neurol.* (Chicago), **12**, 463–467.

Farm Mammals and Artiodactyls

BALCH, C. C. (1955). Sleep in ruminants. *Nature* (London), **175**, 940–941.

BELL, F. R. (1960). The electroencephalogram of goats during somnolence and rumination. *Anim. Behav.*, **8**, 39–42.

DALLAIRE, A. and RUCKEBUSCH, Y. (1974). Sleep patterns in the pony with observations on partial perceptual deprivation. *Physiol. Behav.*, **12**, 189–196.

DALLAIRE, A. and RUCKEBUSCH, Y. (1974). Sleep and wakefulness in the housed pony under different dietary conditions. *Can. J. Comp. Med.*, **38**, 65–71.

DALLAIRE, A. and RUCKEBUSCH, Y. (1974). Rest-activity cycle and sleep patterns in captive foxes (*Vulpes vulpes*). *Experientia*, **39**, 59–60.

DALLAIRE, A., TOUTAIN, P. L. and RUCKEBUSCH, Y. (1974). Sur la periodicite du sommeil paradoxal: faits et hypotheses. *Physiol. Behav.*, **13**, 395–400.

HAFEZ, E. S. E. (1969). *The Behaviour of Domestic Animals*, London: Bailliere, Tindall and Cassell.

IMMELMAN, K. and GEBBING, H. (1962). Schlaf bei Giraffiden. *Z. Tierpsychol.*, **19**, 84–92.

JOUVET, M. and VALATX, J. L. (1962). Etude polygraphique du sommeil chez l'agneau. *C. r. Soc. Biol.* (Paris), **156**, 1411–1414.

KLEMM, W. R. (1966). Sleep and paradoxical sleep in ruminants. *Proc. Soc. Exp. Biol. Med.* USA, **121**, 635–638.

KRISTAL, M. B. and NOONAN, M. (1979). Note on sleep in captive giraffes (*Giraffa camelapardis reticulata*). *S. Afr. J. Zool.*, **14**, 108.

MERRICK, A. W. and SHARP, D. W. (1971). Electroencephalography of resting behaviour in cattle with observations on the question of sleep. *Am. J. Vet. Res.*, **32**, 1893–1897.

MUNRO, J. (1957). Sleep in sheep. *Proc. Br. Soc. Anim. Prod.*, **71**, 75.

RUCKEBUSCH, Y. (1962). Activite corticale au course du sommeil chez le chevre. *C. r. Soc. Biol.,* **156**, 867–871.

RUCKEBUSCH, Y. (1962). Evolution post-natale du sommeil chez les Ruminants. *C. r. Soc. Biol.* (Paris), **156**, 1869–1873.

RUCKEBUSCH, Y. (1963). Etude polygraphique et comportementale et l'evolution post-natale du sommeil physiolgique chez l'agneau. *Arch. Ital. Biol.*, **101**, 111–132.

RUCKEBUSCH, Y. (1963). Etude EEG et comportementale des alternances veille-sommeil Chez l'ane. *C. r. Soc. Biol.*, **157**, 840–844.

RUCKEBUSCH, Y. (1970). Les animaux revent-ils? *Revue med. vet.*, **121**, 713–718.

RUCKEBUSCH, Y. (1972). The relevance of drowsiness in the circadian cycle of farm animals. *Anim. Behav.*, **20**, 637–643.

RUCKEBUSCH, Y. (1972). Comparative aspects of sleep and wakefulness in farm animals. In: M. H. CHASE (Ed.) *The Sleeping Brain*, pp. 23–28 (Brain Information Service — Brain Research Institute, Los Angeles).

RUCKEBUSCH, Y. and MARQUET, (1964). Etat physique des aliments et niveau de vigilance chez les Ruminants. *J. Physiol.* (Paris), **56**, 438–439.

RUCKEBUSCH, Y. and MOREL, M. T. (1968). Etude polygraphique du sommeil chez le porc. *C. r. Soc. Biol.* (Paris), **162**, 1346–1354.

RUCKEBUSCH, Y., BARBEY, P. and GUILLEMOT, P. (1970). Les etats de sommeil chez le cheval (*Equus caballus*). *C. r. Soc. Biol.* (Paris), **164**, 658–665.

RUCKEBUSCH, Y. and BELL, F. R. (1970). Etude polygraphique et comportementale des etats de vieille et de sommeille chez la vache (*Bos taurus*). *Ann. Rech. veter.*, **1**, 41–62.

RUCKEBUSCH, Y. (1971). Activite electro-corticale chez le foetus de la brebis (*Ovis aries*) et de la vache (*Bos taurus*). *Rev. Med. Vet.*, **34**, 483–510.

RUCKEBUSCH, Y. and BARBEY, P. (1971). Les etats de sommeil chez le foetus et le nouveau-ne de la vache (*Bos taurus*). *C. r. Soc. Biol.* (Paris), **165**, 1176–1184.

RUCKEBUSCH, Y. (1972). Development of sleep and wakefulness in the foetal lamb. *Electroenceph. Clin. Neurophysiol.*, **32**, 119–128.

RUCKEBUSCH, Y., DALLAIRE, A. and TOUTAIN, P. L. (1974). Sleep patterns and environmental stimuli (cattle). In: P. LEVIN and W. P. KOELLA, (Eds.) *2nd Europ. Congr. Sleep. Res.*, Rome, pp. 273–276. Basel: Karger.

STEINHART, P. (1937). Der Schlaf des Pferdes. *Z. Veterinark*, **49**, 145–157, 193–232.

STROMBERG, M. W. and USENIK, E. A. (1962). Electrocorticographic patterns in normal pigs and burros. *Amer. J. Vet. Res.*, **23**, 734–743.

TRIBE, D. E. (1970). The behaviour of the grazing animal, a critical review of present knowledge. *J. Brit. Grassland Soc.*, **5**, 209–224.

Rabbits

FAURE, J., VINCENT, D., LENOVENNE, J. and GEISSMANN, P. (1963). Sommeil lent et stade paradoxal chex le Lapin des deux sexes: role du milieu. *C. r. hebd. Seanc. Soc. Biol.*, **157**, 799–804.

NAREBSKI, J., TYMICZ, J. and LEWOSZ, W. (1969). The circadian sleep of rabbits. *Acta Biol. exp.*, **29**, 185–200.

SPIES, H. G., WHITMOYER, D. I. and SAWYER, C. H. (1970). Patterns of spontaneous and induced paradoxical sleep in intact and hypophysectomized rabbits. *Brain Res.*, **18**, 155–164.

Elephants

HARTMANN, E., BERNSTEIN, J. and WILSON, C. (1967). Sleep and dreaming in the elephant. *Psychophysiol.*, **4**, 389.

KURT, F. (1960). Le sommeil des elephants. *Mammalia*, **0**, 259–272.

Carnivores

COPLEY, M. P., JENNINGS, D. P. and MITTLER, M. M. (1976). A study of continous forty-eight hour sleep-waking recording in five dogs. *Sleep Research*, **5**, 94.

DELORME, F., VINCENT, P. and JOUVET, D. (1964). Etude statistique du cycle Vieille-sommeil chez le chat. *C. r. Soc. Biol.* (Paris), **158**, 2128–2130.

FOLK, G. E., jun. (1960). Day-night rhythms and hibernation. *Bull. Mus. Comp. Zool.*, **124**, 209–232.

HARRISON, R. and RIDGEWAY, S. (1972). Seals, dolphins and diving. *New Scientist*, **55**, 283–285.

LATASH, L. P. and GALINA, G. S. (1975). Polygraphic characteristics of the dog's sleep. *Sleep Research*, **4**, 145.

LUCAS, E. A., POWELL, E. W. and MURPHEE, O. D. (1976). A comparison of dog and cat baseline sleep-wake patterns. *Sleep Research*, **5**, 98.

LUCAS, E. A. (1978). A study of the sleep and waking patterns of the laboratory cat. *Sleep Research*, **7**, 142.

NELSON, R. A. (1973). Winter sleep in the black bear. *Mayo. Clin. Proc.*, **48**, 733–737.

NELSON, R. A., WAHNER, H. W., JONES, J. D., ELLOFSON, R. D. and ZOLLMAN, P. E. (1973). Metabolism of bears before, during and after winter sleep. *Am. J. Physiol.*, **224**, 491–496.

RUCKEBUSCH, Y. and GANJOUX, M (1976). Sleep patterns of the laboratory cat. *Electroenceph. Clin. Neurophysiol.*, **41**, 483–490.

STERMAN, M. B., KNAUSS, T., LEHMANN, M. D. and CLEMENTE, C. D. (1965). Circadian sleep and waking patterns in the laboratory cat. *Electorenceph. Clin. Neurophysiol.*, **19**, 509–517.

URSIN, R. (1968). The two stages of slow wave sleep in the cat and their relation to REM sleep. *Brain Res.*, **11**, 347–356.

URSIN, R. (1970). Sleep stage relations within the sleep cycles of the cat. *Brain Res.*, **20**, 91–97.

ZEPELIN, H. (1970). Sleep of the jaguar and the tapir: a prey-predator contrast. *Psychophysiology*, **7**, 305–306.

Cetaceans

FLANIGAN, W. F. (1975). More nocturnal observations of captive, small cetaceans: 1. The killer whale, *Orcinus orca*. *Sleep Research*, **4**, 139.

FLANIGAN, W. F. (1975). More nocturnal observations of captive, small cetaceans: 2. The pacific white-sided dolphin, *Lagenorhynchus obliquidens*. *Sleep Research*, **4**, 140.

FLANIGAN, W. F. (1975). More nocturnal observations of captive small cetaceans: 3. Further study of the beluga whale, *Delphinapterns leucas*. *Sleep Research*, **4**, 141.

McBRIDE, A. F. and HEBB, D. O. (1948). Behaviour of the captive bottle nose dolphin, *Tursiops truncatus*. *J. Comp. Physiol. Psychol.*, **41**, 111–123.
McCORMICK, J. G. (1969). Relationship of sleep, respiration and anaesthesia in the porpoise — a preliminary report. *Proc. nat. Acad. Sci.* USA, **62**, 697–703.
PILERRI, G. (1979). The blind Indus dolphin, *Palanista Indi*. *Endeavour*, **3**, 48–56.
SERAFETINIDES, E. A., SHURLEY, J. T. and BROOKS, R. E. (1972). Electroencephalogram of the pilot whale in wakefulness and sleep: lateralisation aspects. *Int. J. Psychobiol.*, **2**, 129–135.
SHURLEY, J. T., SERAFETINIDES, E. A., BROOKS, S. E., ELSNER, R. and KENNEY, D. W. (1969). Sleep in cetaceans: 1. The pilot whale, *Globicephala scammoni*. *Psychophysiol.*, **6**, 230.

Bats

BREBBIA, D. R. and PAUL, R. C. (1969). Sleep pattern in two species of bat, *Myotis lucifugus* (little brown) and *Eptesicus fuscus* (big brown). *Psychophysiol.*, **6**, 229.
BREBBIA, D. R. and PYNE, E. T. (1972). Environmental hypothermia and cerebral electrical activity of the little brown bat, *Myotis lucifugus*. *Psychophysiol.*, **9**, 122.

Rodents

ADOLPH, E. F. and LAWROW, J. W. (1951). Acclimatization to cold air; hypothermia and heat production in the golden hamster. *Am. J. Physiol.*, **166**, 62–74.
ALLISON, T., GERBER, S. D., BREEDLOVE, S. M. and DRYDEN, G. L. (1977). A behavioural and polygraphic study of sleep in the shrews *Suncus murinus*, *Blarina brevicauda* and *Cryptatis parva*. *Behav. Biol.*, **20**, 354–366.
BARTHOLOMEW, G. A. and CADE, T. J. (1957). Temperature regulation, hibernation, and aestivation in the little pocket mouse, *Perognathus longimembris*. *J. Mammal.*, **38**, 60–72.
COHEN, H., GUILLENMINAULT, C. and DEMENT, W. (1972). Sleep and REM deprivation in the hamster. *Psychophysiology*, **9**, 121.
CROWCROFT, P. (1953). The daily cycle of activity in British shrews. *Proc. zool. Soc.*, London, **123**, 715–729.
ESTEP, D. Q., FISCHER, R. B. and GORE, W. T. (1978). Effects of enclosure size and complexity on the activity and sleep of the eastern chipmunk, *Tamias striatus*. *Behav. Biol.*, **23**, 249–253.
ESTEP, D. Q., CANNEY, E. L., COCHRAN, C. G. and HUNTER, J. L. (1978). Components of activity and sleep in two species of chipmunks, *Tamias striatus* and *Eutamias dorsalias*. *Bull. Psychonomic. Soc.*, **12**, 341–343.
FLORANT, G. L., TURNER, B. M. and HELLER, H. C. (1978). Temperature regulation during wakefulness, sleep, and hibernation in marmots. *Am. J. Physiol.*, **235**, R82–R88.
FOLK, M. A. (1963). The daily distribution of sleep and wakefulness in the arctic ground squirrel. *J. Mammal.*, **44**, 575–577.
FRIEDMANN, J., ESTEP, D., HUNTLEY, A., DEWSBURY, D. and WEBB, W. (1975). On the validity of using laboratory mice versus wild mice for sleep research. *Sleep Research*, **4**, 142.
HARRIS, D. V., WALKER, J. M. and BERGER, R. J. (1979). Torpor in the pocket mouse (Perognathus longimembris): a continuation of the sleep process. *Sleep Research*, **8**, 133.
HASKELL, E. H., WALKER, J. M., BERGER, R. J. and HELLER, H. C. (1977). Effects of acute cold stress on sleep patterns of a hibernator (*Citellus lateralis*). *Sleep Research*, **6**, 103.
JOUVET-MOUNIER, D. and ASTIC, L. (1966). Etude du sommeil chez le Cobaye adulte et nouveau-ne. *C. r. Soc. Biol.* (Paris), **160**, 1453–1457.

KASTANIOTIS, C. and KAPLAN, P. F. (1976). Sleep and wakefulness in the mongolian gerbil, *meriones unguiculatus. Sleep Research*, **5**, 96.

KILDUFF, T. S. and DUBE, M. G. (1976). Sleep characteristics of the cotton rat (*sigmodon Hispidus*). *Sleep Research*, **5**, 97.

NICHOLLS, E. E. (1922). A study of spontaneous activity in the guinea pig. *J. Comp. Psychol.*, **2**, 303–330.

PELLET, J., BERAUD, G. and PAILLARD, J. (1966). Un probleme controverse: l'insomnie du Cobaye. *Rev. Neurol.* (Paris), **115**, 535–537.

PELLET, J. and BERAUD, G. (1967). Organisation nycthemerale de la veille et du sommeil chez le cobaye (*Cavia porcellus*). *Physiol. Behav.*, **2**, 131–137.

PELLET, J. and BERAUD, G. (1970). Organisation nycthemerale de la vieille et du sommeille chez le Corbaye (*Cavia porcellus*). Comparaisons interspecifiques avec le Rat et le Chat. *Physiol. Behav.*, **2**, 131–137.

ROLDAN, E., WEISS, T. and FIFKOVA, E. (1963). Excitability changes during the sleep cycle of the rat. *Electroenceph. Clin. Neurophysiol.*, **15**, 775–785.

SOUTH, F. E., BREAZILE, J. E., DELLMAN, H. D. and EPPERLY, A. D. (1969). Sleep, hibernation and hypotheria in the yellow-bellied marmot (*M. flaviventris*). In: MUSACCHIA and J. F. SAUNDERS (Eds.), *Depressed Metabolism*. Proc. 1st Int. Congr. on depressed metabolism, pp. 277–312, New York: Elsevier.

TIMO-IARA, C., NEGRAO, N., SCHMIDEK, W. R., HASHINO, MENZES, C. and ROCHA, T. L. (1970). Phases and states of sleep in the rat. *Physiol. Behav.*, **5**, 1057–1062.

VAN TWYVER, H. (1969). Sleep patterns of five rodent species. *Physiol. Behav.*, **4**, 901–905.

VAN TWYVER, H. and ALLISON, T. (1969). EEG study of the shrew (*Blarina brevicauda*): a preliminary report. *Psychophysiology*, **6**, 231.

WALKER, J. M., GLOTZBACH, S. F. BERGER, R. J. and HELLER, H. C. (1977). Sleep and hibernation in ground squirrels (*Citellus* spp.): Electrophysiological observations. *Am. J. Physiol.*, **233**, R213–R221.

WALKER, L. E., HARRIS, D. V., WALKER, J. M. and BERGER, R. J. (1980). Sleep patterns and respiration rate in the pocket mouse (Perognathus longimembris) at different temperatures. *Sleep Research*, **9**, 113.

WEISS, T. and ROLDAN, E. (1964). Comparing study of sleep cycle in rodents. *Experientia*, **20**, 280–283.

Insectivores

ALLISON, T. and VAN TWYVER, H. (1969). Notes from underground: sleep in the moles, *Scalopus aquaticus* and *Condylura cristata. Psychophysiol.*, **6**, 229.

ALLISON, T. and VAN TWYVER, H. (1970). Sleep in the moles, *Scalopus aquaticus* and *Condylura cristata. Exp. Neurol.*, **27**, 564–579.

BERGER, R. J. and WALKER, J. M. (1972). A polygraphic study of sleep in the tree shrew (*Tupaia glis*). *Brain. Behav. Evol.*, **5**, 54–69.

FOURRE, A. M., RODRIGUEZ, F. L. and VINCENT, J. D. (1974). Etude polygaphique de la vieille et du sommeil chez le Herisson (*Erinaceus europeanus*). *Soc. de Biol. de Bordeaux*, **168**, 959–964.

KARADZIC, W. (1967). Polygraphisches Studium des Tatigkeitsrhythmus der Westblindmaus *Spalax leucodon* Nordman, 1840. *Saugetierkundliche Mitteilungen*, **2**, 167–170.

SAVIC, J. and MIKES, K. (1967). Zur Kenntnis des 24 Stunden Rhytmus' von *Spalax leucodon. Z. Saugetierk.* (Hamburg–Berlin), **32**, 232–238.

TAUBER, E. S., MICHEL, F. and ROFFWARG, H. P. (1968). Preliminary note on the sleep and waking cycle in the desert hedgehog (*Paraechinus hypomelas*). *Psychophysiol.*, **5**, 201.

TOUTAIN, P. L. and RUCKEBUSCH, Y. (1975). Arousal as a cyclic phenomenon during sleep and hibernation in the hedgehog (*Erinaceus europeanus*). *Experientia*, **31**, 312–314.

VAN TWYVER, H. and ALLISON, T. (1969). EEG study of the shrew (*Blarina brevicauda*): preliminary report: *Psychophysiol.*, **6**, 231.

Edentates

AFFANNI, J. M., LISOGORSKY, E. and SCARVALLI, A. M. (1972). Sleep in the giant South American Armadillo *Priodontes giganteus* (*Edentata mammalia*). *Experientia.*, **28**, 1046–1047.

ALLISON, T. and VAN TWYVER, H. V. (1972). Sleep in the armadillo, *Dasypus novemcinctus*. *Psychophysiol.*, **9**, 123.

BEEBE, W. (1926). The three-toed sloth (*Bradypus cuculliger cuculliger Wagler*). *Zoologica*, (New York), **7**, 1–67.

HOWARTH, S. T. and TOOLE, J. F. (1973). Some observations on the circadian rhythm of *Choloepus hoffmanni*, the two-toed sloth. *Laboratory Animal Science*, **23**, 377–379.

PRUDOM, A. E. and KLEMM, W. R. (1973). Electrographic correlates of sleep behaviour in a primitive mammal, the armadillo, *Dasypus novemcinctus*. Physiol. Behav., **10**, 275–282.

SUNQUIST, M. E. and MONTGOMERY, G. G. (1973). Activity patterns and rates of movement of two-toed and three-toed sloths (*Cholopus hoffmanni* and *Bradypus infuscatus*). *J. Mammal.*, **54**, 946–954.

Marsupials

AFFANI, J. (1972). Observations on the sleep of some South American marsupials and edentates. In: M. H. CHASE (Ed.) *The Sleeping Brain*, pp. 21–23 (Brain Information Service — Brain Research Institute, Los Angeles).

AFFANI, J. M. and VACCAREZZA, O. L. (1964). Observaciones sobre el sueno del marsupial *Didelphis azarae*. Rev. Soc. argent. Biol., **40**, 2–8.

CICALA, G. A., ALBERT, I. B. and ULMER, F. A. (1970). Sleep and other behaviours of the red kangaroo (*Megaleia rufa*). *Anim. Behav.*, **18**, 786–790.

LOPRESTI, R. W. and MCGINTY, D. J. (1970). Sleep in the Phalanger (*Trichosurus vulpecula*): an Australian marsupial. *Psychophysiol.*, **7**, 304.

VAN TWYVER, H. and ALLISON, T. (1970). Sleep in the opossum, *Didelphis* marsupialis. *Electroenceph. Clin. Neurophysiol.*, **29**, 181–189.

WALKER, J. M. and BERGER, R. J. (1979). The ontogenesis of sleep states, thermogenesis and thermoregulation in the Virginia opossum. *Develop. Psychobiolog.*

Monotremes

ALLISON, T. and GOFF, W. R. (1968). Sleep in a primitive mammal, the spiny anteater. *Psychophysiol.*, **5**, 200.

ALLISON, T., VAN TWYVER, H. and GOFF, W. R. (1972). Electrophysiological studies of the echidna *Tachyglossus aculeatus*. I — Waking and sleep. *Arch. Ital. Biol.*, **110**, 145–184.

Hyracoidea

SNYDER, F. (1976). Sleep-waking patterns of hyracoidea. *Sleep Research*, **7**, 87.

Mixed

GRZIMEK, B. (1956). Schlaf von Giraffen and Okapi. *Naturwissenschaften*, **43**, 406.

SNYDER, R., BUGBEE, N. and DONTHITT, T. C. (1972). Telemetric studies of 24 hour sleep-waking patterns in some primitive mammals. *Psychophysiol.*, **9**, 122–123.

ZEPELIN, H. (1970). Sleep of the Jaguar and the Tapir: a prey–predator contrast. *Psychophysiol.*, **7**, 305.

Birds

BAKHUIS, W. L. and CORNER, M. A. (1973). Spontaneous motility bursts during sleep in the chick, as related to phasic 'paradoxical' cerebral bioelectric activity. *Brain Res.*, **50**, 200–204.

BERGER, R. J. and WALKER, J. M. (1972). Sleep in the burrowing owl (*Speotyto cunicularia hypugaea*). *Behav. Biol.*, **7**, 183–194.

BERGER, R. J., WALKER, J. M. and SCOTT, T. D. (1970). Characteristics of sleep in the Burrowing Owl and the Tree Shrew. *Psychophysiol.*, **7**, 303.

HISHIKAWA, Y., CRAMER, H. and KUHLO, W. (1969). Natural and melatonin-induced sleep in young chickens — a behavioural and electrographic study. *Exp. Brain. Res.*, **7**, 84–94.

KARADZIC, V. (1972). Sleep in the owl (*Strix Aluce*): a preliminary study. *Eleventh Annual Meeting of APSS*, New York.

KARADZIC, V., KORACEVIK, R., MOMIROV, D. (1973). Sleep in the owl (*Strix Aluco, strigidae*). In: W. P. KOELLA and P. LEVIN (Eds.), *Sleep*, Basel: Karger.

KARMANOVA, I. G., KHOMUTETSKAYA, D. E. and CHURNOSOV. E. V. (1970). Peculiarities of the paradoxical stage of sleep in hens. *J. evol. Biochem. Physiol.*, 252–259.

KARMANOVA, I. G. and CHURNOSOV, E. V. (1971). Electrophysiological investigations of natural sleep and wakefulness of turtles and chickens. *Zhumal Evoliutsionnoi biokhimii i fiziolog*, **8**, 47–53. Paraxoxical sleep in hens. *Neuroscience translations*, published by Federation of American Societies for Experimental Biology for the National Institute of Mental Health, **16**, 21–28.

KARMANOVA, I. G. and CHURNOSOV, E. V. (1974). Electrophysiological study of the circadian rhythm of sleep and wakefulness in owls. *ZH. Evol. Biochem. Fiziol.*, **10**, 48–57.

KEY, J. B. and MARLEY, E. (1962). The effect of the sympathetic amines on behaviour and electrical activity of the chicken. *Electroenceph. Clin. Neurophysiol.*, **14**, 90–105.

KLEIN, M., MICHEL, F. and JOUVET, M. (1964). Etude polygraphique du sommeil chez les Oiseaux. *C. r. Soc. Biol.* (Paris), **158**, 99–103.

OOKAWA, T. and GOTOH, J. (1964). Electroencephalographic study of chickens: Periodic recurrence of low voltage and fast waves during behavioural sleep. *Poultry Sci.*, **43**, 1603–1604.

OOKAWA, T. and GOTOH, J. (1965). Electroencephalogram of the chicken recorded from the skull under various conditions. *J. Comp. Neurol.*, **124**, 1–14.

OOKAWA, T. and TAKAGI, K. (1968). EEG of free behavioural chicks at various developmental levels. *Jap. J. Physiol.*, **18**, 87–99.

OOKAWA, T. (1972). Avian wakefulness and sleep on the basis of recent electrorencephalic observations. *Poultry Sci.*, **51**, 1565–1574.

PETERS, J. J., VONDERAHE, A. R. and SCHMID, D. (1965). Onset of cerebral electrical activity associated with behavioural sleep and attention in the developing chick. *J. Exp. Zool.*, **160**, 255–262.

ROFAS-RAMIREZ, J. A. and TAUBER, E. S. (1970). Paradoxical sleep in two species of avian predator (Falconiformes). *Science*, (New York), **167**, 1754–1755.

SCHADE, J. P., CORNER, M. A. and PETERS, J. J. (1965). Some aspects of the electro-ontongenesis of sleep patterns. In: K. AKERT, C. BALLY, J. P. SCHADE (Eds.), *Progress in Brain Research*, Vol. 18, Amsterdam: Elsevier.

SCHLEHUBER, C. J., FLEMING, D. G., LANGE, G. D. and SPOONER, C. E. (1974). Paradoxical sleep in chickens. *Behav. Biol.*, **11**, 537–546.

SHIBATA, M. and KADONO, H. (1970). Effects of urethane on electrocorticogram in the chicken. *Poultry Sci.*, **49**, 1484–1491.

SILVA, E. E., ESTABLE, C. and SEGUNDO, J. P. (1959). Further observations on animal hypnosis. *Arch. Ital. Biol.*, **97**, 197–177.

SUGIHARA, K. and GOTOH, J. (1973). Depth-electroencephalograms of chickens in wakefulness and sleep. *Jap. J. Physiol.*, **23**, 371–379.

SUSIC, V. T. and KOVACEVIC, R. M. (1973). Sleep patterns in the owl *Strix aluco. Physiol. Behav.*, **11**, 313–317.

TAMISIER, A. (1972). Rythmes nycthemeraux des sarcelles l'hiver pendant 1 eur hivernarge en camargue. *Alauda (Revue Internationale d'Ornithologie)*, **40**, 235–256.

TAMISIER, A. (1973). Etho-ecological studies of Teal. *Wildfowl*, **25**, 123–133.
TRADARDI, V. (1966). Sleep in the pigeon. *Arch. Ital. Biol.*, **104**, 516–521.
TYMICZ, J., NAREBSKI, J., PAZUR, W. and STRAWINSKI, S. (1974). Circadian sleep-wakefulness of the chaffinch (*Fringilla coelebs*). In: W. P. KOELLA and P. LEVIN (Eds.), *Sleep*, Basel: Karger.
TYMICZ, J., NAREBSKI, J. and JURKOWLANIEC, E. (1975). Circadian sleep-wakefulness rhythm of the starling. *Sleep Research*, **4**, 146.
VAN TWYVER, H. and ALLISON, T. (1971). Sleep in the pigeon. *First Int. Congr. APSS*, June, Bruges, Belgium.
VAN TWYVER, H. and ALLISON, (1972). A polygraphic and behavioural study of sleep in the pigeon (*Columba livia*). *Exp. Neurol.*, **35**, 138–153.
WALKER, J. M. and BERGER, R. J. (1972). Sleep in the domestic pigeon (*Columba livia*). *Behav. Biol.*, **7**, 195–203.
WALKER, J. M., WALKER, L. E., PALCA, J. W. and BERGER, R. J. (1980). Nightly torpor in the ringed neck dove: an extension of SWS. *Sleep Research*, **9**, 112.
WEITNAUER, E. (1952). Ubernachtet der Mauer segler, *Apus apus* (L.), in der Luft? *Der Ornithol. Beob.*, **49**, 37–44.

Reptiles

FLANIGAN, W. F., jan. (1972). Behavioural states and electroencephalograms of reptiles. In: M. H. CHASE (Ed.), *Persepectives in the Brain Sciences. I. The Sleeping Brain* Los Angeles: Brain Information Service.
FLANIGAN, W. F., jun. (1973). Sleep and wakefulness in iguanid lizards *Ctenosaura pectinata* and *Iguana inguana*. *Brain. Beh. Evol.*, **8**, 401–436.
FLANIGAN, W. F. jun., WILCOX, R. H. and RECHTSCHAFFEN, A. (1973). The EEG and behavioral continuum of the crocodilian, *Caiman sclerops*. *Electroenceph. Clin. Neurophysiol.*, **34**, 521–538.
FLANIGAN, W. F. jun. (1973). Sleep and wakefulness in chelonian reptiles: I. The red-footed tortoise, *Geochelone carbenaria*. *Sleep Research*, **2**, 82.
FLANIGAN, W. F. jun. (1974). Sleep and wakefulness in chelonian reptiles: II. The red-footed tortoise, *Geochelone carbonia*. *Archs. Ital. Biol.*, **112**, 253–277.
FLANIGAN, W. F. jun., KNIGHT, C. P., HARTSE, K. M. and RECHTSCHAFFEN, A. (1973). Sleep and wakefulness in chelonian reptiles: II. The eastern box turtle, *Terrapene carolina*. *Sleep Research*, **2**, 83.
FLANIGAN, W. F. jun., KNIGHT, C. P., HARTSE, K. M. and RECHTSCHAFFEN, A. (1974). Sleep and wakefulness in chelonian reptiles: I. The box turtle, *Terrapina caralina*. *Archs. Ital. Bio.*, **112**, 227–252.
HERMANN, H., JOUVET, M. and KLEIN, M. (1964). Analyse polygraphique du sommeil de la tortue. *C. r. hebd. Seanc. Acad. Sci.* (Paris), **258**, 2175–2178.
HUNTLEY, A. C., FRIEDMAN, J. K. and COHEN, H. B. (1977). Sleep in an iguanid lizard, *Dipsosaurus dorsarlis*. *Sleep Research*, **6**, 104.
HUNTLEY, A. C. and COHEN, H. B. (1980). Further comments on 'sleep' in the desert iguana, *Dipsosaurus dorsalis*. *Sleep Research*, **9**, 111.
KARMANOVA, I. G., BELEKHOVA, M. G. and TCHURNOSOV, E. V. (1971). Specifics of behavioural and electrographic patterns of natural sleep and wakefulness in reptiles. *Sechenov Physiol. J.* USSR., **57**, 504–511.
KARMANOVA, I. G. and CHURNOSOV, E. V. (1972). Electrophysiological study of natural sleep and wakefulness in turtles and hens. *ZL. Evol. Biokhim. Fiziol.*, **8**, 47–53.
MEGLASSON, M. D. and HUGGINS, S. E. (1979). Sleep in a crocodilian, *Caiman sclerops*. *Comp. Biochem. Physiol.* (A), **63**, 561–567.
PEYRETHON, J. and DUSAN-PEYRETHON, D. (1969). Etude polygraphique du cycle vieille-sommeil chez trois genres de reptiles. *C. r. Soc. Biol.* (Paris), **163**, 181–186.
RECHTSCHAFFEN, A., BASSAN, M. and LEDECKY-JANECEK, S. (1968). Activity patterns in *Caiman sclerops* (Crocodilia). *Psychophysiol.*, **5**, 201.

ROMO, R., CEPEDA, C. and VELASCO, M. (1978). Behavioural and electrophysiological patterns of wakefulness-sleep states in the lizard (*Phrinsoma regali*). *Bol. Estud. Med. Biol.*, **30**, 13–18.

STROPES, S. L. (1975). *Sleep behaviour in reptiles*. PhD thesis, University of Arizona.

SUSIC, V. (1972). Electrographic and behavioural correlations of the rest activity cycle in the sea turtle, *Caretta caretta*, L. (Chelonia). *J. exp. mar. Biol. Ecol.*, **10**, 81–87.

TAUBER, E. S., ROFFWARG, H. P. and WEITSMAN, E. D. (1966). Eye movements and electroencephalogram activity during sleep in diurnal lizards. *Nature* (London), **212**, 1612–1613.

TAUBER, E. S., ROFAS-RAMIRE, J. and HERNANDEZ-PEON, R. (1968). Electrophysiological and behavioural correlates of wakefulness and sleep in the lizard *Ctenosaura pectinata*. *Electroenceph. Clin. Neurophysiol.*, **24**, 424–433.

VAN TWYVER, H. and ALLISON, T. (1973). Polygraphic studies of the American Alligator. *Sleep Research*, **2**, 87.

VASILESCU, E. (1970). Sleep and wakefulness in the tortoise (*Emys orbicularis*). *Rev. Roum. Biol. (ser. zool).*, **15**, 177–179.

WALKER, J. M., BERGER, R. J. and SCOTT, T. D. (1973). Absence of electrophysiological signs of sleep in the tortoise (*Testudo denticulata*). *Sleep Research*, **2**, 88.

WARNER, B. F. and HUGGINS, S. E. (1978). An electroencephalographic study of sleep in young caimans in a colony. *Comp. Biochem. Physiol.*, **59A**, 139–144.

Amphibia

HOBSON, J. A. (1968). Respiration and EEG synchronisation in the frog. *Nature*, **213**, 988–989.

HOBSON, J. A. (1967). Electrographic correlates of behaviour in the frog with special reference to sleep. *Electroenceph. Clin. Neurophysiol.*, **22**, 113–121.

HOBSON, J. A., GOIN, O. B. and GOIN, C. J. (1968). Electrographic correlates of behaviour in the tree frog. *Hyla septentrionalis*. *Psychophysiol.*, **5**, 202.

HOBSON, J. A., GOIN, O. B. and GOIN, C. J. (1968). Sleep behaviour of frogs in the field. *Psychophysiol.*, **5**, 202.

HOBSON, J. A., GOIN, O. B. and GOIN, C. J. (1968). Electrographic correlates of behaviour in tree frogs. *Nature*, **220**, 386–387.

HUNTLEY, A.C., DONELLEY, M. and COHEN, H. B. (1978). Sleep in the western toad, *Bufo. boreas*. *Sleep Research*, **7**, 141.

LAZAREV, S. G. (1978). Electrophysiological analysis of wakefulness and primary sleep in the frog. *Rana temporaria*. *ZL. Evol. Biokhim. Fiziol.*, **14**, 379–384.

LUCAS, E., STERMAN, M. B. and MCGINTY, D. J. (1969). The salamander EEG: a model of primitive sleep and wakefulness. *Psychophysiol.*, **6**, 230.

SEGURA, E. T. (1966). Estudios electroencephalographicos en anfibios. *Acta Physiol. Lat. Amer.*, **16**, (suppl. 2).

Fish

HOBSON, J. A. (1965). Diurnal-nocturnal activity of some inshore fishes in the Gulf of California. *Copeia*, **3**, 291–302.

PEYRETHON, J. and DUSAN-PEYRETHON, D. (1967). Etude polygraphique du cycle veille-sommeil d'un teleosteen (*Tinca tinca*). *C. r. Soc. Biol.* (Paris), **161**, 2533–2537.

SHAPIRO, C. M. and HEPBURN, H. R. (1976). Sleep in a schooling fish, *Tilapa mossambika*. *Physiol. Behav.*, **16**, 613–615.

STARK, W. A. and DAVIS, W. P. (1966). Night habits of fishes of Alligator Reef, Florida. *Ichthyologica*, **38**, 313–356.

TAUBER, E. S. and WEITZMAN, E. D. (1969). Eye movements during behavioural inactivity in certain Bermuda reef fish. *Psychophysiol.*, **6**, 230.

TITKOR, E. S. (1976). Characteristics of the diurnal rhythm of wakefulness and rest in the catfish. *Ictalurus nebulosus*. *Zh. Evol. Biokhim. Fiziol.*, **12**, 335–340.

WEBER, E. (1961). Uber Ruhelagen von Fischen. *Zeitsch. f. Tierpsychol.* **18**, 517–533.
WINN, H. E. (1955). The formation of a mucous envelope at night by parrot fishes. *Zoologica*, **40**, 145–147.

Molluscs

STRUMWASSER, F. (1971). The cellular basis of behaviour in Aplysia. *J. Psychiat. Res.*, **8**, 237–257.

Insects

ANDERSON, F. S. (1968). Sleep in moths and its dependence on the frequency of stimulation in *Anagasta kuehniella*. *Opuscula Entom.*, **33**, 15–24.
BLEST, A. D. (1960). The evolution, ontongeny of quantitative control of some New World saturnid moths. *Behaviour*, **13**, 297–318.
EBERHARD, W. G. (1974). The natural history of *Trigonopsis cameronii*. *Trans. Roy. Entomol. Soc.*, **125**.
EVANS, H. E. and LINSLEY, E. G. (1960). Notes on a sleeping aggregation of solitary bees and wasps. *Bull. S. Calif. Acad. Sci.*, **59**, 30–37.
EVANS, H. E. and EBERHARD, M. J. W. (1970). *The Wasps*, pp. 36–37, 177–178, University of Michigan Press.
LIN, N. (1968). A note on the sleeping behaviour of *Philanthus gibbosus* (fabricus). *Proc. ent. soc. Wash.*, **70**, 10–12.
TSUTSUMI, C. (1968). Studies on the behaviour of the housefly *Musca domestica* L. *Jap. J. Med., Sci. Biol.*, **21**, 195–204.
WIGGLESWORTH, V. B. *Principles of Insect Physiology*, 7th edn., London: Chapman & Hall, pp. 313–314.

CHAPTER 4

Infant Sleep Development

Ronald M. Harper, Zehava Frostig and David Taube

4.1 Introduction

Infant sleep is of interest to both clinical and theoretical researchers. Sleep states dramatically alter physiological functions which are essential for survival, and the extent of this alteration by illness or developmental disturbance has been the object of considerable study. Specifically, the control of respiratory and cardiac activity during sleep and waking, the development of state-related EEG signals, and the establishment of motoric patterns have been of particular clinical significance. A description of the temporal course of development in each of these parameters has been of theoretical interest to investigators of the neurological organization underlying sleep development.

This chapter will outline the principal physiological changes occurring during sleep that are associated with development. A broader view of sleep development, however, must consider the temporal occurrence of various physiological signs constituting 'state', i.e. the time in development when the characteristics of particular states emerge. Rapid eye movements and twitches of peripheral musculature, for example, have historically been associated with a state of sleep called 'active', 'desynchronized', or 'REM' sleep (AS). Both rapid eye movements and peripheral twitches are present during that state in the newborn, and in fact, constitute the definition of 'REM' sleep. Other phenomena, however, such as the presence of 12–14 Hz sleep 'spindle' activity on the EEG, are not present during quiet sleep (QS) in the very young infant. Thus, the constituent physiological components that compose adult sleep require time to develop, and the appearance of these 'signs' of sleep constitute significant neurological markers.

In addition to considering the temporal appearance of sleep-related physiological signs, we must consider whether, during the course of a sleep period, these physiological signs occur together in a 'normal' coalescence, or whether they are temporally dissociated. For example, both rapid eye movements and loss of facial muscle tone are normally characteristic of REM sleep. If facial muscle tone were high during REM sleep, or decreased dramatically during other states, then a failure of those neural mechanisms regulating state integration might be suspected. We shall see that these integrative mechanisms require a period of time to develop, and that deviations from normal coalescence development may be sufficiently large to be indicative of pathology.

A final consideration in sleep state development is the knowledge that sleep states are periodic in the infant, that this periodicity requires a period of time to develop, and that disturbances in state development may be indicative of risk. This aspect of development related to assessment of periodic activity is closely related to the coalescence aspect described earlier, since activity in physiological parameters which are periodic are frequently oscillating together, or in a certain phase relationship with other physiological parameters.

It is the purpose of this chapter to illustrate these developmental considerations in the study of infant sleep, utilizing the contributions from a large number of international investigators. We will also draw upon recordings and data from our own infant sleep studies for particular examples. Our own data were gathered from a long-term study of sleep in 25 control infants and 25 infants at risk for the Sudden Infant Death Syndrome (SIDS). These studies were 12-h all night (19.00–07.00) sleep recordings from full-term infants recorded in the newborn period (1–6 days) and at 1, 2, 3, 4 and 6 months of age. The recordings included standard physiological monitoring of heart and respiratory rate and variability, body movement, eye movement, muscle activity from facial muscles, and bilateral EEG channels (sites C3–T3 and C4–T4) (Harper *et al.*, 1976; Hofmann *et al.*, 1977). All data were digitized onto computer tape for later analysis. Minute-by-minute estimates of median heart and respiratory rate and variability, integrated EMG and somatic activity, and band pass filtered EEG at 12–14 Hz, 4–7 Hz and 0–3 Hz were estimated using a PDP–12 computer. In addition, spectral estimates of all EEG bands during selected portions of QS and AS were calculated. Sleep states were encoded on a minute-by-minute basis by observers trained to an 80% reliability and values for physiological parameters by state were estimated.

4.2 Physiological Changes during Sleep Development

Obtaining developmental curves for basic physiological measures during each sleep state is a principal need for both basic researchers and clinical practitioners. A principal aim of sleep researchers should thus be establishing quantitative values for physiological measures of EEG, cardiac, respiratory and somatic activity such that deviations from control values can be readily noted. Although this seems to be a trivial need, it was not until the early 1970s that inexpensive computer technology provided access to such a capability; before that time, much of our knowledge was derived from qualitative or spotty temporal observations.

Developmental parametric assessments of physiology have recently emerged, and the powerful modulation of virtually all physiological parameters by sleep has been documented. These parametric values change dramatically, and not always in a linear fashion, with development. This can be illustrated with plots of heart-rate and variability trends in Fig. 4.1, which describes the effect of sleep–waking states on heart-rate and variability parameters, and demonstrates the absurdity of attempting to establish normative physiological values without knowledge of state influence. This figure demonstrates the reduced cardiac rates during QS and AS, the relatively large variability during AS and AW, the decline in variability in QS at 1 month, and a rise in heart-rate during the first month of life followed by a decline from the 1–6 month period during sleep states (Harper *et al.*, 1976, 1982a). Watanabe *et al.* (1973) have shown similar changes in low birth weight infants, and Katona *et al.* (1980) have demonstrated that the decline in rate continues over the first year of life. Heart rate and variability constitute a primary definition of state in the infant; values of these parameters change with age, and these changes must be considered in the quantification of state. The characteristics of both heart-rate and variability

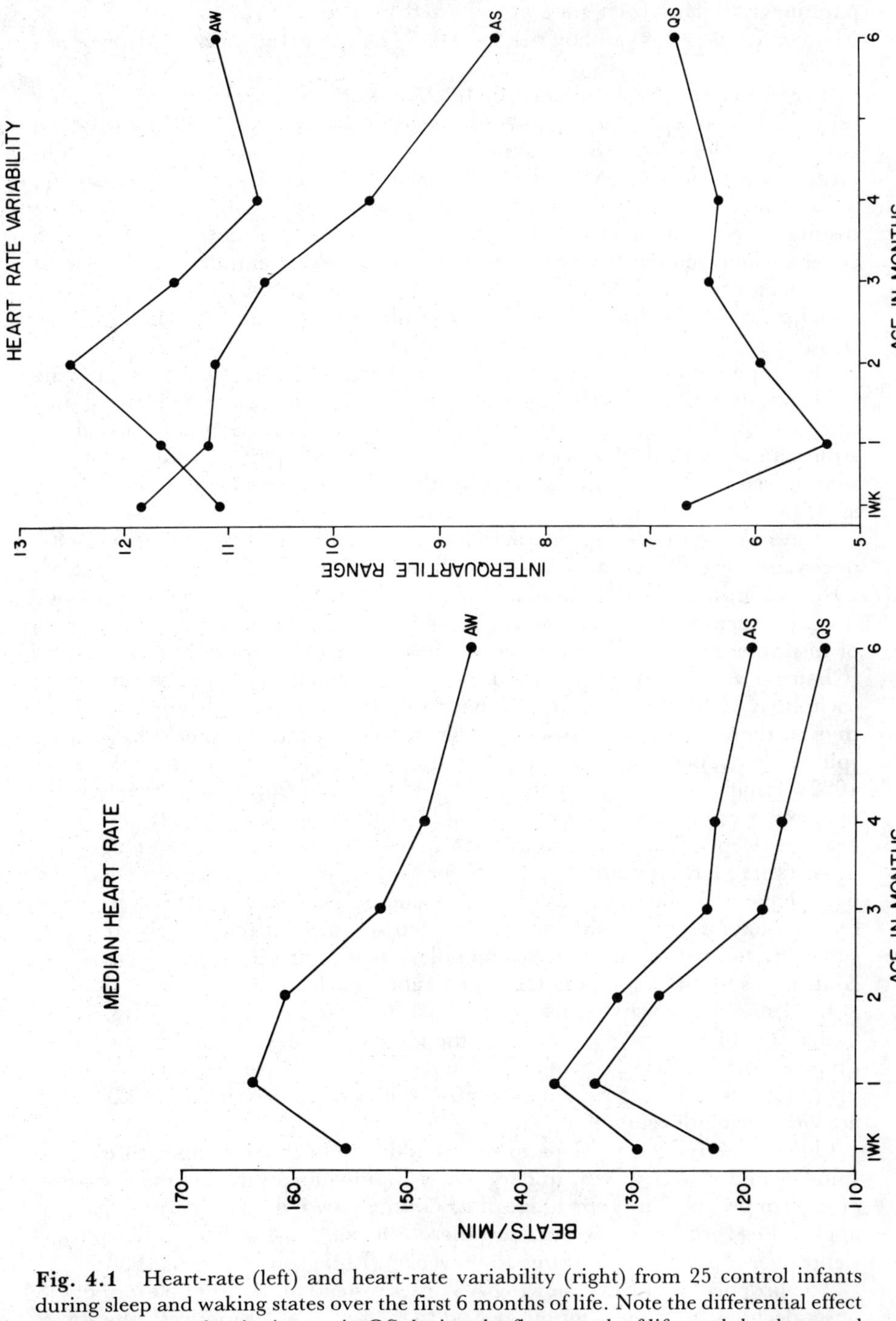

Fig. 4.1 Heart-rate (left) and heart-rate variability (right) from 25 control infants during sleep and waking states over the first 6 months of life. Note the differential effect on rate by state, the rise in rate in QS during the first month of life, and the decreased variability at 1 month in QS. This figure demonstrates the necessity for recognition of state in determining cardiac rate and variability values.

parameters during each state are affected by illness (Watanabe *et al.*, 1973; Miyazaki *et al.*, 1979) and by risk for SIDS (Leistner *et al.*, 1980; Harper *et al.*, 1982a).

The presence of sleep spindles, or 1–3 bursts of 12–14 Hz rhythmical activity on the EEG, is also a principal component of the definition of sleep states in adults and older infants. Sleep spindles require 1–2 months post-term in the full-term infant to develop (Metcalf, 1964, 1970; Lenard, 1970; Curzi-Dascalova, 1977; Ellingson & Peters, 1980). Spindles associated with sleep should be distinguished from other spindle activity observed in premature infants which cover a wider frequency range (8–24 Hz), and appear over different brain areas than sleep spindles (Ellingson, 1982). Sleep spindle activity can be quantified with time series spectral techniques by examining EEG activity in the 12–14 Hz band.

Development of EEG activity in the spindle band during QS (essentially the only condition in which this activity is prominent in the young infant) is shown in Fig. 4.2b. This figure, which is derived from spectral EEG estimates, demonstrates a rise in 12–14 Hz activity over the 1–3 month period, with a relatively sharper rise over 2–3 months, and a relative stabilization thereafter (Sterman *et al.*, 1977).

Disturbances in sleep spindle activity, such as abnormally prominent bursts, or reduced or abolished activity, are indicative of pathology in infants (Lenard, 1970; Ellingson, 1982). Spindle activity is enhanced in certain metabolic diseases, such as phenylketonuria (Gross & Schulte, 1969; Schulte *et al.*, 1973) or histidinemia (Woody *et al.*, 1965) and after certain types of brain damage (Chatrian *et al.*, 1963). Sleep spindle activity is reduced in hypothyroid infants (Schultz *et al.*, 1968), a symptom that can be at least partially corrected with thyroid therapy. Both an absence of sleep spindles and extremely large sleep spindles have been observed in mentally retarded children (Shibagaki *et al.*, 1982). Finally, spectral estimates of 12–14 Hz activity are increased at 8 weeks of age in a group of siblings of SIDS victims (Sterman *et al.*, 1982).

Since sleep spindles have so frequently been associated with pathology, it is important to have quantitative values for such activity with age. Sleep physiologists have traditionally relied on the presence of sleep spindle activity to define QS in adults and older infants. Since sleep spindles reflect, or help to define state, the temporal occurrence of spindles, as well as the amount of activity, contributes to understanding the organization of sleep.

EEG slow wave activity also increases in QS with development (Fig. 4.2a). Unlike 12–14 Hz activity, however, the increase in slow wave activity is continuous from the first week of life through 3 months of age. Activity in the 4–7 Hz (approximate theta range) during AS follows a course similar to 12–14 Hz activity during development (Fig. 4.2c).

Other state-related EEG patterns, in addition to the development of sleep spindles and slower waves, undergo very rapid changes during the 4–8 week post-term period. The percentage of EEG time showing tracé alternant pattern approaches zero by 6–7 weeks, and there is a rapid loss of frontal sharp transients over a parallel time frame (5–8 weeks) (Ellingson & Peters, 1980).

The proportion of EEG showing AS onset instead of the adult pattern of QS onset declines from the 1 month period to near zero at 2 months (Ellingson & Peters, 1980). Food intake plays a role in this sleep transition, with food intake being more frequently accompanied by onset of AS (Harper *et al.*, 1977).

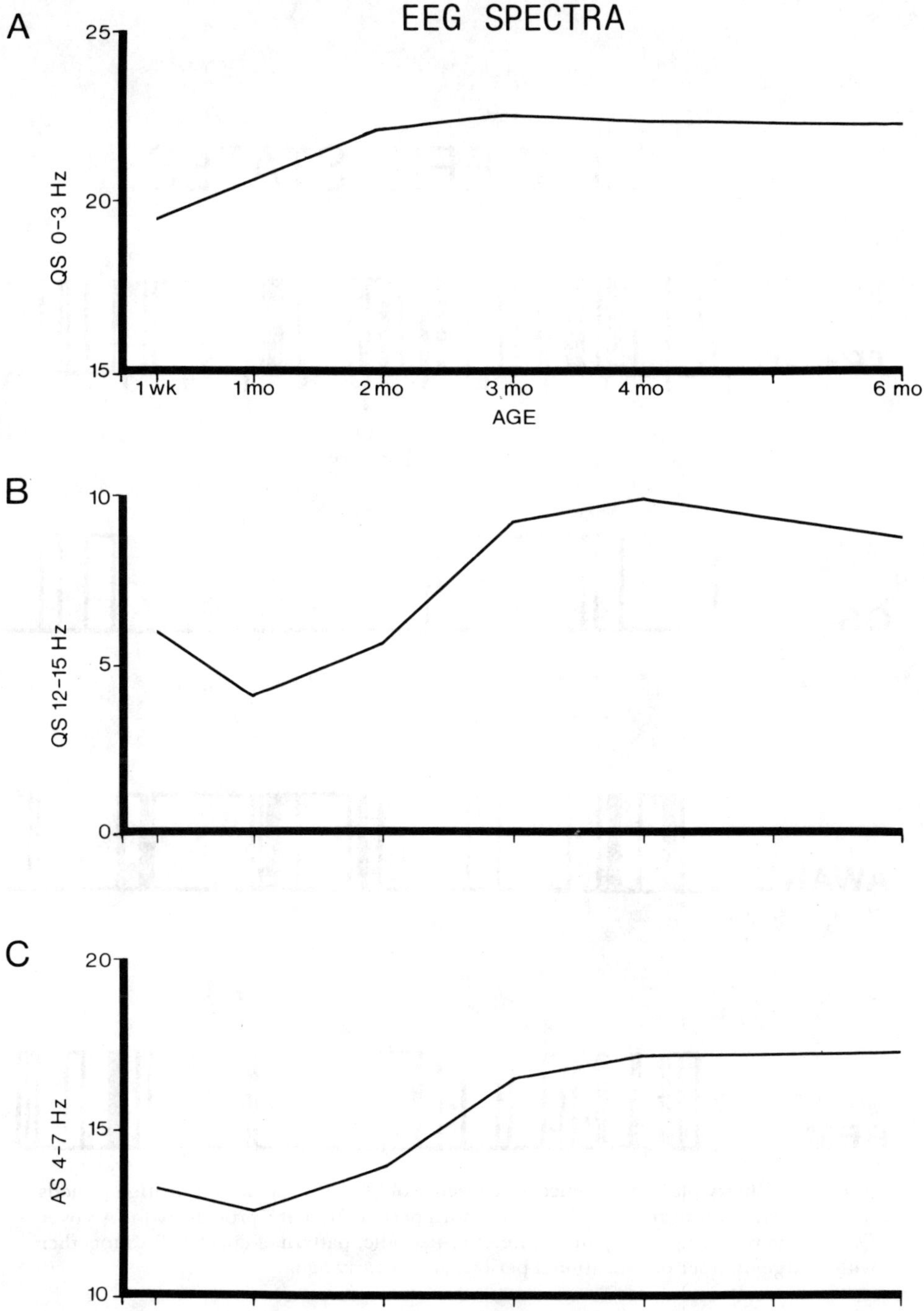

Fig. 4.2 This figure plots trends in power (assessed by spectral activity) in 0–3 Hz, 12–14 Hz and 4–7 Hz EEG with development. The 0–3 Hz and 12–14 Hz activity were obtained in QS, 4–7 Hz activity was obtained in AS. (Redrawn from M. B. Sterman *et al*. (1982) *Electroencephalography and Clinical Neurophysiology* **53**, 166–181, by permission.)

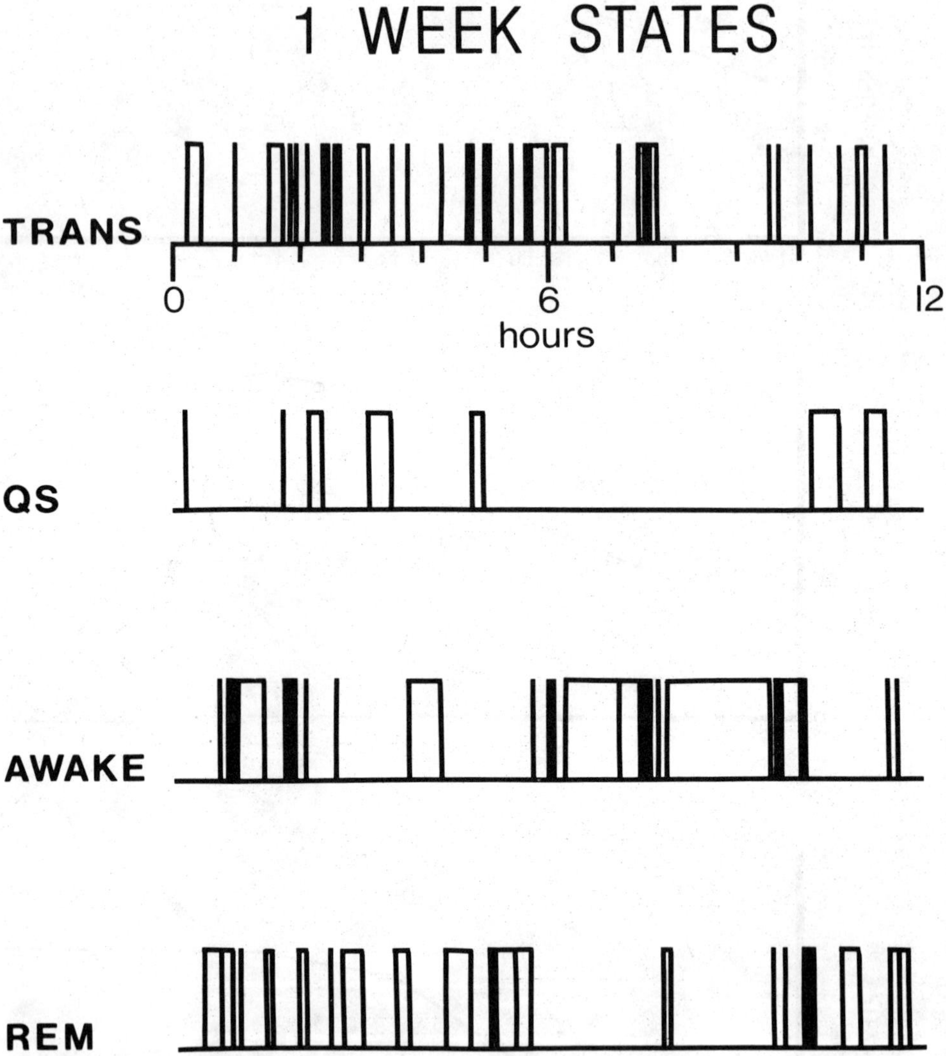

Fig. 4.3 Binary plots of presence and absence of QS, AS, AW and transition periods from a healthy full-term infant in the newborn period. Note the propensity for AS over QS and the relatively disorganized, i.e. non-periodic, pattern of epochs of AS together with a large number of transitional periods at this early age.

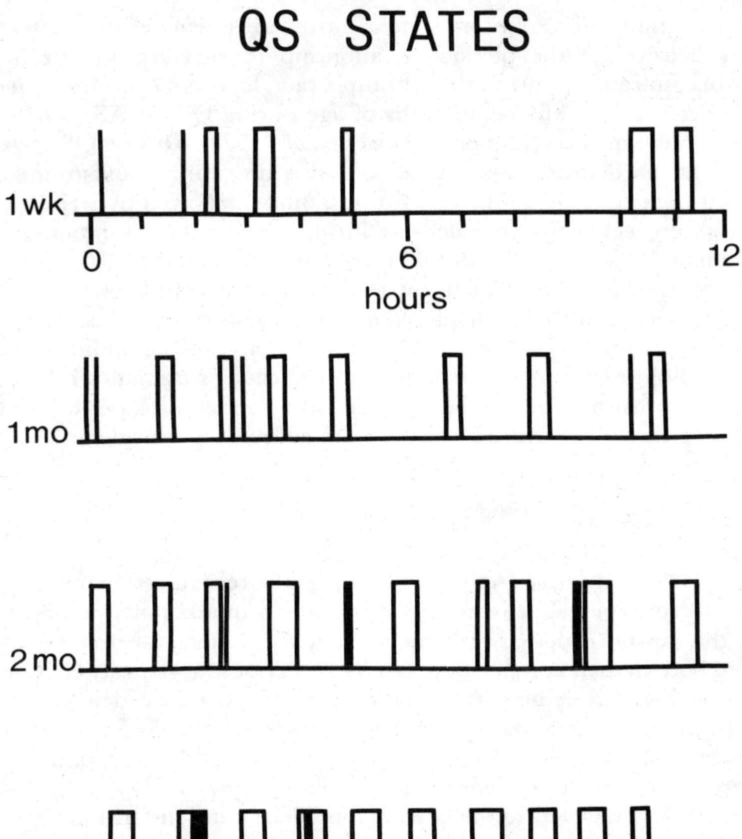

Fig. 4.4 Plots of epochs of QS from 1 week to 6 months of life. Several characteristics of QS development can be noted; there is a relative paucity of QS early in life compared to older infants, epochs of QS become more sustained later in life, and QS epochs become rather periodic at 1 cycle/h by 3 months.

The development of respiratory control during sleep is of principal interest to clinicians because of the obvious relationship to survival. One principal measure of respiratory control, that of simple rate, follows a continuous decline from the first week of life to 3 months of age during QS; in AS, the decline continues until 6 months (Hoppenbrouwers *et al.*, 1978). During QS there is a decline in apnea density (the number of >6 s breathing pauses/number of minutes in each state × 100) from 1 to 4 months, followed by stabilization; there is a sharp decline in apnea density during AS over the first month, with a more gradual decline until 3 months (Hoppenbrouwers *et al.*, 1977).

These trends in respiratory activity describe a maturation of motor control. When such motor control is considered in the framework of sleep state, a valuable developmental index is obtained. All of the physiologic findings demonstrate that absolute levels of physiological activity change dramatically with age. The changes must also be described within the context of state, or within a temporal organization of variables which are collectively considered.

4.3 State Periodicity

Both quiet (QS) and active (AS) sleep states can be recognized in the full-term newborn. QS occupies approximately 20% and AS approximately 45% of total time in the newborn period. In this period, these states are relatively disorganized both in their composition and in the periodic organization of successive epochs. Fig. 4.3 demonstrates the pattern of observer-coded sleep states derived from a 4-day-old infant. There is a preponderance of AS over QS time, a relatively high proportion of unclassifiable, or transition time, and a rather large number of state transitions evident in this record.

This chapter is devoted to the description of sleep in full-term infants. It is often useful to examine the development of sleep in premature infants to study the ontogeny of neural control, although this topic is outside the scope of this chapter. Descriptions of EEG and state development in prematures, and the relationship of developmental abnormalities to later risk have been well described elsewhere (Dreyfus-Brisac, 1964, 1968, 1970; Parmelee *et al.*, 1968).

The developmental course for establishing a stable periodic sequence in sleep state is both valuable for describing state development, and useful for indicating neurological deficits. A sequence of QS epochs from a normal full-term infant has been plotted over the first 6 months in Fig. 4.4. A progressive increase in periodic organization of sleep states over the first 3 months of life is observed. By 3 months, QS epochs are highly repetitive and have an hourly organization. QS time progressively increases over the 6 month period, with sustained periods being present at 6 months.

With appropriate attention to signal conditioning, periodic organization of sleep states can be quantified with time series spectral techniques, and such procedures have been applied to these data (Harper *et al.*, 1974, 1981b; Fig. 4.5). Spectral analysis provides a measure of periodic activity over a set of frequencies, and any single band can be followed over time. We examined the development of periodicity at 1 cycle/h in each sleep state, since the hourly influence on infant state organization is particularly dominant. Trends of that activity are shown in Fig. 4.6. Periodic activity at 1 cycle/h rises rapidly from the newborn period, and nearly asymptotes by 3 months of age; similar curves

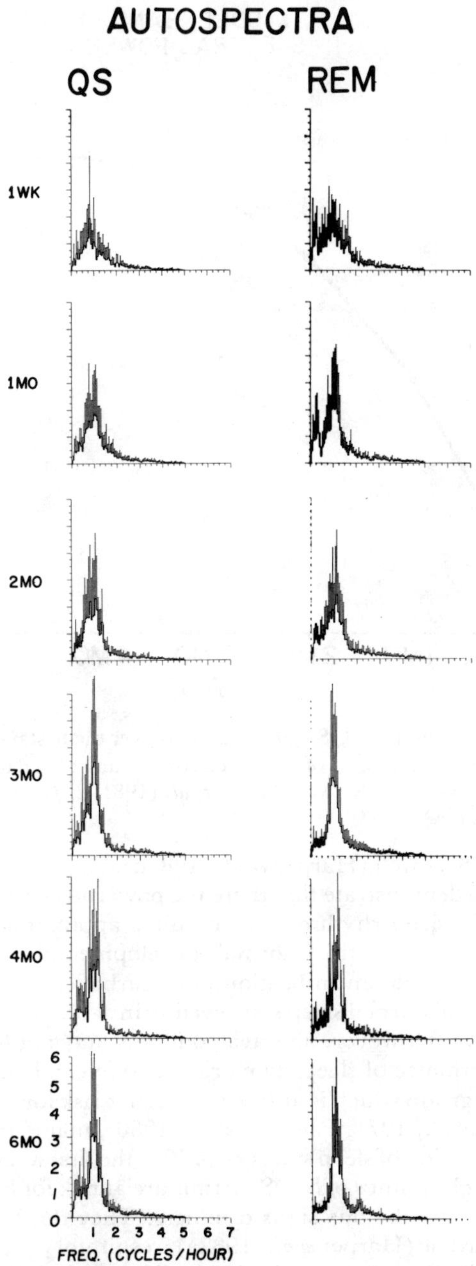

Fig. 4.5 This figure applies quantitative values to assessment of periodicity for data such as those shown in Figs 4.2 and 4.3. The binary epochs of QS that we have obtained in Figs 4.2 and 4.3, as well as binary epochs of AS periods, have been subjected to spectral analysis, and averages of those spectral estimates from 20 control infants have been plotted, together with variability values (fine vertical lines). Note the wide spread of frequencies at 1 week and the gradual consolidation to a narrow band centered at 1 cycle/h with development. Trends at that frequency are seen in Fig. 4.5.

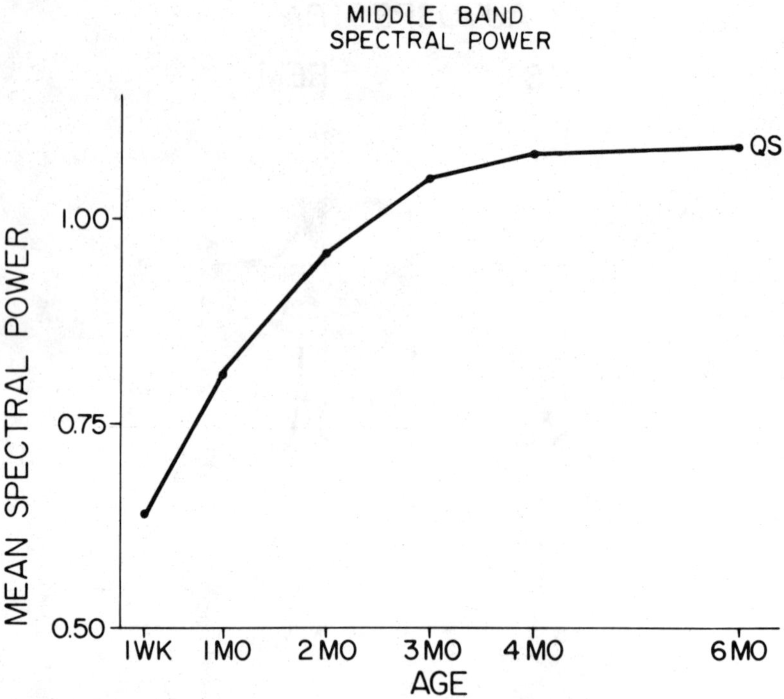

Fig. 4.6 Power at 1 cycle/h for QS states is plotted over the first 6 months of life. Note the very rapid rise until 3–4 months of age. Such curves can be used to chart normal state development. (Redrawn from R. M. Harper *et al.* (1981) *Experimental Neurology* **72(2)** 294–307, by permission.)

are observed for AS as well (Harper *et al.*, 1981b).

Figs 4.5. and 4.6 demonstrate that there is a powerful central nervous system organizer of hourly sleep rhythms that requires approximately 3 months to develop. Deviations from this normal developmental curve of periodic organization may provide an indication of disturbance in CNS maturation. There is evidence of disturbed sleep state cycling in acute stages of severe illness (Monod *et al.*, 1967). However, aggravated illness may not be the only condition in which disturbance of sleep state organization can be noted. Siblings of victims of SIDS, a group which is at five-fold higher risk for the syndrome than controls (Froggatt *et al.*, 1971; Petersen *et al.*, 1980), manifest a disturbance in the periodic organization of sleep states as early as the first week of life (Harper *et al.*, 1981c). Although siblings of SIDS victims are at risk for SIDS, they appear 'healthy' and show no obvious signs of illness. They do, however, exhibit a variety of subtle cardiac (Harper *et al.*, 1982a), respiratory (Hoppenbrouwers *et al.*, 1978), and EEG (Sterman *et al.*, 1982) differences from control infants. Thus, the quantitative assessment of the development of state periodicity may be useful as an index of pathology, even when the particular neurological signs may be subtle.

Although the finding of disturbed periodic organization of sleep states is of theoretical interest since these results point to CNS pathology, few clinical situations can warrant the enormous cost of observer classification of the long sleep records required for adequate statistical assessment of state periodicities. Moreover, in addition to the obvious circular argument of defining sleep states by particular physiological signs, and then relating disorders of physiology with reference to these states, there are severe problems of observation repeatability and human observer reliability. It would be desirable, instead, to move towards a description of sleep that depends entirely on objective, quantifiable assessments of those physiological measures which constitute state. For this purpose, we will consider two aspects of sleep physiology: coalescence of physiological variables, and periodic organization of activity.

Sleep states are not entirely determined by absolute levels of physiological activity such as heart-rate or respiratory variability; such values change dramatically with age, as Figs 4.1 and 4.2 show. Instead, the coalescence of relative amounts of activity in a set of physiological variables is used to describe a particular state. One object of describing the development of state in the infant should thus be the quantification of this clustering of levels of activity. Prechtl (1974) has pioneered the utilization of multivariate procedures for demonstrating the development of coalescence with age; he has also demonstrated a loss of coalescence in severely ill infants.

We have utilized two additional measures for assessing state organization, both of which are related to time series analysis techniques. The first procedure, assessment of periodic activity at particular ultradian frequencies in each of the physiological measures that are used to define sleep state, has already been demonstrated for binary sleep states. We have shown that sleep states are periodic in the infant, and that this periodicity requires some time to develop. Measurement of this developmental periodicity could thus provide a quantifiable indicator of the temporal organization of sleep states, and provide a 'marker' for neurological assessment.

Sleep states are defined by the clustering of various levels of activity in selected physiological parameters. Direct examination of physiological activity can contribute to the assessment of state. Fig. 4.7 demonstrates the development of an hourly periodicity in two parameters for a normal full-term infant over the first 6 months of life. The first parameter is minute-by-minute respiratory variability, the second is minute-by-minute integrated 13 Hz activity in the EEG. Although there is little hourly periodic organization in the newborn period, a well-organized rhythm with fewer faster transients has emerged on each of the records by 2–3 months of age. In the case of integrated 13 Hz activity, an hourly periodicity is present by 1 month, although a great deal of transient activity is also prominent (Harper *et al.*, 1981a). Respiratory variability also demonstrates some hourly organization at 1 month, but this activity is intermixed with both slower and faster rhythms. The developmental course of an hourly periodicity in 13 Hz activity over the first 6 months of life is seen in Fig. 4.8, which demonstrates a rapid rise to 3 months of age, followed by stabilization or decline of activity. Measurement of this physiological activity and assessment of associated periodic activity can provide an objective indication of state organization. This assessment is relatively simple with modern microcomputers, which can continuously acquire physiological activity and assess components of periodic activity.

A second measure for assessing state characteristics is coherence, which describes the degree of coupling between two variables at particular periodic frequencies (Harper *et al.*, 1974; Orr & Naitoh, 1976). This procedure is

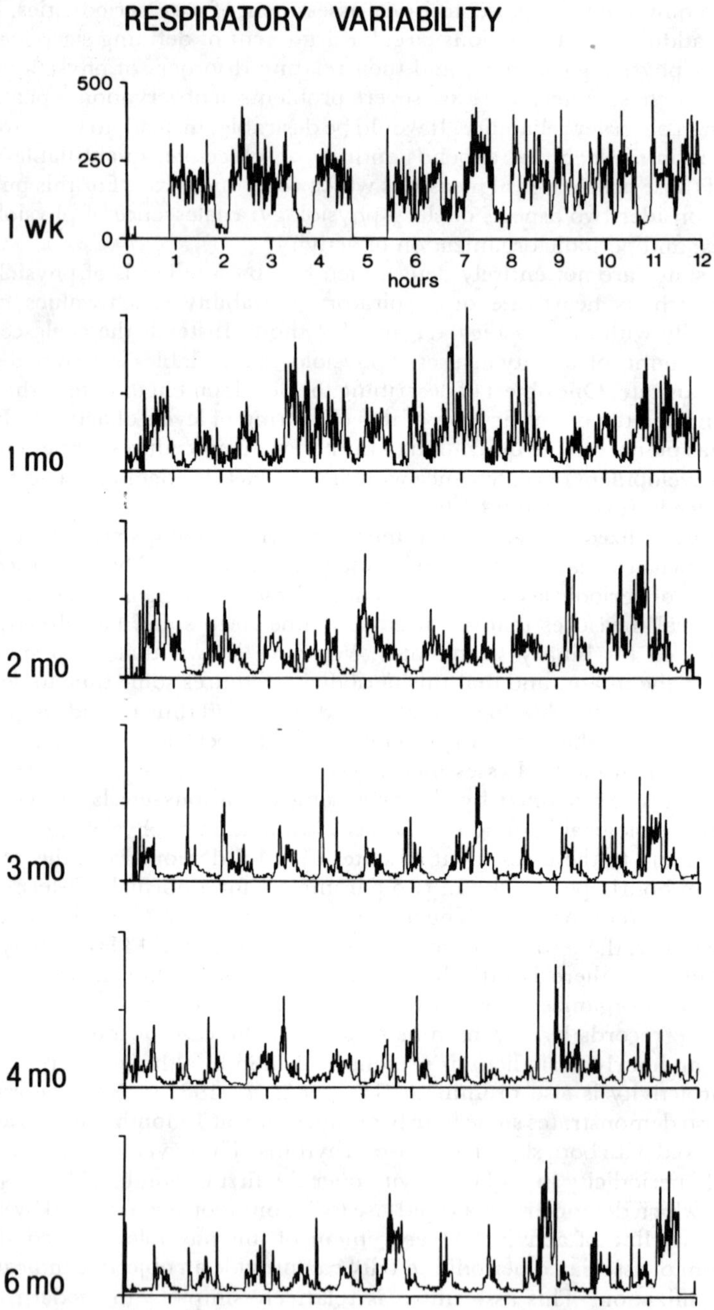

Fig. 4.7 Plots of minute-by-minute values of respiratory variability (assessed by interquartile range) and integrated activity in the 13 Hz (12–14 Hz) band of EEG for 720-min recording periods over the first half year of life. Recordings were from a full-term control infant. (There is a 43-min gap in the 1 week recording near the fifth hour.) Several developmental points can be observed. There appears to be less high-frequency activity

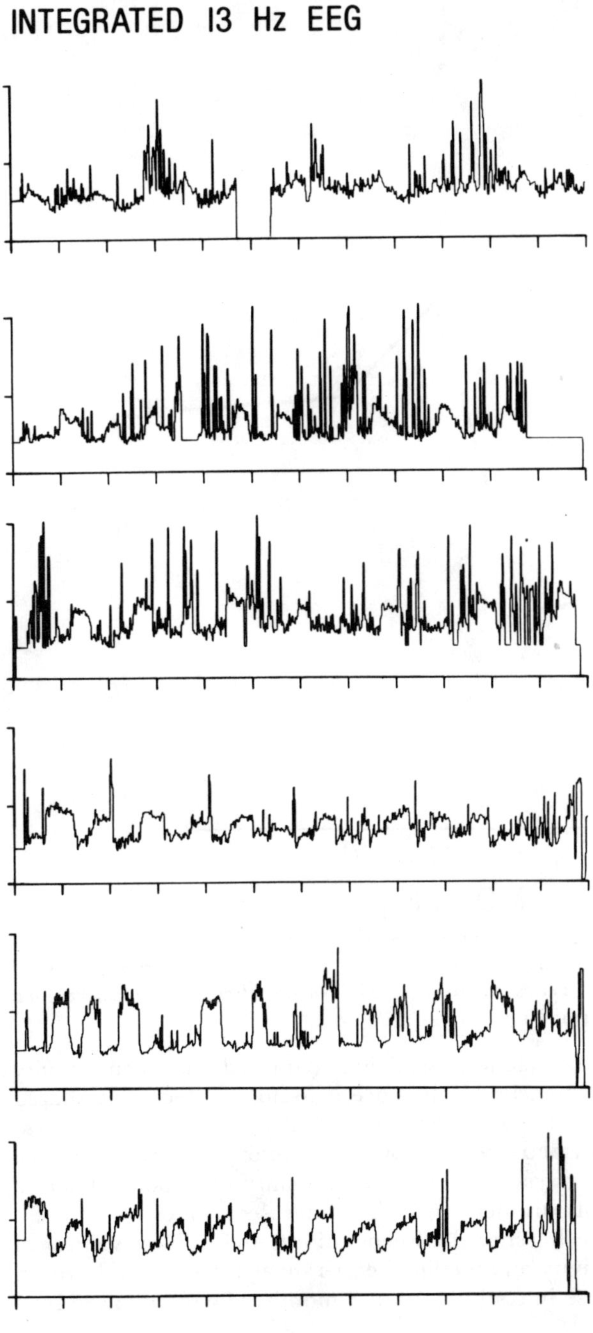

in later ages (represented here by spike-like artifacts on the record). This is especially the case on the EEG plots. There is little hourly periodicity at 1 week, although there is a slower rhythm, particularly on the EEG plot. The near-hourly rhythm becomes quite prominent by 3 months of age on both records.

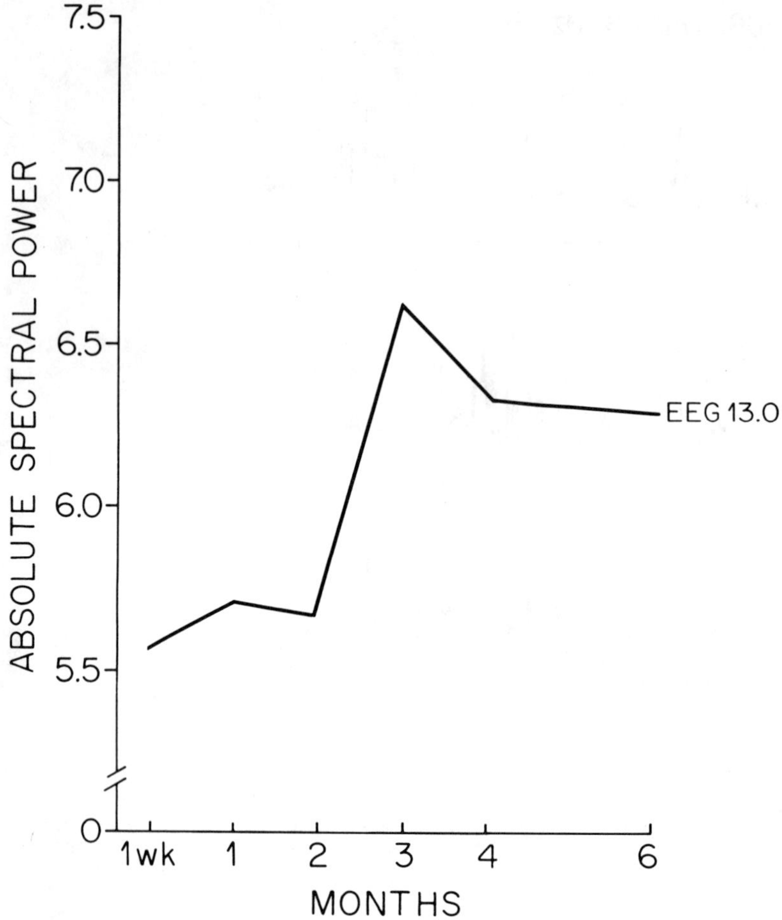

Fig. 4.8 Development of spectral power at 1 cycle/h. Plot of hourly periodic development in integrated 13 Hz activity over the first half year of life. Note the very rapid rise of activity to 3 months of age. (Redrawn from R. M. Harper *et al.* (1981) *Experimental Neurology* **73**, 127–143, by permission.)

analogous to assessing a correlation coefficient (squared) between activity measured at particular frequencies. Coherence is useful in describing shared activity between variables, i.e. higher coherence results if activity in one parameter varies together with activity in another parameter. Since coherence assesses 'coupling' between variables, it is a useful quantitative tool to describe the coalescence of the set of parameters which defines sleep state.

The development of coherence between minute-by-minute values of integrated 13 Hz EEG activity and median heart-rate at 1 cycle/h is shown in Fig. 4.9. Note the rapid rise in coupling until 3 months of age, followed by a stabilization.

Fig. 4.9 describes the development of coalescence at 1 cycle/h, which, as we have observed from the state periodic data, underlies the principal sleep cycle frequency. For this reason, quantitative assessment of coherence between variables at 1 cycle/h, such as sleep spindle EEG and heart-rate, may be useful

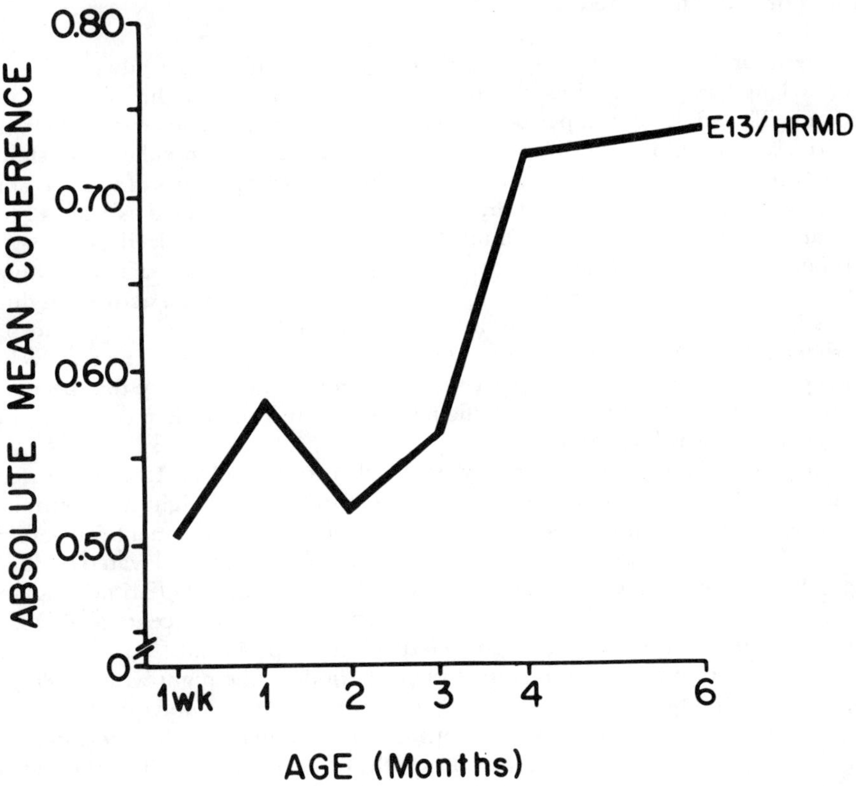

Fig. 4.9 Plot of the development of coherence between integrated 13 Hz activity and median heart-rate over the first half year of life. Note again the rapid rise in activity between 2 and 3 months. (Redrawn from R. M. Harper *et al.* (1981) *Experimental Neurology* **73**, 127–143, by permission.)

for defining state. We are not limited to activity at 1 cycle/h, however, and it now appears that the reduction in high frequency activity, or developmental changes in slower periodicities, may be as important a marker for quantitative state maturation as the hourly periodicity. As trends in these other periodic components become apparent, we can look forward to statistical descriptions of state coalescence on a number of temporal dimensions.

Monod *et al.* (1965, 1967, 1972) have described the dissociation of normally coalescing physiological variables during episodes of acute illness. They describe such dissociations as absence of chin muscle activity during QS, or fewer eye movements during AS. Respiratory and cardiac rhythms were often dissociated from the sleep cycle. Thus, lack of integration, or coalescence of physiological variables that normally constitute state, may be associated with acute illness. More subtle disturbances may also be indicated by assessing that lack of coalescence. Indeed, siblings of SIDS victims exhibit a disturbance in such organization with development (Harper *et al.*, 1982b).

4.4 Time of Night Effects

The temporal organization of AS and QS states in adults is periodic, with the period length approximating 90 min rather than the hourly rhythm observed in infants. The adult 90-min period is not stable across a night, however. There is relatively more QS earlier in the night, with a more stable oscillation of state sequence later in the sleep period. In addition, the components of QS are not uniform across a night in the adult. Four distinct stages, classified as Stages 1 to 4, can be distinguished within adult QS. Stage 4 is characterized by a large proportion of very high amplitude, low frequency 'delta' waves. The relative amount of each stage of QS does not remain constant in the adult across a night; there is relatively more high amplitude, low frequency EEG, i.e. Stage 4 sleep, earlier in the night relative to other QS stages (Feinberg, 1974). The relatively high proportion of Stage 4 sleep early in the night has given rise to the speculation that such sleep reflects metabolic processes which underlie recovery from the need for sleep (Feinberg, 1974).

Sleep in infants tends toward a nocturnal distribution by 15 days of age (Monod & Pajot, 1965). There is also a differential time of night distribution, but this effect is not manifested until the first month of life (Hoppenbrouwers *et al.*, 1982). The percentage of QS in the first half of the night is elevated by that age; this is a transient effect, but at 3 months the percentage of QS time is again elevated earlier in the night. By 4–6 months, an even higher percentage of QS is present in the first half of the night, relative to later periods.

The distribution of AS also shifts to later periods in the night with development. This shift begins at 1 month with an increase in the second quarter of the night, levels during the second month, and then composes a higher percentage of sleep in the third quarter at 3 months of age. Finally, all of the last 3 quarters of the night show an increase in AS relative to QS by 4–6 months (Hoppenbrouwers *et al.*, 1982). An increase in low frequency activity early in the night is also observed in developing infants, but this increase, as measured by EEG spectral analysis, is limited to the 2–3 month period (Sterman *et al.*, 1977).

Several principles of state organization can be discerned from these findings. Superimposed upon the hourly state cycling is a developing tendency for QS epochs to appear earlier in the night and AS periods to be more prominent later. At particular ages, there is a tendency for large slow waves to occur earlier in the night. The beginnings of adult sleep organization, which has an enhanced Stage 4 occurring earlier in the night, a greater overall percentage of QS, and a greater percentage of AS occurring later in the night can be observed at particular developmental stages.

4.5 Summary

Analysis of infant sleep stage organization is now entering an exciting period with recent technological capabilities which allow the assessment of long-term physiological recording at low cost. The assessment of sleep state and of the physiological components that comprise state has always been hindered by the enormous cost and unreliability of observer state classification and observer determination of qualities such as EEG parameters. The advent of inexpensive signal processing devices permits the easy measurement of physiological components such as cardiac and respiratory parameters, and components of EEG and somatic activity for both clinical and research use.

The ability to assess the temporal organization of physiological components defining state without requiring human scoring is critical for establishing the feasibility of using sleep as a diagnostic tool. We have seen that long-term recording of physiological activity allows the determination of ultradian rhythms that underlie sleep states, that this temporal organization requires a period of time to develop, and that deviations from this developmental curve are indicative of risk. Moreover, viewing the organization of physiological variables in periodic terms allows us to assess the coalescence of variables at particular frequencies using time series techniques. Determination of the coalescence of variables can assist in the automatic definition of state. Clinical observations demonstrate that lack of coalescence in variables that normally constitute state is indicative of illness, and we have demonstrated that even subtle developmental differences can be discerned by such coalescence disturbances.

The current status of infant sleep development can thus be summarized as (1) bringing recognition to the essential nature of determining physiological activity in terms of the temporal coalescence of other physiological variables, i.e. state, and (2) recognizing that the temporal organization of clusters of physiological variables is itself indicative of development. Quantitative assessment for both aspects of physiology are essential for insights into infant sleep development.

Acknowledgements

A large number of investigators made contributions to these studies, including Drs. T. Hoppenbrouwers and J. Hodgman, Los Angeles County-USC Women's Hospital, Drs. M. B. Sterman and D. J. McGinty of the Sepulveda Veterans' Administration Medical Center, and Dr. B. Leake of UCLA. E. Hofmann, S. Geidel and J. Mason provided valuable technical assistance. This research was supported by NIH-NICHD HD-1-4608-02. Data collection efforts were previously supported by HD-4-2810 and HD-2-2777.

References

CHATRIAN, G. E., WHITE, L. E. and DALY, D. (1963). Electroencephalographic pattern resembling those of sleep in certain comatose states after injuries to the head. *Electroencephalography and Clinical Neurophysiology*, **15**, 272.

CURZI-DASCALOVA, L. (1977). EEG de veille et de sommeil du nourrisson normal avant 6 mois d'age. *Revue D'Electroencephalographie et de Neurophysiologie Clinique*, **7(3)**, 316–326.

DREYFUS-BRISAC, C. (1964). The electroencephalogram of the premature infant and full-term newborn. Normal and abnormal development of waking and sleeping patterns. In: P. KELLAWAY and I. PETERSEN (Eds.), *Neurological and Electroencephalographic Correlative Studies in Infancy*, pp. 186–207.

DREYFUS-BRISAC, C. (1968). Sleep ontogenesis in early human prematurity from 24 to 27 weeks of conceptional age. *Developmental Psychobiology*, **1(3)**, 162–169.

DREYFUS-BRISAC, C. (1970). Ontogenesis of sleep in human prematures after 32 weeks of conceptional age. *Developmental Psychobiology*, **3(2)**, 91–121.

ELLINGSON, R. J. and PETERS, J. F. (1980). Development of EEG and daytime sleep patterns in nòrmal full-term infants during the first 3 months of life: Longitudinal observations. *Electroencephalography and Clinical Neurophysiology*, **49**, 112–124.

ELLINGSON, R. J. (1982). Development of sleep spindle bursts during the first year of life. *Sleep*, **5(1)**, 34–46.

FEINBERG, I. (1974). Changes in sleep cycle patterns with age. *Journal of Psychiatric Research*, **10**, 283–306.

FROGGATT, P., LYNAS, M. A. and MACKENZIE, C. (1971). Epidemiology of sudden unexpected death in infants ('cot death') in Northern Ireland. *British Journal of Preventive and Social Medicine*, **25**, 119–134.

GROSS, H. P. and SCHULTE, F. J. (1969). Uber Vermehrte Spindelaktivitat in Schlaf-EEG bei Kindern mit Phenylketonurie. *Zeitschrift fuer Kinderheilkunde*, **105**, 324–333.

HARPER, R. M. SCLABASSI, R. J. and ESTRIN, T. (1974). Time series analysis and sleep research. *IEEE Transactions on Automatic Control*, AC–**19(6)**, 932–943.

HARPER, R. M., HOPPENBROUWERS, T., STERMAN, M. B., MCGINTY D. J., and HODGMAN, J. (1976). Polygraphic studies of normal infants during the first six months of life: I. Heart rate and variability as a function of state. *Pediatric Research*, **10(11)**, 945–951.

HARPER, R. M., HOPPENBROUWERS, T., BANNETT, D., HODGMAN, J., STERMAN, M. B. and MCGINTY, D. J. (1977). Effects of feeding on state and cardiac regulation in the infant. *Developmental Psychobiology*, **10(6)**, 507–517.

HARPER, R. M., LEAKE, B., MIYAHARA, L., HOPPENBROUWERS, T., STERMAN, M. B. and HODGMAN, J. (1981a). Development of ultradian periodicity and coalescence at 1 cycle/hr in electroencephalographic activity. *Experimental Neurology*, **73**, 127–143.

HARPER, R. M., LEAKE, B., MIYAHARA. L., MASON, J., HOPPENBROUWERS, T., STERMAN, M. B. and HODGMAN, J. (1981b). Temporal sequencing in sleep and waking states during the first 6 months of life. *Experimental Neurology*, **72(2)**, 294–307.

HARPER, R. M., LEAKE, B., HOFFMAN, H., WALTER, D. O., HOPPENBROUWERS, T., HODGMAN, J. and STERMAN, M. B. (1981c). Periodicity of sleep states is altered in infants at risk for the Sudden Infant Death Syndrome. *Science*, **213**, 1030–1032.

HARPER, R. M., LEAKE, B., HODGMAN, J. E. and HOPPENBROUWERS, T. (1982a). Developmental patterns of heart rate and heart rate variability during sleep and waking in normal infants and infants at risk for the Sudden Infant Death Syndrome. *Sleep*, **5(1)**, 28–38.

HARPER, R. M., FROSTIG, Z., HOPPENBROUWERS, T., STERMAN, M. and HODGMAN, J. (1982b). Developmental organization of physiological variables at 1 cycle/hour in infants at risk for the Sudden Infant Death Syndrome. In: M. H. CHASE, D. F. KRIPKE and P. L. WALTER (Eds.), *Sleep Research*, in press.

HOFMANN, E., HAVENS, B., GEIDEL, S., HOPPENBROUWERS, T. and HODGMAN, J. E. (1977). Long-term continuous monitoring of multiple physiological parameters in newborn and young infants. *Acta Paediatrica Scandinavica Supplement*, **266**.

HOPPENBROUWERS, T., HODGMAN, J. E., HARPER, R. M., HOFMANN, E., STERMAN, M. B. and MCGINTY, D. J. (1977). Polygraphic studies of normal infants during the first six months of life: III. Incidence of apnea and periodic breathing. *Pediatrics*, **60(4)**, 418–425.

HOPPENBROUWERS, T., HARPER, R. M., HODGMAN, J. E., STERMAN, M. B. and MCGINTY, D. J. (1978). Polygraphic studies of normal infants during the first six months of life: II. Respiratory rate and variability as a function of state. *Pediatric Research*, **12**, 120–125.

HOPPENBROUWERS, T., HODGMAN, J. E., HARPER, R. M. and STERMAN, M. B. (1982). Temporal distribution of sleep states, somatic activity, and autonomic activity during the first half year of life. *Sleep*, *5(2)*, 131–144.

KATONA, P. G., FRASZ, A. and EGBERT, J. (1980). Maturation of cardiac control in full-term and pre-term infants during sleep. *Early Human Development*, **4(2)**, 145–159.

LEISTNER, H. L., HADDAD, G. G., EPSTEIN, R. A., LAI, T. L., EPSTEIN, M. A. F. and MELLINS, R. B. (1980). Heart rate and heart rate variability during sleep in aborted Sudden Infant Death Syndrome. *Journal of Pediatrics*, **97**, 51–55.

LENARD, H. G. (1970). The development of sleep spindles in the EEG during the first two years of life. *Neuropadiatrie*, **1(3)**, 264–276.

METCALF, D. R. (1964). The effect of extrauterine experience on the ontogenesis of EEG sleep spindles. *Psychosomatic Medicine*, **31**, 393–399.

METCALF, D. R. (1970). EEG sleep spindle ontogenesis. *Neuropadiatrie,* **1**, 428–433.

MIYAZAKI, S., WATANABE, K., and HARA, K. (1979). Heart rate variability in full-term, normal and abnormal newborn infants during sleep. *Brain and Development*, **1(1)**, 57–60.

MONOD, N., ELIET-FLESCHER, J. and DREYFUS-BRISAC, C. (1967). Le sommeil du nouveau-né èt du premature: III. Les troubles de l' organisation du sommeil chez le nouveau-né pathologique: Analyse des études polygraphiques. *Biology of the Neonate*, **11**, 216–247.

MONOD, N. and PAJOT, N. (1965). Le sommeil du nouveau-né et du premature: I. Analyse des études polygraphiques (mouvements oculaires, respiration et EEG) chez le nouveau-né à terme. *Biology of the Neonate*, **8**, 281–307.

MONOD, N., PAJOT, N. and GUIDASCI, S. (1972). The neonatal EEG: statistical studies and prognostic value in full-term and pre-term babies. *Electroencephalography and Clinical Neurophysiology*, **32**, 529–544.

ORR, W. C. and NAITOH, P. (1976). The coherence spectrum: an extension of correlation analysis with application to chronobiology. *International Journal of Chronobiology*, **3**, 171–192.

PARMELEE, A. H., SCHULTE, F. J., AKIYAMA, Y., WENNER, W. H., SCHULTZ, M. A. and STERN, E. (1968). Maturation of EEG activity during sleep in premature infants. *Electroencephalography and Clinical Neurophysiology*, **24**, 319–329.

PETERSON, D. R., CHINN, N. M. and FISHER, L. D. (1980). The Sudden Infant Death Syndrome: repetitions in families. *Journal of Pediatrics*, **97(2)**, 265–267.

PRECHTL, H. F. R. (1974). The behavioural states of the newborn infant: a review. *Brain Research*, **76**, 185–212.

SCHULTZ, M. A., SCHULTE, F. J., AKIYAMA, Y. and PARMELEE, A. H. (1968). Development of electroencephalographic sleep phenomena in hypothyroid infants. *Electroencephalography and Clinical Neurophysiology*, **25**, 351–358.

SHIBAGAKI, M., SIGEHIRO, K. and WATANABE, K. (1982). Spindle evolution in normal and mentally retarded children: a review. *Sleep*, **5(1)**, 47–57.

STERMAN, M. B., HARPER, R. M., HAVENS, B., HOPPENBROUWERS, T., MCGINTY, D. J. and HODGMAN, J. E. (1977). Quantitative analysis of infant EEG development during quiet sleep. *Electroencephalography and Clinical Neurophysiology*, **43**, 371–385.

STERMAN, M. B., MCGINTY, D. J., HARPER, R. M., HOPPENBROUWERS, T. and HODGMAN, J. E. (1982). Developmental comparison of sleep EEG power spectral patterns in infants at low and high risk for sudden death. *Electroencephalography and Clinical Neurophysiology*, **53**, 166–181.

WATANABE, K., IWASE, K. and HARA, K. (1973). Heart rate variability during sleep and wakefulness in low-birthweight infants. *Biology of the Neonate*, **22**, 87.

WOODY, N. C., SNYDER, C. H. and HARRIS, J. A. (1965). Histidinemia. *American Journal of Diseases of Children*, **110**, 606–613.

CHAPTER 5

A Life Span Perspective on Sleep

Harold Zepelin

Changes in sleep with advancing age have been well documented, but their functional consequences, apart from the discomfort known to be associated with sleep disturbance in the later years, remain in doubt. Better understanding of these changes, and of stable features of sleep, would help to solve the puzzle of sleep's still unexplained purpose, and perhaps would also help to alleviate sleep-related distress. With these possibilities in mind, this chapter will review present knowledge and relevant theoretical controversy in this area.

5.1 Maturation of Sleep

Neither in humans nor in other species is it possible to define a single maturational end-point of the sleep process or a single point that marks the onset of its senescence. Different aspects of sleep have different timetables, which is evidence of sleep's regulation by multiple mechanisms. An overview of maturational timetables therefore seems useful as a backdrop for discussion of senescence. More detailed examination of sleep's maturation appears in Chapter 4.

With variation in timing from species to species, the sleep–wakefulness cycle in mammals and birds emerges from the primordial foetal condition either late in foetal life or shortly after birth (Ellingson & Rose, 1970; Ellingson, 1972). This is followed by maturation of sleep's structural and temporal organization. Structural organization refers to the constellations of physiological variables that distinguish sleep from the waking state, the REM sleep state from the non-REM (NREM) state, and the sleep stages that make up NREM sleep (Stages 1–4) from each other. A fundamental structural element is the EEG. In humans most of the EEG waveforms that characterize sleep take shape by 10 weeks post-term (Ellingson, 1975), but about 1 year of age may be required before the EEG can be used confidently with other sleep signs (eye movements and muscle tone) for the classification of sleep stages as in adults (Dreyfus-Brisac, 1979). (See Fig. 5.1 for descriptions of waveforms and stages.) Modifications in sleep spindles (Lenard, 1970; Tanguay *et al.*, 1975) and K-complexes (Metcalf *et al.*, 1971), which are important signs of NREM sleep, occur after this age. EEG amplitude, which rises from birth on, continues to increase. This is especially true for delta activity, which reaches its maximum amplitude sometime between the ages of 3 and 5 (Feinberg *et al.*, 1977). Judged by its amplitude in combination with its waveforms, the EEG is mature at this point.

As the EEG develops, the different states attain their mature identities. REM and NREM sleep respectively evolve from active sleep (AS) and quiet sleep

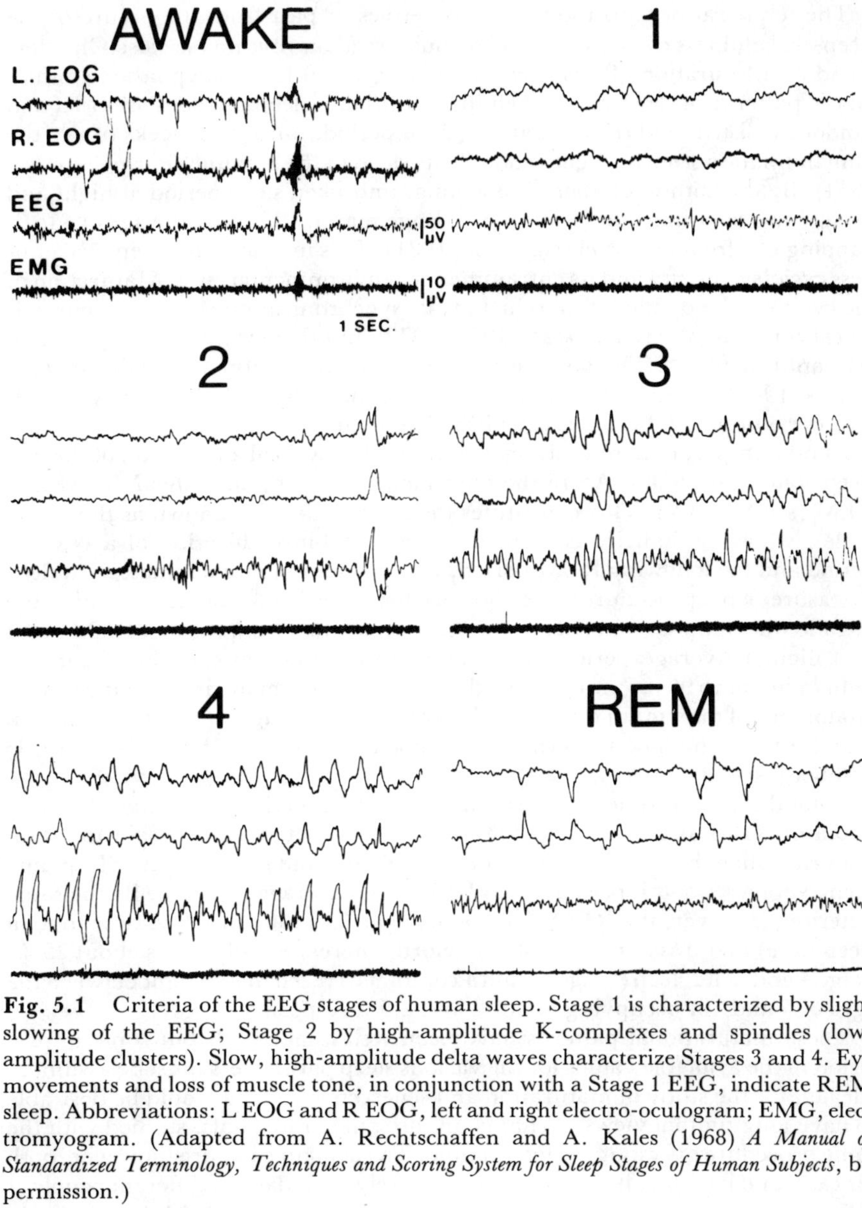

Fig. 5.1 Criteria of the EEG stages of human sleep. Stage 1 is characterized by slight slowing of the EEG; Stage 2 by high-amplitude K-complexes and spindles (low-amplitude clusters). Slow, high-amplitude delta waves characterize Stages 3 and 4. Eye movements and loss of muscle tone, in conjunction with a Stage 1 EEG, indicate REM sleep. Abbreviations: L EOG and R EOG, left and right electro-oculogram; EMG, electromyogram. (Adapted from A. Rechtschaffen and A. Kales (1968) *A Manual of Standardized Terminology, Techniques and Scoring System for Sleep Stages of Human Subjects*, by permission.)

(QS) — so termed because they are based on loosely associated behavioural criteria (Anders *et al.*, 1971). REM sleep is then characterized by a distinct constellation of variables consisting of a Stage 1 EEG, rapid eye movements, chin muscle atonia, irregular respiration and heart rate, and relatively frequent body movements and twitching, while NREM sleep is characterized by spindling, K-complexes, and slow waves in the EEG, along with regular heart-rate and respiration. The maturity of these states seems likely to precede the EEG's attainment of peak amplitude.

The temporal organization of sleep derives in part from the nature of the sleep–wakefulness cycle as an endogenous circadian rhythm (see also Chapters 1 and 2). Maturation of this rhythm involves a shift from polyphasic to monophasic patterns of sleep and wakefulness. Initially, sleep episodes are brief and randomly distributed throughout the 24-h period, but by 16 weeks of age the human infant's sleep at night is double its sleep in the daytime (Parmelee *et al.*, 1964). By the 26th week there is one long, unbroken sleep period at night and usually two daytime naps (Kleitman & Engelmann, 1953). By the age of 4 to 5, napping is infrequent (Webb & Dube, 1981). This indicates the sleep–wakefulness cycle's maturity and its entrainment to environmental cues. Maturation of the cycle can be defined also to include its synchronization with other physiological rhythms (Weitzman *et al.*, 1975, 1979), but there is little information on relevant timetables. The body temperature rhythm in humans attains mature form at 10–11 months (Abe *et al.*, 1978). Its synchrony with the sleep–wakefulness cycle probably becomes established at about the same time.

Another aspect of temporal organization is the cyclical alternation of the two sleep states — QS and AS in the foetus and newborn, and later NREM and REM (see Fig. 5.2). This constitutes the sleep cycle (also known as the REM cycle), whose periodicity is defined by the combined duration of a NREM period and the following REM period, with intervening wakefulness excluded. (Measurement procedures are not well-standardized. Some investigators include wakefulness; some begin counting cycles only from the first REM onset of a night.) Average periodicity gradually increases from 50–60 min in the human infant to 90–95 min in the adult. If the cycle's maturity is defined by its attainment of maximum duration, the available data suggest that this occurs in middle or late childhood (Sterman & Hoppenbrouwers, 1971; Feinberg, 1974; Feinberg & Floyd, 1979).

Total daily sleep time decreases dramatically in early life, as does the daily quota of REM sleep (see Fig. 5.3). These parameters can be said to attain maturity when they achieve fairly stable levels at about the age of 20. Sleep time then averages 7.5–8 h per day, and REM sleep averages 1.5–2 h. By the same criterion, however, the REM sleep percentage (the ratio of REM time to total sleep time) matures at the age of 5 or shortly thereafter, when it is about 25%. Stage 4 and delta sleep (Stages 3 and 4 combined) reach their height between the ages of 5 and 10, occupying about 2 and 2.5 h respectively.

These maturational patterns have been well established, but some imprecision in the available values for the various sleep parameters must be assumed. Ideally, for the study of maturation and senescence alike, it would be desirable to have longitudinal views of change in the same individuals, studied with the same procedure over long periods of time. The available picture, however, both for early and later life, is derived almost entirely from data on different people at different age levels, usually studied in different laboratories with incompletely standardized procedures. Although there is considerable variability between individuals, the research samples have been small in virtually all laboratory studies (typically, 10–20 per age level). Not surprisingly, therefore, there is some disagreement, especially regarding daily amounts and percentages of sleep stages (Roffwarg *et al.*, 1966; Feinberg *et al.*, 1967; Williams *et al.*, 1974).

Studies in other species have disclosed developmental sequences like those in humans (Ellingson, 1972). In all species, AS and REM sleep are the initially predominant states, indicating that they are ontogenetically primitive sleep.

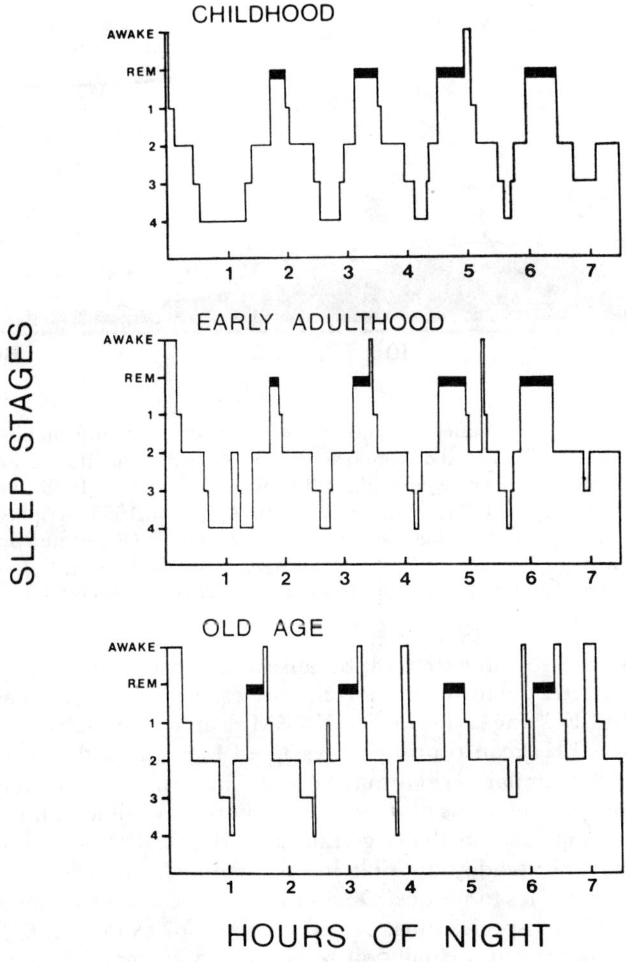

Fig. 5.2 Schematic representation of the cycling of human sleep stages at different times of life, with childhood broadly defined to include early adolescence, and old age including the period from the mid-50s to the early 70s. This is a composite representation of data drawn from Feinberg (1974), Williams *et al.* (1974), Feinberg and Floyd (1979), and Zepelin (data on file). (Reprinted by permission of Roche Products Inc. from Figure 4 in *Roche Seminars on Aging* No. 9 — Section 1: *Aging in Sleep*, Zepelin, copyright © 1982 by Roche Products Inc. All rights reserved.)

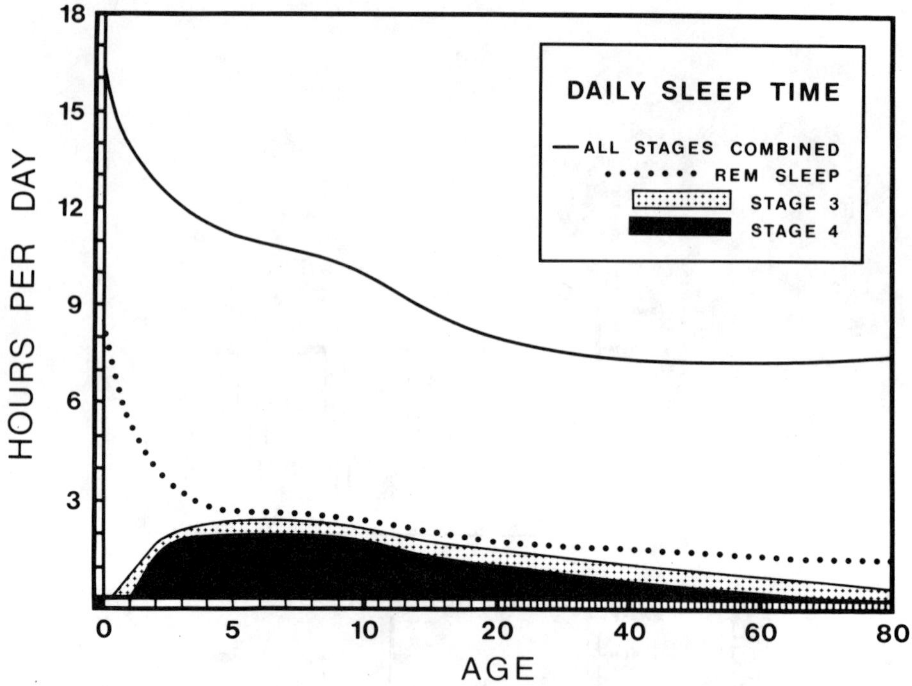

Fig. 5.3 Changes in daily sleep quotas over the human life span from birth to the age of 80 years. Estimates are based on rough averaging of results from the following studies, which include surveys: Parmelee *et al.*, 1964; Roffwarg *et al* ., 1966; Tune, 1969a; Zepelin, 1973; Feinberg, 1974; Williams *et al.*, 1974; Webb, 1975; Kripke *et al.*, 1979; Zepelin (data on file). Note changes in scale at ages 10 and 20. (Reprinted by permission of Roche Products Inc. from *Roche Seminars on Aging* No. 9 — Section 1: *Aging in Sleep*, Zepelin, copyright © 1982 by Roche Products Inc. All rights reserved.)

(The echidna may be an exception because adult specimens lack REM sleep; Allison *et al.*, 1972). However, not all species, when mature, have equally differentiated EEG stages. Periods of NREM sleep with a high density of delta activity (0.5–3.0 Hz) constituting Stages 3 and 4 are characteristic of primates (Pegram, 1972). Similar periods may be found in carnivores, since subdivision of NREM sleep on the basis of slow wave activity is possible in the cat (Ursin, 1968) and perhaps also in the dog (Latash & Shlyk, 1975). In other species NREM sleep is not readily divisible in this manner. Maturational timetables also differ from species to species. Obviously, relative to the human's, the timetables of short-lived species must be accelerated. For example, the laboratory rat's sleep is mature in virtually all respects by the age of 30 days (Jouvet-Mounier *et al.*, 1968). More surprisingly, although the proportion of REM sleep declines with maturation in all species, the extent of this decline is governed by a 'maturity law' (Verley & Garma, 1975), as Fig. 5.4 illustrates. In precocial species, whose sensory and motor abilities are fairly mature at birth (e.g. guinea pig, sheep), the sleep states are also well developed, and the subsequent change in their proportions is slight. In altricial species, whose immaturity at birth also characterizes their sleep (e.g. rat, cat), maturation

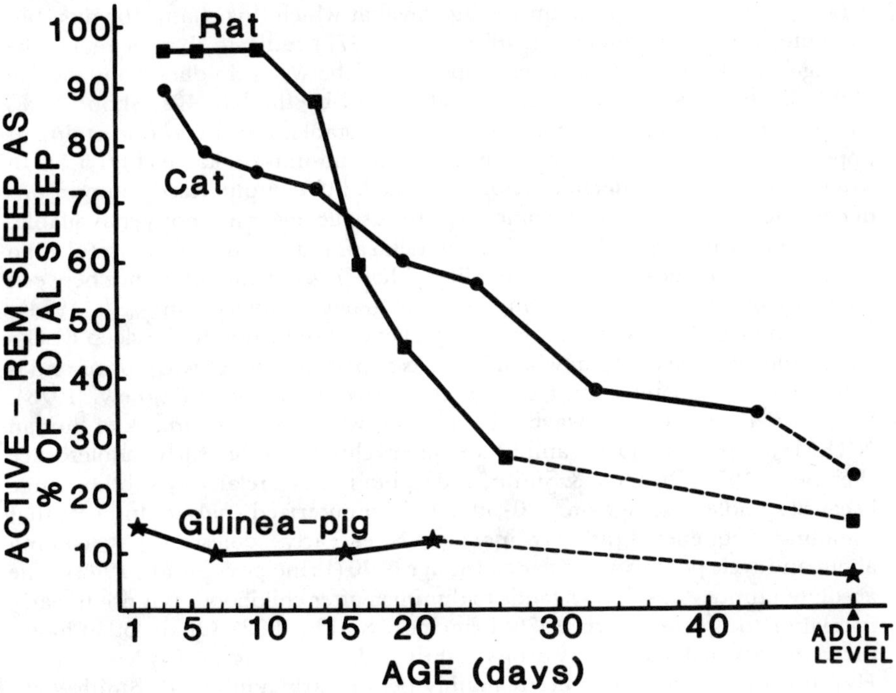

Fig. 5.4 Maturational changes in REM sleep as a percentage of total sleep time in two altricial species (rat and cat) and a precocial species (guinea pig). (Reproduced from D. Jouvet-Mounier, L. Astic and D. Lacote (1970) *Developmental Psychobiology*, **2**, 216–239, © John Wiley & Sons, Inc., by permission.)

involves a drastic decline from a high proportion of REM sleep. Finer gradations on the altricial–precocial dimension are also reflected in these proportions, so that the REM sleep percentage in humans has less room for decline after birth than it does in rats or cats, who are born relatively immature (see Fig. 5.3). On the other hand, the initial REM sleep quota in humans is higher than in the rhesus monkey, which is born relatively mature (Meier & Berger, 1965). A further consequence of the 'maturity law' is a fairly strong relationship between degree of maturity at birth and the REM sleep quota in adulthood; the less mature a species is at birth, the more time it tends to spend in REM sleep as an adult (Zepelin, 1980).

5.2 Senescent Change in Human EEG Stages

Senescent change becomes evident in the human sleep EEG even before daily sleep quotas reach their mature level. Reversing its maturational trend, the amplitude of delta activity begins to diminish during childhood. Some delta waves in early childhood may attain an amplitude of a millivolt or more (peak to peak), while averaging 200–250 uV (Feinberg *et al.*, 1977). Though measurable with careful visual techniques, the amplitude decline is easily recognized only when sleep EEGs of adults are compared with those of children. The available data are too sparse to pinpoint the age level at which this change begins, but computerized measurements (Smith *et al.*, 1977) indicate that in males the average amplitude of delta waves drops by 30% between childhood and the age of 13. By the 30s this drop reaches 60%, and by the late 40s, about 75%. Thereafter delta amplitude may remain fairly stable, but this is uncertain. At upper age levels in men the effect is dramatic and unmistakable (Fig. 5.5). In women the amplitude decline is not as marked, but computerized comparisons of delta activity in men and women at various age levels are not yet available. Since women are longer-lived than men, delta amplitude may seem useful as an index of physiological age, but more likely there is a lifelong difference between the sexes with respect to EEG amplitude in general (Buchsbaum *et al.*, 1974).

This change in delta activity is part of a general reduction in the sleep EEG's amplitude over the life span which is not as apparent in other waveforms and is detectable for the most part only with electronic methods (Agnew, 1973). Spindling activity (sigma waves; 12–15 Hz), which is the hallmark of human NREM sleep, also loses amplitude after childhood or early adolescence (Feinberg, 1976; Principe & Smith, 1982), but this is a relatively subtle change because spindles average only 20–30 uV. Computerized analyses indicate that spindling frequency gradually increases after early adolescence, becoming about one cycle per second faster by the age of 70 (Principe & Smith, 1982). The absolute number of spindles tends to diminish after childhood, but not linearly in relation to age (Feinberg, 1976; Principe & Smith, 1982). On the other hand, the frequency of delta activity drops slightly with increasing age (by less than 0.2 Hz); this slowing seems to occur mainly before early adulthood (Smith *et al.*, 1977; Feinberg *et al.*, 1980).

Directly related to the reduction of delta amplitude is a gradual decrease in the amount of delta sleep. Standardized scoring of Stages 3 and 4 requires minimum amounts of delta activity in each scoring epoch, and this activity must reach a minimum amplitude (Rechtschaffen & Kales, 1968). Even when the amplitude requirement is reduced to allow for age-related decline, the decrease in delta sleep, particularly Stage 4, is ultimately drastic. Estimates of the daily amounts of Stages 3 and 4 at upper age levels vary widely. For men and women aged 70 and above, the estimates at one extreme are 6–7% of daily sleep time for Stage 4 and 23–24% for delta sleep (Feinberg *et al.*, 1967; Prinz, 1977). At the other extreme, Stage 4 and delta values 50% lower than these have been reported for women in their 70s, and virtual absence of delta sleep has been reported for men at that age level (Williams *et al.*, 1974). Fig. 5.3 presents an approximate average of the available estimates for men and women combined. It is generally recognized that the absence of Stage 4 at upper age levels, especially in men, is not uncommon. Because Stage 3 in older sleepers to some extent represents degraded Stage 4, it accounts for an increasing percentage of delta sleep. There is one report of more Stage 3 in elderly sleepers than in the young (Feinberg *et al.*, 1967). (See also Kahn & Fisher, 1969; Kales *et al.*, 1967; Miles & Dement, 1980.)

Computerized analyses (Smith *et al.*, 1977) have demonstrated that loss of delta amplitude is primarily responsible for reduced Stage 4 and delta sleep, 70% of the delta waves in men aged 43–79 falling under 20 uV peak amplitude (which is below the criteria usually employed for visual scoring of delta activity in studies of ageing) as opposed to 5% in children aged 3–5. A reduction in the absolute number of delta waves probably also contributes to the lowered per-

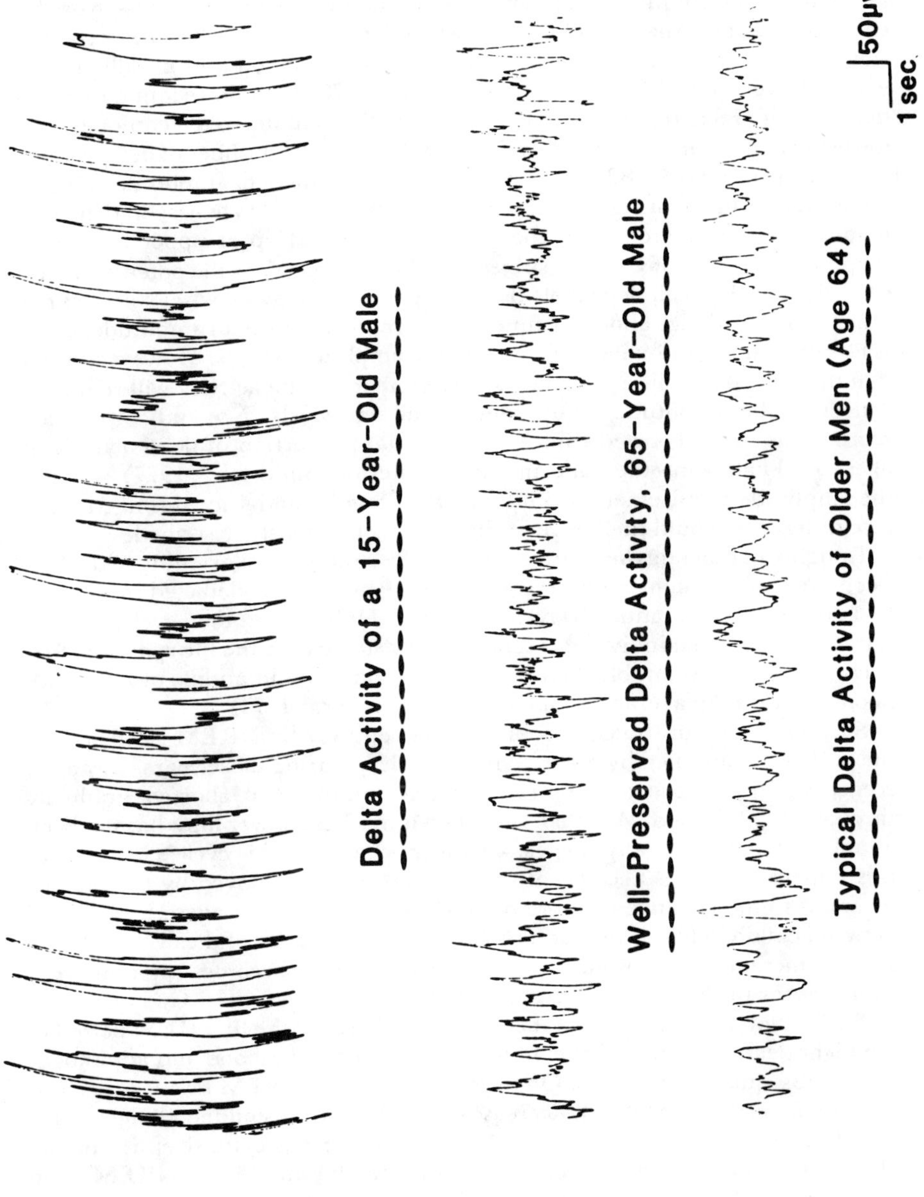

Fig. 5.5 Recordings of human delta activity at its peak amplitude from F_4–A_1 derivations in sleeping males of different ages. (Reprinted by permission from Figure 1, page 433; in *Sleep Disorders: Basic and Clinical Research* by M. H. Chase and E. D. Weitzman (eds.) Copyright 1983, Spectrum Publications, Inc., Jamaica, New York.)

centages of Stage 4 and delta sleep, but there is a disagreement on this point. Smith *et al.* reported that the number of waves exceeding 5 uV peak amplitude remained constant across the life span, but this is questionable because their statistical analyses appear inadequate. (While tests between five successive age levels showed only minor differences, it seems there were no tests across the entire age range. Analyses of the published data by the present author show a statistically significant 12% reduction between childhood and middle age in waves above 5 uV.) Moreover, Feinberg *et al.* (1978; 1980) have found reduced delta activity related to aging in two studies with computerized techniques. On the other hand, emphasizing the relative stability of the number of delta waves, Webb and Dreblow (1982) have advocated abandonment of amplitude requirements for visual scoring of sleep at upper age levels. When scored in this manner, they have reported, the amount of delta sleep at upper age levels 'approximates that of younger subjects'. This approach has the potential merit of giving weight to all detectable delta activity. This may be wise, since, in the absence of knowledge about the functional significance of delta amplitude, there is no compelling rationale for ignoring low-amplitude waves. However, proof that there is no age difference in visually scoreable delta activity will require a waiver of the amplitude requirement at all age levels. No study with such scoring has been reported. Since a substantial proportion of delta activity at ages 25–34 falls below the usual amplitude criterion (Smith *et al.*, 1977), waiving the amplitude requirement should increase Stages 3 and 4 for this age range. Age differences could then remain the same as previously described.

Roughly paralleling the changes in delta sleep there is a shortening of the first sleep cycle of the night (Feinberg & Floyd, 1979). This is depicted in Fig. 5.2 and summarized quantitatively in Fig. 5.6. Unlike the other cycles, whose durations in normal individuals remain fairly stable over the life span, the first cycle changes considerably. It attains its peak duration in middle or late childhood when it may average about 130 min (Feinberg, 1974).

Such extreme durations, occupied almost entirely by NREM sleep, reflect the peak levels attained by Stage 4 and delta sleep during those years. By adolescence this cycle becomes shorter, and it continues to shorten gradually throughout adulthood. Whether and when it reaches a lower limit has not been established. (Fig. 5.6 may suggest an abrupt change in this cycle's length, but this impression arises because of the age groupings employed by the investigators. As much change or more occurs gradually between ages 16 and 65 as between childhood and early adulthood.) That shortening of the cycle involves some reduction in the absolute amount of delta activity becomes apparent from comparisons of the cycle's components at different age levels. Change in the REM fraction is not a factor in the shortening because the first REM period of the night decreases only a little in duration between childhood and adulthood, and it subsequently increases. On the other hand, the NREM fraction, according to Feinberg's data (1974), decreases about 50% from childhood (ages 4–11) to old age (ages 67–96), i.e. from 115 to 55 min. Since delta sleep is initially about 85% of the NREM fraction (98 min), the 60 min loss of NREM sleep must mean a loss of delta activity. (This loss could not come just from the 17 min of non-delta sleep.) As opposed to an outright loss, the possibility of an age-related shift of delta activity from the early to the latter part of the night has been raised (Keane *et al.*, 1977), but this was not confirmed by another study from the same laboratory (Smith *et al.*, 1977) or by Feinberg *et al.* (1978, 1980).

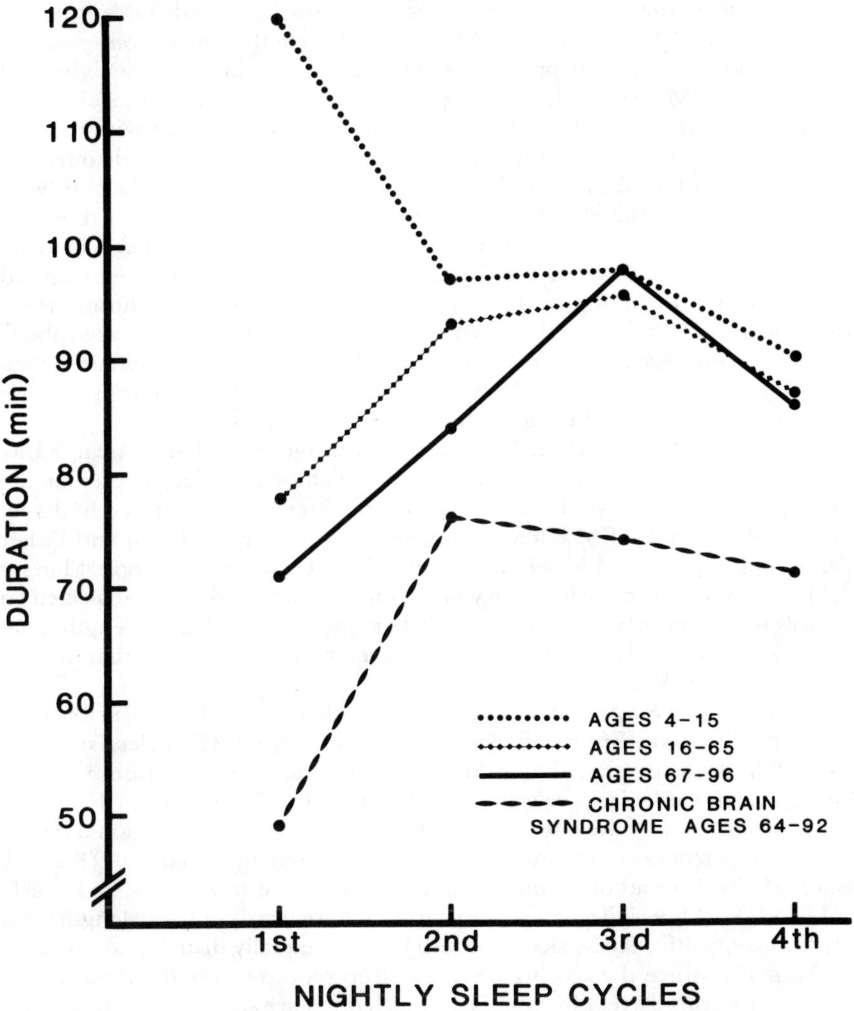

Fig. 5.6 Durations of the first four sleep cycles (NREM–REM) of the night at three age levels and in one group with chronic brain syndrome of old age. Males predominated in all groups. Durations were measured from NREM onset to the end of the succeeding REM period, not counting intrusions of wakefulness. Cycles beyond the fourth are not shown because of sparse data at upper age levels. (Copyright © 1979, The Society for Psychophysiological Research. Reprinted with permission of the publisher from 'Systematic trends across the night in human sleep cycles' by I. Feinberg and T. C. Floyd, *Psychophysiology*, 1979, **16**, 283–291.)

Other cycles of the night do not change like the first because delta sleep is concentrated early in the sleep period. Moreover, the lengthening of young adults' REM periods as the night progresses compensates for lost delta activity and shortened NREM sleep in the later cycles. This helps to maintain stability in cycle lengths. However, if sleep cycles are defined as beginning with the first REM period, there is a curvilinear, umbrella-shaped pattern of cycle duration across the night for all three of the normal age groups listed in Fig. 5.6, with cycle durations for the elderly tending to be intermediate between those for children and younger adults (Feinberg & Floyd, 1979). Changes in delta activity are not well-reflected by this definition. If cycle durations are measured in real time (i.e. including intrusions of wakefulness), almost all durations for elderly sleepers, whatever definition of the cycle is employed, are elevated above those of the other age levels. Only the first NREM–REM cycle in children then lasts longer than cycles of the elderly (Feinberg & Floyd, 1979). This is because wakefulness is common during sleep periods of the elderly.

Shortening of the first NREM period means an age-related decrease in REM latency, which is most commonly defined as the amount of sleep preceding the first REM period of the night. In addition to the previously described findings, evidence of reduced REM latency has come from studies by Kahn and Fisher (1969), and Zepelin and McDonald (1981). These studies also suggest longer REM latency at upper age levels in women than in men, as could be expected on the basis of women's better-preserved delta activity. As with cycle length, age-related decreases in REM latency are obscured by measurements that include wakefulness (e.g. Williams *et al.*, 1974).

Compared with Stage 4 and delta sleep, REM sleep is relatively stable over most of the life span. From childhood to early adulthood REM sleep occupies about 25% of sleep time, though its absolute duration drops from 3 to 2 h. During adulthood it declines gradually, falling below 1.5 h per day (less than 20% of sleep time) by the late 60s or early 70s (see Fig. 5.3). Additional reductions in the percentage and amount of REM are likely in the late 80s (Kahn & Fisher, 1969). Instead of becoming longer as the night progresses, as in early adulthood, REM periods in the later years are more nearly equal in length (Fig. 5.2). Consequently, REM sleep tends to be more equally distributed throughout the night. Since the scoring of REM sleep requires only the intermittent appearance of rapid eye movements — which often are sparse — the frequency of eye movements is an additional parameter of interest. Over most of adulthood the number of eye movements decreases only slightly, but from the 60s onward there is evidence of a sharper decline (Feinberg, 1976).

5.3 Daily Sleep Quotas

Whether total daily sleep time decreases markedly in old age, as commonly believed, is a question still awaiting resolution. Overnight laboratory studies tend to reinforce this impression (see reviews by Roffwarg *et al.*, 1966; Miles & Dement, 1980). However, some laboratory studies which strongly suggest a decrease in sleep time are of limited value with respect to this issue because they lack comparisons of elderly sleepers with young adults under identical conditions (e.g. Lairy *et al.*, 1962; Passouant, 1963; Kahn & Fisher, 1969; Prinz, 1977). One study that failed to give evidence of an age difference (Feinberg *et al.*, 1967) must be discounted because young sleepers were allowed less time in bed than the elderly. Studies of elderly sleepers have also varied in the age ranges covered, which have been extremely broad (e.g. 65–96; 71–95). This gives a diffuse picture of age differences but makes it impossible to pinpoint the extent of decline at any particular stage in later life. With these considerations in mind, the study by Williams *et al.* (1974), spanning most of adulthood decade by decade, must be judged the most definitive. Allowing the sleepers unlimited time in bed, this study found an average reduction in sleep time of half an hour from the 20's to the 70's, but with a greater reduction for men than for women (see Table 5.1). On the basis of tests between adjacent decades, the authors concluded that there were no significant age differences. However, a significant decline might have been detected by testing across the entire age range. With about the same laboratory procedures, Kales *et al.* (1967) reported a greater difference (1.2 h) between young adults and people aged 64–87. This difference appears significant; its size could be related to the higher age levels that were represented.

Aside from procedural and statistical shortcomings in the available data, laboratory studies cannot give wholly satisfactory estimates of age differences because they do not take napping into account. Ultimately, EEG recordings by means of portable devices worn by sleepers in their usual environments will provide satisfactory measures of daily sleep quotas. An intriguing example in this respect is a 24-h study with portable cassette recordings from five men and five women past the age of 90 in Vilcabamba, Ecuador, a community famous for extreme longevity (Okudaira *et al.*, 1981). Nocturnal sleep time averaged 422 min, but total sleep time for the 24 h, including naps for some individuals, averaged 458 min. The 36 min of sleep obtained by napping would be overlooked in a laboratory study, but could be sufficient to influence conclusions about the effects of ageing.

Despite imprecision in subjective estimates of sleep time, surveys on sleep habits are an indispensable supplement for laboratory studies because they can provide information on napping and lend themselves to the study of large samples. Not all surveys have dealt with napping, but only surveys that ignored it in the calculation of daily sleep quotas have indicated reduced sleep time in old age. (See McGhie & Russell, 1962; Gerard *et al.*, 1978.) That sleep time may increase with age even aside from napping has been suggested by the most extensive survey on record. This was a health study by the American Cancer Society, with questionnaires completed by 823,065 participants who had no prior history of cardiovascular disease or diabetes (Kripke *et al.*, 1979). Along with questions about insomnia and use of sleeping pills, the questionnaire inquired, 'How many hours of sleep do you usually get at night?' With increasing age, more men and women alike reported short sleep durations (less than 6 h), but an even greater number reported long durations (9 h or more). The long: short ratio rose dramatically with age, especially for men (Table 5.2). From the early 30s to the age of 70 women's sleep time did not change (averaging slightly less than 8 h), and men's increased somewhat (from 7.8 to 8.1 h). From 70 to 90, however, as could be expected with the dramatic increase in the percentage of long sleep durations, average sleep time increased to 8.8 h for men and 8.6 h for women.

Surveys that have included naps when estimating daily sleep quotas have found little or no change in old age. In Britain 509 people kept 24 h sleep charts

Table 5.1 Estimates of Total Daily Sleep Time During Adulthood Obtained by Three Different Procedures

Age group	Overnight laboratory recordings (Williams *et al.*, 1974) (Mean sleep time, min)[1]		24-hour charts (Tune, 1969a, b) (Mean sleep time, min)[2]	Questionnaires: sleep + napping (Zepelin, 1973 & data on file) (Mean sleep time, min)[3]	
	Men	Women	Men and women combined	Men	Women
20–29	419 (15)* ($n = 11$)	430 (22) ($n = 10$)	460 (25 men, 35 women)	454 (51) ($n = 40$)	—[4]
30–39	421 (22) ($n = 10$)	426 (31) ($n = 10$)	462 (36 men, 27 women)	434 (48) ($n = 90$)	443 (60) ($n = 34$)
40–49	389 (47) ($n = 10$)	425 (23) ($n = 11$)	445 (63 men, 39 women)	430 (50) ($n = 102$)	436 (44) ($n = 46$)
50–59	390 (49) ($n = 12$)	431 (35) ($n = 11$)	435 (77 men, 55 women)	432 (58) ($n = 110$)	425 (47) ($n = 57$)
60–69	407 (45) ($n = 10$)	405 (56) ($n = 11$)	455 (46 men, 52 women)	444 (59) ($n = 70$)	431 (56) ($n = 59$)
70–79	373 (87) ($n = 11$)	413 (37) ($n = 10$)	453 (24 men, 30 women)	477 (47)[5] ($n = 13$)	480 (60) ($n = 18$)

* Standard deviations that were available are in parentheses.

[1] The authors concluded there were no age differences but reported no statistical tests across the entire age range.

[2] For a subsample of this data ($n = 240$) with similar sleep times the author reported that analysis of variance showed a significant effect for age ($p < .05$) but not for sex.

[3] With ages 20–29 excluded, two-way analysis of variance (age × sex) showed a significant effect for age ($p < .05$). This effect was not significant when the analysis was confined to people employed full-time or if ages 70–79 were excluded because of small sample size.

[4] Data not collected.

[5] Includes two men aged 80–81.

Table 5.2 Percentages of Men and Women with Long and Short Nightly Sleep Durations

	Men		Women	
Age group	Short durations (< 6 h)	Long durations (≥ 9 h)	Short durations (< 6 h)	Long durations (≥ 9 h)
30–34	2.50	6.55	2.51	8.49
35–39	2.52	5.73	2.32	7.56
40–44	2.38	5.70	2.21	7.59
45–49	1.95	6.32	2.48	7.36
50–54	1.92	7.06	2.97	7.05
55–59	1.89	7.96	3.42	7.35
60–64	2.04	10.05	3.87	8.75
65–69	2.36	14.01	4.35	10.57
70–74	2.62	17.75	5.16	10.02
75–79	3.17	20.44	5.98	15.44
80–84	3.56	26.31	6.16	22.71
85–89	4.00	38.80	6.03	30.72
≥ 90	4.70	49.80	5.10	43.90

Adapted from Kripke *et al.* (1979)

for an average of 52 days and scored every half-hour period for the occurrence of sleep (Tune, 1969a). From the 20s to the 70s there was only a 7 min decrease in daily sleep quotas. The shortest sleep time was in the 40s and 50s. This decline in mid-life was the basis of statistically significant change (Tune, 1969b) (see Table 5.1). Questionnaires about napping and sleep at night that were completed by 720 university graduates in the US gave similar results (Zepelin, 1973). For men and women combined, the shortest daily sleep time was in the 50s and the longest was in the 70s. A drop in mid-life was again the basis of statistically significant change, but the effect of age was not significant when the analysis was confined to people employed full-time (see Table 5.1). This was because average sleep time in the 70s dropped when retirees were excluded. Other surveys suggest stability of sleep quotas into the early 80s, especially if napping is taken into account (Clement & Bourliere, 1961; Strauch & Wollschlager, 1973; Olivier-Martin *et al.*, 1975).

The survey findings make it seem unlikely that sleep time decreases in later life, but there remains sufficient uncertainty to keep this an open question. The findings by Tune and Zepelin are strikingly in accord in suggesting a saucer-shaped, curvilinear pattern, with sleep quotas in the 70s equalling or surpassing those in early adulthood. However, this pattern could be peculiar to certain populations, since it was not present in the Cancer Society findings, which were based on more representative sampling. Moreover, although most survey findings make it seem that napping is responsible for reports of increased sleep time in the 70s, the Cancer Society study indicates that it is not the crucial factor, and is perhaps not even essential. Gerard *et al.* (1978) also reported increased daily sleep from the 70s to the 90s aside from napping, as did Laird

(1931). Based on Tune's (1968) figures for nap time as a percentage of daily sleep, only about 4 min of the 20-min increase he found from the 50s to the 60s could be accounted for by napping. Similarly, in Zepelin's findings (data on file), only 4 min of the 33-min increase in men's sleep time from the 60s to the 70s and only 11 min of the 49-min increase for women during the same time period could be accounted for by reports of increased napping. Obviously, other factors must be considered. In surveys people may not distinguish sufficiently between time spent asleep and time spent in bed; elderly people may report more sleep time simply because they spend more time in bed. Another possibility is suggested by the dramatic age-related increase in the percentage of people reporting long sleep durations in the Cancer Society study: perhaps long sleep durations promote survival into and during old age. This could be true even though the same study found that both high and low daily sleep quotas (at all age levels) were associated with relatively high mortality rates. A survivor effect remains possible because of the increase with age in the long: short ratio (see Table 5.2). Resolution of these issues will require not only more precise measurement of sleep time, but also longitudinal studies to check interrelationships of age, sleep time, and survivorship.

5.4 Sleep Disturbance

There is relatively little ambiguity about the increase of sleep disturbance in the later years. In the laboratory, middle-aged and elderly sleepers awake spontaneously during the night considerably more often than younger people, and they lie awake longer. The number of awakenings per night varies from study to study, depending in part on the length of time allowed in bed and on the investigator's criterion for scoring awakenings. Samples containing sleepers aged 80 and above have averaged as many as 10 awakenings (40 s or more in duration) during about 8 h in bed (Kales *et al.*, 1967). Typically, for sleepers in their 60s or 70s, three to six awakenings can be expected, which is still double or triple the number for young sleepers. Elderly sleepers spend significantly more total time awake because they also have greater difficulty returning to sleep after an awakening (Webb & Campbell, 1980). These disruptions of sleep become increasingly severe with advancing age, as indicated within elderly samples by substantial, positive correlations of age with the number of awakenings per night and with time spent lying awake (Feinberg *et al.*, 1967; Kahn & Fisher, 1969). Underscoring this trend are reports of extremely frequent awakenings in samples containing individuals aged 90 and above (Hayashi *et al.*, 1979; Okudaira *et al.*, 1981). An additional indicator of disturbed sleep related to ageing is an increase in the amount and percentage of Stage 1 NREM sleep, which is a transitional stage associated with arousals (Kales *et al.*, 1967; Williams *et al.*, 1974).

Sleep efficiency, which is calculated as the percentage of time in bed spent asleep, declines from 95% or better in early adulthood to 80–85% and less in the 70s and beyond, the downward trend becoming manifest in the 40s and accelerating in the 60s (Williams *et al.*, 1974; Miles & Dement, 1980). Two factors contribute to this loss of efficiency: more time in bed in the later years, and more time spent lying awake. With time in bed equated for young and elderly sleepers, efficiency for sleepers in their 60s is still less (Zepelin &

McDonald, 1981), and the difference rises along with the elderly sleepers' ages (Kales *et al.*, 1967). Since sleep latency (time taken initially to fall asleep) does not increase substantially in the laboratory until the 70s (Williams *et al.*, 1974), the loss of efficiency seems to be based almost entirely on wakefulness after sleep onset. However, survey data on this point must also be considered.

Surveys have provided much additional evidence of sleep disturbance at upper age levels, especially increased complaints of frequent awakenings accompanied by difficulty in returning to sleep (see review by Miles & Dement, 1980). However, surveys also indicate that laboratory studies may overstate the frequency of awakenings in old age. Although Tune (1969a) found that the frequency of awakenings increased linearly with age, they averaged only about three per week in the 70s. Another British survey found an average of only 1.6 awakenings per night for sleepers aged 65–98 (Gerard *et al.*, 1978). Undoubtedly amnesia for awakenings from sleep at home helps to explain these low frequencies, while laboratory procedures probably induce some awakenings and exaggerate the importance of brief arousals. The age difference in the number of awakenings in laboratory studies may also be magnified by an age differential in the reaction to laboratory procedures. In contrast to laboratory findings, some surveys indicate an age-related increase in the time required for initial sleep onset (Gerard *et al.*, 1978; Bixler *et al.*, 1979), but they leave the impression that this may occur only in women, as found by McGhie and Russell (1962). Other surveys found no age difference in this respect in either sex (Zepelin, 1973; Karacan *et al.*, 1976). Most surveys show a general increase in the use of sleeping pills (Miles & Dement, 1980) which could indicate increased difficulty in falling asleep, but the use of pills may also be prompted by increased difficulty of sustaining sleep throughout the night.

Surveys have also shown dramatic age-related increases in non-specific sleep complaints. In the American Cancer Society study, the percentage of men and women who checked 'insomnia' as a complaint increased linearly from about 8 and 14% respectively in the 30s to 17% of men in their early 80s and 31% of women in their 60s and beyond (Hammond, 1964). In other words, the percentage of respondents with this complaint doubled. The results were strikingly similar for an urban population in the state of Florida, USA, where the percentage of respondents that complained of 'trouble with sleeping' either 'often' or 'sometimes' also increased linearly during adulthood from 25 to 49% for men and women combined (Karacan *et al.*, 1976). Generally the age-related complaints disclosed by surveys are more common in women than in men (Strauch & Wollschlager, 1973; Miles & Dement, 1980), but laboratory studies have not sustained the impression that women have poorer sleep as they age. On the contrary, it seems that if there is any sex difference, men are at a disadvantage (Williams *et al.*, 1974). Evidence on this point is tenuous since men and women differ consistently only with respect to delta activity. Measures of sleep latency, sleep efficiency, and number of awakenings do not consistently distinguish between them in middle age and the later years. For the time being it is necessary to conclude that the greater frequency of women's complaints constitutes a difference only in the perception of sleep experience.

As previously noted, napping assumes importance in the later years because it may compensate for reduced nocturnal sleep. Increased napping could therefore be a sign of sleep disturbance and of possible change in sleep's temporal organization. Although surveys generally suggest that napping becomes increasingly prominent (Miles & Dement, 1980), the degree to which it is characteristic of old age is sometimes exaggerated. About 70–80% of people aged 70 and above are at least occasional nappers (Tune, 1969a; Gerard *et al.*, 1978), but napping appears just as common among college students (Lawrence & Shurley, 1971). This indicates that napping is to some extent situational and may increase in old age simply because of retirement and the availability of free time. Survey findings are consistent in showing that from age 30 onwards the length of naps increases with age, as does the percentage of daily sleep time obtained through napping, but even in the 70s naps account for only about 5% of daily sleep (Tune, 1969b; Zepelin, data on file). How much difference there is between the 70s and the 20s is uncertain: Tune reported napping was at a minimum during the 20s (about 3 min per day; less than 1% of sleep time), but Zepelin found almost as much in men in their 20s (20 min per day; 4% of sleep time) as in 70-year-olds (27 min per day; 5% of sleep time). In any event, the amount of napping in the later years is not sufficient to constitute a change in sleep's temporal organization. More impressive in this respect is a shift by older people to earlier bedtimes and earlier times of arising in the morning (Tune 1969a; Gerard *et al.*, 1978). There is limited evidence that napping compensates for sleep disturbance. Tune (1969a) found a significant but small correlation between the frequency of napping and nocturnal awakenings ($r = 0.19$). Zepelin (data on file) found similar correlations of napping by elderly men with self-reported sleeping pill use and difficulty of resuming sleep after an awakening.

5.5 Sources of Senescent Change

Satisfactory explanation of the senescent changes in sleep requires a distinction between normal ageing of the sleep process and alterations of sleep that are secondary to other manifestations of ageing. By definition, a normal age-related change is universal, or nearly so, within a species, occurring in virtually everyone, given that the individual lives long enough. (Some examples are changes in vision, audition, and muscular strength.) Sleep disturbance is often described as an inevitable accompaniment of ageing, but the available data hardly justify its classification as normal. A substantial percentage of elderly people seems free from such disturbance. An unknown proportion of the sleep disturbance found in old age has its inception earlier in life, and so may not be age-related. Moreover, sleep disturbance that arises in later life is not a unitary phenomenon but springs from a variety of causes. Along with normal ageing of the sleep process, these may include: (1) deterioration of sleep that is secondary to normal ageing in other physiological processes, (2) deterioration that is secondary to disease or mental disorders, (3) outright sleep pathology that is age-related, and (4) situational changes that affect sleep. Without recognition of these factors, normal change in the sleep process is exaggerated and oversimplified. For example, nocturia contributes importantly to the high frequency of awakenings at upper age levels, possibly accounting for 20% of the awakenings in laboratory studies (Feinberg *et al.*, 1967) and an even higher percentage in surveys (Gerard *et al.*, 1978; Zepelin & Morgan, 1981). Such awakenings should properly be ascribed to the normal, age-related reduction of bladder capacity, not to deterioration of the sleep process. Likewise, complaints of difficulty in sustaining sleep at night may be the result of napping, which can lessen the need for nocturnal sleep. In this instance the underlying cause may be situational, that is, the availability of free time owing to retirement.

Some illnesses are a source of sleep disturbance (Johns *et al.*, 1970; Williams *et al.*, 1974; Raskind & Eisdorfer, 1977), but there has been no quantitative assessment of the impact illness has on sleep in old age. Undoubtedly, mental distress associated with other problems of ageing is an additional disruptive force, but its impact is also difficult to measure. Complicating the picture is the fact that sleep disturbance may be a cause of illness as well as a consequence. The American Cancer Society survey found that mortality rates for some illnesses were associated with both long and short daily sleep quotas, but cause–effect relationships were not clear (Kripke *et al.*, 1979). Retired peoples' complaints of sleep disturbance are associated with self-ratings of poor health and poor morale, but it is uncertain whether sleep disturbance is consequence or cause (Zepelin & Morgan, 1981). Depression, which is the most prominent mental health problem in old age, is characterized by sleep disturbance (Kupfer *et al.*, 1978), but disorders of sleep are possible causal factors in some types of depression (Wehr *et al.*, 1979; Vogel *et al.*, 1980). There is a need for longitudinal research to identify antecedent–consequent sequences by tracking relationships over extended periods of time between health status on the one hand and sleep patterns on the other.

Recent research has disclosed sleep disorders that cannot be considered normal or secondary to illness but whose prevalence increases with age. The prime example of such outright age-related pathology is sleep apnea (periodic cessation of breathing during sleep). Some apnea (cessation of airflow lasting at least 10 s) or hypopnea (shallow breathing of similar duration) is normal at all age levels, mainly in REM sleep and in NREM Stages 1 and 2 (Phillipson, 1978). Relatively common in REM sleep, which is characterized by irregular breathing, are *central* apneas (marked by absence of respiratory effort), often in association with bursts of eye movements. Apneas may also be *obstructive* (marked by blockage of airflow), or *mixed* (part central, part obstructive). Multiple obstructive or mixed apneas associated with loud snoring and excessive daytime sleepiness lead to a diagnosis of sleep apnea syndrome (Association of Sleep Disorders Centers, 1979).

Disturbed breathing during sleep increases with age, especially in men (Webb, 1974; Block *et al.*, 1980), but the extent of this increase is not yet certain. Several studies have suggested that perhaps 30% of the elderly population has five or more apneas per hour of sleep, which would be considered pathological if associated with excessive daytime sleepiness (Ancoli-Israel *et al.*, 1981; Carskadon & Dement, 1981; Smyth *et al.*, 1981). However, one equally extensive study found a zero percentage with this many apneas (Bixler *et al.*, 1982). Since breathing disturbances during sleep do not typically depend on state of health or on respiratory abnormalities in the waking state, they must be sleep-induced, but why they increase with age remains to be ascertained. One possible cause is change in the respiratory passages. This could also explain why snoring (which is caused by inspiratory effort) increases with age until the 60s, by which time 60% of men and 40% of women are habitual snorers (Lugaresi *et al.*, 1980). A possible additional or alternative cause is change in the control of respiration during sleep. The deterioration of delta sleep, in which apnea is ordinarily rare, may also allow increased respiratory disturbances (Ware *et al.*, 1981).

Severe sleep apnea in clinical populations causes serious drops in blood oxygen saturation, which in turn causes cardiopulmonary stress that is a threat to health. Whether apnea arising in the later years has comparable effects, and whether it is a cause of other sleep disturbance, is not yet clear. If apnea is an important source of age-related sleep disturbance it should be associated with subjective complaints regarding sleep or excessive daytime sleepiness, but this is not the case, since elderly sleepers with breathing disturbances are typically asymptomatic (Ancoli-Israel *et al* ., 1981; Carskadon & Dement, 1981). One report suggesting that apnea causes increased daytime sleepiness in elderly people (Carskadon *et al.*, 1980) can be discounted on the basis of another finding in the same laboratory that daytime sleepiness does not vary with age (Carskadon *et al.*, 1981). Oxygen desaturation associated with apnea arising late in life may simply not be as severe as in clinical cases. However, one study indicates that apnea reduces REM sleep and increases wakefulness and Stage 1 in elderly sleepers (Ancoli-Israel *et al.*, 1981). Although less prevalent and less worrisome as a potential health problem, nocturnal myoclonus (also known as leg jerks or periodic movements during sleep) can also be classified as a sleep pathology that increases with age and may contribute to sleep disturbance (Ancoli-Israel *et al.*, 1981).

5.6 Normal Age-Related Changes

5.6.1 Delta Activity

Because of its prominence and because it qualifies as a normal change, the deterioration of delta activity (especially its loss of amplitude) commands attention as a major consequence of normal ageing in human sleep, but it cannot be assumed to mirror change in the sleep process. Both the initial development of delta activity and its later deterioration could reflect changes in the brain that are independent of sleep, namely, maturation and subsequent deterioration or loss of cortical neurons. This would be consistent with the principal theories of the EEG, which either hold that brain waves represent summated post-synaptic potentials in sub-populations of cortical neurons that are modulated by subcortical pacemakers (Elul, 1973) or attribute EEG activity to the cortex as a whole, with EEG patterns determined by structural features of the cortex and the extracerebral tissues (Nunez, 1981). In either view, degeneration and loss of cortical neurons (which are non-dividing) would cause loss of delta amplitude. Especially striking, in view of the importance attached to dendrites in cortical electrogenesis (Purpura, 1959), is the ageing pattern of dendritic atrophy and loss that recapitulates the maturational steps of the perinatal period, but in reverse order (Scheibel & Scheibel, 1975). This parallels the change in delta sleep.

Highlighting the possible importance of neuronal loss are findings that delta activity in aged albino rats gives no sign of reduced amplitude that can be reliably detected by either visual or electronic measurement (Zepelin *et al.*, 1972; Rosenberg *et al.*, 1979). This difference between species (see Fig. 5.7 for comparison with Fig. 5.5) could be related to stability in the rat's population of

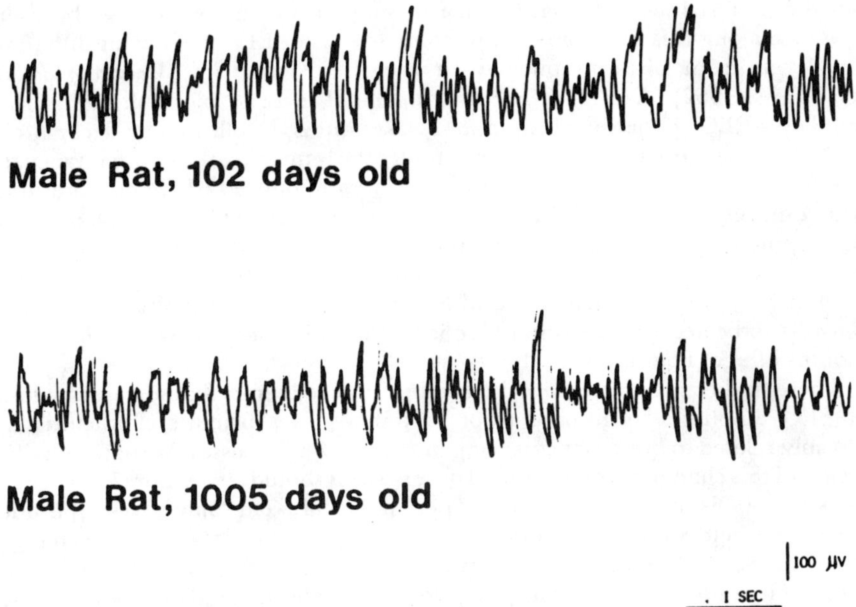

Fig. 5.7 EEG recordings during NREM sleep in albino rats at different age levels, obtained from screw electrodes threaded through the skull. (Reprinted by permission from Figure 4, page 441 in *Sleep Disorders: Basic and Clinical Research* by M. H. Chase and E. D. Weitzman (eds.) Copyright 1983, Spectrum Publications, Inc., Jamaica, New York.)

cortical neurons (Brizzee *et al.*, 1978; Diamond & Connor, 1981), as contrasted to severe neuronal loss in some cortical areas during human adulthood (Brody, 1978). Since the rat is not exempt from neuronal atrophy (Feldman & Dowd, 1975), the stability of its delta activity requires additional explanation. (Either neuronal atrophy does not seriously affect the EEG, or stability of the rat's neuronal population compensates for it.) In the laboratory mouse, whose neuronal population is more stable than humans', there is some age-related decline of delta amplitude late in life, but less drastic than in humans (Rosenberg *et al.*, 1978). This decline may require far-reaching neuronal loss which occurs sometime after 24 months of age (Johnson & Erner, 1972). Since human EEGs are recorded from the scalp and rodents' EEGs from the dura, it remains essential to determine whether differences in the findings could be related to this procedural difference. (Conceivably, aging of the human skull could alter its electrical conductivity in a manner that selectively attenuates slow-wave activity.)

Extensive studies of the waking EEG provide additional evidence that decline of delta amplitude occurs independently of changes in the sleep process. In humans between ages 2 and 21 the electronically measured amplitude of waking delta activity declines almost linearly with increasing age, as does the amplitude of some other frequency bands (Matousek & Peterson, 1973; see also John *et al.*,

1980). To what extent this change coincides with the change of delta amplitude during sleep is impossible to judge because similar sleep data are too meagre, but the patterns are sufficiently alike to suggest a common source. Further evidence along this line comes from comparisons of EEG activity at different age levels from birth to puberty in the rhesus monkey (*Macaca mulatta*) (Caveness, 1962). As Fig. 5.8 shows, an initial increase of amplitude in the monkey's EEG, both during sleep and wakefulness, is followed by decline, all within the space of two years. This resembles the human pattern from infancy to adulthood in compressed form and with more pronounced EEG deterioration. The compression reflects the monkey's relative maturity at birth coupled with a developmental rate six times as fast as a human's. Delta deterioration precedes the monkey's old age by 15 years or more (estimated from its maximum life span of 32 years). The likelihood of a similar timetable in the baboon (*Papio papio*) is indicated by a drastic reduction of its delta sleep between 12 and 24 months of age (Pegram *et al.*, 1969).

These findings, generally overlooked in the sleep literature, indicate that loss of EEG amplitude beginning prior to puberty is a primate characteristic, possibly related to brain structure or general growth processes. Perhaps classification of this change as maturational or senescent should await more knowledge of its cause. Distinct pre-pubertal and post-pubertal events may have amplitude decline as their common outcome. Possible prepubertal causes include change in the extra-cerebral tissues, biochemical change affecting EEG activity, and the culmination of maturational processes, whose effects could merge with those of post-pubertal neuronal deterioration and loss. Clearly the rhesus monkey, because of its EEG patterns and other similarities to humans (Ordy, 1981), is the ideal 'animal model' for the study of these issues.

5.6.2 *Intensity of sleep*

A promising measure of normal ageing in the sleep process is the auditory awakening threshold (AAT). Since a basic characteristic of sleep is reduced responsiveness to external stimuli, the level of stimulation required to cause a return to wakefulness provides a measure of sleep's intensity, or depth.

Table 5.3 Auditory Awakening Thresholds at Three Age Levels in Men and Women

Values shown are mean AATs, with sound pressure level expressed in decibels (dB). Standard deviations are in parentheses. Outcomes of statistical analyses are discussed in the text.

	Stage 4 (dB)		Stage 2 (dB)		REM (dB)	
Age Level	Men	Women	Men	Women	Men	Women
18–25 (n = 18)	105 (9)	97 (21)	85 (23)	78 (22)	85 (17)	80 (17)
40–48 (n = 18)	90 (17)	85 (23)	77 (25)	65 (19)	79 (16)	83 (18)
52–71 (n = 18)	73 (11)[1]	69 (23)	66 (14)	57 (11)	62 (9)	70 (20)

[1]The Stage 4 value is for only 3 men.

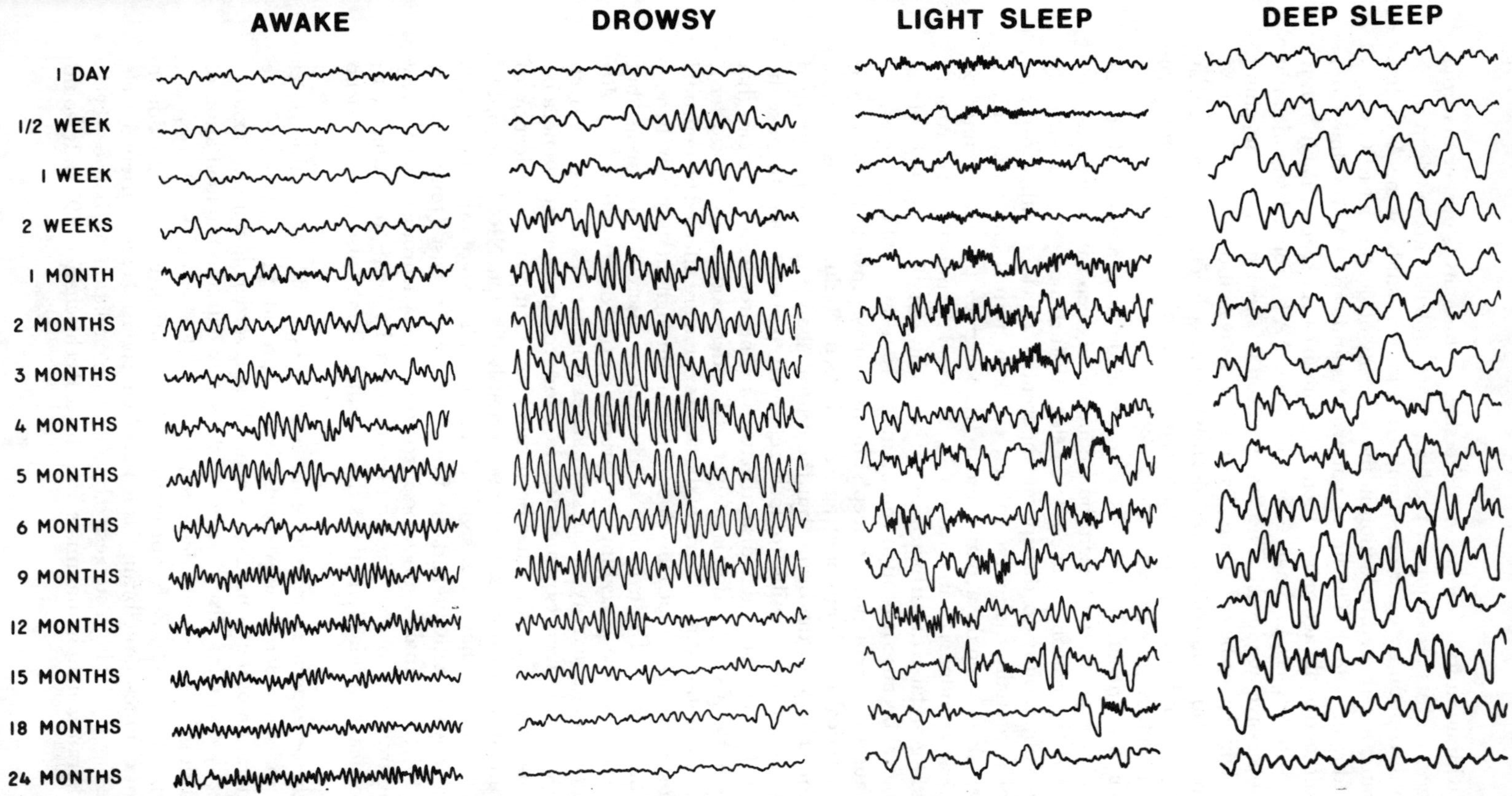

Fig. 5.8 EEG recordings during wakefulness and sleep at successive age levels in the rhesus monkey during the first two years of life. The composite summary is the outcome of longitudinal and cross-sectional comparisons. The recordings were from needle electrodes on the scalp. 'Deep sleep' corresponds to delta sleep, 'light sleep' to Stage 2. (Reproduced from W. F. Caveness (1962), *Atlas of Electroencephalography in the Developing Monkey*, by permission of Addison-Wesley Publishing Co.)

Assessed with auditory stimulation, delta sleep in humans is deeper than the other stages, and its reduction in the later years probably makes sleep more subject to disruption by external stimuli. In addition, study of the AAT has demonstrated age-related reduction in the intensity of sleep in all EEG stages (McDonald *et al.*, 1981). The linear pattern of significant AAT decline from young adulthood to old age in both men and women can be seen in Table 5.3. It is clearest with respect to Stage 4, in which the AAT dropped significantly between successive age levels. The Stage 2 drop was less steep, not reaching statistical significance between the 20s and 40s, as was also true of the REM AAT. Another indication of less deep sleep at upper age levels is the finding that elderly individuals become sensitized to repetitive auditory stimulation, while young sleepers habituate (Zepelin *et al.*, 1981).

Whether lowering of the AAT is a universal phenomenon classifiable as normal ageing remains to be seen, but reduction of sleep's intensity may well be the underlying reason for age-related sleep disturbance. Sleep's normally increasing vulnerability to disruption apparently coincides with a growing number of potentially disruptive influences, both normal and pathological. Who suffers from sleep disturbance and to what degree can be determined by both the basic soundness of an individual's sleep and the pressure of disruptive influences. Age-related disturbance cannot be readily classified as either normal or pathological because it is often compounded from causes of both types.

What causes the reduction of sleep's intensity may prove to be the fundamental theoretical question about aging and sleep. Reduced intensity must reflect some change in the brain, but the critical change cannot be specified because it has not been possible to 'localize' the sleep process, and because the interaction of the widespread neural structures and neurochemical systems that participate in sleep's regulation is not yet well understood (Morgane & Stern, 1974). An assumption that all parts of the sleep system are affected by neuronal loss is unjustified because such loss does not occur throughout the brain (Brody, 1978). What is needed is evidence of changes in discrete brain areas, but relevant data are sparse. Recalling the part that cortical deterioration may play in the decay of delta activity, a question arises whether this also affects sleep intensity. A major influence by such deterioration seems to be ruled out because cortical responsibility for sleep has been ruled out. Complete decortication of the cat eliminates slow wave activity and seriously disrupts NREM sleep, but does not abolish its behavioural signs; if only a small strip of orbital cortex is spared, slow wave activity and NREM sleep both persist (Jouvet, 1962; Moruzzi, 1972). Normally, subcortical structures are synchronized by activity descending from the cortex. This can be considered a sleep-promoting influence. If cortical deterioration affects this circuitry, it may also diminish sleep intensity.

As might be expected, organic brain syndromes of old age (multi-infarct dementia and senile dementia Alzheimer's type) provide the clearest evidence that degeneration of the brain alters sleep. These disorders apparently exacerbate typically occurring disturbance, as shown by extreme fragmentation of sleep, and drastically reduced delta activity and REM sleep (Feinberg *et al.*, 1967; Prinz *et al.*, 1982). Either pronounced brain shrinkage or a reduction in the amount of functioning brain tissue may be responsible for shortened cycle length (see Fig. 5.6). This is suggested by the positive relationship between cycle length and brain weight in mammals (Zepelin & Rechtschaffen, 1974). It would be surprising if sleep intensity were not also seriously affected. The neuronal changes that characterize Alzheimer's type dementia occur in subcortical as well as cortical areas and may directly affect all parts of the sleep system (Ishii, 1966). Since acetylcholine participates in REM sleep regulation (Gillin *et al.*, 1978), deficiency of the cholinergic system, which typifies Alzheimer's dementia (Bartus *et al.*, 1982), could be responsible for reduced REM time. It remains to be seen whether this deficiency is detectable in the brain stem, where REM centres are situated. Similar cholinergic deficiency in normals is possible but not as clear-cut (Bartus *et al.*, 1982). There is also a rough parallel between age-related decline in the REM sleep percentage and the normal loss of norepinephrine-containing cells in the locus coeruleus, which some investigators consider critical for REM sleep (Brody, 1978), but controversy about the role of this brain stem structure (Jones *et al.*, 1977) leaves the significance of this parallel in doubt.

Although there is now serious doubt that serotonin is the primary regulator of NREM sleep, it still appears to play some role (Morgane & Stern, 1974; Gillin *et al.*, 1978). Reduced serotonin concentration, indicating loss of serotonergic neurons in the raphe system, as found in the aged rat's brain (Meek *et al.*, 1977) may affect sleep intensity. An increase of monoamine oxidase (catabolic enzyme of serotonin), as found in the aged human hindbrain (Ordy, 1981), could be a contributing factor. Reduction of cerebral blood flow, which is associated with signs of ageing in the waking EEG, has also been mentioned as an influence on sleep, but the only sleep variable reported to correlate with blood flow is REM time (Prinz *et al.*, 1975). This correlation appears substantial between ages 75 and 90, but it is not clear how dependent it is on the correlation of blood flow and REM time with age. A similar question arises with respect to a suggestion that sleep disturbance increases with age owing to increased plasma norepinephrine, which might elevate sympathetic nervous system activity and cause nocturnal arousal (Prinz *et al.*, 1979). There is no evidence of an independent correlation between plasma norepinephrine and arousal during sleep. A direct comparison of autonomic variables (heart-rate, skin potential) and their relationship to sleep disturbance in young and elderly sleepers found no evidence in support of this hypothesis (Zepelin & McDonald, 1981).

There is widespread belief that change in sleep's biorhythmic properties is a major cause of its deterioration with increasing age (Miles & Dement, 1980). However, this is still largely speculation that relies on analogies with other physiological rhythms. There is a dearth of evidence regarding such change in sleep itself. As previously discussed, increased napping in the later years does not reach proportions that would constitute evidence of basic change in sleep's temporal organization. Data from a small sample of elderly sleepers studied in a free-running situation (without time cues) indicate that the sleep–wakefulness cycle retains its endogenous rhythmicity, with unchanged period length and REM–NREM cycling (Weitzman *et al.*, 1980). The only suggestion of significant change in the alternation of sleep and wakefulness has come from studies of the albino rat, whose cycle is synchronized with light and dark (sleep occurring mainly during the light period). Although still synchronized in this manner, the sleep of aged rats has twice been found more evenly distributed across light and dark periods than young rats' sleep (Rosenberg & Rechtschaffen, 1978; Rosenberg *et al.*, 1979), suggesting some loss of endogenous rhythmicity or of responsiveness to environmental cues. The import of these findings is unclear, however. When their light–dark cycle was reversed, the aged rats who initially showed a rhythm deficiency slept the same as young rats (Rosenberg *et al.*, 1980). Another study of rats found no age difference in the diurnal distribution of sleep (Zepelin *et al.*, 1972), nor was there evidence of such a difference in a comparison of young and aged mice (Rosenberg *et al.*, 1977).

It is noteworthy that in humans the suprachiasmatic nucleus, which seems to be the principal regulator of circadian behavioural rhythms (Webb & Dube, 1981), shows hardly any signs of deterioration in old age (Andrew, 1956). (There are no comparable data on other species.) Observational studies of rest–activity and sleep–wakefulness patterns in institutionalized elderly people indicate no loss of capacity for synchronization of these rhythms with environmental cues (Webb & Swinburne, 1971; Wessler *et al.*, 1976). If sleep suffers from biorhythmic change, it may be a result of altered relationships with other bodily rhythms. Overnight comparisons of sleepers at different age levels have shown that the nightly trough and subsequent upturn of body temperature tend to be reached earlier in older sleepers (Fig. 5.9). With age held constant, this pattern correlated significantly with wakefulness late in the night, especially in older women (Zepelin & McDonald, 1981). This is consistent with findings of short sleep episodes and frequent awakenings on the rising phase of the temperature cycle during sleep in time-free environments (Czeisler *et al.*, 1980).

Deterioration of sleep with advancing age could be related to a diminished sleep requirement. Proof that the daily quota remains stable into old age would not preclude this possibility, since some sleep in the later years, rather than fulfilling a physiological need, could merely 'fill' free time. Even if the quota remains stable, a reduced sleep requirement could be expressed by less intense, lighter sleep. In ecological perspective, stability of the daily quota — with enough flexibility to accommodate day-to-day variation in demands on the organism — would seem to be an adaptive requirement, since the duration and placement of the sleep period is complementary to the duration and timing of wakefulness and activity. In other words, sleep quotas probably remain stable because stability in the temporal pattern of a species' behaviour is essential for its survival. On the other hand, reduction of sleep's intensity, even if it entails sleep disturbance, leaves the temporal framework essentially unchanged. Consistent with these suppositions is the previously discussed evidence that sleep's biorhythmic properties persist in later life.

Because human sleep quotas are subject to social influences (e.g. work schedules, retirement), animal studies are desirable to test this view. Such studies at present are few. Primarily the albino rat has been studied, with findings that are not thoroughly consistent, but the most extensive 24-h study indicates stability of total daily sleep time until late in life, i.e. about 900 days (Rosenberg, 1980). (See also Zepelin *et al.*, 1972; Rosenberg *et al.*, 1979.) A report of drastically reduced sleep time in aged laboratory mice (Eleftheriou *et al.*, 1975) must be discounted because of short recording periods with inadequate time for post-surgical recovery. In humans a striking indication of the sleep quota's persistence is contained in the finding that, despite its fragmentation, total sleep time over 24-h periods in Alzheimer-type dementia patients was virtually identical to sleep time in age-equated normals (Prinz *et al.*, 1982).

Stable sleep quotas notwithstanding, there could be an age-related reduction in the capacity for sleep. This is suggested by a finding that older men (ages

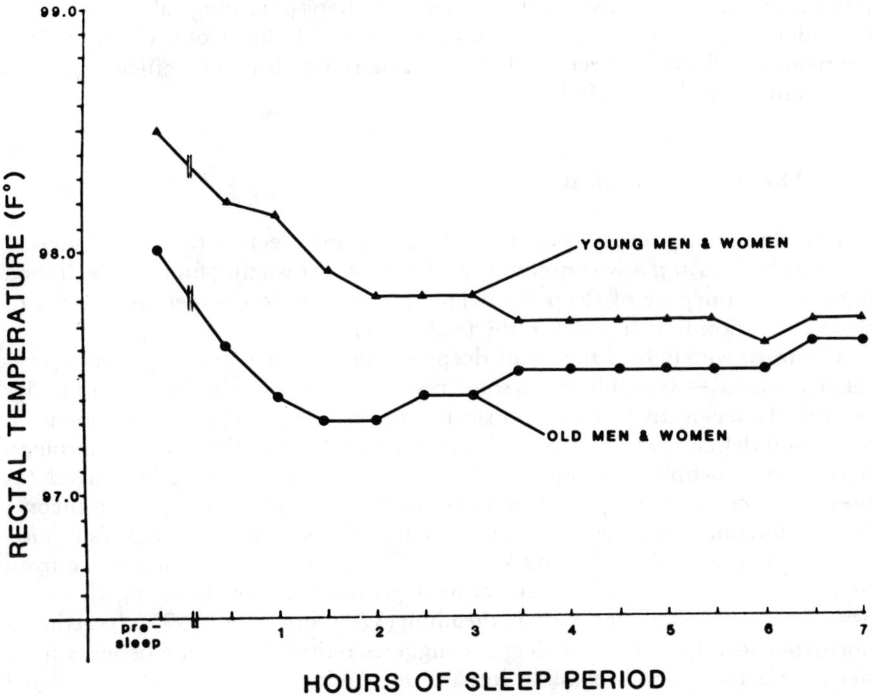

Fig. 5.9 Comparisons of rectal temperature in young sleepers (ages 18–23) and older sleepers (ages 57–71) prior to and during sleep, with averages calculated each half hour and averaged over two nights. (Reprinted by permission from Figure 2, page 438 in *Sleep Disorders: Basic and Clinical Research* by M. H. Chase and E. D. Weitzman (eds.) Copyright 1983, Spectrum Publications, Inc., Jamaica, New York.)

50–60), when asked to sleep as long as possible in the laboratory, slept only 61 min more than usual, while young men (ages 20–29) slept 165 min more (Campbell & Webb, 1980). Increased tolerance for sleep loss — and hence a reduced need for sleep — has been suggested by a survey finding that men aged 35–85 reported fewer ill effects from sleep loss than younger men (Laird, 1931). A contrary impression was reported by Webb and Agnew (1962), who found that 220-day-old rats became exhausted sooner than younger rats on a continuously rotating running wheel that presumably deprived them of sleep. The investigators suggested that the older animals had less tolerance for sleep loss, but this inference is debatable. Independently of their need for sleep, the older animals may have been less able to withstand the stressful procedure. There may be some parallel here with the few findings on sleep deprivation at different age levels in humans. During 66–127 h of sleep deprivation (Vojtechovsky *et al.*, 1969), men in their 40s consistently showed greater decrements of physical strength and energy mobilization than men in their 20s, but for the first 60 h or so the older men showed better emotional tolerance of sleep loss, and their mental efficiency suffered less. As sleep deprivation was prolonged, emotional attitudes and mental efficiency in the older men suffered more. This seemed to occur because of their physical decrements. Perhaps physiological deficits made the older people especially sensitive to the stressful effects of prolonged sleep deprivation. Physical effects could have impaired their mental efficiency. This issue remains to be clarified.

5.7 Theoretical Implications

A guiding assumption in the study of ageing and sleep is that knowledge of normal changes and any consequences they have for waking functions will shed light on the purpose of sleep. To what extent then do competing theories of sleep's function find support in the facts under review?

The most widely held theory of sleep — and the one usually applied to age-related change — is that it serves some restorative purpose in the brain or body, or both. Deteriorative changes in sleep supposedly contribute to physiological or mental deficits; who sleeps well should age relatively little. For example, a finding that people with long daily sleep quotas tend to be long-lived (as previously conjectured) could be claimed as evidence for restorative theory. Despite its common-sense appeal, this theory suffers from a shortage of supporting evidence (see discussion by Webb, 1975a). Some support has come from findings that daily peaks in the secretion of growth hormone in young adults are associated with delta sleep early in the night (Weitzman *et al.*, 1975). Its reduced nocturnal secretion in older sleepers suggests reduced anabolic benefits from sleep, and therefore a possible impact on waking functions. However, the reduced secretion rates are unrelated to the amount of delta sleep (Carlson *et al.*, 1972; Prinz *et al.*, 1976), and there is no evidence of any related functional decrement. Since the capacity for growth hormone secretion seems unaffected by ageing, there may simply be a reduced metabolic need for it (Andres & Tobin, 1977).

An important version of restorative theory applied to ageing is the sleep–cognition hypothesis, which holds that age-related deterioration of sleep represents reduced effectiveness of restorative brain processes that are essential for waking cognitive functions, i.e. acquisition and processing of information (Feinberg *et al.*, 1967; Feinberg, 1974; 1976). According to this hypothesis, delta sleep plays a critical role. This is suggested by (1) the decrease of delta sleep and diminution of delta amplitude during the sleep period, both presumably reflecting consummation or exhaustion of the sleep process, and (2) similar changes when the amount of wakefulness intervening between sleep periods is reduced, presumably lessening production of the 'substrate' necessary for delta activity (Feinberg *et al.*, 1978, 1982). The resemblance between these changes and the effects of ageing is taken as support for the view that age-related change in delta activity is related to cognitive decline. This presumed relationship could mean either reduced need for delta activity or reduced support for waking cognition, but the latter interpretation seems to take priority. In either event, the hypothesis remains speculative. The analogy between change in delta during the sleep period and its change over the life span would be plausible if there was evidence in either case of a relationship with cognitive functions. In the absence of such evidence, the same facts can be used to support a variety of theories (e.g. that sleep is for bodily restoration). Evidence regarding cognition has been sought unsuccessfully in correlations of delta variables with IQ tests in late adulthood (Feinberg *et al.*, 1967; Feinberg, 1976). The narrow range of delta variables in such studies could account for the negative findings. However, prospects for confirmation of the sleep-cognition hypothesis at lower age levels are not promising, since most of the change in delta occurs when people are near their peak of intellectual function, and IQ scores rise or remain stable during most of this period (Botwinick, 1977). The analogy between the life span and the sleep period is questionable also because similar changes in delta activity could stem from a variety of causes, some of them, as previously discussed, not even sleep-related. Moreover, there is no evidence that delta activity makes a unique contribution, distinguishable from the rest of sleep (Johnson, 1973). It is time to consider the possibility that the changes in delta activity, like the greying of the hair, have no consequence for vital functions.

Although Feinberg (1974) has dismissed REM sleep as unimportant for cognition, it correlated significantly with IQ measures in his data (Feinberg *et al.*, 1967). Another study showed that the rate of decline in IQ measures in elderly people over an 18-year period correlated with the amount of REM sleep obtained per day at the end of that period (Prinz, 1977). (REM sleep was measured only at the end of the 18-year period; there was no evidence that REM sleep and IQ scores declined together.) These relationships between REM sleep and IQ could exist because some ageing process (perhaps change in cerebral blood flow) affects both. Before change in REM sleep can be considered a cause of change in cognitive processes there must be evidence of an independent relationship between them. The possibility of such a relationship seems greater for REM sleep than for delta.

An alternative to restorative theory is the view that sleep is simply a state of adaptive immobility or 'non-responding' that is timed in a manner consistent with a species' environmental adaptation (Meddis, 1975; Webb, 1975a). Sleep quotas are presumed to vary with a species' status as prey or predator and with the amount of time required for self-maintenance (foraging, etc.). Since this theory makes daily quotas the critical issue, the principal question regarding the life span that it should be called upon to answer is why sleep quotas in altricial species are so high in early life. This pattern is contrary to Webb's (1975b) prediction that vulnerability to predation and high food requirements will be associated with low quotas. However, 'immobility theorists' typically adjust their reasoning post hoc to suit each circumstance (see Webb, 1975a), making the theory very slippery and essentially untestable in the life span context.

Facts of the life span fit best with theories of sleep that emphasize energy conservation as its purpose. One such theory holds that reduced metabolic rate during sleep offsets the cost of thermoregulation in birds and mammals (Berger, 1975). Another theory, based on the positive correlation between basal metabolic rates and daily sleep quotas in mammals, suggests that sleep is a state of enforced rest whose duration, so to speak, ensures a balanced energy budget. Perhaps animals with high metabolic rates tend to be long sleepers because activity is relatively expensive for them (Zepelin & Rechtschaffen, 1974). The decline of daily sleep quotas during maturation and the apparent reduction of sleep's intensity in adulthood are in accord with both theories, since these changes are paralleled by a decline in metabolic rate. In other words, the need for sleep and its intensity diminish as metabolic rate decreases. Walker and Berger (1980), utilizing overnight laboratory data for males aged 3–79 (Williams *et al.*, 1974) found a significant correlation of 0.98 between sleep time and the corresponding normative values for basal metabolic rate taken from published sources. With age held constant, the correlation of metabolic rate was 0.95 with sleep time and 0.89 with REM time. Zepelin (1982b) extended these analyses, combining data for males and females, and testing for correlations between age and sleep parameters with metabolic rate partialed out. Age then failed to correlate significantly with total sleep time or REM time, suggesting that the decline in metabolic rate could be the key process that reduces the need for sleep. However, delta and Stage 4 percentages and durations correlated significantly with age even when metabolic rate was partialed out ($r = -0.85$ to -0.94), suggesting that delta activity is governed by an age-related factor other than metabolic rate. The foregoing findings lend support to metabolic theories of sleep and refute Meddis' assertion (Chapter 3) that correlations between sleep time and metabolic rate are 'a statistical artifact'.

5.8 Summary

Sleep's biorhythmic character seems to make for stability of the daily sleep quota during adulthood, but within this framework there seems to be either a diminished need for sleep and/or diminished intensity. These changes, which underlie the age-related increase in sleep disturbance, could be caused by decline in metabolic rate, by other, still unsuspected systemic changes, or by alteration of the mechanisms responsible for sleep. Independent of these changes, it seems, is the deterioration of delta amplitude, which has a different time course. It is caused primarily by loss and/or deterioration of cortical neurons, and also perhaps by change in extra-cerebral tissues. Decrease in the number of delta waves suggests alteration in the activity of a pacemaker. Age-related change in the duration of the sleep cycle goes hand in hand with the change in delta activity. Extreme reduction of cycle length in chronic brain syndrome reflects the extensive loss of functioning tissue. Of all the normal changes in sleep parameters, the decline of REM time late in life seems most closely linked with waking functions. But aside from the distress obviously related to sleep disturbance, the functional consequences of the changes in sleep are still obscure.

Acknowledgements

The author's recent research was supported by National Institute on Aging Grant AG00723 and by a Biomedical Research Support Grant and a Research Fellowship from Oakland University. Cathleen S. McDonald collaborated on much of this research and made helpful suggestions for this chapter. The staff of Kresge Library at Oakland University gave valuable bibliographic assistance. Helen K. Poole supervised preparation of the manuscript.

References

ABE, K., SASAKI, H., TAKEBAYASHI, K., FUKUI, S. and NAMBU, H. (1978). The development of circadian rhythm of human body temperature. *J. Interdiscipl. Cycle Res.*, **9**, 211–216.

AGNEW, H. W. (1973). Integrator analysis of the sleep electroencephalogram. *Electroenceph. Clin. Neurophys.*, **34**, 391–397.

ALLISON, T., VAN TWYVER, H. and GOFF, W. R. (1972). Electrophysiological studies of the echidna (*Tachyglossus aculeatus*). *Arch. Ital. Biol.*, **110**, 145–184.

ANCOLI-ISRAEL, S., KRIPKE, D. F., MASON, W. and MESSIN, S. (1981). Sleep apnea and nocturnal myoclonus in a senior population. *Sleep*, **4**, 349–358.

ANDERS, T., EMDE, R. and PARMELEE, A. (1971). *A manual of standardized terminology, techniques and criteria for scoring of states of sleep and wakefulness in newborn infants*, Los Angeles: UCLA Brain Information Service.

ANDRES, R. and TOBIN, J. D. (1977). Endocrine systems. In: C. E. FINCH and L. HAYFLICK, (Eds.), *Handbook of the biology of aging*, New York: Van Nostrand Reinhold, pp. 357–378.

ANDREW, W. (1956). Structural alterations with aging in the nervous system. *J. Chronic Diseases*, **3**, 575–596.

ASSOCIATION OF SLEEP DISORDERS CENTERS (1979). Diagnostic classification of sleep and arousal disorders. *Sleep*, **2**, 1–137.

BARTUS, R. T., DEAN, R. L., BEER, B. and LIPPA, A. S. (1982). The cholinergic hypothesis of geriatric memory dysfunction. *Science*, **217**, 408–417.

BERGER, R. J. (1975). Bioenergetic functions of sleep and activity rhythms and their possible relevance to aging. *Fed. Proc.*, **34**, 97–102.

BIXLER, E. O., KALES, A., SOLDATOS, C. R., KALES, J. D. and HEALEY, S. (1979). Prevalence of sleep disorders in the Los Angeles metropolitan area. *Am. J. Psychiat.*, **136**, 1257–1262.

BIXLER, E. O., KALES, A., SOLDATOS, C. R., VELA-BUENO, A., JACOBY, J. A. and SCARONE, S. (1982). Sleep apneic activity in a normal population. *Res. Comm. Chem. Pathol. Pharm.*, **36**, 141–152.

BLOCK, A. J., WYNNE, J. W. and BOYSEN, P. G. (1980). Sleep-disordered breathing and nocturnal oxygen desaturation in post-menopausal women. *Am. J. Medicine*, **69**, 75–77.

BOTWINICK, J. (1977). Intellectual abilities. In: J. BIRREN, and K. W. SCHAIE, (Eds.), *Handbook of the psychology of aging*, New York: Van Nostrand Reinhold, pp. 580–605.

BRIZZEE, K. R., ORDY, J. M., HOFER, H. and KAACK, B. (1978). Animal models for the study of senile brain disease and aging changes in the brain. In: R. KATZMAN, R. D. TERRY and K. L. BICK (Eds.), *Alzheimer's disease: Senile dementia and related disorders,* New York: Raven Press, pp. 515–553.

BRODY, H. (1978). Cell counts in cerebral cortex and brainstem. In: R. KATZMAN, R. D. TERRY, and K. L. BICK, (Eds.), *Alzheimer's disease: Senile dementia and related disorders*, New York: Raven Press, pp. 345–351.

BUCHSBAUM, M. S. (1974). Age and sex differences in averaged evoked responses in a normal population, with observations on patients with gonadal dysgenesis. *Electroenceph, Clin. Neurophys.*, **37**, 137–144.

CAMPBELL, S. S. and WEBB, W. B. (1980). Sleep length and sleep termination in an aging population. *Sleep Research.*, **9**, 122.

CARSKADON, M. A., VAN DEN HOED, J. and DEMENT, W. C. (1980). Sleep and daytime sleepiness in the elderly. *J. Geriat, Psychiat.*, **13**, 135–151.

CARSKADON, M. A., RICHARDSON, G. S. and DEMENT, W. C. (1981) Twenty-four-hour sleep tendency in elderly and young adult subjects. *Sleep Res.*, **10**, 290.

CARSKADON, M. A. and DEMENT, W. C. (1981). Respiration during sleep in the aged human. *J. Geront.*, **36**, 420–423.

CARLSON, H. E., GILLIN, J. E., GORDEN, P. and SNYDER, P. (1972). Absence of sleep-

related growth hormone peaks in acromegalics and aged normal subjects. *Sleep Research*, **1**, 181.
CAVENESS, W. F. (1962). *Atlas of electroencephalography in the developing monkey*, Reading, Mass: Addison-Wesley.
CLEMENT, T. and BOURLIERE, F. (1961). Le sommeil chez l'adulte et les personnes âgées: Facteurs qui peuvent influer sur cet état. *Colloques internationaux du Centre de la Recherche Scientifique* (Paris), **96**, 155–173.
CZEISLER, C. A., WEITZMAN, E. D., MOORE-EDE, M. C., ZIMMERMAN, J. C. and KNAUER, R. S. (1980). Human sleep: its duration and organization depend on its circadian phase. *Science*, **210**, 1264–1267.
DIAMOND, M. C. and CONNOR, J. R. (1981). A search for the potential of the aging brain. In: S. J. ENNA, T. SAMORAJSKI and B. BEER (Eds.), *Brain neurotransmitters and receptors in aging and age-related disorders*, New York: Raven Press, pp. 43–58.
DREYFUS-BRISAC, C. (1979). Ontogenesis of brain bioelectrical activity and sleep organization in neonates and infants. In: F. FALKNER and J. M. TANNER (Eds.), *Human Growth* (Vol. 3), New York: Plenum Press, pp. 157–182.
ELEFTHERIOU, B. E., ZOLOVICK, A. J. and ELIAS, M. F. (1975). Electroencephalographic changes with age in male mice. *Gerontologia*, **21**, 21–30.
ELLINGSON, R. J. (1972). Development of wakefulness-sleep cycles and associated EEG patterns in mammals. In: C. D. CLEMENTE, D. P. PURPURA and F. E. MAYER (Eds.), *Sleep and the maturing nervous system*, New York: Academic Press, pp. 166–174.
ELLINGSON, R. J. (1975). Ontogenesis of sleep in the human. In: G. C. LAIRY and P. SALZARULO (Eds.), *The experimental study of human sleep: Methodological problems*, New York: Elsevier, pp. 129–146.
ELLINGSON, R. J. and ROSE, G. H. (1970). Ontogenesis of the electroencephalogram. In: W. A. HIMWICH (Ed.), *Developmental neurobiology*, Springfield, Ill: Charles C. Thomas, pp. 441–474.
ELUL, R. (1972). The genesis of the EEG. *Int. Rev. Neurobiol.*, **15**, 227–272.
FEINBERG, I. (1974). Changes in sleep cycle patterns with age. *J. Psychiat. Res.*, **10**, 283–306.
FEINBERG, I. (1976). Functional implications of changes in sleep physiology with age. In: R. D. TERRY and S. GERSHON (Eds.), *Neurobiology of aging*, New York: Raven Press, pp. 23–41.
FEINBERG, I., KORESKO. R. L. and HELLER, N. (1967). EEG sleep patterns as a function of normal and pathological aging in man. *J. Psychiat. Res.*, **5**, 107–144.
FEINBERG, I., HIBI, S. and CARLSON, V. R. (1977). Changes in EEG amplitude with age. In: K. NANDY and I. SHERWIN (Eds.), *The aging brain and senile dementia*, New York: Plenum Press, pp. 85–98.
FEINBERG. I., MARCH, J. D., FEIN, G., FLOYD, T. C., WALKER, J. M. and PRICE, L. (1978). Period and amplitude analysis of 0.5–3c/sec activity in NREM sleep of young adults. *Electroenceph. Clin. Neurophys.*, **44**, 202–213.
FEINBERG, I. and FLOYD, T. C. (1979). Systematic trends across the night in human sleep cycles. *Psychophysiol.*, **16**, 283–291.
FEINBERG, I., FEIN, G. and FLOYD, T. C. (1980). Period and amplitude analysis of NREM EEG in sleep: repeatability of results in young adults. *Electroenceph. Clin. Neurophys.*, **48**, 212–221.
FEINBERG, I., FEIN, G. and FLOYD, T. C. (1982). Computer-detected patterns of electroencephalographic delta activity during and after extended sleep. *Science*, **215**, 1131–1133.
FELDMAN, M. L. and DOWD, C. (1975). Loss of dendritic spines in aging cerebral cortex. *Anat. Embryol.*, **148**, 279–301.
GERARD, P., COLLINS, K. J., DORE, C. and EXTON-SMITH, A. N. (1978). Subjective characteristics of sleep in the elderly. *Age and Ageing*, **7** (Suppl.), 55–59.
GILLIN, J. C., MENDELSON, W. B., SITARAM, H. and WYATT, R. J. (1978). The

neuro-pharmacology of sleep and wakefulness. *Ann. Rev. Pharmacol. Toxicol.*, **18**, 563–579.

HAMMOND, E. (1964). Some preliminary findings on physical complaints from a prospective study of 1,064,004 men and women. *Am. J. Pub. Health*, **54**, 11–23.

HAYASHI, Y., EIICHI, O., SHIRO, E. and WANTANABE, H. (1979). The all-night polygraphies for healthy aged persons. *Sleep Research*, **8**, 122.

ISHII, T. (1966). Distribution of Alzheimer's neurofibrillary changes in the brainstem and hypothalamus of senile dementia. *Acta. Neuropathol.*, **6**, 181–187.

JOHN, E. R., AHN, H., PRICHEP, L., TREPETIN, M., BROWN, D and KAYE, H. (1980). Developmental equations for the electroencephalogram. *Science*, **210**, 1255–1258.

JOHNS, M. W., EGAN, P., GAY, T. J. A. and MASTERSON, J. P. (1970). Sleep habits and symptoms in male medical and surgical patients. *Brit. Med. J.*, **2**, 509–512.

JONES, B. E., HARPER, S. T., and HALARIS, A. E. (1977). Effects of locus coeruleus lesions upon cerebral monoamine content, sleep-wakefulness states and the response to amphetamine in the cat. *Brain Res.*, **124**, 473–496.

JOHNSON, H. A. and ERNER, S. (1972). Neuron survival in the aging mouse. *Exp. Geront.*, **7**, 111–117.

JOHNSON, L. C. (1973). Are stages of sleep related to waking behavior? *Amer. Scient.*, **61**, 326–338.

JOUVET, M. (1962). Recherches sur les structures nerveuses et les mecanismes responsables des different phases du sommeil physiologique. *Arch. Ital. Biol.*, **100**, 125–206.

JOUVET-MOUNIER, D., ASTIC, L. and LACOTE, D. (1968). Ontogenesis of the states of sleep in rat, cat, and guinea pig during the first postnatal month. *Devel. Psychobiol.*, **2**, 216–239.

KAHN, E. and FISHER, C. (1969). The sleep characteristics of the normal aged male. *J. Nerv. Ment. Dis.*, **148**, 477–494.

KALES, A., WILSON, T., KALES, J. D., JACOBSON, A., PAULSON, M. J., KILLAR, E. and WALTER, R. D. (1967). Measurements of all-night sleep in normal elderly persons: effects of aging. *J. Amer. Geriat. Soc.*, **15**, 405–414.

KARACAN, I., THORNBY, J. I., ANCH, M., HOLZER, C. E., WARHEIT, G. J., SCHWAB, J. J. and WILLIAMS, R. L. (1976). Prevalence of sleep disturbance in a primarily urban Florida county. *Soc. Sci. Med.*, **10**, 239–244.

KEANE, B., SMITH, J. and WEBB, W. (1977). Temporal distributions and ontogenetic development of EEG activity during sleep. *Psychophys.*, **14**, 315–321.

KLEITMAN, N., and ENGELMANN, T. G. (1953). Sleep characteristics of infants. *J. Appl. Physiol.*, **6**, 269–282.

KRIPKE, D., SIMONS, R., GARFINKEL, L. and HAMMOND, E. (1979). Short and long sleep and sleeping pills. *Arch. Gen. Psychiat.*, **36**, 103–116.

KUPFER, D. J., SPIKER, D. G., COBLE, P. A., and SHAW, D. H. (1978). Electroencephalographic sleep recordings and depression in the elderly. *J. Amer. Geriat. Soc.*, **26**, 53–57.

LAIRD, D. A. (1931). A survey of the sleep habits of 509 men of distinction. *Amer. Med.*, **26**, 271–275.

LAIRY, G. C., COR-MORDRET, M., FAURE, R. and RIDJANOVIC, S. (1962). Étude EEG du sommeil du vieillard normal et pathologique. *Rev. Neurol.*, **107**, 188–202.

LATASH, L. P. and SHLYK, G. G. (1975). Polygraphic characteristics of the dog's sleep. *Sleep Research*, **4**, 145.

LAWRENCE, B. E. and SHURLEY, J. T. (1971). Napping habits of a college student population. *Psychophysiol.*, **7**, 294.

LENARD, H. (1970). The development of sleep spindles in the EEG during the first two years of life. *Neuropaediatrie*, **1**, 264–276.

LUGARESI, E., CIRIGNOTTA, F., COCCAGNA, G. and PIANA, C. (1980). Some epidemiologic data on snoring and cardiocirculatory disturbances. *Sleep*, **3**, 221–224.

MATOUSEK, M. and PETERSEN, I. (1973). Frequency analysis of the EEG in normal

children and adolescents. In: P. KELLAWAY, and I. PETERSEN (Eds.), *Automation of clinical electroencephalography*, New York: Raven Press.
MCDONALD, C. S., ZEPELIN, H. and ZAMMIT G. K. (1981). Age and sex patterns in auditory awakening thresholds. *Sleep Research*, **10**, 115.
MCGHIE, A. and RUSSELL, S. M. (1962). The subjective assessment of normal sleep patterns. *J. Ment. Sci.*, **108**, 642–654.
MEDDIS, R. (1975). On the function of sleep. *Anim. Behav.*, **23**, 676–691.
MEEK, J. L., BERTILSSON, L., CHENEY, D. L., ZSILLA, G. and COSTA, E. (1977). Aging-induced changes in acetylcholine and serotonin content of discrete brain nuclei. *J. Gerontol.*, **32**, 129–131.
MEIER, G. W. and BERGER, R. J. (1965). Development of sleep and wakefulness patterns in the infant rhesus monkey. *Exp. Neurol.*, **12**, 257–277.
METCALF, D. R., MONDALE, J. and BUTLER, F. K. (1971). Ontogenesis of spontaneous K-complexes. *Psychophysiol.*, **8**, 340–347.
MILES, L. E. and DEMENT, W. C. (1980). Sleep and aging. *Sleep*, **3**, 119–220.
MORGANE, P. J. and STERN, W. C. (1974). Chemical anatomy of brain circuits in relation to sleep and wakefulness. In: E. WEITZMAN (Ed.), *Advances in sleep research* (Vol. 1), New York: Spectrum, pp. 1–130.
MORUZZI, G. (1972). The sleep-waking cycle. *Ergebnisse der Physiol.*, **64**, 1–165.
NUNEZ, P. L. (1981). *Electric fields of the brain: The neurophysics of EEG*, New York: Oxford.
OKUDAIRA, N., FUKUDA, H., OHTANI, K., NISHIHARA, K., ENDO, S. and TORII, S. (1981). Sleep patterns in healthy elderly persons in Vilcabamba, Ecuador. *Sleep Research*, **10**, 116.
OLIVIER-MARTIN, R., CENDRON, H. and VALLERY-MASSON, J. (1975). Le sommeil chez les sujets âgés. *Ann. Medico-Psychol.*, **1**, 77–90.
ORDY, J. M. (1981). Neurotransmitters and aging in the human brain. In: D. DANON, N. W. SHOCK and M. MAROIS (Eds.), *Aging: A challenge to science and society*, New York: Oxford.
PARMELEE, A. H., WENNER, W. H. and SCHULZ, H. R. (1964). Infant sleep patterns: from birth to 16 weeks of age. *J. Pediat.*, **65**, 576–582.
PASSOUANT P. (1963). Influence de l'age sur l'organization du sommeil de nuit et la periode de sommeil avec mouvements oculaires. *J. Psychol. Normals et Pathol.*, **41**, 257–279.
PEGRAM, V., BERT, J. and NAQUET, R. (1969). The ontogeny of EEG sleep patterns in the baboon. *Psychophys.*, **6**, 228.
PEGRAM, V. (1972). Comparison of field vs laboratory sleep in the baboon (*Papio papio*) and developmental sleep patterns in the young baboon. In: M. H. CHASE (Ed.), *The Sleeping Brain*, Los Angeles: Brain Information Service, pp. 33–36.
PHILLIPSON, E. A. (1978). Respiratory adaptations in sleep. *Ann. Rev. Physiol.*, **40**. 133–156.
PRINCIPE, J. C. and SMITH, J. R. (1982). Sleep spindle characteristics as a function of age. *Sleep*, **5**, 73–84.
PRINZ, P. N., OBRIST, W. D. and WANG, H. S. (1975). Sleep patterns in healthy elderly subjects: individual differences as related to other neurobiological variables. *Sleep Research*, **4**, 132.
PRINZ, P., BLENKARN. D., LINNOILA, M. and WEITZMAN, E. (1976). Growth hormone levels during sleep in elderly males. *Sleep Research*, **5**, 87.
PRINZ, P. M. (1977). Sleep patterns in the healthy aged: relationship with intellectual function. *J. Gerontol.*, **32**, 179–186.
PRINZ, P. N., HALTER, J., BENEDETTI, C. and RASKIND, M. (1979). Circadian variation of plasma catecholamines in young and old men: relation to rapid eye movement and slow wave sleep. *J. Clin Endocrin. and Metab.*, **49**, 300–304.
PRINZ, P. N., PESKIND, E. R., VITALIANO, P. P., RASKIND, M. A., EISDORFER, C., ZEMCUZNIKOV, N. and GEBER, C. J. (1982). Changes in the sleep and waking EEGs

of non-demented and demented elderly subjects. *J. Amer. Geriat. Soc.*, **30**, 86–93.
PURPURA, D. P. (1959). Nature of electrocortical potentials and synaptic organizations in cerebral and cerebellar cortex. In: C. C. PFEIFFER and J. R. SMYTHEIS (Eds.), *International review of neurobiology*, New York: Academic Press, pp. 47–163.
RASKIND, M. A. and EISDORFER, C. (1977). When elderly patients can't sleep. *Drug Therapy*. **7**, 44–50.
RECHTSCHAFFEN, A. and KALES, A. (1968). *A Manual of standardized terminology, techniques, and scoring system for sleep stages of human subjects*, Washington, DC: Public Health Service, US Govt Printing Office.
ROFFWARG, H. P., MUZIO, J. N. and DEMENT, W. C. (1966). Ontogenetic development of the human sleep-dream cycle. *Science*, **152**, 604–619.
ROSENBERG. R. S. (1980). *Lifespan changes in the diurnal sleep rhythms of rats*. Unpublished doctoral dissertation, University of Chicago.
ROSENBERG, R. S., ZEPELIN, H. and RECHTSCHAFFEN, A. (1977). Sleep in young and old mice. *Sleep Research*, **6**, 99.
ROSENBERG, R. S. and RECHTSHAFFEN, A. (1978). Lifespan changes in the diurnal sleep pattern of rats. *Soc. Neurosci. Abs.*, **4**, 125.
ROSENBERG, R. S., ZEPELIN, H. and RECHTSCHAFFEN, A. (1979). Sleep in young and old rats. *J. Gerontol.*, **34**, 525–532.
ROSENBERG, R. S., WINTER, J. and RECHTSCHAFFEN, A. (1980). Effects of light cycle phase reversal on sleep rhythms of young and old rats. *Sleep Research*, **9**, 105.
SCHEIBEL, M. E. and SCHEIBEL, A. B. (1975). Structural changes in the aging brain. In: H. BRODY, D. HARMAN and J. M. ORDY (Eds.), *Clinical, morphologic, neurochemical aspects in the aging central nervous system*, New York: Raven Press, pp. 11–37.
SMITH, J. R., KARACAN, I. and YANG, M. (1977). Ontogeny of delta activity during human sleep. *Electroenceph. Clin. Neurophys.*, **43**, 229–237.
SMYTH, M., GIBLIN, E. C. and LEE, K. (1981). Prevalence of apneas and oxygen desaturation during sleep in healthy older men. *Sleep Research*, **10**, 118.
STERMAN, M. D. and HOPPENBROUWERS, T. (1971). The development of sleep-waking and rest-activity patterns from fetus to adult in man. In: M. B. STERMAN, D. J. MCGINTY and A. M. ADINOLFI, (Eds.), *Brain development and behavior*, New York: Academic Press, pp. 203–227.
STRAUCH, I. and WOLLSCHLAEGER, M. (1973). Sleep behavior in the aged. In: U. JOVANOVIC (Ed.), *The nature of sleep*, Stuttgart: Fischer, pp. 129–131.
TANGUAY, P. E. ORNITZ, E. M., KAPLAN, A. and BOZZO, E. S. (1975). Evolution of sleep spindles in childhood. *Electroenceph. Clin. Neurophys.*, **38**, 175–181.
TUNE, G. S. (1968). Sleep and wakefulness in normal human adults. *Brit. Med. J.*, **2**, 269–271.
TUNE, G. S. (1969a). Sleep and Wakefulness in 509 normal human adults. *Br. J. Med. Psychol.*, **42**, 75–80.
TUNE, G. S. (1969b). The influence of age and temperament on the adult human sleep-wakefulness pattern. *Br. J. Psychol.*, **60** 431–441.
URSIN, R. (1968). The two stages of slow wave sleep in the cat and their relation to REM sleep. *Brain Res.*, **11**, 347–356,
VERLEY, R. and GARMA, L. (1975). The criteria of sleep stages during ontogeny in different animal species. In: G. C. LAIRY and P. SALZARULO (Eds.), *The experimental study of human sleep: Methodological problems*, New York: Elsevier, pp. 109–125.
VOGEL, G. W., VOGEL, F., MCABEE, R. S. and THURMOND, A. J. (1980). Improvement of depression by REM sleep deprivation. *Arch. Gen. Psychiat.*, **37**, 247–253.
VOJTECHOVSKY, M., BREZINOVA, V., SIMANE, Z. and HORT, V. (1969). An experimental approach to sleep and aging. *Hum. Devel.*, **12**, 64–72.
WALKER, J. M. and BERGER, R. J. (1980). Sleep as an adaptation for energy conservation functionally related to hibernation and shallow torpor. *Prog. Brain Res.*, **53**, 255–278.

WARE, J. C. MOORAD, P. J. and FRANKLIN, D. B. (1981). Reduction of sleep apnea during Stage 4 sleep. *Sleep Research*, **10**, 241.

WEBB, P. (1974). Periodic breathing during sleep. *J. Applied Physiol.*, **37**, 899–903.

WEBB. W. B. (1975a). *Sleep: The gentle tyrant*, Englewood Cliffs, NJ: Prentice-Hall.

WEBB, W. B. (1975b). The adaptive functions of sleep patterns. In: P. LEVIN and W. P. KOELLA (Eds.), *Sleep 1974*, Basel: Karger, pp. 13–19.

WEBB, W. B. and AGNEW, H. W. (1962). Sleep deprivation, age, and exhaustion time in the rat. *Science*, **136**, 1122.

WEBB, W. B and CAMPBELL, S. S. (1980). Awakenings and return to sleep in an older population. *Sleep*, **3**, 41–46.

WEBB, W. B. and DREBLOW, L. M. (1982). A modified method for scoring slow wave sleep of older subjects. *Sleep*, **5**, 195–199.

WEBB, W. B. and DUBE, M. G. (1981). Temporal characteristics of sleep. In: J. ASCHOFF (Ed.), *Handbook of behavioral neurobiology: Vol. 4, Biological Rhythms*, New York: Plenum Press, pp. 499–522.

WEBB, W. B. and SWINBURNE, H. (1971). An observational study of sleep of the aged. *Percept. Mot. Skills*, **32**, 895–898.

WEHR, T. A., WIRZ-JUSTICE, A., GOODWIN, F. K., DUNCAN, W. and GILLIN, J. C. (1979). Phase advance of the circadian sleep wake cycle as an antidepressant. *Science*, **206**, 710–713.

WEITZMAN, E. D., BOYAR, R. M., KAPEN, S. and HELLMAN, L. (1975). The relationship of sleep and sleep stages to neuroendocrine secretion and biological rhythms in man. *Recent Progr. Hormone Res.*, **31**, 399–446.

WEITZMAN, E. D., CZEISLER, C. A. and MOORE-EDE, M. D. (1979). Sleep-wake, neuroendocrine and body temperature circadian rhythms under entrained and non-entrained (free-running) conditions in man. In: M. SUDA, O. HAYAISHI and H. NAKAGAWA (Eds.), *Biological rhythms and their central mechanisms*, Amsterdam: Elsevier, pp. 199–227.

WEITZMAN, E. D., CZEISLER, C. A. and ZIMMERMAN, J. C. (1980). Sleep-wake organization during 'free-running' in older men. *Sleep Research*, **9**, 279.

WESSLER, R., RUBIN, M. and SOLLBERGER, A. (1976). Circadian rhythm of activity and sleep-wakefulness in elderly institutionalized persons. *J. Interdiscipl. Cycle Res.*, **7**, 333–348.

WILLIAMS, R. L., KARACAN, I. and HURSCH, C. (1974). *Electroencephalography of human sleep: Clinical applications*, New York: John Wiley.

ZEPELIN, H. (1973). A survey of age differences in sleep patterns and dream recall among well-educated men and women. *Sleep Research*, **2**, 81.

ZEPELIN, H. (1980). REM sleep and the altricial-precocial dimension. *Sleep Research*, **9**, 114.

ZEPELIN, H. (1982a). Aging and sleep. In: *Roche seminars on aging* No. 9, Section 1, Nutley, NJ: Roche Products Inc.

ZEPELIN, H. (1982b). *Metabolic rate and the aging of sleep*. Paper presented to 22nd annual meeting, Association for the Psychophysiological Study of Sleep, San Antonio.

ZEPELIN, H. (1983). Normal age-related change in sleep. In: M. H. CHASE and E. D. WEITZMAN (Eds.), *Sleep disorders: Basic and clinical research*, New York: Spectrum.

ZEPELIN, H., WHITEHEAD, W. E. and RECHTSCHAFFEN, A. (1972). Aging and sleep in the albino rat. *Behav. Biol.*, **7**, 65–74.

ZEPELIN, H. and RECHTSCHAFFEN, A. (1974). Mammalian sleep, longevity, and energy metabolism. *Brain Behav. Evol.*, **10**, 425–470.

ZEPELIN, H., MCDONALD, C. S., WANZIE, F. J. and ZAMMIT, G. K. (1981). Age differences in auditory awakening thresholds. *Sleep Research*, **9**, 109.

ZEPELIN, H. and MCDONALD, C. S. (1981). Age and sex differences in physiological variables during sleep. *Sleep Research*, **10**, 119.

ZEPELIN, H. and MORGAN, L. E. (1981). Correlates of sleep disturbance in retirees. *Sleep Research*, **10** 120.

CHAPTER 6

Cellular Mechanisms of Wakefulness and Slow Wave Sleep

M. Steriade

This chapter aims at relating some aspects of wake and sleep states to neuronal events in the rostral brainstem reticular core and thalamocortical systems, leading to the postulation of some cellular mechanisms underlying shifts in the level of vigilance and maintenance of steady wake–sleep behavioural states. I shall thus address the question *how*, leaving the *why* of various sleep stages to other authors in this volume (see also my 1978 paper and commentaries on it).

6.1 Prolegomena to a Cellular Study of Structures Generating Ascending Activation Processes

6.1.1 Tonic Activity, a Major Criterion for Localizing Key Structures Involved in Wake–Sleep States

An approach at a cellular level requires the application of Claude Bernard's strategy of simplification, even if the picture so obtained has to be completed under more complex, natural conditions. Indeed, when the main goal is to search for neuronal candidates of the major components that define states of vigilance, one is obliged to reduce those behavioural conditions to basic aspects. The component(s) chosen to be analysed among various wake–sleep stigmata should be clearly justified. Here, the distinction between tonic and phasic events is of particular importance. While the advantage of phasic events occurring on a time scale of milliseconds is to be stringently correlated to neuronal firing, wake–sleep states are essentially characterized by temporally enduring phenomena implying long-term regulatory processes: 'the criterion of the existence of *tonic activity* is one of major importance in any attempt to localize the key structures involved in the active production of sleep' (Moruzzi, 1972, p. 112). The same criterion holds true for wakefulness (W). In fact, out of three cardinal indicator variables of wake–sleep states (voltage and frequency of EEG rhythms, muscle activity recorded by neck EMG, and saccadic eye movements), the combination of two tonic events (EEG and EMG) can be used to recognize reliably any steady state of the wake–sleep continuum in normal animals.

The experimenter's task is greatly facilitated when investigating neuronal correlates of the sleep state with EEG desynchronization (D) because internally generated phenomena are largely free from interference with sensory inputs and motor activities. The muscular atonia, that defines D sleep, has been successfully investigated. Tonically firing neurons located in the ventromedial bulbar reticular formation and physiologically identified as projecting to the spinal cord were found to be selectively active just prior and during muscular atonia (Kanamori *et al.*, 1980; Sakai *et al.*, 1981). The increased activity of bulbo-spinal cells during D sleep is probably the factor that leads to tonic post-synaptic inhibition of motoneurons. The latter phenomenon was first demonstrated by Pomepeiano and his colleagues (Gassel *et al.*, 1964; Pompeiano, 1967) and was more recently documented intracellularly (Glenn *et al.*, 1978; Morales & Chase, 1978).

The student of the other active state, W, faces tremendous difficulties as he is unable to control and objectively measure all variables of this state at a given instant. Some investigators take postures and gross movements as W indicators. Since decorticated (and, consequently, thalamically degenerated) animals still display a variety of motor behaviours, the puzzling conclusion sometimes emerges in the literature, namely that brainstem projections to the spinal cord are sufficient to explain W phenomena, while ascending systems reaching the forebrain do not play an essential role in the W state. If in Aplysia the 'arousal' state may be defined by food-seeking and is related to an identified serotoninergic neuron (Weiss *et al.*, 1978), the whole repertoire of the W state in mammals is fortunately not organized in the exclusive terms of motor activity. Ascending systems modulate highly complex thalamocortical activities of which overt motor behaviour may be only an ancillary aspect: association processes occur during W without necessarily being accompanied by motor output. Thalamocortical cellular aspects are opposite in behavioural states associated with EEG desynchronization, compared to EEG-synchronized sleep (S). The cellular mechanisms of the tonic event reflected in the EEG rhythms are exposed in this chapter.

The choice of studying the EEG as a physiological correlate of behaviour starts from the assumption that various EEG patterns faithfully indicate changes in the vigilance level during activated and deactivated states, particularly during transitions between W and S.

[A recent paper and open commentaries have evaluated the correlations EEG desynchronization–arousal and EEG synchronization–sleep (Vanderwolf & Robinson, 1981). The critique of the arousal theory in the target article was mainly based on: (a) the presence of EEG desynchronization during D sleep, in which animals are lying in a sleeping posture and are relatively unreactive to stimuli; (b) the presence of EEG rhythmic 'spindle waves' during such waking behaviours as standing immobile, with the eyes open and watching prey; and (c) the abundance of EEG slow waves following administration of atropine, contrasting with a waking behaviour. Concerning point (a), I remarked that D sleep is a state with a high degree of reticular activation, that thalamocortical cellular events are quite similar in W and D states, opposite to S sleep, and there is therefore no surprise that EEG desynchronization accompanies active (dreaming) sleep. As to point (b), Rougeul, Bouyer and Buser commented that the rhythmic activities they have described during waking are completely distinct from slow wave sleep activities; particularly, when the animal is highly alert, immobile and watching prey, it exhibits fast rhythms developing over restricted neocortical foci (see Fig. 6.7). Last, to point (c), Jasper remarked that, if properly tested, significant impairment of behaviour, especially of learning processes, can be detected under the influence of atropine.]

This choice also takes for granted that neuronal events in thalamocortical systems, where EEG is generated, are relevant to complex phenomena occurring during wake and sleep states. Basically, during W output cells should be in an adequate state for a quick response, and inhibitory mechanisms should act properly to provide accurate reception combined with rapid recovery (see Section 6.1.2). Such events are cellular correlates of adaptive behaviour. Thus, EEG desynchronization is associated with cellular phenomena that are prerequisites for active behavioural states. It is unnecessary to emphasize the distinction which should be made between the state of W and EEG desynchronization, or between S and EEG synchronization. None the less, experimental evidence reported below shows that modifications in neuronal firing and related changes in EEG rhythms during transitional periods from W to S and from S to W create necessary conditions to reach genuine manifestations of wake and sleep states. EEG alterations always precede and announce overt behavioural aspects. And most significant neuronal alterations have recently been found to occur in rostral brainstem structures projecting to thalamic nuclei involved in EEG synchronization–desynchronization processes, long before the motor events of behavioural states (see Section 6.3.1). In fact, Moruzzi and Magoun's (1949) pioneering experiments that set the scene for modern investigations of ascending activation phenomena have analysed changes in spontaneous EEG waves that mimicked the alpha-wave blockade during visual stimulation, attention or mental tasks (Berger, 1930). Since experimental evidence at a cellular level has shown that low voltage fast EEG rhythms are associated with true activation of thalamic and cortical long-axon cells (see Section 6.1.2), the terms EEG desynchronization and EEG activation will be used interchangeably. Throughout this chapter, *activation is meant as a tonic state of readiness in thalamic and cortical neuronal networks that creates the basic conditions for some components of arousal, waking and desynchronized sleep*.

The evidence for and against the involvement of various brain structures in the regulation of wake–sleep states, resulting from experiments using transections, lesions and electrical stimulation, has been amply reviewed by Moruzzi (1972) and Jouvet (1972). Below, I will briefly summarize the main conclusions of those early studies and point out different areas of investigations where modern approaches at global and unitary levels support or conflict with traditional views.

6.1.2 Tonic Ascending Activation: Similarities between Wakefulness and Desynchronized Sleep and Some Methodological Consequences

In Moruzzi's views (page references are to his 1972 review), waking is maintained by 'the ascending reticular system and a group of neurons lying in the posterior hypothalamus (that) are endowed with a tonic influence' (p. 114). The hypothesis that the midbrain reticular formation (MRF) actively maintains W is based on two complementary results: 'electrical stimulation (of the MRF) produces EEG and behavioural arousal' (p. 98) and 'mesencephalic lesions, interrupting most of the MRF but sparing the classical ascending pathways, resulted in a synchronized EEG' (p. 59) and a comatose syndrome. However, in *chronic* preparations with precollicular transection 'spontaneous (EEG) desynchronization tended to appear as chronicity progressed' (p. 17). In low, chronic cerveau isolé animals, desynchronization–synchronization cycles were accompanied by corresponding changes in the pupillary diameter (Villablanca's experiments). The conclusion was drawn that 'a genuine state of wakefulness may be maintained in the isolated cerebrum' (p. 21) by activating structures of the diencephalon.

The conclusions of studies using brainstem transections and electrical stimulation of the MRF have been hotly debated. The difficulties in the interpretation of results are due to the methods employed. Electrical stimulation applied to a brain structure is highly abnormal and may disrupt its timing and organization. On the other hand, the severity of large electrolytic lesions destroying the midbrain tegmentum bilaterally prevents immediate observations on behaviour. At post-lesion stages, compensatory phenomena and the possibility of hypersensitivity of the denervated structures introduce insoluble interpretative problems. The greatest drawback with both electrical stimulation and electrolytic lesions of the MRF is that terminal and passing fibres arising in other reticular fields and non-reticular systems are involved. For instance, the site of choice in the MRF used to elicit arousal and tonic EEG desynchronization by applying high-frequency pulses is traversed by noradrenergic (NA) fibres arising in the locus coeruleus complex. This objection was raised to challenge the MRF role in thalamocortical activation and to propose that 'a noradrenergic system issuing from the anterior part of the locus coeruleus complex, ascending through the dorsal NA bundle . . ., appears to be responsible for the *tonic* cortical activation which accompanies waking' (Jouvet, 1972, p. 221). Jouvet also envisaged that 'a dopaminergic mechanism . . . is responsible for the maintenance of behavioral arousal and alertness' (p. 221). At first sight, the role of monoamine systems in mediating arousal and waking seemed to be strengthened by cellular studies: locus coeruleus (Chu & Bloom, 1974; Hobson *et al.*, 1975) and raphe (McGinty, 1973) neurons have highest discharge rates in the W state, lower during S sleep, and virtually absent during D sleep.

Any further discussion on the role of the rostral reticular or monoamine-containing neurons in *tonic* ascending activation processes should: (1) use stimulation–lesion approaches that avoid involvement of fibres en passage; and (2) define thalamocortical activation in cellular terms to see whether activation processes fit with neuronal events elicited by setting in motion one or another of the hypothesized systems. Data relevant to these two points are discussed below.

Fig. 6.1 Histological aspect of a lesion produced by an unilateral (left) injection (2.5 μg) of kainic acid in the MRF. Frontal plane 3.2. The animal was chronically implanted on both sides with guide cannulae into the superior colliculi (vertical arrows in 1) and sacrificed 10 days following kainic injection. The territory of total neuronal loss on the left side is delimitated by dots in 1. The limits of the lesioned area may roughly indicate the limits of the initially excited area. Details at higher magnifications of the left side are depicted in 2 and 3. Oblique arrows indicate blood vessels and permit localization of areas photographed in 1 and 2, and 2 and 3. Arrowheads in 2 indicate normal ganglion-type cells of the mesencephalic trigeminal nucleus, surviving within a completely depopulated region (for details on the selective and absolute resistance of these ganglion-type cells, see Colonnier *et al.*, 1979). The dorso-ventral, medio-lateral and rostro-caudal diameters of the lesion are 4.0 to 4.2 mm. The lesion affected almost the entire MRF, leaving intact only a limited area dorso-lateral to the red nucleus (see 2–3). The lesion encroached upon the lateral part of the central gray and the lateral part of the

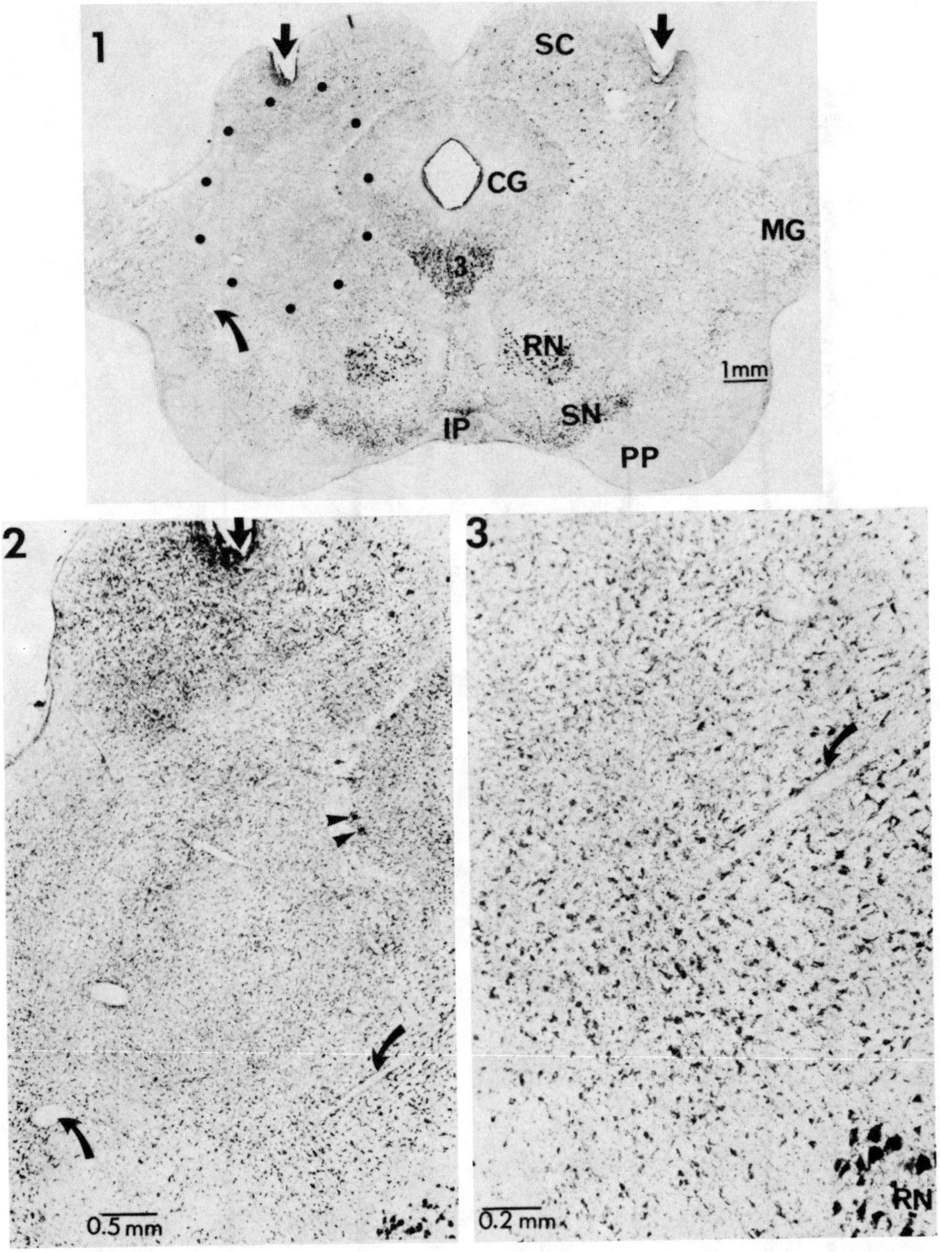

deep layers of superior colliculus. With the exception of ganglion-type trigeminal cells, there was *total loss of neurons* within the lesioned area. Sections stained with unsuppressed Nauta method showed the integrity of axons in fields with complete neuronal depopulation. Abbreviations: SC = superior colliculus; MG = medial geniculate nucleus; CG = central gray; 3 = oculomotor nucleus; RN = red nucleus; IP = interpeduncular nucleus; PP = pes pedunculi. (Reproduced from A. Kitsikis and M. Steriade (1981), *Behavioural Brain Research* **3**, 361–380, by permission.)

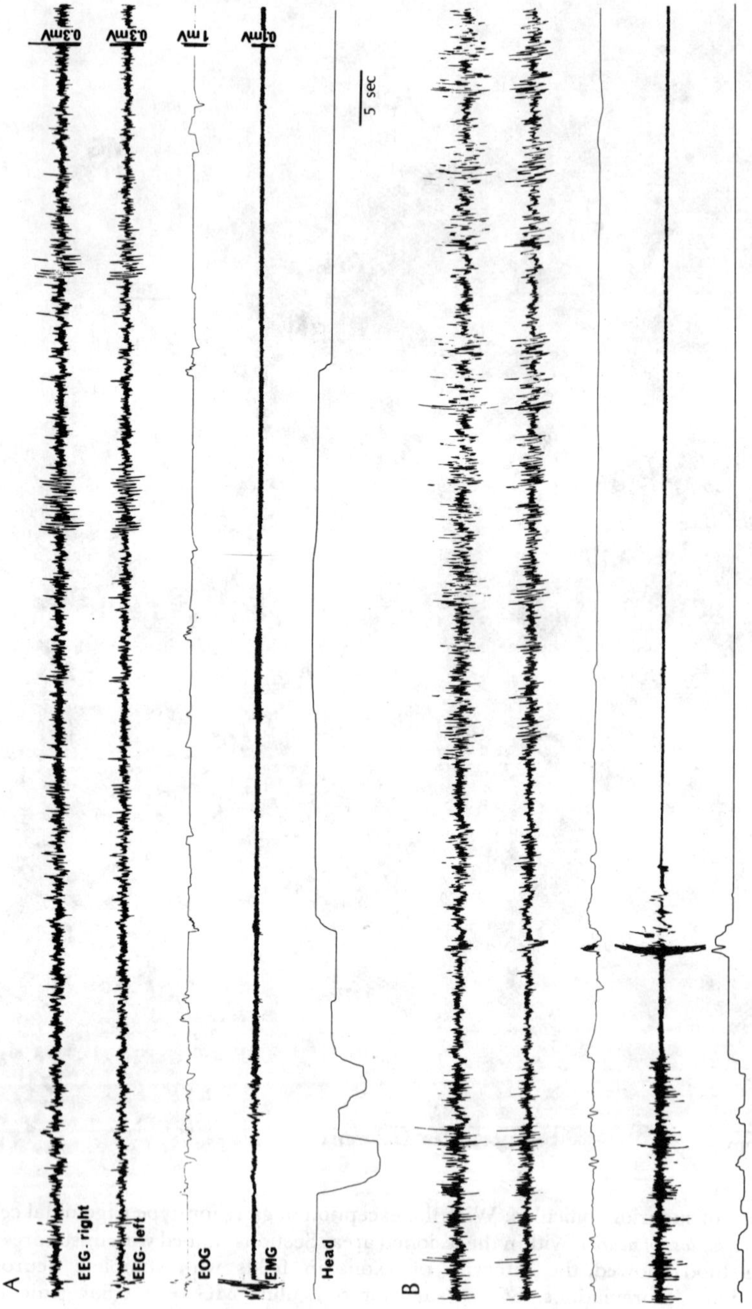
A
EEG-right
EEG-left
EOG
EMG
Head
0.3mV
0.3mV
1mV
0.1mV
5 sec
B

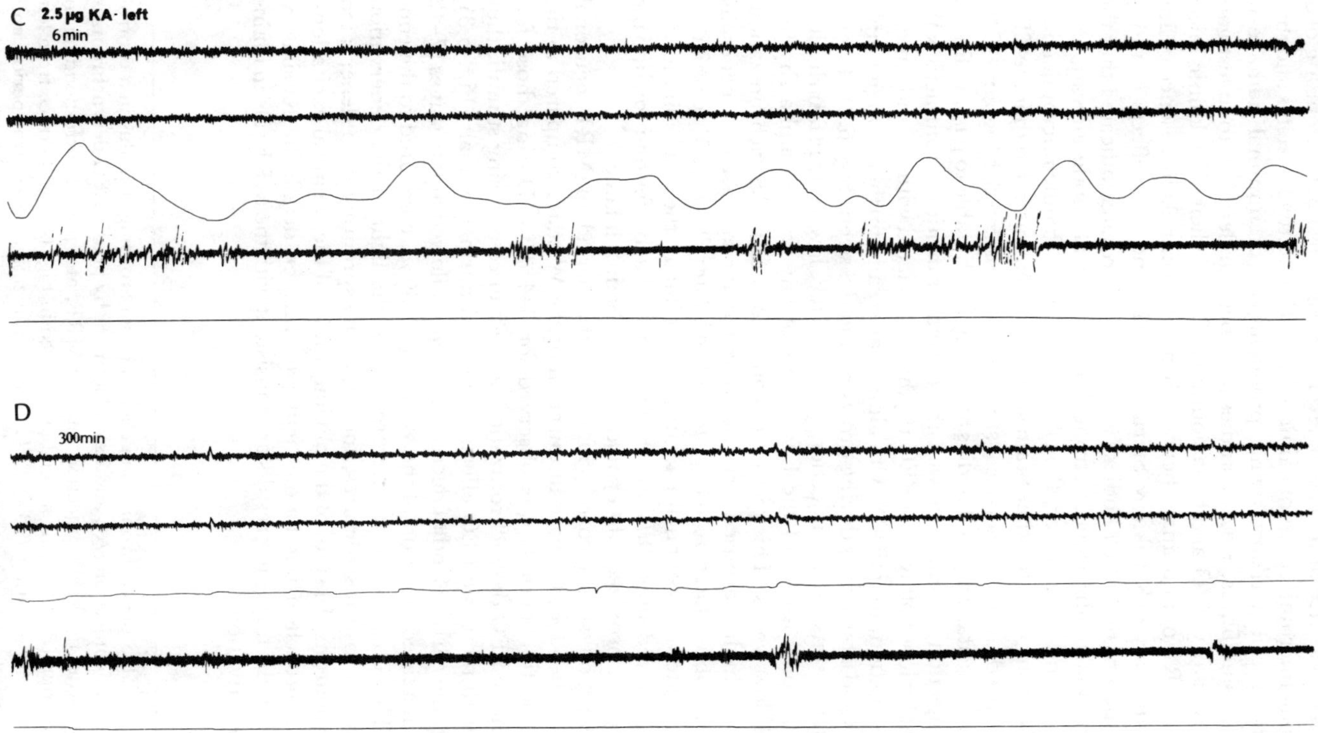

Fig. 6.2 Electrographic signs induced by unilateral (left) injection of 2.5 μg kainic acid into the MRF, in the period of initial excitation. The five ink-written traces depict from top to bottom: surface EEG waves (right and left), ocular movements (EOG), neck EMG and head movements. Note, before injection (A–B), normal fluctuations of EEG desynchronized and synchronized periods. Continuous EEG desynchronization began about 25 s following the onset of injection and lasted for 36 h; it is depicted at 6 min (C) and 5 h (D). During the initial 15 min, slow oscillations were seen on the EOG trace (C), but thereafter such movements disappeared. (Unpublished data)

EEG effects by chemical excitation of the midbrain reticular core. The demonstration of a critical role played by the MRF in tonic EEG activation should come, in addition to the evidence at a cellular level (see Section 6.3.1), from a global approach using microinjections of kainic acid which selectively excites and then rapidly destroys cell perikarya while producing no or minimal damage to terminal or passing fibres. Recent studies have been undertaken to investigate the initial, excitatory EEG and behavioural syndrome elicited by kainic injections into the MRF of non-anaesthetized, behaving animals in absence of any paroxysmal discharge (Kitsikis & Steriade, 1981), and later effects resulting from destruction of nerve cell bodies (Fig. 6.1). The results indicated that the kainate excitation is abnormally strong for a model of subtle alterations in behavioural alertness. However, the effects on EEG by kainic microinjections into the MRF, compared to other brain structures, demonstrated that the EEG activation induced by MRF electrical stimulation (Moruzzi & Mogoun, 1949) is indeed due to excitation of cell bodies and is not attributable to passing fibres. Before the injection, animals showed the normal transitions from active W, characterized by low-voltage fast EEG rhythms associated with eye movements and EMG activation, to quiet W with alpha waves, and further to high amplitude spindles and slow waves during drowsiness and S sleep (Fig. 6.2). Twenty to thirty s after the onset of the injection into the MRF, low-voltage fast rhythms constituted the only aspect of the EEG, without any trace of alpha rhythm, spindles and slow waves. This picture of continuous EEG desynchronization, associated with highly aroused behaviour, lasted for at least 8 h, generally between 12 and 36 h (doses from 0.25 μg to 1μg bilaterally, or 2.5 μg unilaterally). After a bilateral injection of 1 μg in locus coeruleus, the EEG spindles and slow waves recovered after 4 h. After the injection of 1 μl buffer solution into the MRF, a fully synchronized EEG could be seen about 2 h later.

At post-injection stages corresponding to the period of MRF neuronal destruction, a 40–60% decrease in duration of the W state, compared to the control pre-injection period, was observed for 3–4 days. During those few days, only phasic EEG desynchronization accompanied arousing stimuli, thus contrasting with the tonic EEG effects induced in normal animals (Fig. 6.3). Surprisingly, the early period of decreased W was followed at late stages (7–12 days) by an increased duration of the W state (20–50%, compared to the control score). This observation is interpretable in the light of the denervation hypersensivity in rostral structures, including the sprouting onto denervated diencephalic neurons. In spite of the obvious limits of the chemical excitation–destruction approach using kainic acid (see further details in Kitsikis & Steriade, 1981), the foregoing results are consistent with the MRF role in maintaining EEG activation.

Fig. 6.3 Tonic EEG desynchronization elicited by an arousing stimulus in a control period, before kainic injection (A), and its replacement by phasic EEG desynchronization 4 days following the kainic injection into the MRF, at a period corresponding to neuronal destruction (B–C). Same animal as depicted in Fig. 6.2. EEG trace from left hemisphere. Note long-lasting (30 s) EEG desynchronization in control period and much shorter periods of EEG desynchronization (lasting about 3 s) following kainic-induced MRF lesion, in spite of quite similar peripheral signs induced by the arousing auditory stimulus (arrows). (Unpublished data)

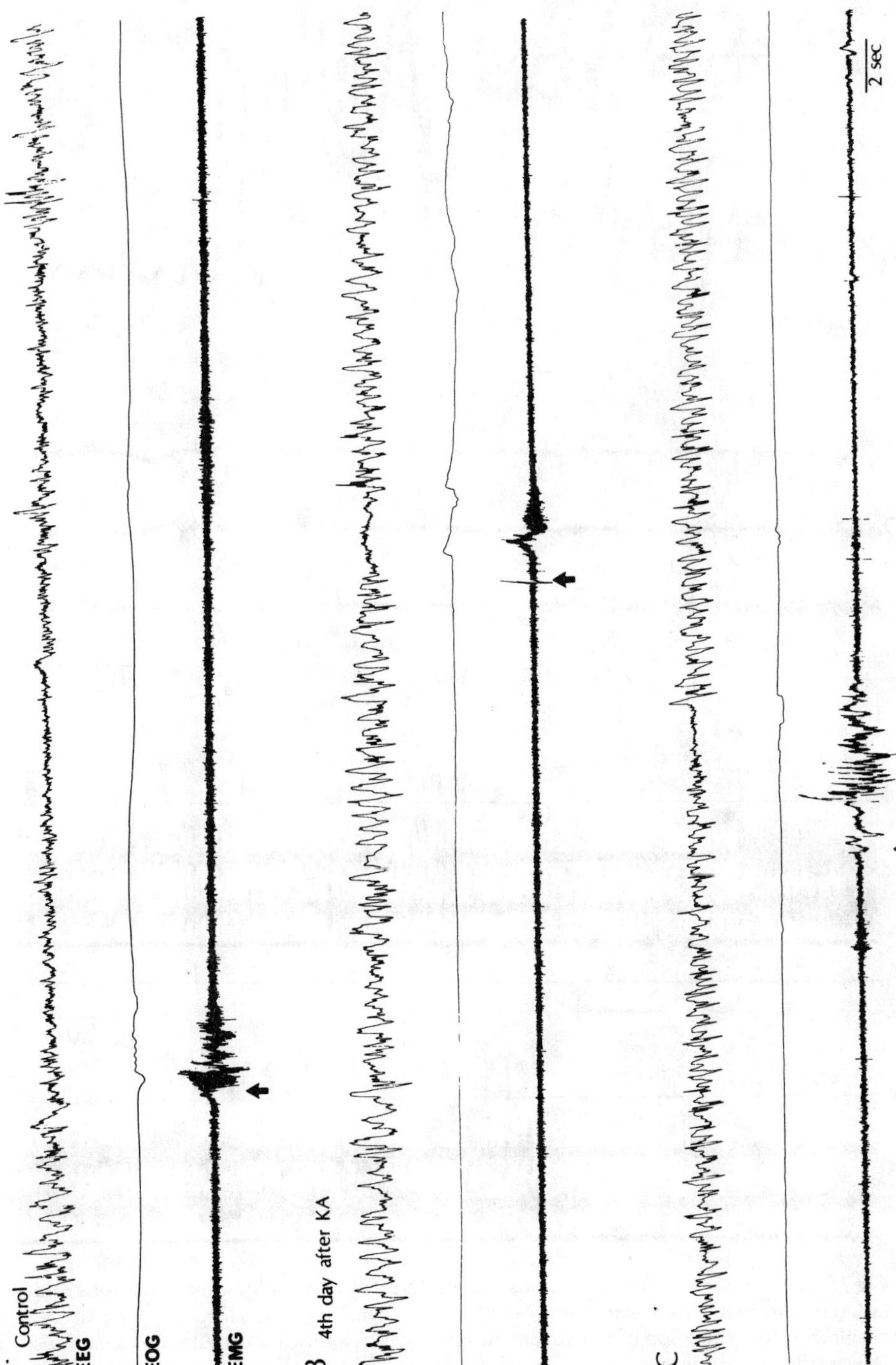
Control
EEG
EOG
EMG
B 4th day after KA
C
2 sec

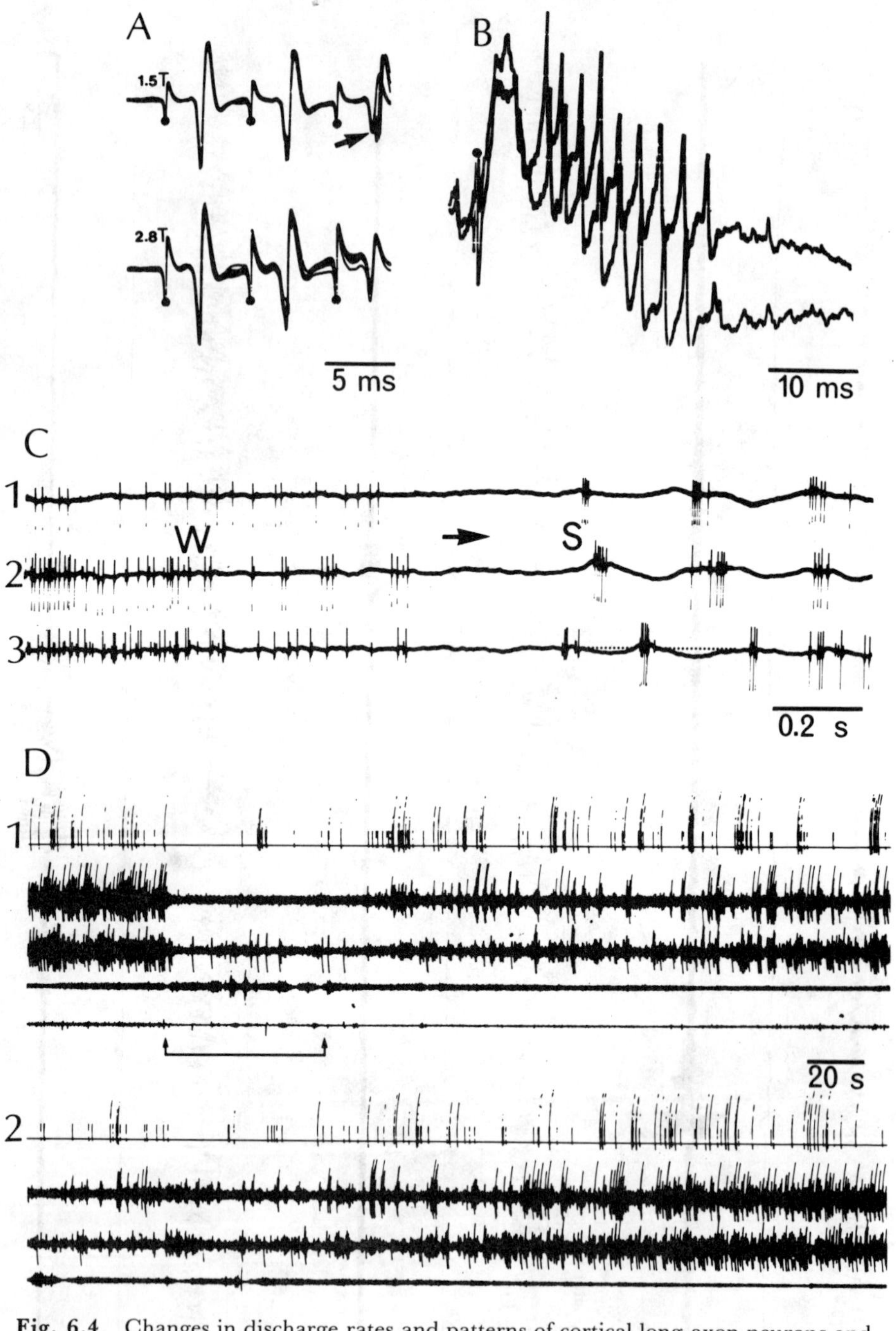

Fig. 6.4 Changes in discharge rates and patterns of cortical long-axon neurons and putative interneurons during waking (W) and synchronized sleep (S) in cat. A: antidromic identification of a cortical neuron in area 5 following stimulation of lateralis intermedius thalamic nucleus (T, threshold, is the intensity eliciting discharges in 50% of the trials); arrow indicates fragmentation between initial segment and somadendritic

Cellular correlates of EEG desynchronization in thalamocortical systems. An attempt to define the cellular processes associated with EEG desynchronization must start with the physiological identification of investigated elements in terms of input–output organization. This is compulsory because of the diversity of thalamic and cortical neuronal classes. Long-axon (thalamocortical and corticofugal) neurons are safely identifiable by antidromic invasion, without intracellular impalement and staining. This is the reason why activation will be characterized here from data on identified long-axon neurons. The investigation of changes in cellular activities at various levels of vigilance should begin with spontaneous activity, but this is only a first step. It must be completed in the same neuron with the analysis of its intrinsic excitability by using testing volleys. The delineation of cellular reactivity should include the whole excitatory–inhibitory sequence of thalamic and cortical events induced by a stimulus. This analysis provides information which sheds light on the accuracy of discrimination and the rapidity of neuronal recovery at different levels of vigilance.

(*a*) *Spontaneous firing* rates of identified thalamocortical, corticothalamic, corticopontine and corticospinal neurons increase during EEG desynchronization induced by MRF stimulation or occurring naturally during both W and D sleep, compared to S sleep (reviewed in Steriade & Hobson, 1976, and Steriade, 1981). The increased firing rate of small-sized, slow-conducting pyramidal tract cells from the very onset of natural arousal in behaving animals (Steriade *et al.*, 1974) was correlated in intracellular studies (Inubushi *et al.*, 1978) to their depolarization during reticular elicited EEG desynchronization. Long-axon thalamic and cortical neurons are characterized by sustained discharge during W and D states, and by a burst-silence pattern during S sleep (Fig. 6.4c). This finding indicates that firing rates and patterns are similar in W and D sleep and, together with other evidence on cellular responsiveness given below, leads to the conclusion that D sleep is *not* an extreme type of S sleep, but a truly activated state. In contrast to long-axon neurons, putative short-axon, local circuit interneurons have very low discharge rates during W, increase discharge rates in S sleep (Fig. 6.4d), and reach highest rates during rapid eye movements in D sleep (Steriade, 1978). Since some experimental evidence suggested that D sleep is important for the consolidation of information acquired during W

---

spikes. B: presumed cortical interneuron in area 5, that could not be backfired from any of the sites of stimulation and responded with a high-frequency burst to a shock applied to the lateralis posterior thalamic nucleus; the spike barrage followed the early slow negative component. C: the big spike represents a neuron in cortical area 5 antidromically identified from the center median thalamic nucleus; three (1 to 3) W → S transitions in successive sleep–waking cycles; increased amplitude of spike from periods 1 to 3, separated by about 70 min; note regular discharge in W and a period of silenced firing preceding the burst-silence pattern in S sleep; dotted line in 3 tentatively indicated the base line. D: presumed cortical interneuron recorded in area 5, driven by lateralis posterior thalamic stimulation with a 500/s spike barrage, as the neuron depicted in B; the five ink-written traces depict unit activity, focal EEG waves, surface EEG waves, EMG and eye movements; note (in 1) striking diminution of spontaneous firing on arousal from S sleep elicited by auditory stimulation (between arrows), and (in 2) progressively increased occurrence of spike bursts with transition from W to S sleep. (Modified from M. Steriade (1978), *Behavioural Brain Sciences*, **3**, 465–514, by permission.)

(Bloch & Fischbein, 1975), the selectively increased firing rates of association cortical interneurons during periods of rapid eye movements in D sleep might indicate that these elements are preferentially involved in maintaining the soundness of a memory trace (Steriade, 1978).

(*b*) *Cellular antidromic and synaptic responsiveness* is best studied with central stimulation, thus preventing unknown modifications at multiple intercalated synapses when using a peripheral stimulus. The responses of thalamic and cortical cells to antidromic stimuli, testing soma excitability, are predictably enhanced during reticular-induced EEG desynchronization and during activated W and D states as compared to slow wave sleep (Fig. 6.5a). The potentiation of antidromic invasion during W and D sleep generally parallels the significantly higher rates of background firing. But facilitation of antidromically elicited discharges is also seen in W when some neurons do not exhibit significantly increased firing rates and even when fast-conducting pyramidal tract neurons cease to discharge spontaneously, at the onset of the arousal reaction (Steriade *et al.*, 1974). In the latter case, the signal-to-noise ratio is obviously further increased. The depression of *secondary* synaptic excitation during activated W and D states should be emphasized as it may explain the obliteration of spindle waves during these states. Different types of spindle waves have a similar polarity and depth-profile to thalamically evoked augmenting and recruiting potentials, and responses of augmenting type originate from an enhancement of secondary synaptic excitation without alteration or even a decrease in the primary component. Augmenting responses and spindle sequences are drastically reduced during behavioural states of W and D sleep, both compared to S sleep (Steriade *et al.*, 1979), and during reticular-induced EEG activation (Steriade & Morin, 1981).

(*c*) *Inhibitory processes* are present throughout the sleep–waking cycle, as appearing from the suppression of spontaneous discharge and the decrease of antidromic or synaptic responsiveness following a testing stimulus. The time-course of inhibition varies, however, with changes in the vigilance level. The duration of the inhibitory period is shorter and cyclic inhibitory-rebound sequences are blocked during MRF stimulation and activated behavioural states, in both thalamic and cortical neurons (Fig. 6.5b). *It follows that the whole sequence of events triggered by a stimulus is telescoped during EEG desynchronization* (Fig. 6.5c). The fact that inhibition is sharp in the W state and recovers much faster than in S sleep provides a mechanism subserving accurate control of thalamic and cortical performances, and allows neurons to follow rapidly recurring activity (Steriade & Deschênes, 1974).

Conclusion: where and how to search for neuronal candidates underlying tonic ascending activation. The foregoing results clearly indicate that thalamic and cortical cellular correlates of adaptive behaviour during natural W are mimicked by MRF stimulation: a state of adequate depolarization proper for a prompt response, and inhibitory mechanisms acting efficiently to provide accurate

---

Fig. 6.5 Responsiveness and inhibitory events in thalamic and cortical neurons during states associated with EEG desyncrhonization and synchronization. A: a cell in parietal association area 5 of chronically implanted cat, antidromically invaded from the center median thalamic nucleus; the antidromic responsiveness was investigated with a

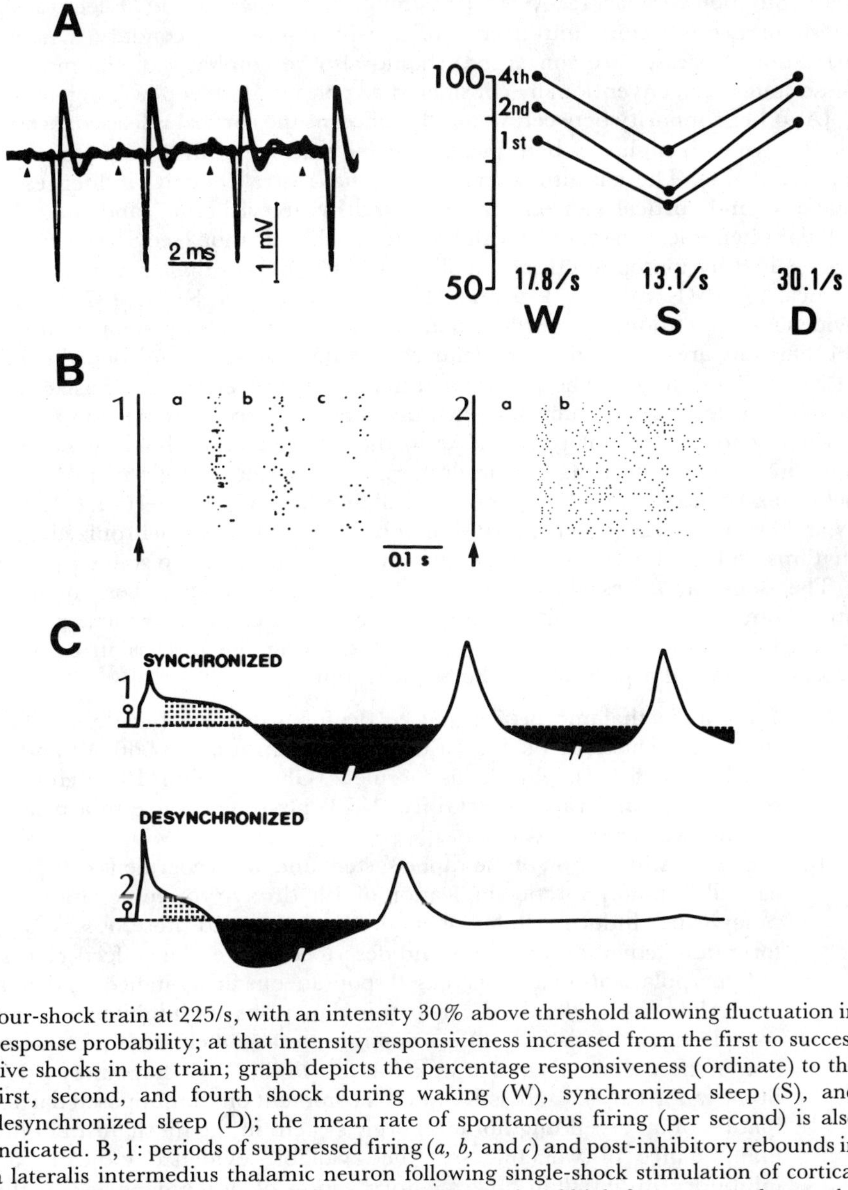

four-shock train at 225/s, with an intensity 30% above threshold allowing fluctuation in response probability; at that intensity responsiveness increased from the first to successive shocks in the train; graph depicts the percentage responsiveness (ordinate) to the first, second, and fourth shock during waking (W), synchronized sleep (S), and desynchronized sleep (D); the mean rate of spontaneous firing (per second) is also indicated. B, 1: periods of suppressed firing (*a, b,* and *c*) and post-inhibitory rebounds in a lateralis intermedius thalamic neuron following single-shock stimulation of cortical area 5 (arrow); and 2: the effect of a preceding train of high-frequency pulses to the midbrain reticular core; note reduced duration of the period of silenced firing and disappearance of the *c* period. C: simplified diagram to show the whole sequence of excitatory-inhibitory events in thalamus and cortex during EEG synchronization and desynchronization; the changes during states characterized by EEG desynchronization consist of: enhanced primary excitation due to antidromic (or monosynaptic) volleys, diminution of the secondary synaptic excitation (dotted part), sharp inhibition but with reduced duration (black part) and blockade of rhythmic inhibitory-rebound sequences. (Modified from M. Steriade (1981) in O. Pompeiano and C. Ajmone-Marsan (Eds.), *Brain Mechanisms and Perceptual Awareness*, by permission of Raven Press.)

discrimination with fast recovery. The similarity between W and D sleep (as far as spontaneous firing, antidromic responsiveness and secondary synaptic excitation processes are concerned) should also be emphasized, the more as these states are conventionally considered as poles in the sleep–waking cycle.

[Another similarity between W and D concerns the cortical release of acetylcholine which is higher in both these activated states than in S sleep (Jasper & Tessier, 1971). There is also good evidence that rostral reticular influences on thalamic and cortical neurons are mediated by acetylcholine, and the basic cellular phenomena associated with EEG desynchronization (see Section 6.1.2) are elicited by iontophoretically applied acetylcholine in thalamic nuclei and cortical areas (Krnjevic, 1974 and 1981; Dingledine & Kelly, 1977). This evidence is mentioned in order to underline the possibility that common mechanisms are involved in reticular ascending activation and both W and D behavioural states. The common traits of W and D are emphasized by deliberately leaving out some diametrically opposite aspects, from the muscular periphery to the mental content. As to the latter, it is probable that quite opposite influences arising in noradrenergic and serotoninergic neurons (see below) and contrasting behaviour of cortical interneurons (see Section 6.1.2) in W and D are superimposed upon a similar background of desynchronized EEG rhythms and similar elementary cellular processes in these two states.]

The question arises concerning the brainstem structure where neurons underlying thalamocortical activation should be searched: reticular in a classical sense or monoamine systems? Restricting the discussion to tonic processes, several aspects should be borne in mind:

(a) Long-axon thalamocortical and corticofugal neurons have essentially the same behaviour during EEG desynchronization in both W and D (see Section 6.1.2), while locus coeruleus (Chu & Bloom, 1974; Hobson *et al.*, 1975) and raphe (McGinty, 1973) neurons behave in a polarly distinct way in these two states.

(b) Electrical stimulation of the raphe system and locus coeruleus complex, as well as iontophoretic application of 5-hydroxytryptamine and norepinephrine, induce cellular phenomena opposite to those observed in forebrain activation processes and described above. The effects consist of hyperpolarization and decreased spontaneous firing in neo- and allocortical neurons; identified corticospinal neurons are inhibited by locus coeruleus stimulation, an effect opposite to that of cholinergric excitation of these elements and to wakefulness (Phillis & Kostopoulos, 1977; Stone *et al.*, 1975). Here is Krnjevic's comment on the supposed participation of an ascending noradrenergic system in the mechanism of the maintenance of wakefulness: 'the available evidence indicates an inhibitory rather than an excitatory action of norepinephrine in the cerebral cortex; this is hardly consistent with an arousing action.' (1974, p. 481).

(c) Last, the failure to induce any change in EEG desynchronization following bilateral destruction of the locus coeruleus complex with 85% to 95% depletion of cortical norepinephrine, together with other experimental data, led to the conclusion that monoaminergic neurons do not mediate tonic EEG activation (Jacobs & Jones, 1978).

While the effects of locus coeruleus stimulation are *not* consistent with what is expected from a presumed *tonic* activating system, the involvement of norepinephrine-containing neurons in specific components of the W state should not be discarded: they function in *phasic* processes rather than in modulation of the tonic arousal level (Aston-Jones & Bloom, 1981), the most intriguing actions probably resulting in an increased signal-to-noise ratio (Foot & Bloom, 1979) or in switching emphasis from one set of inputs to another (Dismukes, 1979).

In view of the above experimental evidence, there are good reasons to concentrate the search for neurons underlying tonic activation at the MRF level and rostral related structures. As related in detail in following sections, MRF neurons are characterized by input properties making them likely candidates to be the site of complex integration processes and give rise to direct routes for transferring excitatory influences to cortically projecting thalamic neurons. The first necessary step in a cellular study of the ascending activation hypothesis consists of the physiological identification of MRF neurons in order to disclose their target(s) and synaptic inputs (Section 6.2.1). The neurons which fulfil discharge criteria making them suitable for subserving ascending influences should be revealed as projecting toward rostral sites involved in activation processes. As the major rostral projection of midbrain reticular neurons proved to be medial-intralaminar thalamic nuclei, the identification step should be completed by recording neurons within these thalamic nuclei to disclose the nature of the direct synaptic input arising in the MRF and reveal their projections toward telencephalic structures (Section 6.2.2). The discharge properties of physiologically identified MRF and medial-intralaminar thalamic neurons with rostral projections should then be studied during states of the natural sleep–waking cycle in behaving animals (Section 6.3).

(a) The first analysis concerns the so-called *steady* states, following the appearance of all electrographic and behavioural signs of W, S and D. To test the hypothesis of a role played by MRF neurons in tonic activation processes characterizing both W and D sleep, firing rates must be measured separately in epochs with and without phasic motor events (W with eye, limb or trunk movements, and quiet, motionless W; and D sleep with or without saccades or rapid eye movements). Movements may actually introduce uncontrolled factors in the evaluation of discharge, due to the proprioceptive feedback generated by movement itself. I shall report firing rates during motionless W with continuous EEG desynchronization (Fig. 6.6a), well-developed S sleep with continuous EEG synchronization, and tonic periods of D sleep. Thus, brief segments of EEG synchronization within the W state (Fig. 6.6b), brief epochs and EEG desynchronization within S sleep, and epochs with rich eye saccades in D sleep should be excluded. Such analyses are required to make correlations between firing properties of neurons hypothesized in maintaining activation processes and purely desynchronized or synchronized EEG patterns over large regions of the neocortical mantle. One should be aware, however, that studies directed to relating various EEG rhythms with changes in the vigilance level have disclosed that, when the cat is hypervigilant and immobile in an attitude of focused attention, fast rhythms in the range of 35–45 Hz develop in distinct neocortical (pericruciate and periansate) foci, while the rest of the cortex is fully desynchronized (Bouyer *et al.*, 1980; Fig. 6.7).

(b) The second type of analyses concern the transitional stats of W, S and D. This is a step required for dealing with the dynamics of change from one

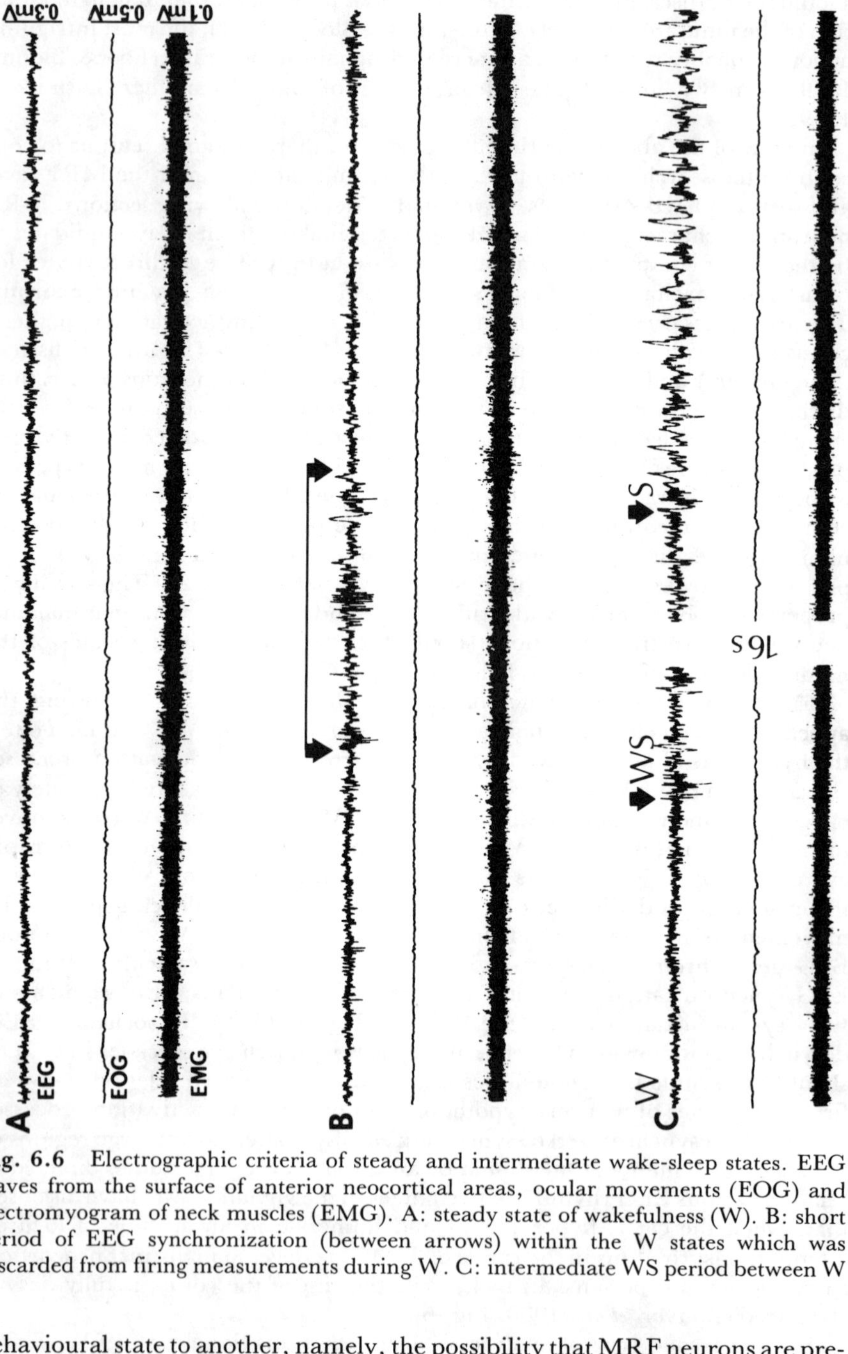

Fig. 6.6 Electrographic criteria of steady and intermediate wake-sleep states. EEG waves from the surface of anterior neocortical areas, ocular movements (EOG) and electromyogram of neck muscles (EMG). A: steady state of wakefulness (W). B: short period of EEG synchronization (between arrows) within the W states which was discarded from firing measurements during W. C: intermediate WS period between W

behavioural state to another, namely, the possibility that MRF neurons are precursors of shifts in states of vigilance. The beginning of the steady W state is

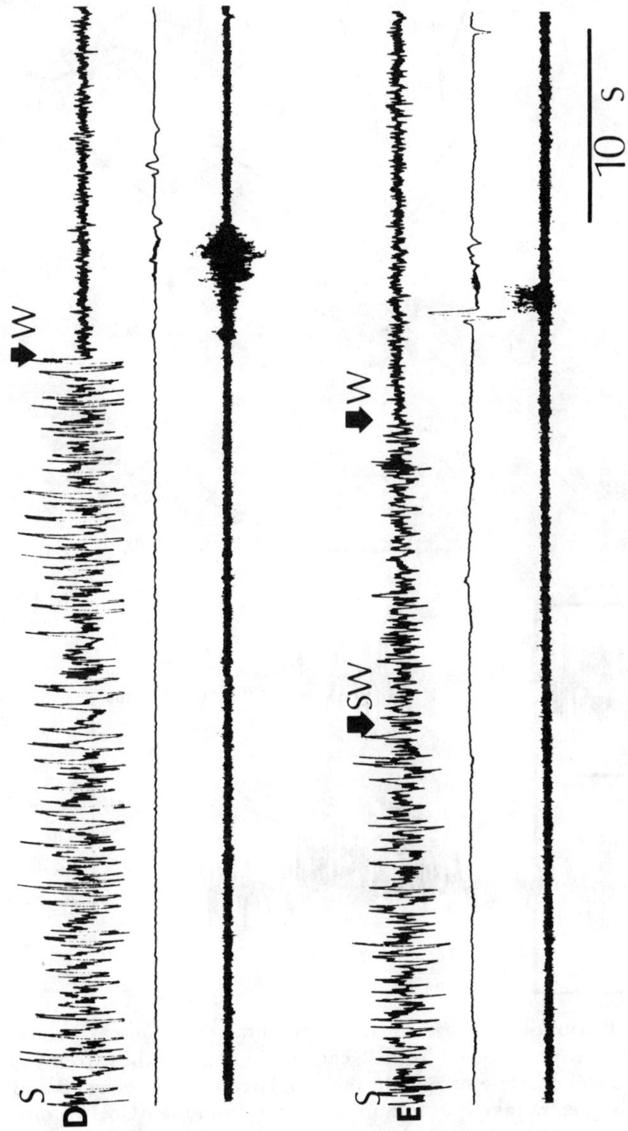

and S steady states. D: abrupt awakening from S sleep. E: intermediate SW period between S and W states. Explanation of different symbols in text. (Reproduced from M. Steriade, G. Oakson and N. Ropert (1982), *Experimental Brain Research*, **46**, 37–51, by permission.)

indicated by overt, generalized EEG desynchronization, associated with increased EMG activity and EOG deflections. Only on rare occasions is W precipitated with all these clear-cut signs (see Fig. 6.6d). More frequently, the

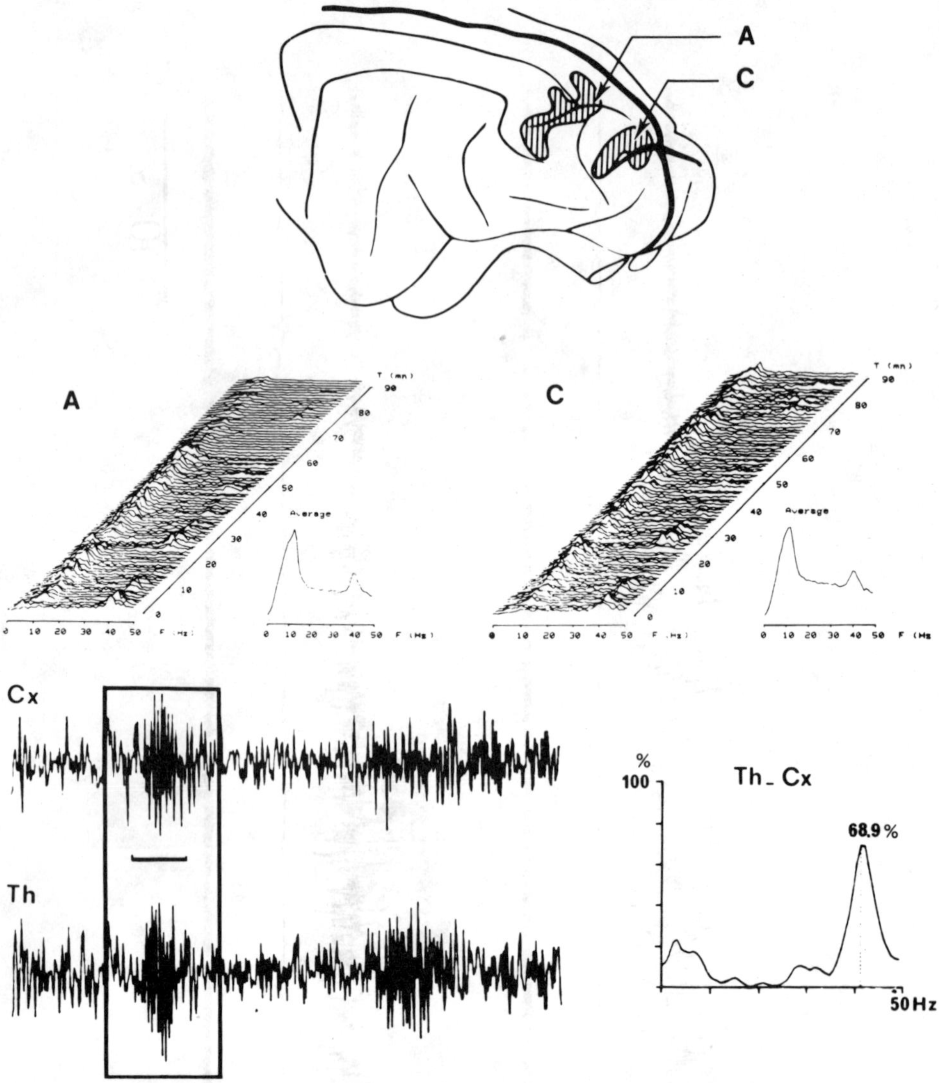

Fig. 6.7 Distribution of fast 35–45 c/s rhythms over the cat anterior cortex. The hatched zones are data pooled from 20 cats, encompassing the extreme limits of the two foci, one (C) over cruciate sulcus, the other (A) over ansate sulcus. Below are presented two evolutive spectra taken, at minute intervals, from the ECoG recorded at A and C, with a total recording time of 90 min. Episodes of fast rhythms (around 40 c/s) that accompany high vigilance and immobility can be seen. They alternate with rhythmic activities in the lower ranges, corresponding to quiet vigilance, to drowsiness and then to sleep (notice that in A no sleep spindles developed in this area). Added to each set of evolutive spectra is the average spectrum computed over the 90 min recording time. Below, fast hypervigilance rhythms simultaneously recorded over the parietal cortex (Cx) and in the posterior thalamic group (Th). Time scales: 0.5 s. Lower right: coherence values vs. frequency between Cx and Th, within the 0–50 Hz band. (Reproduced from J. J. Bouyer, M. F. Montaron and A. Rougeul (1981), *Electroencephalography and Clinical Neurophysiology*, **51**, 244–252, by permission.)

behavioural (EMG and EOG) events follow by several seconds the EEG desynchronization, and the EEG alteration is not abrupt. The beginning of this intermediate epoch between S and W, conventionally termed SW (or between S and D, termed SD), that is the end of S state, is defined as the most precocious of changes consisting of decreased amplitude and increased frequency of rhythms on neocortical or hippocampal leads on a background of a fully synchronized EEG during S sleep. This first EEG change should consequently lead to a generalized unambiguous EEG activation and a complete development of W or D behavioural states (Fig. 6.6e). The beginning of the transitional state between W and S (WS) is the first distinct sign of EEG synchronization (a spindle sequence on anterior leads, a burst of posterolateral slow waves) occurring on a background of fully desynchronized EEG during W and eventually leading to S state (Fig. 6.6c). Thus, the firing rates computed during transitional epochs refer to periods (SW and SD) lasting between the first sign of EEG activation on a background of fully synchronized EEG during S and the onset of completely developed W and D activated states, or to the period (WS) between the first sign of EEG synchronization on a background of fully desynchronized rhythms and the time at which the EEG synchronization is no longer interrupted by transient periods of desynchronization.

6.1.3 *Active Hypnogenic Structures or Deactivation?*

Many possible generators of S sleep have been proposed following stimulation and lesion experiments. Three of them have gained a popular place in sleep physiology: the brainstem medullary region around the solitary tract, the preoptic area of the basal forebrain, and the raphe system (reviewed by Moruzzi, 1972; Jouvet, 1972; Bremer, 1977). Several desiderata should be met by a sleep 'centre': its selective stimulation should produce increased incidence and duration of sleep behaviour; its selective destruction should produce insomnia; and changes in cellular discharge should be highly correlated with, and predictably precede in time, EEG and behavioural signs of S sleep. The results of electrical stimulation and electrolytic lesions are questionable since they might have been due to involvement of fibres en passage. For instance, the hyposomnia or insomnia after the lesion of raphe nuclei (Jouvet, 1972) may be interpreted as possibly due to interruption of ascending axons arising in the hypothesized hyponogenic medullary area and crossing in the pons (Moruzzi, 1972). It is likely that the raphe system is a heterogenous ensemble of nuclei. A more recent paper (Cespuglio *et al.*, 1979) revisited this system by both means of stimulation and localized moderate cooling of rostral and caudal raphe nuclei. Only arousing effects were elicited with electrical stimulation, regardless of nucleus. With reversible cooling of rostral raphe nuclei, S sleep followed by D sleep was induced; cooling the caudal raphe magnus elicited wakefulness. Instead of raphe nuclei, there is a tendency to relate the effects of serotonin with area postrema and the adjacent nucleus of the solitary tract (Puizillout *et al.*, 1981). In a previous monograph (Steriade & Hobson, 1976), we found no cellular evidence supporting the existence of an active hypnogenic 'centre' among the above mentioned three structures. The only systematic studies at a single-cell level concern the raphe neurons and the results invariably reported that discharge rates diminish from W to S sleep, the activity being virtually absent in D sleep (McGinty, 1973; Jacobs & Jones, 1978).

It is not encouraging to note that no study has provided reliable indications fulfilling the above criteria of a sleep-promoting 'centre'. The most recent abstract in hand (Nakamura *et al.*, 1981) which investigated local cerebral glucose utilization for 74 structures, including more than a dozen that have been suggested as possible hypnogenic structures, gave no support to the notion of a 'centre' that actively triggers and maintains sleep. The conclusion of this 2-deoxyglucose study 'appears to favor a deactivation theory of sleep'. We are presently not very far from Bremer's (1935) and Moruzzi & Magoun's (1949) deafferentation concepts.

6.2 Input–Output Organization of Systems Hypothetically Endowed with Activating Properties: The Midbrain Reticular Core and Related Thalamic Nuclei

Between the late 1940s and the late 1950s, the reticular formation was viewed as an undifferentiated structure. Its neuronal networks were left ill-defined because they were not thought to be amenable to morphological and electrophysiological analyses. This caused temporary neglect of the concept of a reticular activating system. The revived interest in the reticular formation during recent years is due to the advent of morphological methods which largely circumvent the problem of passing fibres, and of electrophysiological techniques which allow the recording of identified neurons in behaving animals.

6.2.1 Input–Output Organization of the Midbrain Reticular Core

The MRF is the territory of nucleus cuneiformis and its ventrorostral extension, the central tegmental field. The MRF is considered here distinct from the rostral raphe group, interpeduncular nucleus, ventral tegmental area and substantia nigra. This is justified by the differential histology, input–output organization, discharge properties and chemical signature of these structures.

In contrast to the heterogenous pontine reticular field which includes giant cells ($>60\ \mu m$) interspersed with a large proportion of moderately sized ($\simeq 30\ \mu m$) end small elements ($\simeq 20\ \mu m$), the MRF neurons are homogenously small, generally between 15 and 20 μm (Fig. 6.8b and c). Golgi studies show that MRF neurons belong to the isodendritic type commonly seen in the reticular core and characterized by long, straight and poorly ramified dendrites, generally devoid of spines, and with a considerable degree of dendritic overlap (Fig. 6.8d). The specific feature of very long, overlapping dendrites, which may offer an optimal substratum for integration of multiple converging inputs (Ramon-Moliner & Nauta, 1966), characterizes not only large but also exceedingly small neurons (Ramon y Cajal, 1955).

Fig. 6.8 Morphological features of midbrain and pontine reticular neurons in cat. Nissl (A to C) and Golgi-stained (D) sections. A, sagittal section; PRF = pontine reticular formation; PG = pontine gray; LC = locus coeruleus; IC and SC = inferior and superior colliculi; CG = periaqueductal central gray; MRF = midbrain reticular formation; RN = red nucleus; SN = substantia nigra; 3 = third nerve; RFB = retroflex bundle. B and C = details from typical areas of pontine (B) and midbrain (C)

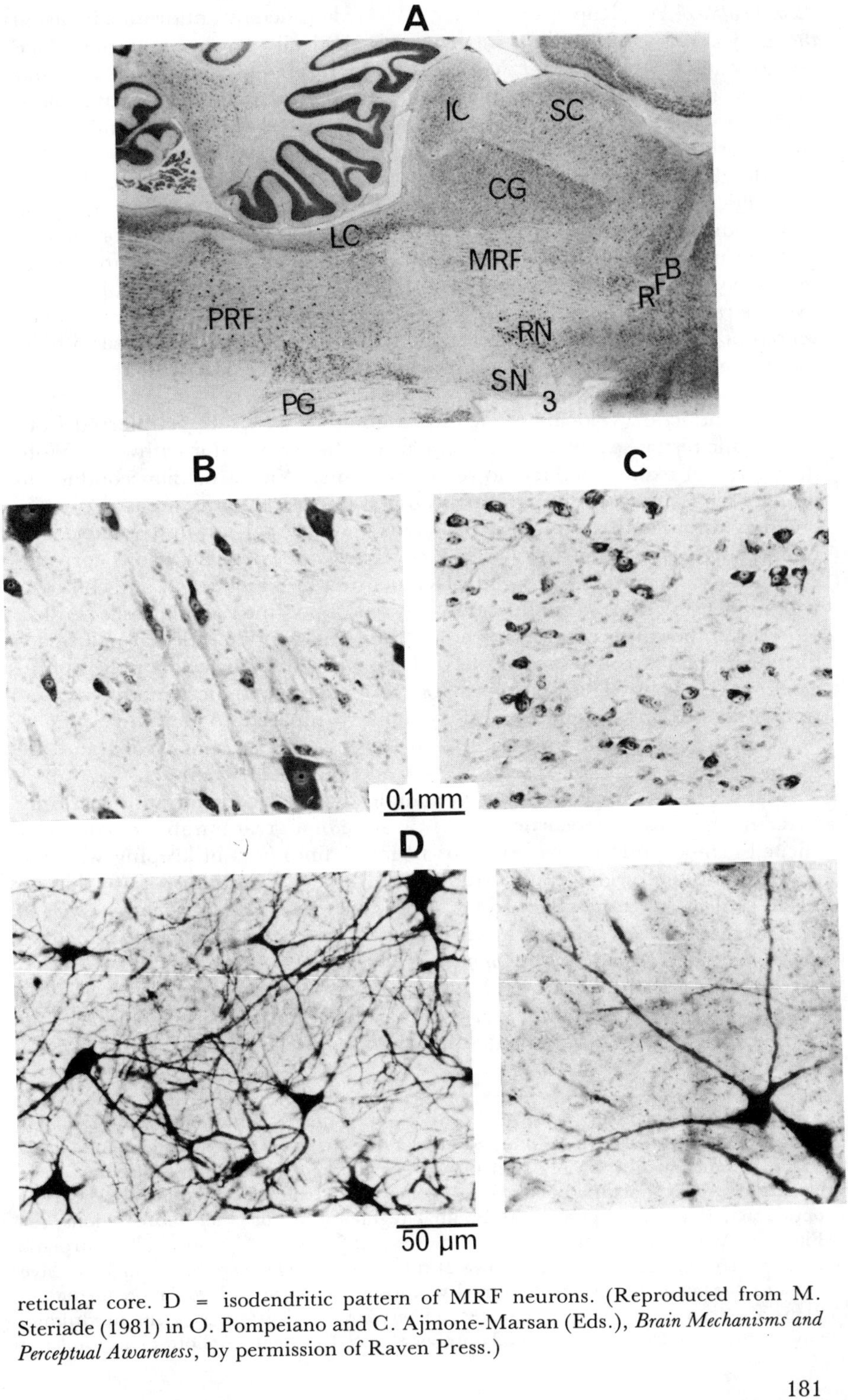

reticular core. D = isodendritic pattern of MRF neurons. (Reproduced from M. Steriade (1981) in O. Pompeiano and C. Ajmone-Marsan (Eds.), *Brain Mechanisms and Perceptual Awareness*, by permission of Raven Press.)

Axonal outflow. We (Ropert & Steriade, 1981) identified by antidromic invasion the projections of individual neurons histologically localized in the MRF territory and established that their three major targets are medial-intralaminar thalamic nuclei, the subthalamic zona incerta field, and the pontine paramedian reticular area (Fig. 6.9). It is interesting that the main rostral targets contain isodendritic neurons characterized by long, radiate processes with a considerable degree of dendritic overlap, very similar to the archetype of brainstem reticular neurons (Ramon-Moliner & Nauta, 1966). A minor neuronal population was activated from the preoptic area and negligibly from lateral thalamic nuclei. About 90% of all antidromically identified MRF neurons were selectively activated from either a rostral or a caudal site; neurons projecting to two rostral targets or giving rise to a descending and an ascending branch represent small fractions. These electrophysiological findings fit in well with the ascending and descending projections of the dorsal MRF described by means of autoradiography methods (Edwards & De Olmos, 1976).

The conduction velocities of axons originating in MRF, as inferred from antidromic response latencies, are similar for the three major pathways. More than 70% of axons conduct slower than 7 m/s. With a median conduction velocity from 3.5 to 4.6 m/s towards both main rostral target areas and pons, one may estimate that a majority of axons measure <1 μm in diameter. The remarkably homogenous, slow conduction velocities of MRF axons corroborate the homogenous, small-sized MRF neurons (see Fig. 6.8c), and contrasts with higher and diverse conduction velocities of pontine reticular cells (Fuller, 1975). Another difference between midbrain and pontine reticular neurons is the much heavier rostral projections of the former. This may explain the significant role played by MRF neurons in the maintenance of tonic ascending activation processes in thalamocortical systems, compared to pontine reticular neurons that project mainly to cranial nerve nuclei or spinal cord and are involved in phasic motor operations (see Section 6.3.1).

It should be finally stressed that we completely failed to invade antidromically MRF neurons from neocortical areas, in spite of a great number of cortically elicited orthodromic responses. This negative finding is in keeping with the conclusion of autoradiographic studies (Edwards & De Olmos, 1976) that no MRF projections are evident to the cerebral cortex. *The synaptic interruption of MRF axons in quite distinct diencephalic nuclei, in their route toward the cortex, contrasts with direct and widespread cortical projections of monoaminergic systems.*

Synaptic inputs. The major afferent systems to MRF arise in the medullary and pontine reticular formation, medial-intralaminar thalamic nuclei, zona incerta,

---

Fig. 6.9 Antidromically identified projection neurons in the midbrain reticular formation (MRF) of cat. IP = interpeduncular nucleus; FTC = central tegmental field; PP = pes pedunculi; CM-Pf and CL = centrum medianum-parafascicularis and centralis lateralis thalamic nuclei; ZI = zona incerta; POA = preoptic area; OT = optic tract; P and B = pontine and bulbar tegmentum. For other abbreviations, see Fig. 6.8. At top, a typical microelectrode descent in the FTC; two small electrolytic lesions (arrows) above (1) and below (2) the recorded cells were found in successive sections; the beginning of two other tracks, more lateral (arrow in 1) and more medial (in 2) are also seen in SC. The percentages indicated in the diagram represent antidromically identified neurons from the total number of tested elements. At bottom, examples of

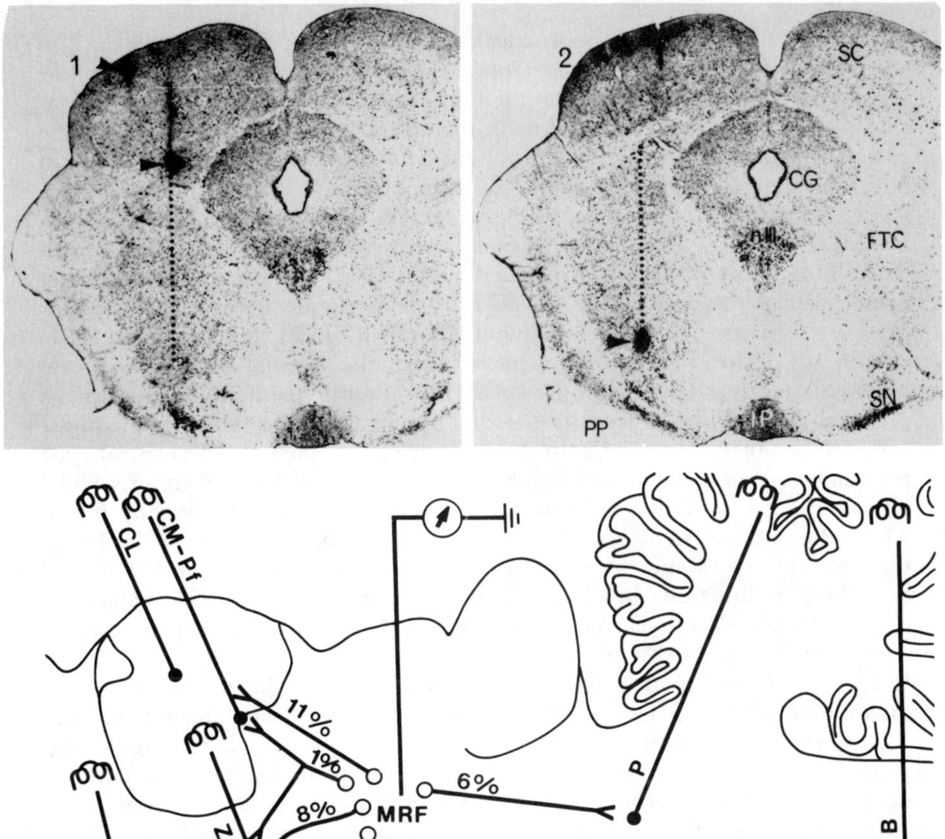

CM-evoked and ZI-evoked antidromic responses in three neurons; note fixed latency, collision with a spontaneously (S) occurring discharge, and ability to follow fast stimuli. (Modified from M. Ropert & M. Steriade (1981), *Journal of Neurophysiology*, **46**, 17–31; and M. Steriade, G. Oakson and N. Ropert (1982), *Experimental Brain Research*, **46**, 37–51, by permission.)

preoptic area and anterior neocortical areas (Ropert & Steriade, 1981). The short-latency, probably monosynaptic, excitations elicited from the bulbar tegmentum and the preoptic area cast doubt on the hypothesis of a direct inhibition exerted by these presumed synchronizing and hypnogenic structures on the rostral reticular core (see Section 6.1.3). The above projections disclosed in electrophysiological investigations are supported by morphological studies (Graybiel, 1977; Mizuno *et al.*, 1969; Scheibel & Scheibel, 1967; Steriade *et al.*, 1982b) (Fig. 6.10). In addition to these sources of afferent fibres, a powerful descending input to MRF was revealed by retrograde tracer experiments using horseradish peroxidase (HRP) to arise in the periaqueductal-periventricular grey and in the dorsolateral hypothalamus (Parent & Steriade, 1981) (Fig. 6.10). The main difference between the medial and the lateral hypothalamic-subthalamic projections to the midbrain tegmentum consists of a preferential distribution from the medial hypothalamus to the periaqueductal grey. Axons originating in both medial and lateral parts of the central grey terminate within the adjacent MRF, as already described by Ramon y Cajal (1955) and constantly found in our retrograde labelling studies (see Fig. 6.10). Thus, the entire system of reciprocal connections between the medial hypothalamic structures and the periaqueductal grey has access to the MRF and, therefore, its functions involving defensive aggression instinctive behaviour and the sleep–waking cycle may affect different types of MRF neurons provided with ascending and descending axons.

The responses elicited in MRF single neurons by many distant structures, the dissimilar discharge patterns and temporal evolutions of excitatory–inhibitory sequences evoked in the same neuron by several testing volleys (Fig. 6.11a) recall the heterogenous afferentation and variation in convergence patterns described by Scheibel *et al.* (1955) in lower brainstem reticular neurons.

In spite of the fact that the same structures appeared to be most effective in inducing both synaptic and antidromic responses, as a rule antidromic activation of a neuron was not accompanied by its synaptic excitation from the same site. The rarity of antidromic identification among synaptically driven neurons (Fig. 6.11b) suggests a relative dichotomy between two groups of neurons: those receiving synaptic inputs from structures outside the midbrain reticular core and those projecting to other areas. Actually, 88% of synaptically driven neurons could not be identified by backfiring, while 72% of antidromically identified elements were neither excited synaptically nor was their spontaneous firing silenced from all stimulated sites. The relative segregation between non-projection and projection elements in terms of the degree of synaptic inputs (Fig. 6.11c) is significant at $p<0.001$. This dichotomy suggests that recipients of synaptic inputs from areas outside the MRF are local elements; they perform intrinsic reticular operations and transfer the result to projection neurons which further process it toward rostral or caudal structures.

Fig. 6.10 Drawings of frontal sections through the midbrain and diencephalon of two cats (A–B) with HRP injections into the MRF. The solid black indicates the main injection site, while the heavy and lighter stippled areas represent the diffusion zone and the halo, respectively. Note massive labelling in zona incerta following HRP injection

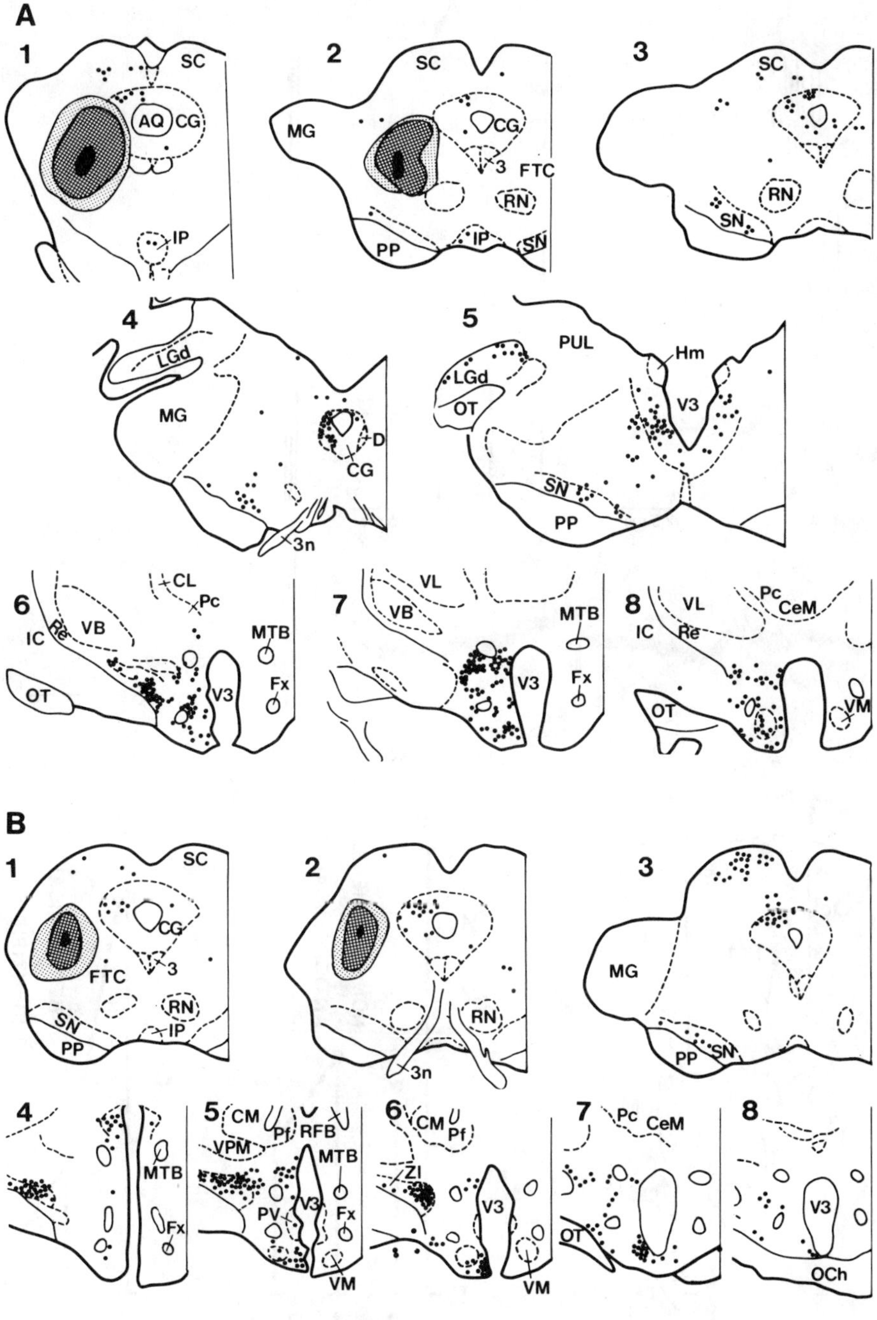

restricted to the MRF (in B), and intense labelling in the medial hypothalamus following HRP injection that encrouched upon the periaqueductal grey (in A). (Modified from A. Parent and M. Steriade (1981), *Brain Research Bulletin*, **7**, 411–418, and M. Steriade *et al.* (1982b), *Brain Research*, **238**, 13–28, by permission.)

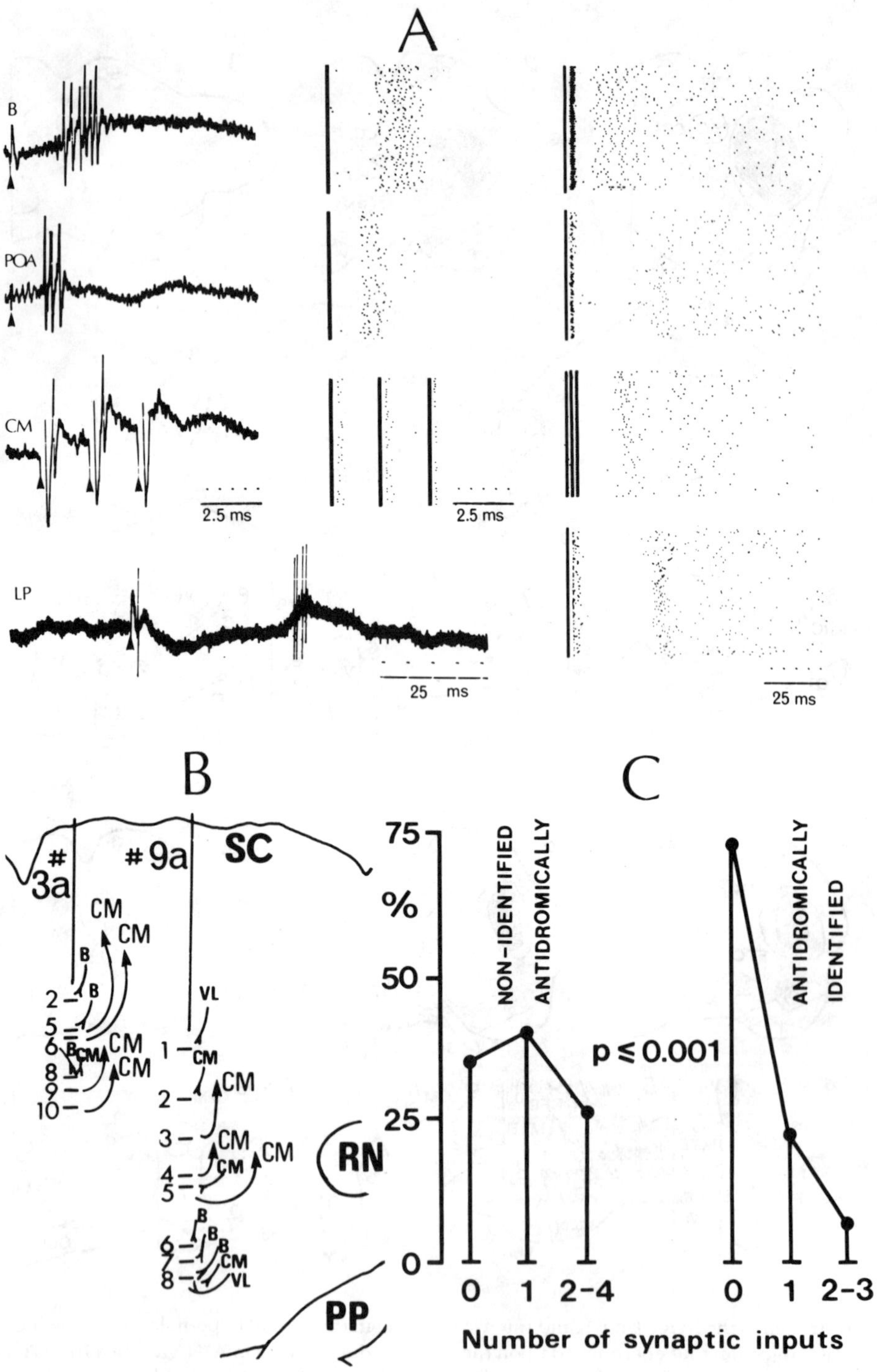
A
B
POA
CM
LP
2.5 ms
2.5 ms
25 ms
25 ms
B
#3a
#9a
SC
CM
CM
B
B
2
5
6
B
CM
CM
8
9
10
CM
VL
1
CM
2
CM
3
CM
CM
4
CM
5
CM
RN
B
B
6
B
7
CM
8
VL
PP
C
75
%
50
25
0
NON-IDENTIFIED
ANTIDROMICALLY
p ≤ 0.001
ANTIDROMICALLY
IDENTIFIED
0
1
2-4
0
1
2-3
Number of synaptic inputs

6.2.2 *Neocortical Projections of Medial-Intralaminar Thalamic Nuclei and their Synaptic Excitation from the Midbrain Reticular Core*

The foregoing section indicated that medial-intralaminar thalamic nuclei are major targets of the MRF. In their pioneering study of ascending pathways in the brainstem reticular formation, Nauta and Kuypers (1958) stated that further experiments need to 'identify beyond hypothesis the final corticipetal link in the anatomical substratum of the phenomenon of diffuse cortical arousal' (p. 27). At that time, no structures other than the specific thalamic nuclei had been shown to project to the neocortex. With the advent of retrograde and anterograde tracing methods, several medial and intralaminar thalamic nuclei were demonstrated to connect directly with widespread neocortical regions. Thus, the reticulocortical link was implicated by these experiments to lie in the medial and intralaminar thalamic nuclei. Especially, neurons in the lateral intralaminar thalamic wing, consisting of centralis lateralis (CL) and paracentralis (Pc) nuclei, were retrogradely labelled following HRP injections into sensorimotor, parietal association and extrastriate neocortical areas (see Hendry *et al.*, 1979; Jones & Leavitt, 1974). The actual identification of individual intralaminar thalamic neurons that relay afferents from the upper brainstem reticular core to the cerebral cortex remained to be achieved by electrophysiological methods and is reported below. As the electrophysiological thalamic exploration was mainly directed to nuclei with widespread cortical projections (CL-Pc and ventromedial, VM), I feel it necessary to present briefly their topography and boundaries.

Systematization and some morphological features of medial-intralaminar thalamic nuclei (Fig. 6.12). In cat, at frontal plane 7, around the retroflex bundle, lies the centrum medianum-parafascicularis (CM-Pf) complex, which projects densely to striatum (Jones & Leavitt, 1974), is a major source of a descending pathway to the MRF (Parent & Steriade, 1981), but has few if any direct projections to cortical areas. The heavier accumulation of Nissl substance in Pf cells usually contrasts with the less dense staining of the CM neurons, mainly located

---

Fig. 6.11 Convergent synaptic excitation of midbrain reticular neurons in cat. A, a neuron in nucleus cuneiformis was excited synaptically following stimulation of bulbar reticular formation (B), preoptic area (POA), centre median (CM) and lateralis posterior (LP) thalamic nuclei; original spikes (left), and fifty-sweep dotgrams at fast (middle) and slow speed (right) to show dissimilar latencies, discharge patterns and suppressed firing-rebound sequences following stimulation of different sites; three-shock train to CM. B, two descents (3a and 9a) in the MRF drawn from sagittal sections (lateral plane 3); target structures (oblique arrows) were identified by antidromic invasion, while excitatory inputs (forked symbols) were recognized from synaptically elicited discharges at short latencies; VL = ventrolateral thalamic nucleus; for other abbreviations, see Fig. 6.9. The graph in C depicts the percentage (ordinate) of cells with various degrees of synaptic convergence in two neuronal populations (which could not be or have been antidromically identified from structures outside the midbrain reticular formation); 0 indicates neurons which have not been synaptically excited, and 1 to 4 indicates the number of stimulated sites which induced synaptic excitation. (Reproduced from M. Steriade *et al.* (1980) in J. A. Hobson and M. A. B. Brazier (Eds.), *The Reticular Formation Revisited*, by permission of Raven Press; and N. Ropert and M. Steriade (1981), *Journal of Neurophysiology*, **46**, 17–31, by permission.)

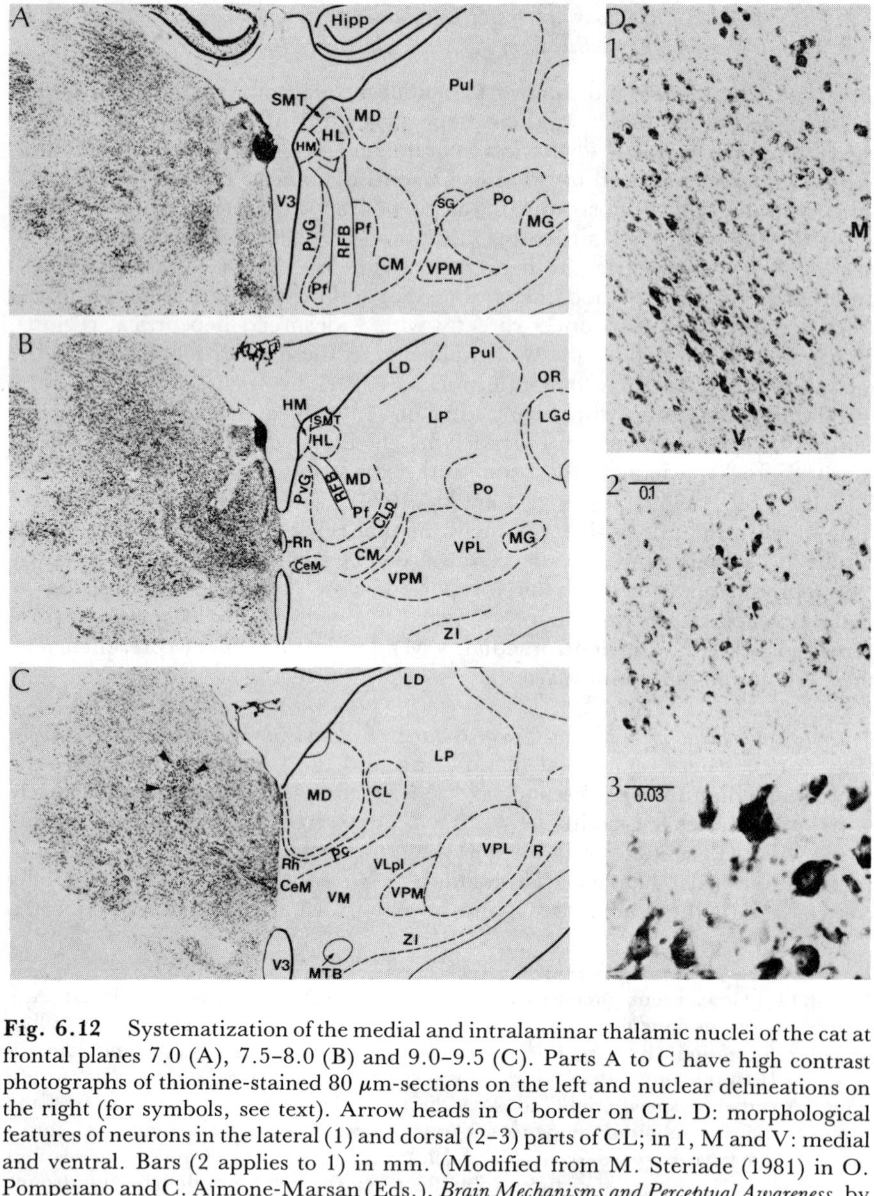

Fig. 6.12 Systematization of the medial and intralaminar thalamic nuclei of the cat at frontal planes 7.0 (A), 7.5–8.0 (B) and 9.0–9.5 (C). Parts A to C have high contrast photographs of thionine-stained 80 μm-sections on the left and nuclear delineations on the right (for symbols, see text). Arrow heads in C border on CL. D: morphological features of neurons in the lateral (1) and dorsal (2–3) parts of CL; in 1, M and V: medial and ventral. Bars (2 applies to 1) in mm. (Modified from M. Steriade (1981) in O. Pompeiano and C. Ajmone-Marsan (Eds.), *Brain Mechanisms and Perceptual Awareness*, by permission of Raven Press.)

lateroventrally (Fig. 6.12a). More rostrally, the Pf nucleus diminishes in size and the CM-Pf complex is broken by the appearance of a lamina where lies the posterior part of CL (Fig. 6.12b). The CL-Pc intralaminar wing fully develops anteriorly to the frontal plane 9.0, ventrolateral to the medialis dorsalis (MD) nucleus, dorsal to the VM, and medial to the lateralis posterior (LP) and ventralis lateralis (VL) nuclei (Fig. 6.12c). The only feature that can demarcate CL from Pc is a loosely organized zone between them. The CL nucleus consists of two major cell populations. Small-size neurons predominate in its ventromedial part, fusing with the Pc and merging posteriorly with the CM-Pf, but larger cells are seen in its lateral and dorsal districts. Fig. 6.12d shows the lateral, deeply Nissl-stained neurons, elongated along the ventromedial–dorsolateral axis of the CL wing, with the long diameter of 30 to 40 μm (D_1), and the oval-polygonal cells in the dorsal part of the CL, 20 to 28 μm in diameter (D_{2-3}). These medium to large-sized cells contrast with the smaller elements (12–18 μm) in the remaining parts of the CL. A distinct class of CL neurons projecting with fast conduction velocities to parietal area 5 and synaptically driven from the MRF was recorded in the region of the relatively large, deeply stained neurons (Steriade & Glenn, 1982).

The VM nucleus, easily distinguishable in sagittal sections, is poorly defined in frontal sections at its dorsolateral limit adjacent to the VL nucleus. It is not usually possible to distinguish between VM and VL solely on a cytoarchitectonic basis. Thus VM is not defined according to cytoarchitectonic criteria, but according to hodologic criteria based on recent studies. The nigral input can be used as a criterion of VM borders. Hendry *et al.* (1979) found that amino acid isotope injections in the middle or lateral parts of the substantia nigra resulted in heavy autoradiographic labeling through the VM and the most medial part of VL, as these nuclei are defined on cytoarchitectonic grounds. The label was quite sparse and patchy in the intralaminar nuclei. In particular, Hendry *et al.* (1979) showed that this nigra-related VM and medial VL region also receives a projection from the entopeduncular nucleus but not from the interpositus-dentate cerebellar nuclei, unlike the ventralis anterior (VA) and VL, which suggests that VM should be defined to include the very medial VL area. This agrees with the fact that nigral neurons are antidromically activated from both the VM and the medial portion of VL (Anderson & Yoshida, 1980). The medial VL region, which is located between the centralis lateralis (CL) and the VM, was named VL paralaminaris (VL pl).

Cortical projections of intralaminar (CL-Pc) thalamic neurons relaying MRF excitatory impulses. Since HRP studies indicated that CL-Pc nuclei project to widespread cortical regions and particularly to sensorimotor and parietal association areas, we (Steriade & Glenn, 1982) covered these areas with a large number of stimulating electrodes to determine by antidromic invasion whether individual axons of CL-Pc origin project to widely separated regions or to quite distinct foci (Fig. 6.13a and e). As to the direct inputs from the MRF to intralaminar neurons, without adequate experimental precautions the interpretation of electrically elicited synaptic responses from the MRF (Fig. 6.13c and d) is questionable because fibres en passage arising at more caudal reticular fields and in extra-reticular aggregates can also be stimulated. The rostral pontine tegmentum was therefore lesioned (Fig. 13b) and time was alloted for the anterograde degeneration of spinothalamic pathways, fibres arising in pontomedullary reticular fields, locus coeruleus axons and other ascending systems.

In view of the hypothesized role of intralaminar nuclei in controlling activities of widespread forebrain regions, the expectation was that intralaminar neurons

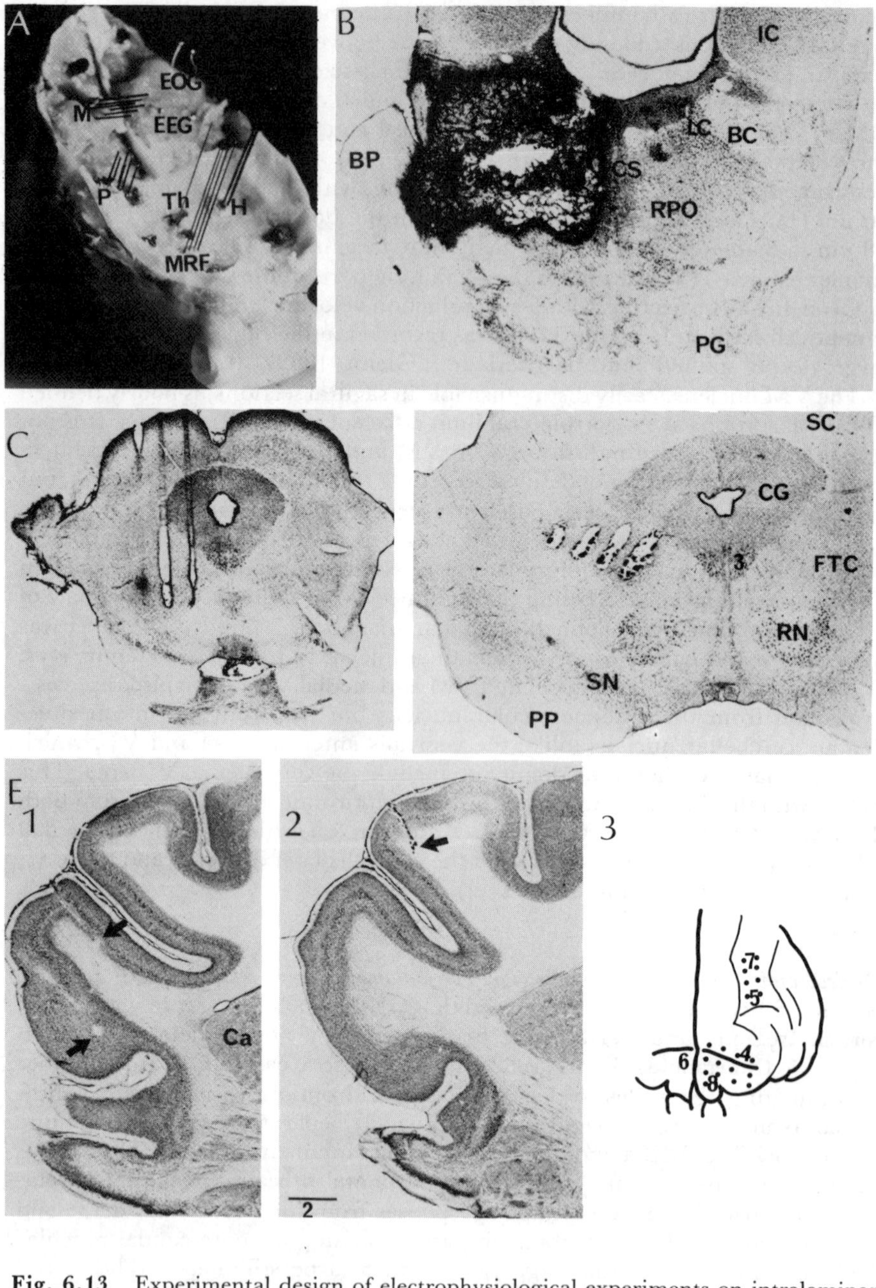

Fig. 6.13 Experimental design of electrophysiological experiments on intralaminar thalamic nuclei (A), pontine lesion (B), and location of stimulating electrodes in MRF (C–D) and cortex (E). Calvarium with chronically implanted stimulating electrodes and the last recording thalamic microelectrode (A), and thionine-stained frontal (B–D) and sagittal (E_{1-2}) sections. In C, the array of stimulating electrodes was inserted vertically into the ventral MRF at plane A 1.5; the most lateral electrode track was found in an anterior section. In D, the stimulating array was inserted obliquely through the contra-

diffusely project to widely separated cortical areas and striatum. CL-Pc *nuclei* do indeed project to numerous motor, sensory and association areas of the cerebral cortex, but only one neuron projected to both the sensorimotor (pericruciate) and parietal association (anterior suprasylvian) cortices in our study, despite the fact that 236 neurons projected to one or the other. The lack of bifurcating neurons to these regions implies that the projection of CL-Pc neurons to the cortex is discrete. Additional evidence was provided by the distribution of cortical points from which antidromic invasions could be evoked. In over 85% of the cases, CL-Pc neurons were backfired from a cortical territory restricted to the distance between two adjacent electrodes (see Fig. 6.13e). Neurons with two active regions separated by an interjacent region of higher threshold were much less frequently encountered. As inferred from antidromic latencies and conduction distances, the CL-Pc projection to suprasylvian area 5 consists of smaller axons than the projection to pericruciate area 4 or 6. The segregated conduction velocities between the pericruciate and suprasylvian projections corroborates the point that CL-Pc projections to different areas of cortex arise from different neurons. In addition, we never antidromically activated an individual CL or Pc unit from both a cortical site and the caudate nucleus in 170 tested neurons. This negative finding might be insignificant if it were not for the fact that over half the tested neurons did have identified projections to one structure or the other. The conduction velocity of CL neurons projecting to the caudate was significantly slower (3.8 m/s) from those projecting cortically (7.1–11.1 m/s) This difference also supports a segregation within CL-Pc nuclei, consisting of neurons with neocortical or caudate projections. Altogether, this evidence indicates that *what we used to call in the past the 'nonspecific' thalamic system consists, in fact, of neurons with highly localised projections towards the telencephalon.*

Eighty-four neurons localized in CL-Pc nuclei were synaptically activated by MRF stimulation at latencies shorter than 5 ms, 36 of which were driven at latencies (<1.5 ms) below which a response can be safely considered to be monosynaptic, taking also into account the slow conduction velocities (3.5–4.6 m/s) of MRF ascending axons. Out of 84 neurons driven synaptically by MRF stimulation at <5 ms, 35 could be identified as projecting to cortical areas 4, 6, 5, or the caudate nucleus (Fig. 6.14). The histogram in Fig. 6.14c shows the relation between the latency of MRF-evoked synaptic activation and the projections of CL-Pc units. These results provide the first indication at a cellular level that *a rapid, bisynaptic route relayed in the CL-Pc intralaminar nuclei transfers excitatory influxes from the MRF toward the caudate nucleus and neocortical areas.*

---

lateral hemisphere. Arrows in E_{1-2} indicate the location of stimulating electrode tips within deep layers of the medial parts of cortical cytoarchitectonic areas 8 and 6 (E_1) and within white matter below the postcruciate part of area 4 (E_2). Bar in E is in mm. Black dots in E3 indicate the location of cortical stimulating electrodes in relation to certain cytoarchitectonic areas. In A, M: stimulation array in the motor (pericruciate) cortex; P: stimulation array in the parietal association (suprasylvian) cortex; MRF: stimulation array in the midbrain reticular formation; Th: recording microelectrode in the intralaminar thalamic nuclei; EOG and EEG: silver balls for recording eye movements and frontal EEG; H: electrodes for recording hippocampal rhythms. (Reproduced from M. Steriade and L. L. Glenn (1982), *Journal of Neurophysiology*, **48**, 352–371, by permission.)

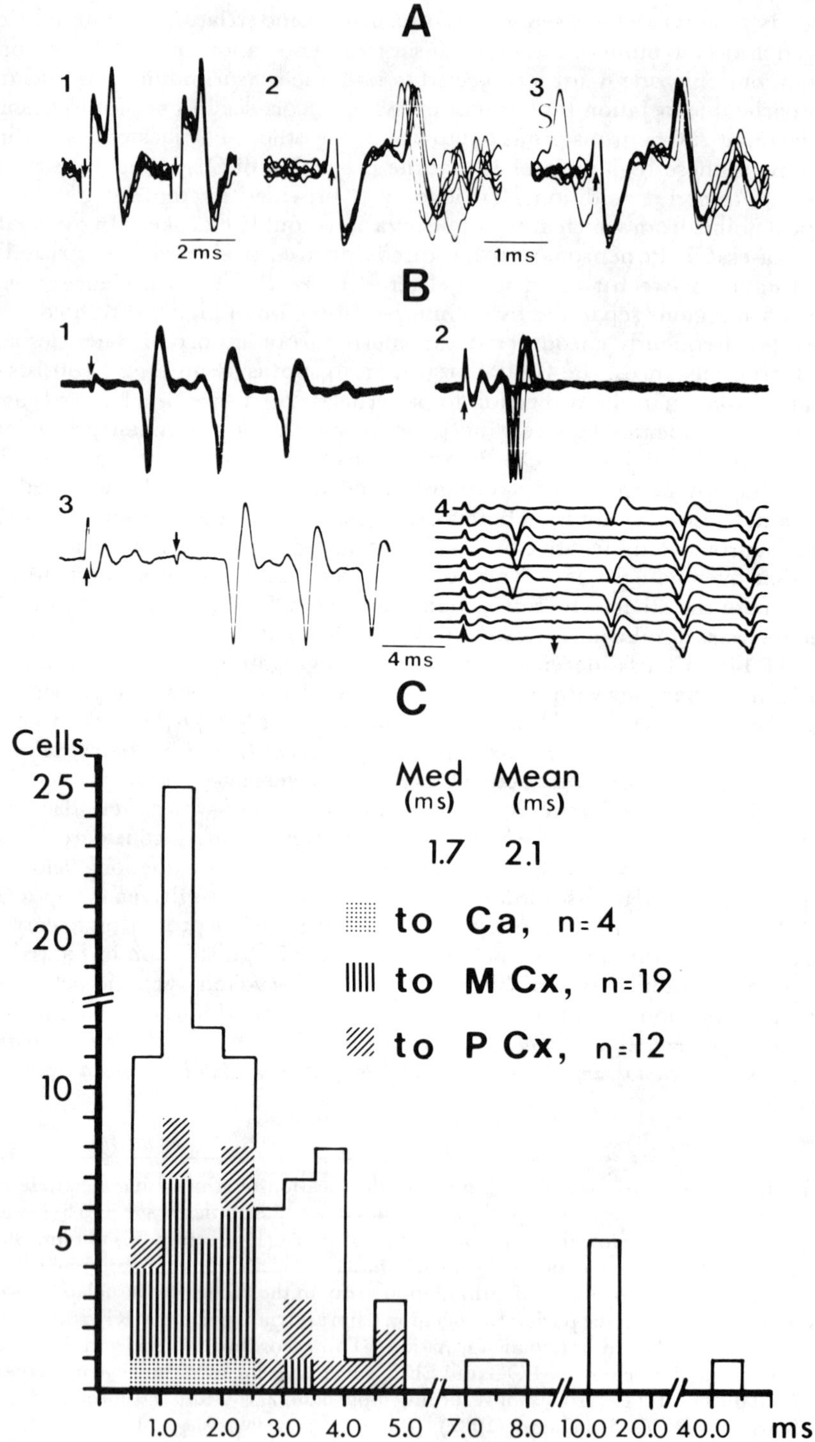

A
1
2
3
S
2 ms
1 ms
B
1
2
3
4
4 ms
C
Cells
25
20
10
5
Med (ms)
Mean (ms)
1.7
2.1
to Ca, n=4
to M Cx, n=19
to P Cx, n=12
1.0
2.0
3.0
4.0
5.0
7.0
8.0
10.0
20.0
40.0
ms

The superficial cortical projection of the VM thalamic nucleus. In 1938 Lorente de No introduced a dual thalamocortical concept by showing a distinct laminar termination of two classes of thalamic afferents, from specific nuclei to mid-layers (III–IV) of the cerebral cortex and from 'nonspecific' nuclei to outer and inners layer (I and VI). The disclosure of a superficial cortical projection from thalamic nuclei relaying MRF ascending influences would be important since intracellular studies (Inubushi et al., 1978a–b) have shown that cortical activation processes begin in the most superficial layer and are than conveyed downward. Autoradiographic studies in rat have disclosed a superficially projecting thalamocortical system arising from the VM thalamic nucleus and terminating in the most superficial quarter of layer I (Herkenham, 1979). The VM-cortical system was thought to subserve the widespread recruiting (superficial) responses elicited by medial thalamic nuclei stimulation. Since electrophysiological studies on recruiting responses have been almost exclusively conducted in cats and structural information of the VM projection is lacking in this species, we (Glenn *et al.*, 1982) undertook experiments using HRP as an anterograde as well as retrograde tracer, and a laminar field potential analysis.

VM projects almost exclusively to layer I of the neocortex (Fig. 6.15). This projection is restricted to motor, premotor and frontal regions, i.e. cytoarchitectonic areas 4, 6, 8 and 12. A number of observations support this. First, HRP transported anterogradely from the VM was found in neocortex anterior, and not posterior, to the dorsal bank of the cruciate sulcus (Fig. 6.16). Second, HRP deposits in precruciate cortex resulted in the retrograde labelling of VM neurons, whereas deposits in the primary somatosensory, auditory, visual or parietal association cortex did not result in VM neuron labelling. Third, clear field potentials evoked by single pulse stimulation of VM could be found in precruciate cortex, but not posteriorly. Fourth, retrogradely labelled layer VI neurons, the spatial distribution of which paralleled that of the layer I projection (Fig. 6.15), was not found posterior to the cruciate sulcus. Lastly, VM neurons were antidromically activated from the anterior sygmoid and proreus gyri, but not from the anterior suprasylvian gyrus. Importantly, there was an agreement between findings from all the above techniques that the projection was the most dense in the medial 2 mm of the crown of the anterior sygmoid gyrus (areas 6 and 8).

The almost exclusive projection of VM to the most superficial quarter of layer I was further supported by the reversal of the VM-evoked surface-negative

---

Fig. 6.14 Intralaminar (CL–Pc) thalamic neurons projecting to the cerebral cortex and synaptically activated from the MRF. Two different neurons that were antidromically identified from cortical area 4 (A_1) and area 6 (B_1) were synaptically driven from the MRF at minimum latencies of 1.1 ms (A_{2-3}) and 2.2 ms (B_2). The latencies of MRF-elicited discharges sometimes fluctuated widely (A_2) or hardly at all (A_3), but was clearly synaptic in nature because the response did not collide with preceding spontaneous spikes (S in A_3). In B, three antidromic volleys at 250/s (only the first pulse is indicated; the second artifact can be seen in the multiple sweep display of B_4 when the response to the first cortical pulse collided with an evoked synaptic activation); both MRF and cortical stimuli were applied successively in B_{3-4}. In C, histogram of the minimum latency of synaptic responses evoked in CL–Pc neurons by MRF stimulation. Neurons antidromically identified to project towards rostral sites are specially indicated. (Modified from M. Steriade and L. L. Glenn (1982), *Journal of Neurophysiology*, **48**, 352–371, by permission.)

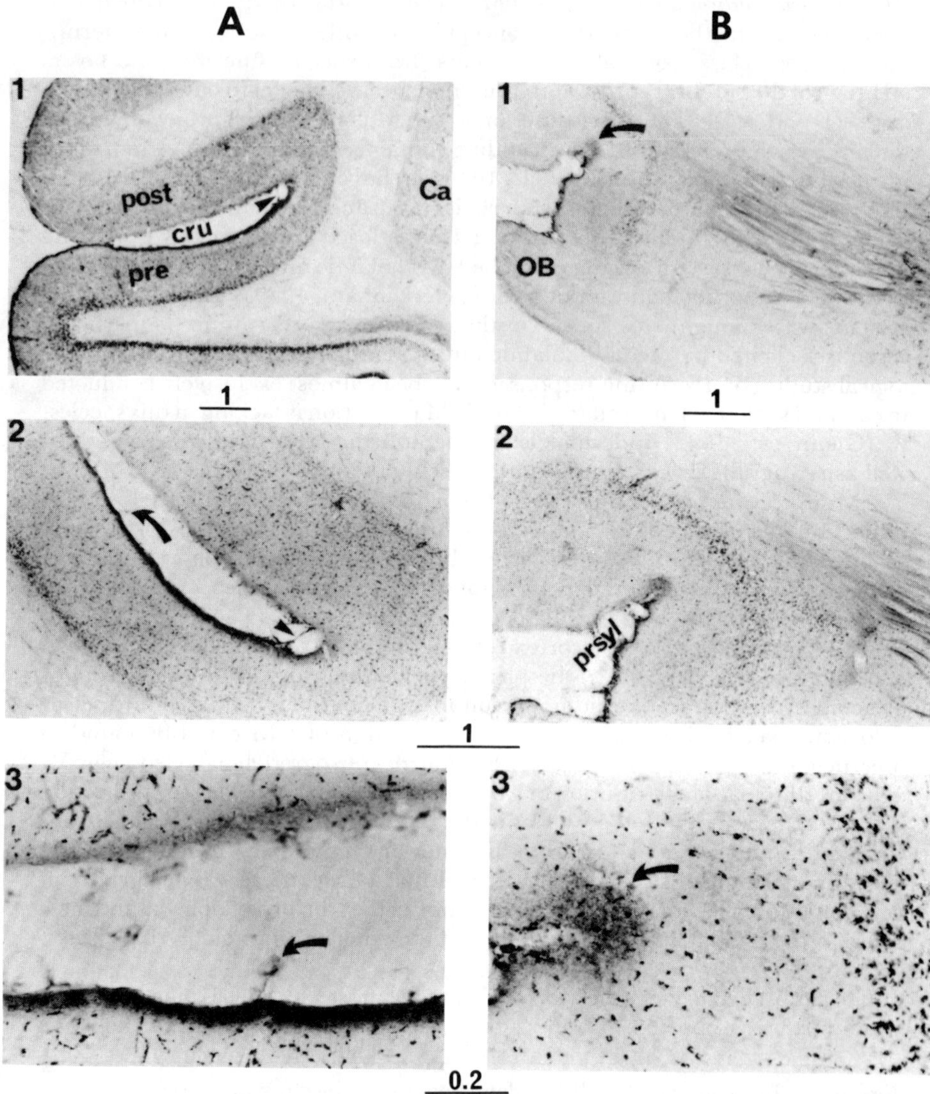

Fig. 6.15 Anterograde and retrograde transport of HRP 48 h after an injection in the ipsilateral VM nucleus. Sagittal sections at $\simeq$ 1.9 mm (A) and $\simeq$4.3 mm (B) from midline. The same region is shown at successively increasing enlargements, going from photos 1 to 3. In A_3, note the reaction product was localized in a dense sharply defined, superficial band 55–60 μm wide in precruciate area 6, whereas a much lighter grain was found in the postcruciate area 4 (arrows mark reference points throughout photos). The heavy band of anterograde labelling in layer I of area 6 (see A_1) was paralleled by retrogradely labelled neurons in layer VI. Anterograde labelling in layer I extended ventrally up to the olfactory bulb (OB), paralleled by retrograde labelling in layer VI. Oblique arrows in B indicate the enlargement of both layer I and the VM terminals in the fundus of the presylvius sulcus (prsyl). Ca: caudate nucleus, cru: cruciate sulcus. (Reproduced from L. Glenn *et al.* (1982), *Neuroscience*, **7**, 1861–1877, by permission.)

waves at depths of only 0.15–0.30 mm and by the quick suppression of the wave after cortex superfusion with manganese. A surface-negative wave can be generated by either a depolarization of superficial elements or hyperpolarization of deep elements. However, an additional observation was made: manganese superfusion greatly reduced the surface-negative, depth-positive VM-evoked wave, without altering the depth-positive wave induced by peduncular stimulation which reflects layer V recurrent inhibitory postsynaptic potentials (IPSPs) (Fig. 6.17). Thus, we can conclude that VM stimulation elicits a depolarization in superficial structures. A candidate for the recipient of VM afference would be the apical dendrites of pyramidal tract neurons.

Morison and Dempsey (1942), in their classic study, found a relation between the sign of stimulus-evoked cortical responses and their distribution. Surface-positive responses were localized to a more restricted cortical focus than surface-negative responses. The surface-positive waves arise from electrical events in layers III–IV, while surface-negative waves arise from events in layers I–II. Numerous recent anatomical studies have provided an important foundation for the greater tendency of outer tier responses to distribute widely. Frost and Caviness (1980) found that projections from thalamic nuclei to the middle tier were generally more localized than those of the outer tier, and that the projections to the middle tier were generally found amidst a much wider projection to the outer tier. This can explain why surface-positive responses are immersed in and surrounded by a larger region of surface-negative responses (Morison & Dempsey, 1942; Schlag & Villablanca 1967). Donoghue & Ebner (1981) found that the central intralaminar nucleus, which projects to the outer tier of the opossum parietal cortex, had a wider termination area than the VB or VL projection to the middle tier. Ferster & Levay (1978) demonstrated that individual afferent fibres terminating in the middle tier of the striate cortex have much more restricted regions of arborization than those that terminate in the outer tier. Thus, the widespread nature of surface-negative potentials and the focal nature of surface-positive potentials can be explained on the basis of recent anatomical findings.

Functional implications. One of the major functions related to the superficial cortical projections arising in the VM (see above) and probably also in intralaminar CL-Pc nuclei (Jones & Leavitt, 1974; Foster, 1980) concerns the EEG desynchronization and tonic activation of cortical processes. Moruzzi & Mogoun (1949) originally found the most effective points for eliciting anterior cortex desynchronization in the medial diencephalon, brainstem reticular formation, and fastigial nuclei. Lesions of the fastigial nuclei or reticular formation can lead to EEG synchronization (reviewed by Moruzzi, 1972). This may be significant in light of the demonstrated fastigial and reticular afference to VM (Herkenham, 1979), and the abundant collaterals sent to the MRF by ascending fastigial fibres (Kievit & Kuypers, 1972). The VM may be a rostral continuation of the upper reticular core, sharing this function with the CL-Pc intralaminar nuclei, and distribute reticular influences to the superficial layers of wide neocortical regions. Support for this view comes from the intracellular studies of Inubushi *et al.* (1978a–b), who concluded that motor cortex activation events are processed from superficial to deep layers. Furthermore, Hyvärinen *et al.* (1980) found an influence of variations in attention on cortical cells in superficial layers but to a lesser degree in middle layers.

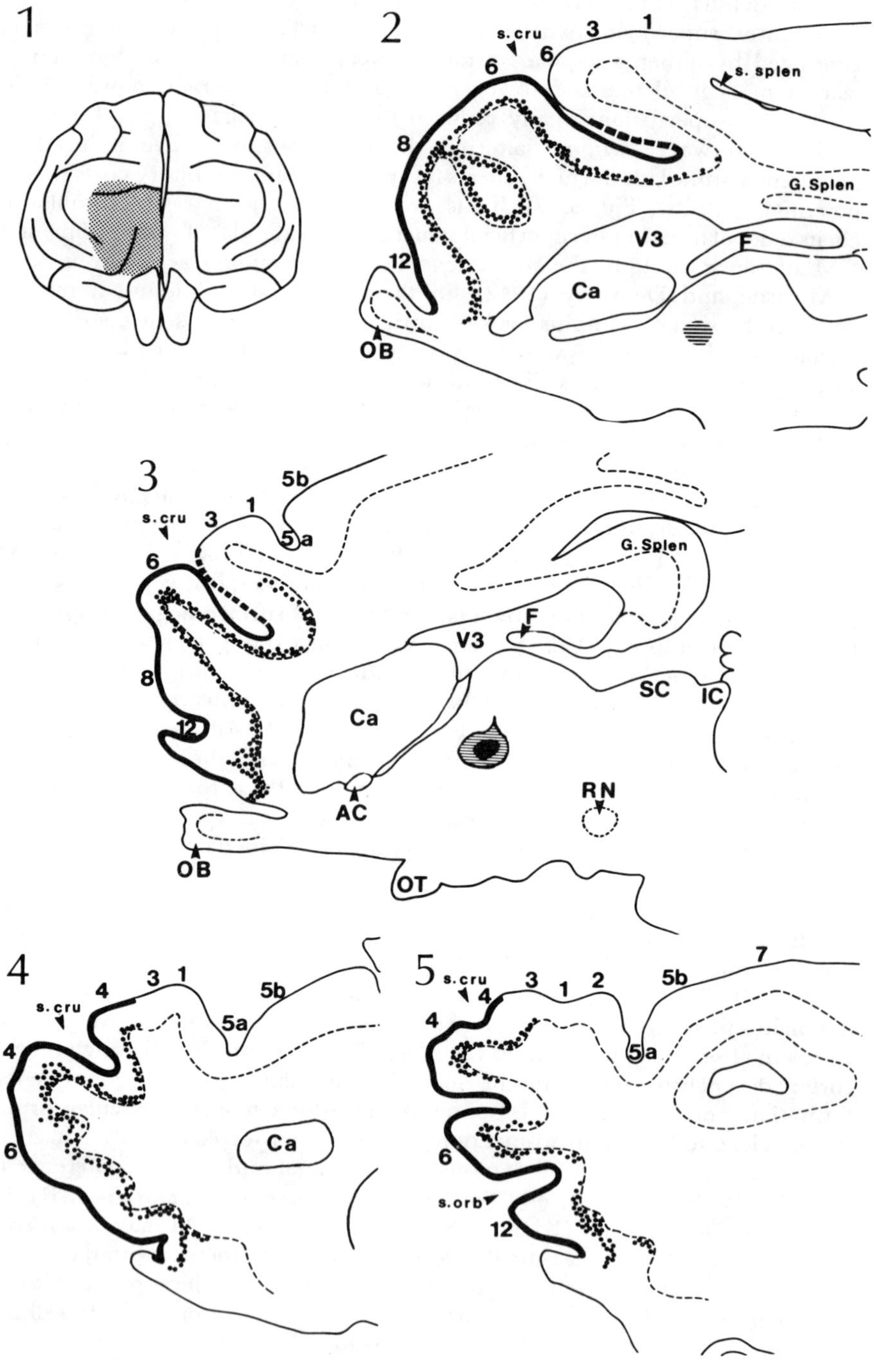
1
2
s. cru
3
1
6
6
s. splen
8
G. Splen
V3
F
12
Ca
OB
3
5b
1
s. cru
3
5a
6
G. Splen
F
V3
8
SC
IC
Ca
12
AC
RN
OB
OT
4
3
1
5b
4
s. cru
5a
4
Ca
6
5
s. cru
3
1
2
5b
7
4
4
5a
6
s. orb
12

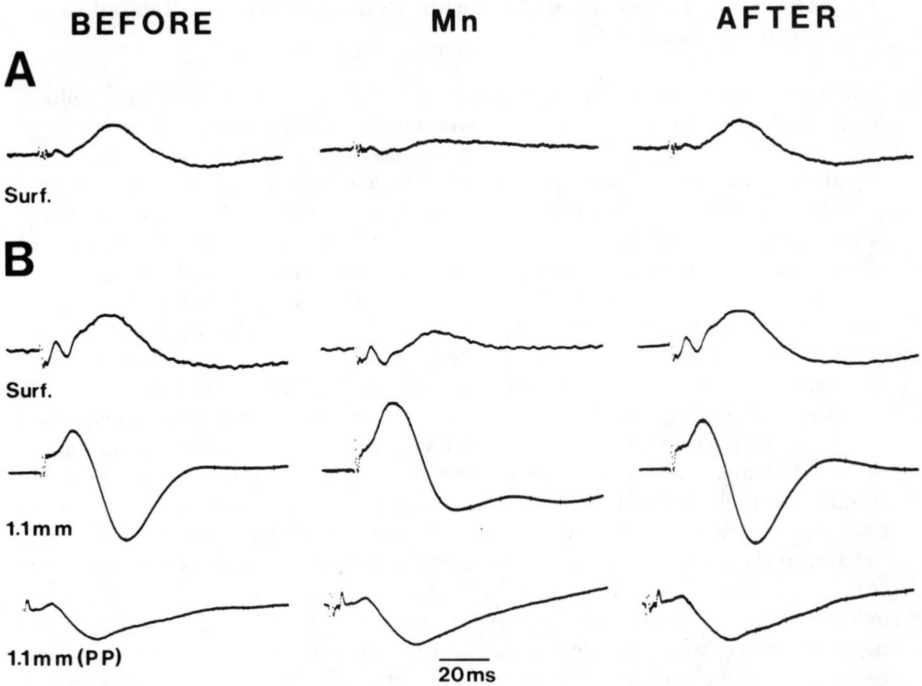

Fig. 6.17 Alteration of VM-invoked responses in area 6 by superfusion of the cortex with Mn^{2+}. Surface (A) and depth (1.1 mm) field potentials were recorded simultaneously. The deep field potentials evoked from the pes pedunculi (PP) were not altered by the Mn^{2+}. (Reproduced from L. Glenn *et al.* (1982), *Neuroscience*, **7**, 1861–1877, by permission.)

Fig. 6.16 Drawings of anterogradely and retrogradely labelled structures after ipsilateral VM injection (size and location shown in part 3). *1*: dorsal view of cortex; stippled area indicates the cortical extension of intense granular reaction in layer I. *2, 3, 4* and *5*: sagittal sections at ≃ 1.0, 2.3, 5.0 and 6.7 mm from midline. HRP reaction product indicative of anterogradely transported HRP in layer I is indicated by a heavy continuous line; heavy dashed lines indicate a liminal grain density. Dots indicate the presence of retrogradely labelled neurons; the density of dots was drawn in close proportion to the density of labelled neurons, but the number of dots is drastically lower than the number of neurons. The light dashed lines indicate the border between the grey and white matter. The location of cytoarchitectonic areas is indicated. Ca: caudate nucleus; V3: third ventricle; F: fornix OB: olfactory bulb; OT: optic tract; RN: red nucleus; CG: central grey; s. cru: cruciate sulcus; G. splen: splenial gyrus; s. orb: orbital sulcus; IC: inferior colliculus; SC: superior colliculus; AC: anterior commissure. (Reproduced from L. Glenn *et al.* (1982), *Neuroscience*, **7**, 1861–1877, by permission.)

6.3 Discharge Properties of Midbrain Reticular Neurons Related to Tonic Activation Processes

The lesion-stimulation approach (Section 6.1.2) cannot resolve, at a cellular level, the hypothetical elements endowed with ascending activating influences. The expectation was that MRF neurons would exhibit an increase in firing rates during W compared to S sleep. Instead, divergent results have been published reporting a decreased (Huttenlocher, 1961) or increased (Kasamatsu, 1970; Manohar *et al.*, 1972) firing rate during W. It is likely that the discrepancy in results is due to the heterogeneity of investigated neurons and the fact that they were not physiologically identified in former studies. I report below the result of experiments relating the rate change of MRF neurons during the sleep–waking continuum to their anatomical localization and input–output characteristics (Steriade *et al.*, 1980; Steriade, 1981; Steriade *et al.*, 1982a). It will be shown that rostrally projecting MRF neurons exhibit tonic discharge patterns and increased firing rates during periods of W and D sleep without phasic motor events. But any attempt to test the hypothesis of reticular ascending activation should also include the dynamics of neuronal activity changes from one state to another, which could reveal whether changes in firing rates precede overt behavioural aspects and the most precocious electrographic signs that announce shifts in the states of vigilance (see Fig. 6.6c, d and e). Our experiments provide evidence that a statistically significant increase in discharge rate of MRF neurons occurs prior to overt behavioural signs of activated states, and also before any change in the fully synchronized EEG rhythms of S sleep epochs developing into awakening.

6.3.1 Discharge Rates and Patterns of MRF Neurons Compared to Other Reticular Elements

MRF neurons increase firing rates during steady W and D activated states. Table 6.1 shows that the median of firing rates in MRF neuronal samples increases by more than two times in both W and D states compared to S sleep. It should be emphasized that the level of spontaneous discharge in MRF neurons is high in both W and D, in spite of the fact that the experiments were conducted on head-restrained animals and that measurements were derived from epochs without phasic motor events. The change in firing rate from S sleep to behavioural states characterized by EEG activation has further implications when it is analysed as a function of (a) rate magnitude, (b) input–output organization, and (c) localization of different neurons within the MRF.

(a) Within the maximized 60-cell sample investigated in W and S states, 45 neurons increased firing rates in W (73% of them discharged above 4/s in S) and 15 neurons decreased firing rates in W (73% of them discharged below 4/s in S). The difference in discharge rate during S between these two groups with opposite behaviour in W and S states is significant at $p < 0.0001$. The rate relation is also valid when comparing S sleep with D sleep. Thus, *the increased firing rate, during activated states, in the investigated MRF neuronal samples is essentially due to cells exhibiting relatively high discharge levels.*

(b) The rates were examined as a function of the degree of input convergence, and were related to the axonal projection in antidromically identified neurons. We divided the 60 cell sample into two subgroups: 43 neurons in

Table 6.1 Firing Rates of Midbrain Reticular Neurons during Wake and Sleep Steady States without Motor Events

N = number of neurons. 26 neurons were recorded during one or several complete sleep-waking cycles. Maximized samples were used for neurons which could be investigated in only two steady states (W and S, D and S). Mean and median indicate impulses per second for each neuronal sample. The weighted pooled rate was computed for each cell for all epochs in a given state; then the non-weighted rate for all cells was computed in each state. SD = standard deviation. Significance levels are from Wilcoxon paired signed-rank tests. * = below our limit of significance (p <0.05).

		Median	Mean	SD	Significance levels	
	W	19.92	20.66	18.78	W > S	$p < 0.0008$
$N = 26$	S	7.89	14.30	14.02	D > S	$p < 0.0001$
	D	18.57	25.68	25.39	W - D	$p < 0.06$*
	W	13.63	18.36	21.05		
$N = 60$					W > S	$p < 0.0001$
	S	6.74	13.28	15.50		
	D	13.95	21.93	24.48		
$N = 32$					D > S	$p < 0.0001$
	S	6.79	11.94	13.60		

which there was an absence or only one excitatory synaptic input, and 17 neurons which received two to four excitatory inputs. The latter subgroup discharged in W at a significantly higher rate than the former (p <0.04). Concerning the axonal projections, we examined 27 neurons projecting selectively to a rostral (thalamus or subthalamus) or a caudal (pons) site. Neurons projecting to the paramedian pons had significantly lower firing rates than those with rostrally projecting axons (p <0.03). More than 80% of neurons projecting selectively to rostral sites increased firing rates in W.

(c) During recording, we had the impression, based on micrometer depth recordings that the discharge rates of successively encountered neurons were higher at deeper levels in the midbrain core. This observation was later histologically verified on 139 neurons found within the MRF territory. Of them, the most important group (n = 62) was found at the plane depicted in Fig. 6.18a. The impression was confirmed that cells found at levels ventral to the depth coordinate zero discharged at higher rates than dorsally located cells (Fig. 6.18a). When firing rates were precisely measured and processed statistically, the relation between firing rate during quiet W and the dorso-ventral localization within the MRF was tested in 44 cells discharging spontaneously above 0.1/s (Fig. 6.18b). The Spearman rank correlation coefficient between high discharge rate and ventral location of neurons (rs = 0.42) was found significant at p <0.005.

These data, showing that *the increase in firing rate of MRF neurons in activated states is essentially due to highly discharging elements (> 4/s), with rostral projections, a great*

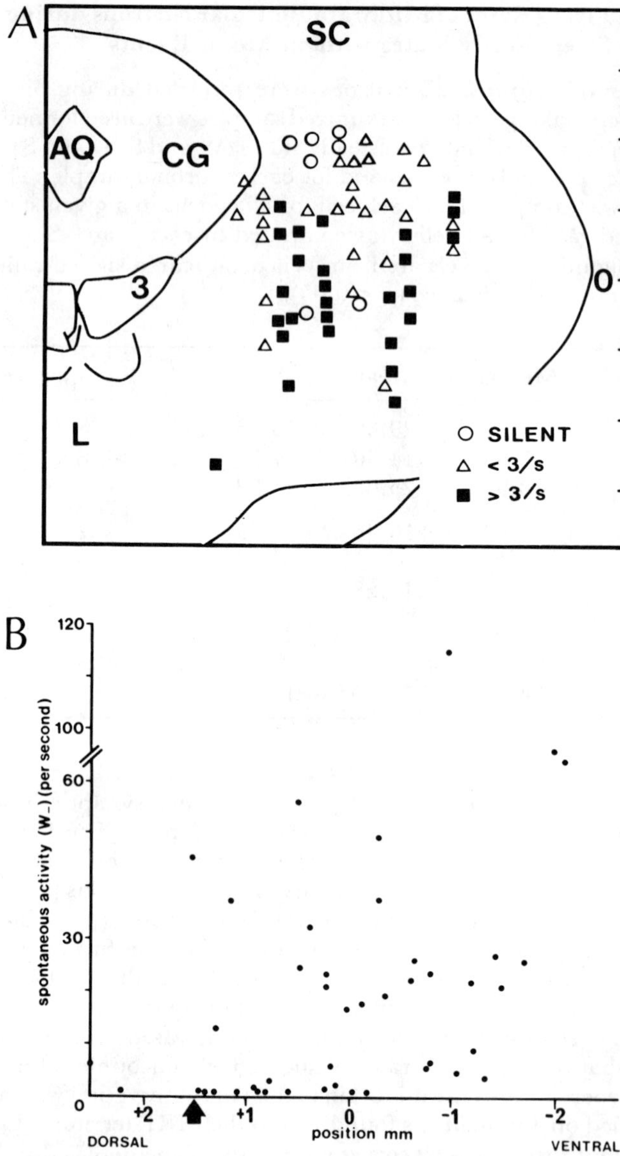

Fig. 6.18 Rate level as a function of dorso-ventral localization in the MRF. A: location at frontal plane 2.5 of neurons whose firing rates were rougly estimated during recording and divided into three classes: silent, below 3/s and above 3/s. B: dorso-ventral position of 44 MRF neurons whose firing rates during quiet W were precisely measured; Spearman rank correlation between high discharge rate and ventral location ($r_s = 0.42$) significant at $p < 0.005$. The arrow in B indicates the limit between deep layers of SC and MRF. (Reproduced from M. Steriade, G. Oakson and N. Ropert (1982), *Experimental Brain Research*, **46**, 37–51, by permission.)

majority of which were found at relatively ventral levels in the midbrain core, may help to explain the unexpected findings of Huttenlocher (1961) reporting higher discharge rates in 88% of MRF neurons during S sleep. Examining his Table 1 (median firing rates in quiet W and S: 1.6/s and 3.2/s, respectively), it is clear that an overwhelming majority discharged below 3/s. Such low discharging neurons were generally found 'in the lower layers of superior colliculus and in the dorsal portions of reticular formation' (p. 462). As suggested by our identification results, some of these elements could be neurons with axons projecting to the paramedian pontine reticular formation. Only a few units with sustained, high levels of discharge were recorded by him at more ventral levels because of technical difficulties due to brain pulsations.

MRF neurons exhibit tonic patterns. We asked whether the discharge patterns of MRF neurons are consistent with their presumed role in maintaining EEG activation. If so, one would hypothesize that rapidly discharging neurons which are responsible for the increased firing rate observed during activated states exhibit a sustained or *tonic* discharge, relatively evenly spread over time, as opposed to the spike clusters interspersed with periods of silence that characterize generators of phasic events. The observation of oscillographic and ink-written records gave us indeed the impression that MRF neuronal firing is sustained in all wake–sleep states (Fig. 6.19a and c). Only a few units exhibited long-duration spike clusters during S, as opposed to tonic discharge in W and D (Fig. 6.19b).

The analysis of interspike interval histograms (ISIHs) and autocorrelation functions (ACFs) affords more precise answers to the question of discharge patterns. It is expected that, if tonic, the ISIHs of MRF neurons consist mainly of medium intervals with relatively few short intervals (<10 ms) and long pauses (>250 ms), and tend towards a symmetric shape. Truly symmetric ISIHs of computer-simulated neurons (Segundo *et al.*, 1968) have a sharp mode with small spread and therefore a small coefficient of variation; their corresponding ACFs are highly periodic with peaks at multiples of the ISIH mode. Both ISIH and ACF analyses in a 15-cell sample showed that highly discharging MRF elements are characterized by tonic discharge patterns, firing features that are commonly seen in small-size neurons (see Fig. 6.8c). *The highest degree of tonicity was found during W*, as expressed in a great proportion of MRF cells by symmetric ISIHs, great interval density around the mode, smallest coefficient variation values, and periodic ACFs (Steriade *et al.*, 1982a). The regular, 'pacemaker' patterns during the W state (Fig. 6.20) should be emphasized since the W state is commonly viewed as a poorly defined, 'dirty' mixture of heterogenous behavioural components that could have destabilized the neuronal firing. The sustained, regular discharge revealed in our study is probably due to the elimination of epochs with phasic motor events and of short period of EEG synchronization during the W state (see Section 6.1.2 and Fig. 6.6b). This was done because our analysis did not bear on the behavioural sphere of vigilance states, but was conducted to test the possible role played by MRF neurons in triggering and maintaining the tonic process of EEG activation. Tonic discharge patterns are peculiar for MRF neurons not only during W, but also during D sleep when the first-order measures were found in many respects to be closer to W than to S sleep. This is in keeping with similar cellular

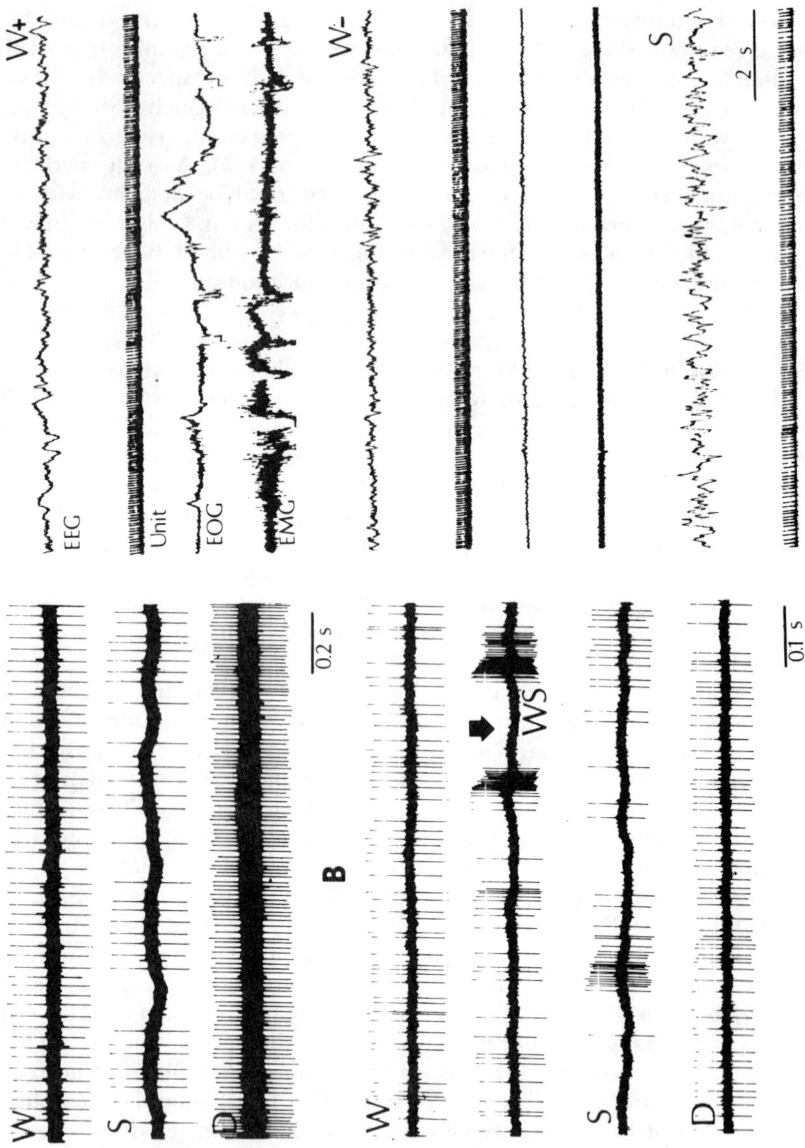

Fig. 6.19 Discharge features of MRF neurons during wake-sleep states. W = wakefulness (with, W + , and without, W – , movements); S = synchronized sleep; D = desynchronized sleep; WS = intermediate state between W and S. A and B: two cells adjacent in a descent, both driven synaptically from CM-Pf and paramedian pons. C: a cell antidromically identified from zona incerta and synaptically driven from preoptic area and paramedian pons. Note sustained, regular firing especially in C, regardless of movement (W +) or quiet (W –) epochs in W, or of rate changes from W to S. (Reproduced from M. Steriade, G. Oakson and N. Ropert (1982), *Experimental Brain Research*, **46**, 37–51, by permission.)

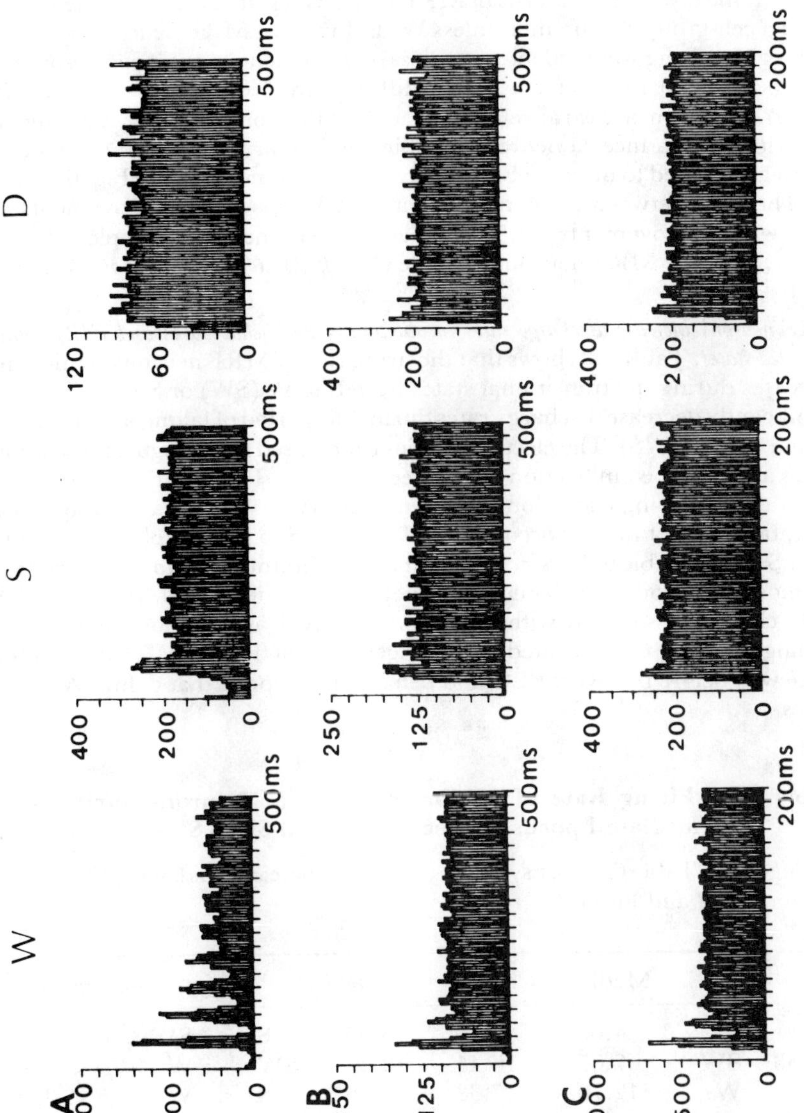

Fig. 6.20 Autocorrelations (ACFs) of three MRF neurons, identified as having a rostrally projecting axon (in A) and multiple excitatory inputs (B–C). ACFs were computed with resolutions of 5 or 2 ms over time ranges of 500 or 200 ms. Note regular peaks, near the modal interval, for three or more cycles during W, contrasting with flat contours in S and D. (Reproduced from M. Steriade, G. Oakson and N. Ropert (1982), *Experimental Brain Research*, **46**, 37–51, by permission.)

processes in thalamocortical systems during W and D, as opposed to S sleep. All these findings support the suggestion that rostrally projecting MRF neurons exert similar activating influences on thalamocortical and corticofugal cells during both W and D states (Steriade, 1978).

The tonic discharge patterns of MRF neurons resulted from statistical analyses of a cell-group during motionless W. But in most MRF neurons, sustained and regular firing was evident regardless of movement or quiet epochs of the W state (see Fig. 6.19c). This aspect is different from other reticular fields (see below) and from a rostral-related structure, the zona incerta. Actually, the majority of zona incerta neurons exhibit spectacular rises in firing frequency, phasically related to increase EMG activity and eye movements (Fig. 6.21a and b). The ratio between median firing rates in W epochs with movements and those without movements is 2.50 in the zona incerta neuronal sample, while it is only 1.15 in the MRF neuronal sample (Fig. 6.21c) (Steriade *et al.*, 1982b).

MRF neurons increase discharge rates in advance of any behavioural and EEG signs of activated states. Table 6.2 shows that the firing rate of MRF neurons significantly increases during the transitional states from S to W (SW) or S to D (SD), and significantly decrease discharge rates during the period of falling asleep between W and S states (WS). The electrographic criteria used to distinguish transitional states are described in Section 6.1.2 (See Fig. 6.6). The changes in firing rates operate fully during transitions between S and W or vice versa, and significant alterations do not further occur from SW and WS to the completely developed W or S states (Table 6.2). Since we define the beginning of transitional states by the most precocious EEG sign and the beginning of steady states by generalized EEG changes associated with or followed by typical behavioural events, the findings in Table 6.2 indicated that changes in the activity of MRF neurons take place well before the overt EEG and behavioural aspects that define W, S or D states.

Table 6.2 Firing Rate of Midbrain Reticular Neurons during Intermediate Epochs between Wake and Sleep States.

See legend to Table 6.1. For symbols of intermediate epochs (SW, WS, SD), see Section 6.1.2 and Fig. 6.6.

		Median	Mean	SD	Significance levels	
	S	4.06	12.10	14.65	S < SW	$p < 0.004$
$N = 33$	SW	7.07	16.41	18.59	SW - W	$p < 0.5$*
	W	12.70	17.33	18.24	S < W	$p < 0.0001$
	W	11.38	16.27	16.98	W > WS	$p < 0.0002$
$N = 52$	WS	7.39	12.87	14.59	WS - S	$p < 0.2$*
	S	6.50	12.19	13.25	W > S	$p < 0.0001$
	S	6.50	11.54	14.05	S < SD	$p < 0.0007$
$N = 26$	SD	8.39	16.94	20.20	SD < D	$p < 0.003$
	D	12.38	21.23	24.75	S < D	$p < 0.0001$

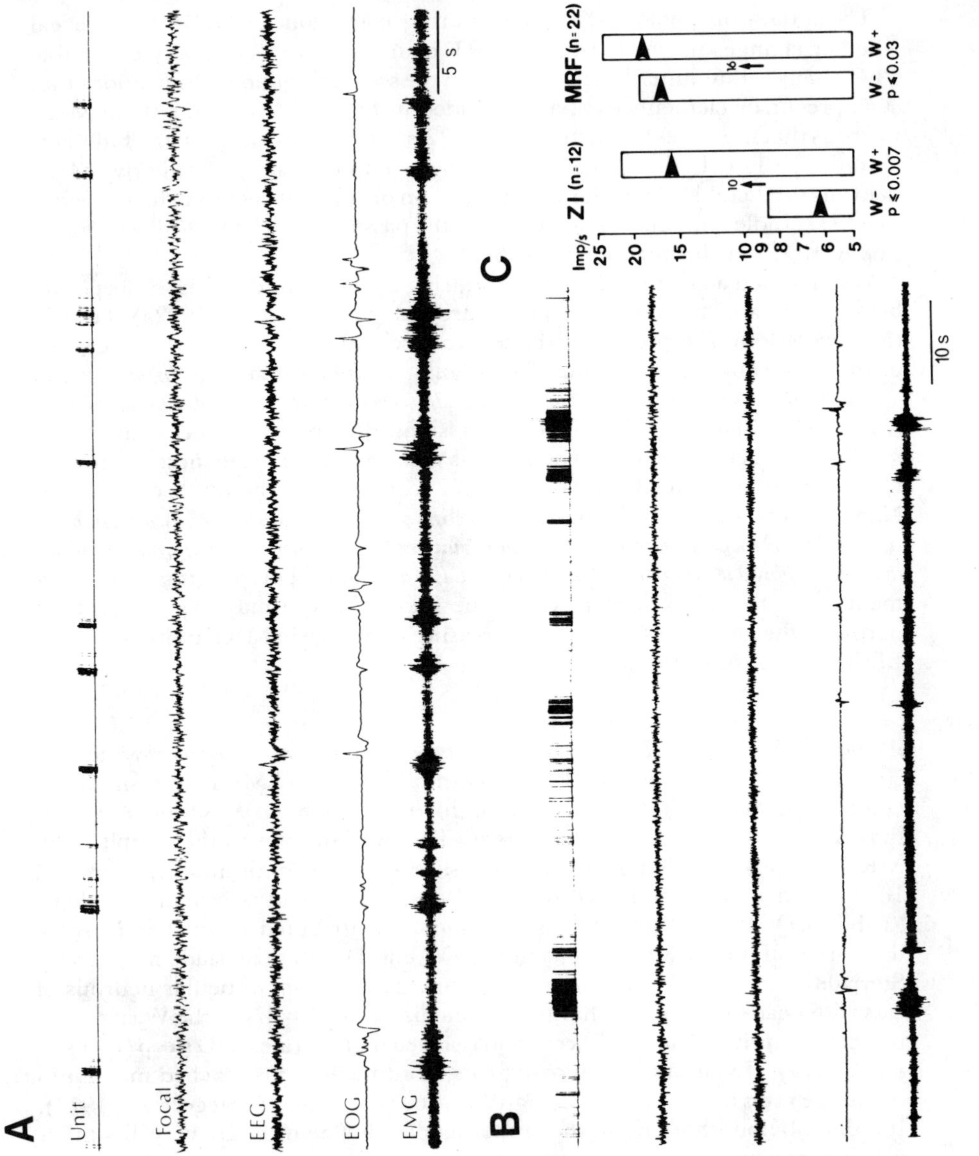

Fig. 6.21 Discharge of zona incerta (ZI) neurons during wake periods with (W +) and without (W −) movements. A and B, two different ZI neurons, antidromically identified by MRF stimulation. The five ink-written traces depict from top to bottom: unit discharge, focal slow waves simultaneously recorded by the microelectrode in the ZI and adequately amplified, EEG waves from the cortical surface, eye movements (EOG) and electromyogram (EMG) of neck muscles. Note in both cases phasic increases in firing rate related to increased EMG activity and EOG deflections. In C, firing rates in a ZI neuronal sample during epochs of W + and W −, compared to those in a MRF neuronal sample during the same substrates of W + and W −. Note that ZI cells showed a greater increase in firing rates during W +. (Reproduced from M. Steriade *et al.* (1982b), *Brain Research*, **238**, 13–28, by permission.)

These data on pooled firing rates during transitional states cannot reveal whether changes in firing rates of MRF neurons occur before any detectable EEG change, thus announcing the shift in the state of vigilance. Indications that such precursor elements exist are provided in Fig. 6.22 depicting three MRF neurons that increase their firing rates 8–22 s before any change in the fully synchronized EEG rhythms, that is prior to the end of S sleep. Similarly, MRF neurons predictably show marked diminution or complete arrest of firing before the first spindle sequence that announces the passage from EEG desynchronization to EEG synchronization (Fig. 6.23).

We analysed a group of 25 neurons during the last minute of the S sleep state before EEG and behavioural signs of arousal (Steriade *et al.*, 1982a). Four of them were found to project selectively to a rostral site and ten were receivers of multiple converging inputs. *A statistically significant increase in firing rate was demonstrated to occur 15 s before the end of S sleep epochs that developed into the W state* (Fig. 6.24). Such long-lead precursor signs do not characterize all MRF neurons. In fact, a proportion of neurons with spectacular rate increase in the S to W transition (such as those in Fig. 6.22) could distort the whole cell sample. None the less, the existence of such neurons suggests that *the increased excitability in some MRF elements eventually leads to recruitment of other neurons in the midbrain core that finally play a leading role in the process of EEG activation*. This progressive recruitment by collateral excitation within the midbrain core may explain, at least partially, the long time ($\simeq 15$ s) of increasing discharge in MRF units before the EEG desynchronization.

A comparison between MRF and other brainstem reticular neurons during the sleep–waking cycle. The high discharge rates found in a great majority of MRF units should be emphasized as they indicate a striking difference between MRF neurons and those located in pontine reticular areas. The median rates in the sample of 26 MRF neurons recorded throughout the sleep–waking continuum were around 18–20/s during both activated states of W and D without phasic motor events (Table 6.1). Body, limb or eye movements contributed to further increase discharge rates of MRF neurons in both W and D states (Steriade *et al.*, 1980; Steriade *et al.*, 1982b). In contrast, paramedian pontine reticular neurons of cats with head-restraint discharged at a median rate of $\simeq 1$/s in the W state, did not significantly change in S sleep, and reached highest rates in D sleep (Hobson *et al.*, 1974). Even in freely moving cats, pontine neurons reached maximum discharge rates of only $\simeq 2$/s during W without movements (Siegel *et al.*, 1977). It is thus obvious that, in cat, the properties of MRF neurons are very dissimilar to those of pontine reticular neurons recorded in either restrained or freely behaving animals. Pontine reticular neurons that discharged at high levels during quiet W represent 16% of the investigated sample in the freely moving rat (Vertes, 1979). It should be mentioned that, for all MRF samples in Table 6.1, 65–80% of neurons discharged above 4/s in quiet W or D sleep without REMs, and 55–60% of neurons discharged above 10/s in the same activated states.

The phasic or clustered discharge patterns of pontine reticular neurons (McCarley & Hobson, 1975a) make it improbable that these elements are involved in tonic ascending activation processes. Rather they seem related to phasic motor phenomena during W and D sleep. Actually, the increase in firing

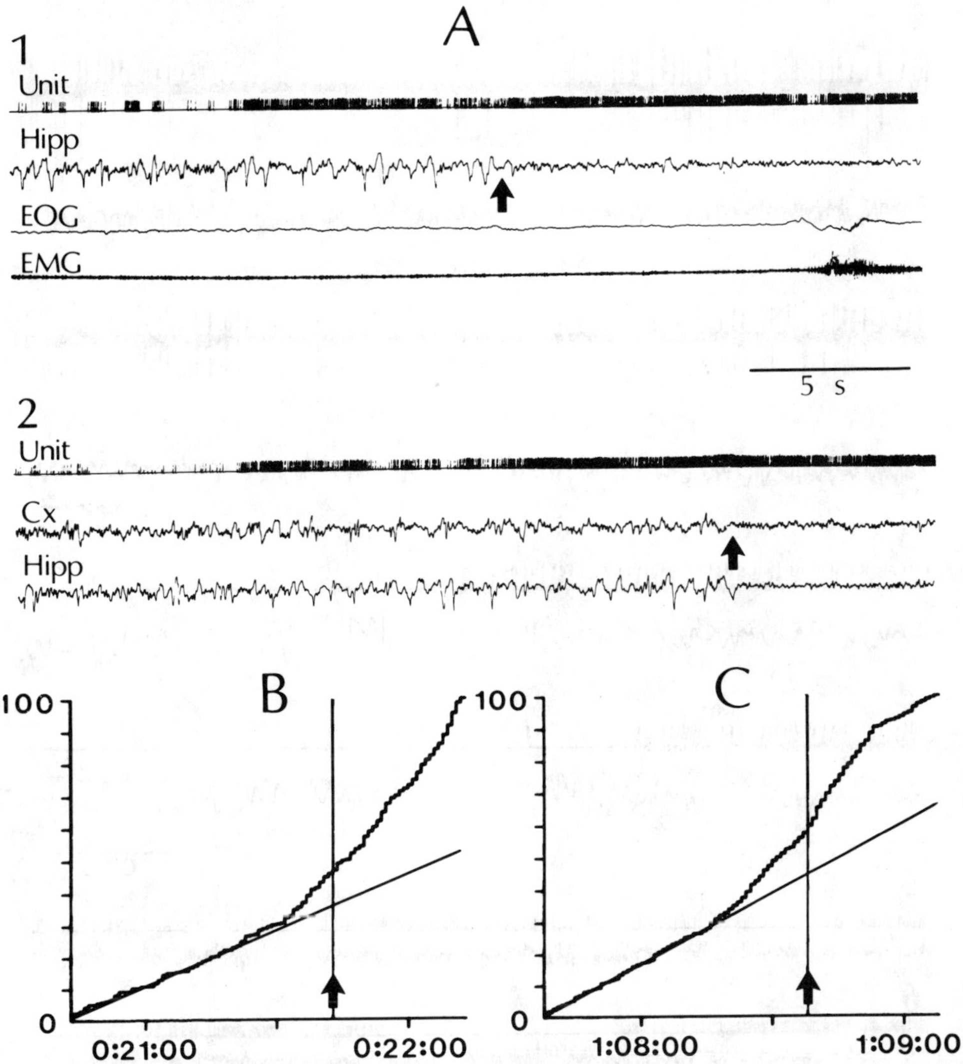

Fig. 6.22 Time course of midbrain reticular discharge during transitions from S sleep to W state. A to C, three different neurons (A and B synaptically driven from CM-Pf and pons, and C antidromically identified from CM-Pf). In A, records depicting two transitions from S to W (arrows indicate the beginning of EEG desynchronization on neocortical, Cx, and hippocampal, Hipp, leads). In B and C, percent cumulative histograms (1s-bins); abscissae indicate the real time of recording; arrows and vertical lines indicate the most precocious signs of reduced amplitude and/or increased frequency of neocortical or hippocampal slow waves; the slope (oblique line) indicates the mean discharge rate during S sleep; inflection points are seen to occur 10 to 22 s in advance of any change in the EEG; behavioural signs of the W state (eye movements and increased muscular tone) occurred several seconds after the arrows (as in A). (Reproduced from M. Steriade, G. Oakson and N. Ropert (1982) *Experimental Brain Research*, **46**, 37–51, by permission.)

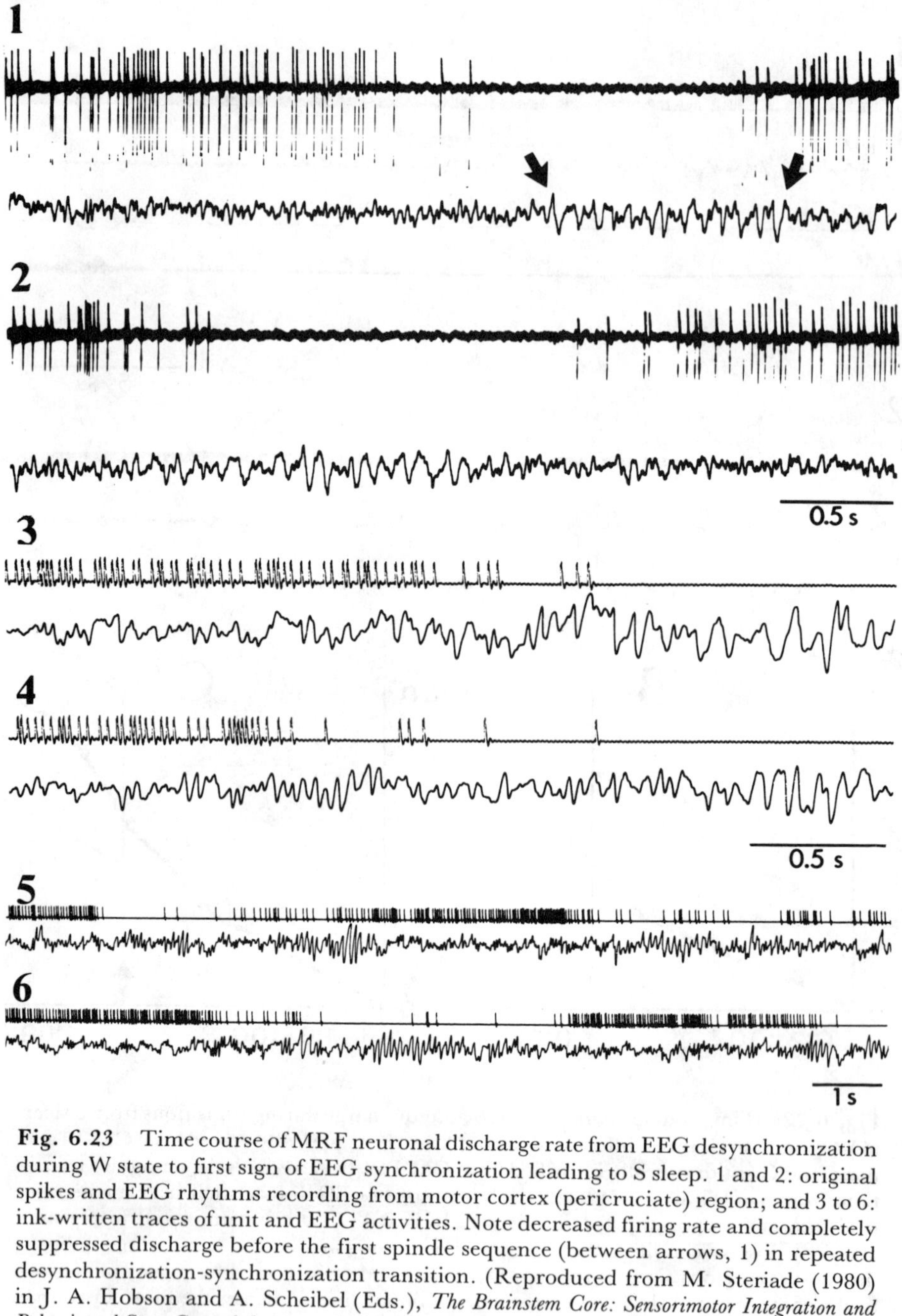

Fig. 6.23 Time course of MRF neuronal discharge rate from EEG desynchronization during W state to first sign of EEG synchronization leading to S sleep. 1 and 2: original spikes and EEG rhythms recording from motor cortex (pericruciate) region; and 3 to 6: ink-written traces of unit and EEG activities. Note decreased firing rate and completely suppressed discharge before the first spindle sequence (between arrows, 1) in repeated desynchronization-synchronization transition. (Reproduced from M. Steriade (1980) in J. A. Hobson and A. Scheibel (Eds.), *The Brainstem Core: Sensorimotor Integration and Behavioural State Control*, by permission of MIT Press.)

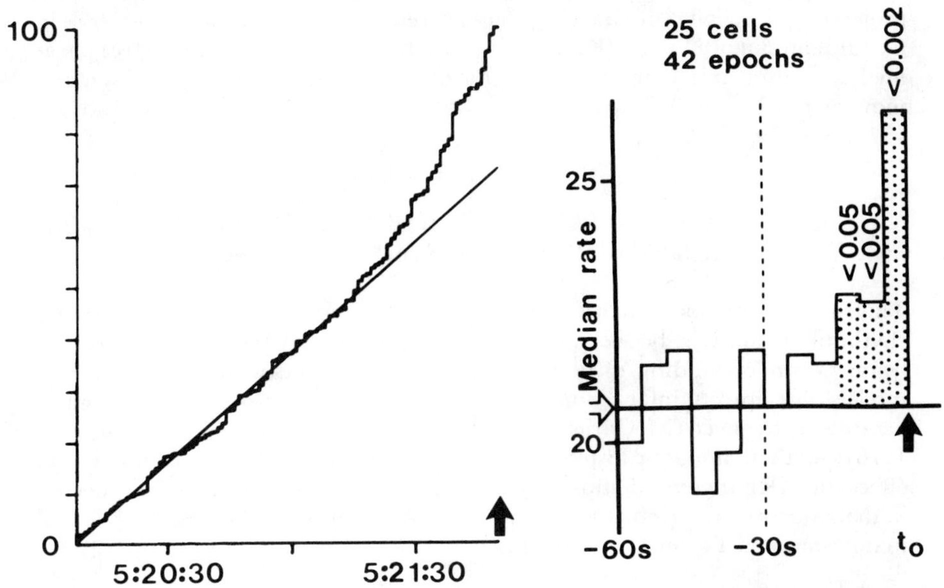

Fig. 6.24 Increase in firing rate of midbrain reticular neurons of cat before the end of synchronized sleep (S) epochs developing into the waking state. At left, percent cumulative histogram of a neuron belonging to the sample analysed in the graph depicted at right. Arrows indicate the first change in the fully synchronized EEG waves (see also Fig. 6.22). At right, 25 cells whose global mean rates in S sleep was at least 4/s were analysed during the last minute of S in 42 epochs leading to the transitional SW state or directly to waking. The Mann–Whitney test was used to compare the reference rate during the first 30 s for all cells with their respective rates in the last six 5 s-bins. Note significantly increased rates in the three 5 s-bins before the end of S sleep (arrow), compared to the discharge rate in the first 30 s. (Reproduced from M. Steriade, G. Oakson and N. Ropert (1982), *Experimental Brain Research*, **46**, 37–51, by permission.)

rate of paramedian pontine neurons during D sleep was entirely related to REMs (Hobson *et al.*, 1974). In the study by Siegel *et al.* (1977), 85% of pontine reticular neurons discharged only during movements in W and REMs in D sleep. In contrast, MRF neurons are characterized by tonic discharge patterns (see Section 6.3.1) associated with high rates, firing features that are commonly seen in relatively small-size neurons. Actually, the remarkably homogenous and small size of MRF neurons, mostly with somata between 15 and 20 μm, and their slow conduction velocities (Ropert & Steriade, 1981; Steriade, 1981) are very dissimilar to the larger size and higher conduction velocities of pontine reticular cells (Fuller, 1975).

In the light of the available data from single unit brainstem recordings during behavioural states of vigilance, it is probable that: (a) receivers of multiple excitatory inputs and rostrally projecting MRF cells with high discharge rates are involved in tonic activation process related to EEG desynchronization during W and D (Steriade, 1981; Steriade *et al.*, 1982a); rostrally projecting bulbar reticular neurons may provide an additional source of EEG activation especially during D sleep (Sakai & Steriade, in preparation); (b) caudally projecting, tonically discharging bulbar reticular neurons are involved in postural atonia of D sleep (Kanamori *et al.*, 1980; Sakai *et al* ., 1981); (c) paramedian pontine reticular neurons are mostly involved in phasic eye and somatic movements during D sleep and W (Hobson *et al.*, 1974; McCarley & Hobson, 1975; Siegel *et al.*, 1977; Vertes, 1979).

6.4 Some Mechanisms of Thalamocortical Activation and Deactivation Processes Related to Waking and Synchronized Sleep

This final section does not attempt to propose different mechanisms underlying rhythmic oscillations between behavioural states of vigilance. We are still far from the understanding of neural timing in sleep state sequences. Different models of reciprocal interactions between specialized brainstem cell aggregates have been advanced (McCarley & Hobson, 1975b; Pompeiano & Valentinuzzi, 1976) and they should be tested intracellularly. Rather, I will discuss the rostral effects of MRF increased and decreased activity in W and S states, as reflected in thalamocortical systems, with some consequences which favour behavioural manifestations of arousal and sleep.

6.4.1 Wake to sleep

At present, the active or passive mechanisms responsible for switching off MRF neurons at sleep onset are not known. As discussed in Section 6.1.3, none of the hypothesized active inhibitory mechanism has been yet supported by firm experimental evidence. Instead, we can start with the decreased MRF neuronal activity that reliably precedes the onset of electrographic signs characterizing S sleep (see Section 6.3.1) and examine the effects exerted at the next synaptic junction. Let me recall that monosynaptic excitatory influences are exerted by MRF ascending axons at their thalamic targets (Section 6.2.2 and Fig. 6.14). The sudden withdrawal of the tonic reticulofugal excitatory barrage of impulses results in disfacilitation of neurons located in thalamic nuclei and corresponding cortical areas. This is seen by striking depression of spontaneous discharge or even complete silencing of firing in intralaminar CL-Pc thalamic neurons, preceding overt signs of EEG synchronized rhythms (Glenn & Steriade, 1982), and by similar events in lateral thalamic (Steriade *et al.*, 1971) and cortical neurons (Fig. 6.4c).

The disfacilitation of, and/or active inhibitory actions upon, thalamic neurons at the W → S transition is most probably the crucial factor behind appearance of inhibitory-rebound sequences in thalamic cells and related rhythmic EEG spindle waves. Recent intracellular analyses *in vitro* (Llinas & Jahnsen, 1982) and *in vivo* (Deschênes *et al.*, 1982) have established the nature of the post-inhibitory rebound excitation. It was found that thalamic neurons have a special voltage-sensitive calcium conductance which is normally inactivated at the resting membrande potential and which is de-inactivated by membrane hyperpolarization. This is a low-threshold calcium spike similar to that described in the inferior olive (Llinas & Yarom, 1981), and it can sustain repetitive firing via sodium-dependent action potentials. Thus, at the resting membrane potential the response evoked in a thalamic relay cell by a depolarizing synaptic potential consists of an early EPSP with occasional single spike discharge, and the response to a depolarizing current pulse is a sustained discharge. Under background hyperpolarization by injecting current, the response pattern becomes a slow rising depolarization which triggers a burst of high-frequency action potentials. Such burst discharges could also be seen during spontaneously occurring hyperpolarizations of the cell membrane which indicates that this mechanism is normally operative in thalamic cells (Deschênes *et al.*, 1982b). In fact, the bursts of high-frequency action potentials obtained in these experimental conditions are identical to those occurring naturally during behavioural slow wave sleep. *It is therefore probable that slightly hyperpolarized neurons, such as thalamic cells suddenly deprived of an excitatory influence from the MRF prior to overt signs of sleep (see Fig. 6.23), exhibit oscillations consisting of brief increases in excitability followed by long-lasting inhibitory phases.*

The overt effect of long-lasting inhibitory potentials in thalamic neurons as the direct consequence of MRF decreased excitability at W → S transition is a powerful blockade of synaptic transmission of impulses travelling in ascending pathways. This may provide a mechanism for closing sensory channels. Actually, testing the excitability of lateral nuclei during the sleep–waking cycle revealed that monosynaptic responses to afferent volleys are inhibited from the first stage of drowsiness, in spite of an unchanged presynaptic deflection (Steriade *et al.*, 1969). In the cerebral cortex too, powerful inhibitory phenomena that appear from the very onset of drowsiness, preceding overt signs of sleep (Steriade *et al.*, 1974b), are attributable to removal of excitatory impulses along thalamocortical projections. Such deafferentation in thalamocortical projections is a necessary prelude for attaining the critical level at which genuine manifestations of sleep occur. It is conceivable that by cutting off the ascending drive of thalamic origin one would create favourable conditions for deactivation processes. A bilateral vascular lesion in humans that mainly involved medial-intralaminar thalamic nuclei induced a lethargic syndrome, with hypersomnia lasting for three years (Façon *et al.*, 1958). This was confirmed by a similiar anatomo-clinical case (Castaigne *et al.*, 1962).

6.4.2 Sleep to Wake

The cellular processes associated with the natural transition from S to W (and S to D) in behaving animals are also elicited by MRF stimulation and essentially consist of increased rates of spontaneous firing in long-axon neurons, increased responsiveness of antidromic and monosynaptic volleys, and blockade of cyclic inhibition-rebound sequences (Steriade, 1981; see Section 6.1.2 and Fig. 6.4 and 6.5 in the present chapter). By setting in motion MRF ascending projections, the increased probability of antidromically elicited discharges is combined with a simultaneous disappearance of the post-inhibitory rebound that takes the pattern of high-frequency spike clusters and is peculiar for slow wave sleep (Steriade *et al.*, 1977). Studies of Krnjevic *et al.* (1971) combining intracellular recording of cortical neurons with extracellular iontophoresis of acetylcholine (ACh), the probable transmitter of the ascending reticular projections, have shown that the depolarizing effect induced by ACh is exerted most clearly with cells relatively deep in the cortex, nearly all pyramidal tract neurons. This excitatory action is accompanied by an increase in membrane resistance, probably due to a reduction in K conductance (Krnjevic, 1974, 1981). Krnjevic (1978) commented that in many central neurons there are two possible states: 'one in which there is a high resting potassium conductance that makes the cell insensitive to excitatory inputs [and is most probably behind the appearance of hyperpolarization-rebound sequences, M. S.; see above, Section 6.4.1] and another characterized by a low potassium conductance, induced by ACh, and therefore a high degree of responsiveness to even small inputs' (p. 497). The former state is likely the stage of sleep with EEG rhythmic synchronized waves and decreased probability of antidromic and synaptic responsiveness, in view of the occurrence of overwhelmingly long periods of hyperpolarization (100 ms) compared to brief (20 ms) subsequent periods of increased excitability. The latter type of state is that characterized by EEG activation, increased responsiveness to incoming messages, and blockade of long-lasting inhibitory phases.

Acknowledgements

This work was supported by the Medical Research Council of Canada (grant MT-3689).

References

ANDERSON, M. E. and YOSHIDA, M. (1980). Axonal branching patterns and location of nigrothalamic and nigrocollicular neurons in the cat. *J. Neurophysiol.*, **43**, 883–895.

ASTON-JONES, G. and BLOOM, F. E. (1981). Norepinephrine-containing locus coeruleus in behaving rats exhibit pronounced responses to non-noxious environmental stimuli. *J. Neurosci.*, **1**, 887–900.

BERGER, H. (1930). Uber das Elektrenkephalogram des Menschen. Zweite Mitteilung. *J. Psychol. Neurol.*, **40**, 160–179.

BLOCH, V. and FISCHBEIN, W. (1975). Sleep and psychological functions: memory. In: G. C. LAIRY and P. SALZARULO (Eds.), *Experimental Study of Human Sleep: Methodological Problems,* Amsterdam: Elsevier, pp. 157–173.

BOUYER, J. J., MONTARON, M. F. and ROUGEUL, A. (1981). Fast fronto-parietal rhythms during combined focused attentive behaviour and immobility in cat: cortical and thalamic localizations. *Electroenceph. Clin. Neurophysiol.*, **51**, 244–252.

BREMER, F. (1935). Cerveau 'isolé' et physiologie du sommeil. *C. R. Soc. Biol.* (Paris), **118**, 1235–1241.

BREMER, F. (1977). Cerebral hypnogenic centers. *Ann. Neurol.*, **2**, 1–6.

CASTAIGNE, P., BUGE, A., ESCOUROLLE, R. and MASSON, M. (1962). Ramollissement pédonculaire médian, tegmento-thalamique avec ophtalmoplégie et hypersomnie. *Rev. Neurol.* (Paris), **106**, 357–367.

CESPUGLIO, R., GOMEZ, M. E., WALKER, E. and JOUVET, M. (1979). Effets du refroidissement et de la stimulation des noyaux du système du raphé sur les états de vigilance chez le chat. *Electroenceph. Clin. Neurophysiol.*, **47**, 289–308.

CHU, N. S. and BLOOM, F. E. (1974). Activity patterns of catecholamine-containing pontine neurons in the dorso-lateral tegmentum of unrestrained cats. *J. Neurobiol.*, **5**, 527–544.

COLONNIER, M., STERIADE, M. and LANDRY, P. (1979). Selective resistance of sensory cells of the mesencephalic trigeminal nucleus to kainic acid-induced lesions. *Brain Research*, **172**, 552–556.

DESCHÊNES, M., ROY, J. P. and STERIADE, M. (1982). The bursting discharges of thalamic ventrolateral cells: demonstration of a voltage-sensitive conductance deinactivation. *Brain Research*, **239**, 289–293.

DINGLEDINE, R. and KELLY, J. S. (1977). Brain stem stimulation and the acetylcholine-evoked inhibition of neurons in the feline nucleus reticularis thalami. *J. Physiol.* (London), **271**, 135–154.

DISMUKES, R. K. (1979). New concepts of molecular communication among neurons. *Behav. Brain Sci.*, **2**, 409–448.

DONOGHUE, J. P. and EBNER, F. F. (1981). The laminar distribution and ultrastructure of fibers projecting from three thalamic nuclei to the somatic sensory-motor cortex of the opossum. *J. Comp. Neurol.*, **198**, 389–420.

EDWARDS, S. B. and DE OLMOS, J. S. (1976). Autoradiographic studies of the projections of the midbrain reticular formation: ascending projections of nucleus cuneiformis. *J. Comp. Neurol.*, **165**, 417–432.

FAÇON, E., STERIADE, M. and WERTHEIM, N. (1958). Hypersomnie prolongée engendrée par des lésions bilatérales du systéme activateur mèdial. Le syndrome thrombotique de la bifurcation du tronc basilaire. *Rev. Neurol.* (Paris), **98**, 117–133.

FERSTER, D. and LEVAY, S. (1978). The axonal arborizations of lateral geniculate neurons in the striate cortex of the cat. *J. Comp. Neurol.*, **182**, 923–944.

FOOTE, S. L. and BLOOM, F. E. (1979). Activity of norepinephrine-containing locus coeruleus neurons in the unanesthetized squirrel monkey. In: E. USDIN (Ed.), *Catecholamines: Clinical-Basic Interactions*, New York: Pergamon Press, pp. 625–627.

FOSTER, J. A. (1980). Intracortical origin of recruiting responses in the cat cortex. *Electroenceph. Clin. Neurophysiol.*, **48**, 639–653.

FROST D. O. and CAVINESS, V. S. (1980). Radial organization of thalamic projections to the neocortex in the mouse. *J. Comp. Neurol.*, **194**, 369–393.

FULLER, J. H. (1975). Brain stem reticular units: some properties of the course and origin of the ascending trajectory. *Brain Research*, **83**, 349–367.

GASSEL, M., MARCHIAFAVA, P. L. and POMPEIANO, O. (1964). Tonic and phasic inhibition of spinal reflexes during deep, desynchronized sleep in unrestrained cats. *Arch. Ital. Biol.*, **102**, 471–449.

GLENN, L. L., FOUTZ, A. S. and DEMENT, W. C. (1978). Membrane potential of spinal motoneurons during natural sleep in cat. *Sleep*, **1**, 199–204.

GLENN, L. L., HADA, J., ROY, J. P., DESCHÊNES, M. and STERIADE, M. (1982). Anterograde tracer and field potential analysis of the neocortical layer I projection from nucleus ventralis medialis of the thalamus in cat. *Neuroscience*, **7**, 1861–1877.

GLENN, L. L. and STERIADE, M. (1982). Discharge rate and excitability of cortically projecting intralaminar neurons during waking and sleep states. *J. Neurosci.*, **2**, 1387–1404.

GRAYBIEL, A. M. (1977). Direct and indirect preoculomotor pathways of the brainstem: an autoradiographic study of the pontine reticular formation in the cat. *J. Comp. Neurol.*, **175**, 37–78.

HENDRY, S. H. C., JONES, E. G. and GRAHAM, J. (1979). Thalamic relay nuclei for cerebellar and certain related fiber systems in the cat. *J. Comp. Neurol.*, **185**, 679–714.

HERKENHAM, M. (1979). The afferent and efferent connections of the ventromedial thalamic nucleus in the rat. *J. Comp. Neurol.*, **183**, 487–518.

HOBSON, J. A., MCCARLEY, R. W., PIVIK, R. T. and FREEDMAN, R. (1974). Selective firing by cat pontine brainstem neurons in desynchronized sleep. *J. Neurophysiol.*, **37**, 497–511.

HOBSON, J. A., MCCARLEY, R. W. and WYZINSKI, P. (1975). Sleep cycle oscillation: reciprocal discharge by two brain stem neuronal groups. *Science*, **189**, 55–58.

HUTTENLOCHER, P. R. (1961). Evoked and spontaneous activity in single units of medial brainstem during natural sleep and waking. *J. Neurophysiol.*, **24**, 451–468.

HYVÄRINEN, J., PORANEN, A. and JOKINEN, Y. (1980). Influence of attentive behavior on neuronal responses to vibration in primary somatosensory cortex of the monkey. *J. Neurophysiol.*, **43**, 870–882.

INUBUSHI, S., KOBAYASHI, T., OSHIMA, T. and TORII, S. (1978a). Intracellular recordings from the motor cortex during EEG arousal in unanesthetized brain

preparations of the cat. *Jap. J. Physiol.*, **28**, 669–688.
INUBUSHI, S., KOBAYASHI, T., OSHIMA, T. and TORII, S. (1978b). An intracellular analysis of EEG arousal in cat motor cortex. *Jap. J. Physiol.*, **28**, 689–708.
JACOBS, B. L. and JONES, B. A. (1978). The role of central monoamine and acetylcholine systems in sleep-wakefulness states: mediation or modulation? In: L. L. BUTCHER (Ed.), *Cholinergic-Monoaminergic Interactions in the Brain*, New York: Academic Press, pp. 271–290.
JASPER, H. H. and TESSIER, J. (1971). Acetylcholine liberation from the cerebral cortex during paradoxical (REM) sleep. *Science*, **172**, 601–602.
JONES, E. G. and LEAVITT, R. Y. (1974). Retrograde axonal transport and the demonstration of non-specific projections to cerebral cortex and striatum from thalamic intralaminar nuclei in the rat, cat and monkey. *J. Comp. Neurol.*, **154**, 349–378.
JOUVET, M. (1972). The role of monoamines and acetylcholine-containing neurons in the regulation of the sleep-waking cycle. *Ergebn. Physiol.*, **64**, 166–307.
KANAMORI, N., SAKAI, K. and JOUVET, M. (1980). Neuronal activity specific to paradoxical sleep in the ventromedial medullary reticular formation of unrestrained cats. *Brain Research*, **189**, 251–255.
KASAMATSU, T. (1970). Maintained and evoked unit activity in the mesencephalic reticular formation of the freely behaving cat. *Exp. Neurol.*, **28**, 450–470.
KIEVIT, J. and KUYPERS, H. G. J. M. (1972). Fastigial cerebellar projections to the ventrolateral nucleus of the thalamus and the organization of the descending pathways. In: T. FRIGYESI *et al.* (Eds.), *Corticothalamic Projections and Sensorimotor Activities*, New York: Raven Press, pp. 91–111.
KITSIKIS, A. and STERIADE, M. (1981). Immediate behavioural effects of kainic acid injections into the midbrain reticular core. *Behav. Brain Res.*, **3**, 361–380.
KRNJEVIC, K. (1974). Chemical nature of synaptic transmission in vertebrates. *Physiol. Rev.*, **54**, 418–540.
KRNJEVIC, K. (1978). Cholinergic control of excitability in the sleep-waking cycle. *Behav. Brain Sci.*, **1**, 496–498.
KRNJEVIC, K. (1981). Transmitters in motor systems. In: J. M. BROOKHART, V. B. MOUNTCASTLE and V. B. BROOKS (Eds.), *Handbook of Physiology*, Vol. II, part 1, Bethesda: American Physiological Society, pp. 107–154.
KRNJEVIC, K., PUMAIN, R. and RENAUD, L. (1971). The mechanisms of excitation by acetylcholine in the cerebral cortex. *J. Physiol.* (London), **215**, 247–268.
LLINAS, R. and JAHNSEN, H. (1982). Electrophysiology of mammalian thalamic neurones *in vitro*. *Nature*, **297**, 406–408.
LLINAS, R. and YAROM, Y. (1981). Electrophysiology of mammalian inferior olivary neurones *in vitro*. Different types of voltage-dependent ionic conductance. *J. Physiol.* (London), **315**, 549–567.
LORENTE DE NO, R. (1938). Cerebral cortex: architecture, intracortical connections, motor projections. In: J. FULTON (Ed.), *Physiology of the Nervous System*, New York: Oxford Press; pp. 291–340.
MANOHAR, S., NODA, H. and ADEY, W. R. (1972). Behavior of mesencephalic reticular neurons in sleep and wakefulness. *Exp. Neurol.*, **34**, 140–157.
MCCARLEY, R. W. and HOBSON, J. A. (1975a). Discharge patterns of cat pontine brain stem neurons during desynchronized sleep. *J. Neurophysiol.*, **38**, 751–766.
MCCARLEY, R. W. and HOBSON, J. A. (1975b). Neuronal excitability modulation over the sleep cycle: a structural and mathematical model. *Science*, **189**, 58–60.
MCGINTY, D. J. (1973). Neurochemically defined neurons: behavioural correlates of unit activity of serotonin-containing cells. In: M. T. PHILLIPS (Ed.), *Brain Unit Activity during Behavior*, Springfield, Ill: Thomas, pp. 244–267.
MIZUNO, N., CLEMENTE, C. D. and SAUERLAND, E. K. (1969). Fiber projections from rostral basal forebrain structures in the cat. *Exp. Neurol.*, **25**, 220–237.
MORALES, F. and CHASE, M. (1978). Intracellular recording of lumbar motoneuron membrane potential during sleep and wakefulness. *Exp. Neurol.*, **62**, 821–827.

MORISON, R. S. and DEMPSEY, E. W. (1942). A study of thalamocortical relations. *Amer. J. Physiol.*, **135**, 281–292.
MORUZZI, G. (1972). The sleep-waking cycle. *Ergebn. Physiol.*, **64**, 1–165.
MORUZZI, G. and MAGOUN, H. W. (1949). Brain stem reticular formation and activation of the EEG. *Electroenceph. Clin. Neurophysiol.*, **1**, 445–473.
NAKAMURA, R. K., KENNEDY, C., GILLIN, J. C., SUDA, S., ITO, M., STORCH, F., MENDELSON, W., MISHKIN, M. and SOKOLOFF, L. (1981). Hypnogenic-center theory of sleep: no support from 2- deoxiglucose studies in monkeys. *Abstr. Soc. Neurosci.*, **7**, 234.
NAUTA, W. J. H. and KUYPERS, H. G. J. M. (1958). Some ascending pathways in the brain stem reticular formation. In: H. H. JASPER *et al.*, (Eds.), *Reticular Formation of the Brain*, Boston–Toronto: Little, Brown, pp. 3–30.
PARENT, A. and STERIADE, M. (1981). Afferents from the periaqueductal gray, medial hypothalamus and medial thalamus to the midbrain reticular core. *Brain Res. Bull.*, **7**, 411–418.
POMPEIANO, O. (1967). The neurophysiological mechanisms of the postural and motor events during desynchronized sleep *Proc. Ass. Res. Nerv. Ment. Dis.*, **45**, 351–423.
POMPEIANO, O. and VALENTINUZZI, M. (1976). A mathematical model for the mechanism of rapid eye movements induced by an anticholinesterase in the decerebrate cat. *Arch. Ital. Biol.*, **114**, 103–154.
PUIZILLOUT, J. J., GAUDIN-CHAZAL, G., SAYADI, A. and VIGIER, D (1981). Serotoninergic mechanisms and sleep. *J. Physiol.* (Paris), **77**, 415–424.
RAMON-MOLINER, E. and NAUTA, W. J. H. (1966). The isodendritic core of the brain stem. *J. Comp. Neurol.*, **126**, 311–336.
RAMON Y CAJAL, S. (1955). *Histologie du système nerveux de l'homme et des vertébrés.* Consejo superior de investigaciones cientificas, Madrid, t. II, 933 pp.
ROPERT, N. and STERIADE, M. (1981). Input-output organization of the midbrain reticular core. *J. Neurophysiol.*, **46**, 17–31.
SAKAI, K., SASTRE, J. P., KANAMORI, N. and JOUVET, M. (1981). State specific neurons in the pontomedullary reticular formation with special reference to the postural atonia during paradoxical sleep in the cat. In: O. POMPEIANO and C. AJMONE-MARSAN (Eds.) *Brain Mechanisms and Perceptual Awareness*, New York: Raven Press, pp. 405–429.
SCHEIBEL, M. E. and SCHEIBEL, A. B. (1967). Structural organization of nonspecific thalamic nuclei and their projection toward cortex. *Brain Research*, **6**, 60–94
SCHEIBEL, M., SCHEIBEL, A., MOLLICA, A. and MORUZZI, G. (1955). Convergence and interaction of afferent impulses on single units of reticular formation. *J. Neurophysiol.*, **18**, 309–331.
SCHLAG, J. and VILLABLANCA, J. (1967). Cortical incremental responses to thalamic stimulation. *Brain Research*, **6**, 119–142.
SEGUNDO, J. P., PERKEL, D. H., WYMAN, H., HEGSTAD, H. and MOORE, G. (1968). Input-output relations in computer-simulated nerve cells. *Kybernetic*, **4**, 157–171.
SIEGEL, J. M., MCGINTY, D. G. and BREEDLOVE, S. M. (1977). Sleep and waking activity of pontine giganto cellular field neurons. *Exp. Neurol.*, **56**, 553–573.
STERIADE, M. (1978). Cortical long-axoned cells and putative interneurons during the sleep-waking cycle (with commentaries). *Behav. Brain Sciences*, **3**, 465–514.
STERIADE, M. (1980). State-dependent changes in the activity of rostral reticular and thalamocortical elements. In: J. A. HOBSON and A. SCHEIBEL (Eds.), *The Brainstem Core: Sensorimotor integration and Behavioral State control*, Boston, Mass: MIT Press, pp. 83–91.
STERIADE, M. (1981). Mechanisms underlying cortical activation: neuronal organization and properties of the midbrain reticular core and intralaminar thalamic nuclei. In: O. POMPEIANO and C. AJMONE-MARSAN (Eds.) *Brain Mechanisms and Perceptual Awareness*, New York: Raven Press, pp. 327–377.
STERIADE, M., APOSTOL, V. and OAKSON, G. (1971). Control of unitary activities in

cerebellothalamic pathway during wakefulness and synchronized sleep. *J. Neurophysiol.*, **34**, 384–413.

STERIADE, M. and DESCHÊNES, M. (1974). Inhibitory processes and interneuronal apparatus in motor cortex during sleep and waking. II Recurrent and afferent inhibition of pyramidal tract neurons. *J. Neurophysiol.*, **37**, 1093–1113.

STERIADE, M., DESCHÊNES, M. and OAKSON, G. (1974a). Inhibitory processes and interneuronal apparatus in motor cortex during sleep and waking. I Background firing and responsiveness of pyramidal tract neurons and interneurons. *J. Neurophysiol.*, **37**, 1065–1092.

STERIADE, M., DESCHÊNES, M, WYZINSKI, P. and HALLÉ, J. P. (1974b). Input-output organization of the motor cortex and its alterations during sleep and waking. In: O. PETRE-QUADENS and J. SCHLAG (Eds.), *Basic Sleep Mechanisms* New York: Academic Press, pp. 144–200.

STERIADE, M. and GLENN, L. L. (1982). The neocortical and caudate projections of intralaminar thalamic neurons and their synaptic excitation from the midbrain reticular core. *J. Neurophysiol.*, **48**, 352–371.

STERIADE, M. and HOBSON, J. A. (1976). Neuronal activity during the sleep-waking cycle. *Progr. Neurobiol.*, **6**, 155–376.

STERIADE, M., IOSIF, G. and APOSTOL, V. (1969). Responsiveness of thalamic and cortical motor relays and during arousal and various stages of sleep. *J. Neurophysiol.*, **32**, 251–265.

STERIADE, M., KITSIKIS, A. and OAKSON, G. (1979). Excitatory-inhibitory processes in parietal association neurons during reticular activation and sleep-waking cycle. *Sleep*, **1**, 339–355.

STERIADE, M., and MORIN, D. (1981). Reticular influences on primary and augmenting responses in primary somatosensory cortex. *Brain Research*, **205**, 67–80.

STERIADE, M., OAKSON, G. and DIALLO, A. (1977). Reticular influences on lateralis posterior thalamic neurons. *Brain Research*, **131**, 55–71.

STERIADE, M., OAKSON, G. and ROPERT, N. (1982a). Firing rates and patterns of midbrain reticular neurons during steady and transitional states of the sleep-waking cycle. *Exp. Brain Res.*, **46**, 37–51.

STERIADE, M., PARENT, A., ROPERT, N. and KITSIKIS, A. (1982b). Zona incerta and lateral hypothalamic afferents to the midbrain reticular core of cat — an HRP and electrophysiological study. *Brain Research*, **238**, 13–28.

STERIADE, M., ROPERT, N., KITSIKIS, A. and OAKSON, G. (1980). Ascending activating neuronal networks in midbrain reticular core and related rostral systems. In: J. A. HOBSON and M. A. B. BRAZIER (Eds.), *The Reticular Formation Revisited* New York: Raven Press, pp. 125–167.

VANDERWOLF, C. H. and ROBINSON, T. E. (1981). Reticulo-cortical activity and behavior: a critique of the arousal theory and a new synthesis (with commentaries). *Behav. Brain Sciences*, **4**, 459–514.

VERTES, R. P. (1979). Brain stem gigantocellular neurons: patterns of activity during behavior and sleep in the freely moving rat. *J. Neurophysiol.*, **42**, 214–228.

WEISS, K. R., COHEN, J. and KUPFERMAN, I. (1978). Modulatory control of buccal musculature by a serotonergic neuron (metacerebral cell) in Aplysia. *J. Neurophysiol.*, **41**, 181–203.

CHAPTER 7

REM Sleep Control Mechanisms: Evidence from Lesion and Unit Recording Studies

J. M. Siegel

7.1 General Considerations

This chapter will summarize some recent evidence concerning how the state of REM sleep is generated. The two approaches that have contributed most to our understanding of REM sleep generation are the surgical approach of removing or separating parts of the brain and the recording approach of observing single unit activity within the brain. We will discuss each in turn. But first we must be aware of the limitations and benefits of each approach. The lesion technique has produced most of our current knowledge about the workings of the brain. The logic is simply that if one wants to understand the functions of a brain region, one removes that region and observes the behavioural deficit. The removed area is assumed to have mediated the lost behavioural function. However it has long been recognized that this is a risky inference. The loss of a behavioural function as a result of a brain lesion should not be taken as proof that one has localized the centre for the behaviour in question to the ablated area. Instead the lesion may have produced a disruption of the input or output to a critical area located elsewhere, may have altered the animal's motivational state or may have made the animal too ill to express the behavioural function. These caveats are especially important in REM sleep studies, since it is well known that this state is quite sensitive to any conditions that disturb normal bodily functions.

A more conservative and reliable interpretation of lesion and transection studies relies on positive evidence. Any behavioural function which survives the destruction of a certain brain area does not require that area. Thus if REM sleep can occur after removal of the neocortex, it is clear that the neocortex is not required for REM sleep generation (Jouvet, 1962). This *does not* mean, as some have implied, that the neocortex plays no active role in REM sleep generation in the intact animal, only that it plays no *essential* role in the generation of this state. It is known that while forebrain regions are not required for REM sleep generation, even small lesions of these areas produce gross changes in the structure of REM sleep (Gadea-Ciria, 1976).

A more subtle problem in the interpretation of lesion studies investigating REM sleep control lies in the definition and description of behavioural states existing after the lesion. In the intact animal REM sleep is readily recognized as a constellation of physiological signs including (1) EEG desynchrony, (2) neck muscle atonia, (3) rapid eye movements, (4) PGO spikes, (5) respiratory and cardiac irregularity, (6) diminished behavioural responsiveness to external stimuli. These phenomena are manifestations of dramatic changes in neuronal activity in most regions of the brain. A central feature of sleep is the regular recurrence of these neuronal changes in a cycle lasting approximately 30 min in the cat and 90 min in humans. This basic rest–activity cycle is also apparent in waking behaviour. A variety of experiments have established that activity levels, attention, food ingestion and other variables vary in intensity in waking in this regular rhythm (Kripke, 1972; Lavie *et al.*, 1974; Orr & Hoffman, 1974), although in humans this cycle can be obscured by external demands. It has been proposed that REM sleep is merely the sleeping brain's expression of this more basic oscillation in behavioural state (Kleitman, 1963).

After some brain lesions we can see all of the signs of REM sleep in reasonably normal configuration. The interpretation of such experiments is easy. However, other brain manipulations disrupt certain aspects of REM sleep while leaving others intact. For example, small lesions in the dorso-lateral pons prevent the atonia of REM sleep while leaving its other phenomena intact, producing a state in which the cat appears to be 'acting out a dream' or more objectively described, performs various behavioural activities while unresponsive to the external world and while manifesting all the physiological signs of REM sleep except for atonia (Jouvet & Delorme, 1965). Sleep researchers have generally agreed that this state is a variant of REM sleep.

A more difficult state to interpret is one resulting from the injection of carbachol into the pons. After this procedure an atonic state with rapid eye movements occurs. This state may have a much longer duration than the normal REM sleep state (Amatruda *et al.*, 1975). Some investigators report that cats in this state move their eyes to track objects in the external world, indicating that they are conscious (Mitler & Dement, 1974). Is this a state of REM sleep in which the cat retains a partial-responsiveness to the external world but loses behavioural cyclicity and state duration regulation, or is it an abnormal waking state with loss of motor tone?

Ultimately, labelling a state as REM or non-REM sleep after brain manipulation is not the critical issue. It is more important to describe the states that exist and determine which if any elements of REM sleep remain. Such a data-oriented approach is heuristically more valuable than the sterile approach of trying to decide what to label a state. This descriptive approach permits one to decide which elements of the REM state are tightly coupled and which can be dissociated. It opens new areas for further focused research on each mechanism. This is the approach we shall use in interpreting lesion studies of the REM sleep mechanism.

Unit recording allows us to observe the brain activity of the intact animal. The principal limitation of this technique is that unit data are essentially correlational. Assuming one could establish that certain neuronal groups are selectively active or inactive in REM sleep, it would not follow that these groups are REM sleep generators or even that they are involved in REM sleep control. They might merely be passively driven by other neurons more centrally involved in REM sleep control, or they might be related to one of the minor phenomena of REM sleep.

One approach often used in neurophysiological studies is the study of latency relationships. For example, a neuronal group can be determined to elicit mono- or polysynaptically certain motor effects. However, such approaches must be applied with great caution to unit studies of REM sleep generation. The change of physiological signs from the non-REM sleep pattern to the REM sleep pattern takes place over a period of a minute or more. Indeed it is best described as a gradual process with only arbitrarily defined transition points. Not surprisingly most brain units show a similar activity cycle. Therefore defining the lead or lag between the neuronal activity change and the state change becomes an exercise in justifying and comparing arbitrarily defined points of unit activity increase with equally arbitrary points of state transition. Points of detectable change in unit activity may be influenced more importantly by the variability of the units baseline discharge rate than by the magnitude of its rate change during the SWS–REM sleep transition. A better approach would be to compare entire cycles of unit activity to the REM cycle and compute the phase lag between these measures. This would allow one to formulate hypotheses about the sequence in which different neuronal groups are changing activity throughout the cycle. In contrast to 'onset' or offset' points, the peak rate and shape of the neuronal discharge profile can be accurately measured. However, this more difficult approach has not been widely used.

We are left with two imperfect techniques with which to examine REM generation processes. However, when used in concert, the lesion and recording techniques can provide considerable insight into the anatomical localization and dynamics of the mechanisms of REM sleep control.

7.2 Lesion and Transection Studies

Transection studies, in which one totally separates forebrain and brainstem systems, provide a means of rapidly localizing the areas critical to REM sleep. Severing the brainstem at the midbrain level does not interfere with the manifestations of REM sleep in structures caudal to the cut (Fig. 7.1) (Jouvet, 1962; Villablanca, 1966). These animals have a REM sleep state consisting of atonia, rapid eye movements and PGO activity. Therefore neural structures caudal to the midbrain are sufficient to generate this state. The spinal cord and cerebellum can also be separated from the brainstem without disturbing REM sleep (Adey *et al.*, 1968; Jouvet, 1962). Therefore the medulla and pons appear to be sufficient to generate the REM sleep state. There is little disagreement among sleep researchers on this point. However, consensus on a more precise localization of REM sleep generation mechanisms *within* this area has not been achieved.

A critical experiment aimed at further defining the minimum area required for REM sleep was performed by Jouvet, who divided the brainstem at the caudal pontine level (1962). He reported no atonia in muscles controlled by caudal brainstem systems and therefore concluded that there was no REM sleep state being generated in this region. Jouvet also described three states in the forebrain of this preparation. One was a waking-like state in which the cat had a desynchronized EEG and tracking eye movements. The second was a non-REM sleep-like state in which the forebrain EEG was synchronized. The third was termed a 'difficult to interpret' state. This state was similar to the first state, except that only spontaneous non-tracking eye movements occurred and pupils were constricted as in REM sleep. Unfortunately PGO spikes and unit activity were not recorded in these preparations, so the identification of this state as

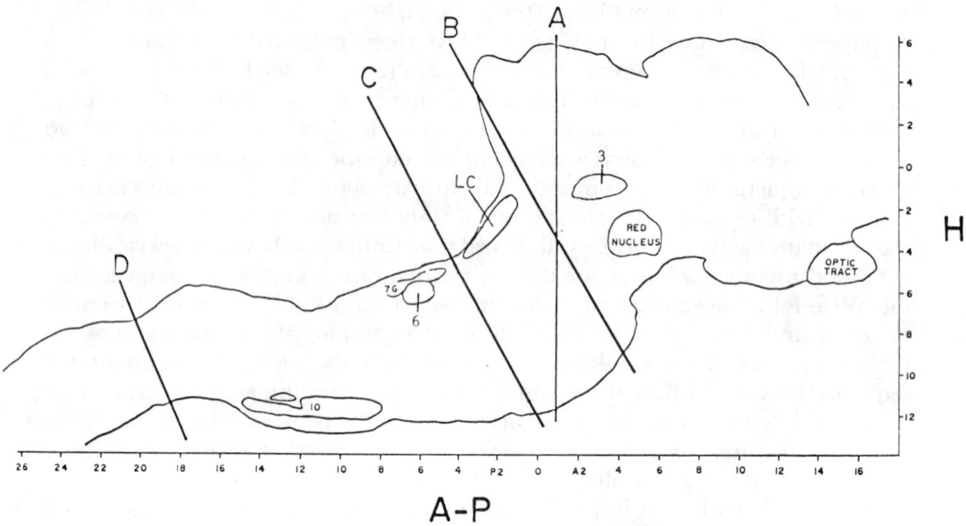

Fig. 7.1 Outline of sagittal section of cat brainstem. A and B midbrain transections, C caudal pontine transection, D spinal cord transection. 3, occulomotor nucleus; LC, locus coeruleus, 6, abducens nucleus; 7G, genu of the facial nerve; 10, inferior olive. Coordinates are from the Berman (1968) atlas.

REM sleep is speculative. Similarly, in light of the factors discussed in the first part of this chapter, the absence of atonia is not sufficient to rule out the existence of some elements of REM sleep in more caudal portions of this preparation. Since this preparation is so critical to current ideas on the localization of REM sleep control mechanisms, we have studied it in some detail (Siegel *et al.*, 1981). In addition to EEG and EMG variables we have recorded unit activity in both the forebrain and brainstem areas. We have made a special effort to record PGO activity in the forebrain and EKG and respiratory activity controlled by the brainstem. We also developed a surgical technique that permits us, by cutting the third nerve on one side, the sixth nerve on the other side and the fourth nerves on both sides, to restrict forebrain-generated eye movement to one eye and brainstem-generated eye movement to the other eye. This allows us to determine which half of the preparation is generating any observed eye movements.

Forebrain. After the transection, forebrain and brainstem states are independent of each other. We saw three states in the isolated forebrain (Fig. 7.2). (1) A state with desynchronized EEG and no PGO spikes. Tracking eye movements could be induced in this state. (2) A state with intermittent synchronized EEG and no PGO spikes. This state looked similar to the drowsy state of the intact cat. (3) A state with continuous synchronized EEG and isolated high amplitude PGO spikes. This state resembled the state of transitional SWS seen in the intact cat. No state with PGO spikes and desynchronized EEG was seen. Sleep states in the forebrain were much longer than those seen in intact animals. No ultradian rhythm of sleep cycles was observed. We saw no regularly recurring periods of

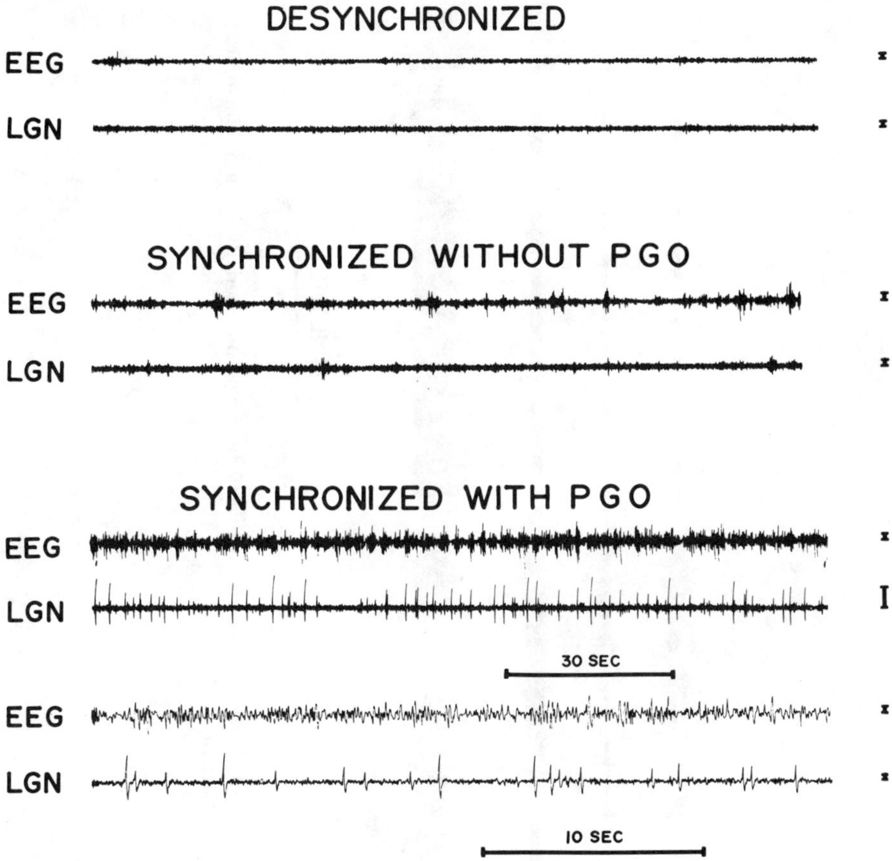

Fig. 7.2 Forebrain states. EEG, sensorimotor electroencephalogram, LGN, lateral geniculate nucleus activity. The bottom two traces show EEG and LGN activity at higher speed during synchronization with PGO.

forebrain-commanded eye movements. Eye movements that did occur were not accompanied by increased unit activity. A total of 80 midbrain units were recorded across all three forebrain states. Mean discharge rates were highest during state 1 (15.6/s), lower during state 2 (14.2/s) and lowest during state 3 (13.5/s). A closer look at rates in individual units revealed that cells that decreased rate in state 3 (Fig. 7.3) had significantly higher ($p<0.006$, U test) rates of spontaneous activity during the desynchronized state than units which increased rate in state 3. A similar finding was made on midbrain units recorded in waking and slow wave sleep (SWS) in the intact cat (Huttenlocker, 1961), thus reinforcing the similarity of this state to normal SWS. In contrast, REM sleep in the intact cat is accompanied by a massive rate increase in virtually all midbrain units.

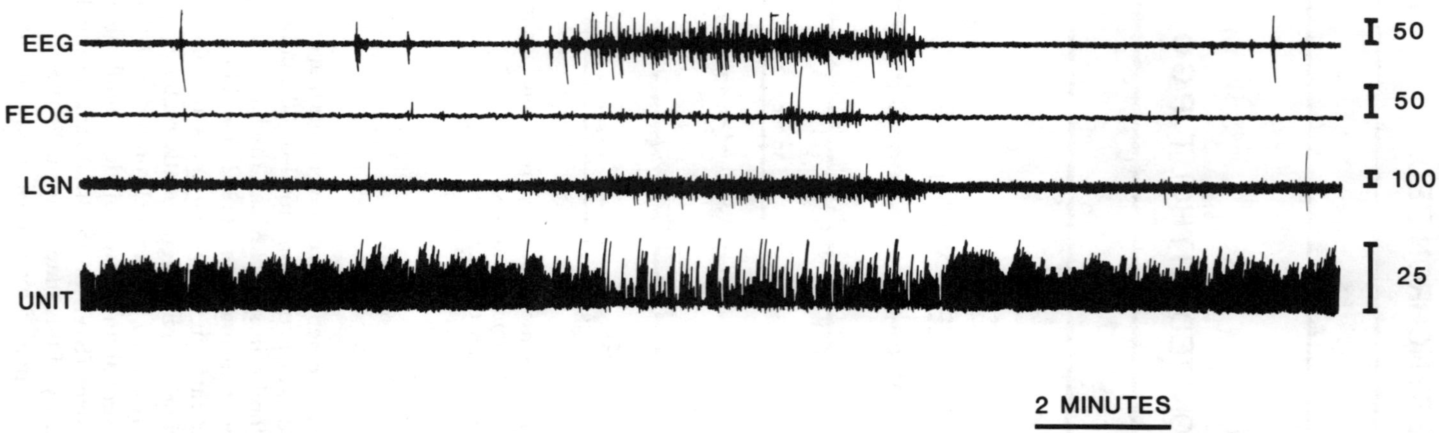

Fig. 7.3 Forebrain unit activity. Unit channel is the output of a resetting counter triggered by single unit activity in midbrain reticular formation. Rate is in spikes/s. FEOG, forebrain triggered EOG activity.

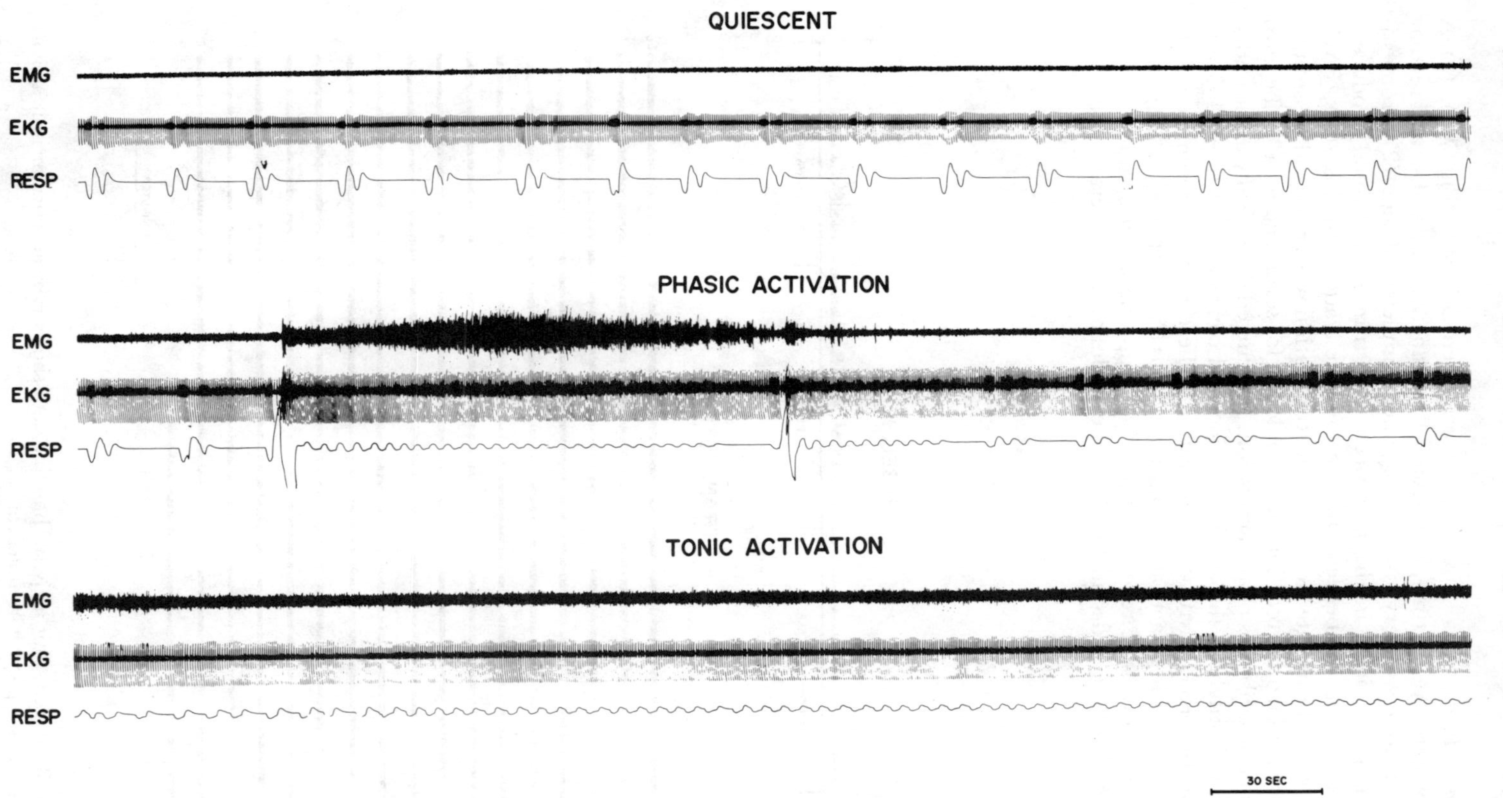

Fig. 7.4 Caudal brainstem states. EMG, dorsal neck muscle activity; Resp, strain gauge indication of chest movement.

Brainstem. Three states were seen in brainstem systems (Fig. 7.4). (1) A quiescent state. At this time, heart-rate and unit activity were slow and regular and muscle tone was very low, although not completely absent. (2) Strong stimulation, particularly in the first week after transection, could produce a second state that can be described as tonic activation. In this state, EMG amplitude and heart rate were all high. Respiration was rapid and gross body movements often occurred. This state could last for several hours. (3) The third state can be described as phasic activation. It occurred periodically in the undisturbed cat throughout the survival period and consisted of a brief, 1–3 min activation of EKG, EMG and respiration. These arousals resembled those reported to occur in intact cats at state transitions (McGinty *et al.*, 1979). In the transected cat this state recurred regularly at approximately 24-min intervals. Unit activity was recorded in 28 cells in the medulla. All accelerated during the

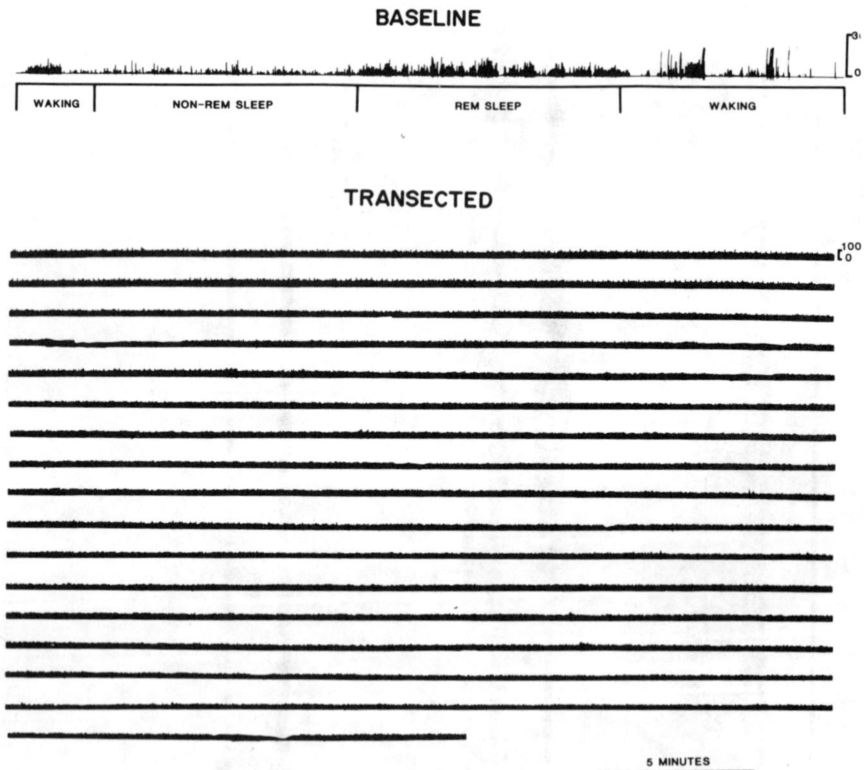

Fig. 7.5 Brainstem unit activity. Baseline data shows typical reticular unit activity pattern during sleep cycle in intact cat.

phasic activation periods. At other times activity was remarkably invariant (Fig. 7.5). Conversely, all periods of increased unit activity were accompanied by increased muscle activity. No dissociation of these variables resembling that seen in REM sleep occurred. No groups of brainstem-commanded rapid eye movements were seen. However, rapid, isolated biphasic EOG deflections were seen. These did not co-vary with any other parameter. Visual observation revealed that they corresponded to nictitating membrane blinks, presumably resulting from activation of the retractor bulbi muscles via the sixth nerve.

We interpret these data to indicate that neither the pons and attached forebrain, nor the medulla and spinal cord are sufficient to generate REM sleep. However each can generate certain aspects of this state. The forebrain can generate isolated PGO spikes which normally occur during the transition to REM sleep. The medulla appears sufficient to generate a massive and sustained activation of EKG, EMG, respiration and reticular unit activity. The medulla, unlike the forebrain, also has a basic rest–activity cycle. This cycle may be responsible for the regular recurrence of REM sleep in the intact cat.

These studies lead us to conclude that a relatively large brainstem region including both pontine and medullary regions is critically involved in generating the REM sleep state. Smaller lesions within the brainstem area reveal certain other aspects of REM sleep control. As described above, small lesions of the dorsal pons can prevent the atonia of REM sleep. Other studies have shown that pathways ascending from lateral pontine regions are critical in conveying PGO spikes rostrally to forebrain regions (Laurent *et al.*, 1974). Lesions in the region of the vestibular nuclei appear to disrupt the eye movement bursts and associated phenomena of REM state while keeping its other manifestations intact (Pompeiano & Morrison, 1965) although the exact locus of the necessary lesion is in some dispute (Perenin *et al.*, 1972). These studies, then, show how certain elements of the REM control mechanisms can be selectively damaged while other aspects of the state remain intact. Large lesions of the pons appear to eliminate most signs of REM sleep. This may be due to a combination of the effects of damage to the specific areas mentioned above and disconnection of medullary areas as occurs in transections.

7.3 Unit Recording Studies

Unit recording studies provide another approach to the localization of REM sleep control mechanisms. One would expect any cell group that was involved in generating REM sleep to do something unusual in this state. This might be to go on, go off or change activity pattern. As discussed above, demonstrating that a cell had such a property would not prove that it generated the REM sleep state. In fact, unit investigations of *most* cell groups have reported changes in activity relatively characteristic of REM sleep. However, cell groups that show little or no unusual change in activity in REM sleep seem to be poor candidates for having an important role in REM sleep control.

The medial reticular formation of the brainstem (nucleus reticularis pontis oralis, caudalis and gigantocellularis) comprises much of the pontomedullary area critical for REM sleep control. Virtually all of the cells in this region show one of three patterns of sleep cycle activity (Siegel, 1979c; Siegel *et al.*, 1976, 1977, 1979). The first type of cell discharges in bursts during waking movement and is silent during sleep (Fig. 7.6). The second type has a high level of tonic activity in quiet waking and non-REM sleep which increases during waking movements and REM sleep. The third type of cell has a low level of tonic activity but also is active in conjunction with waking movements and REM sleep. We have described the specific movement relations of reticular calls elsewhere (Siegel, 1979a, b; Siegel & McGinty, 1977). The discharge rates of reticular cells in waking and REM sleep are positively correlated (Siegel *et al.*, 1979). The activity patterns of these cells can be best understood as being related to motor activation, which occurs in both waking and REM sleep. Since they do not qualitatively alter their discharge rate or pattern in REM sleep these cells do not appear likely to have a central role in REM sleep generation. This conclusion is further supported by recent lesion studies indicating that destruction of medial reticular cells does not disturb REM sleep (Sastre *et al.*, 1979). In looking for cells that discharge selectively in REM sleep it is important to record during normal waking behaviours. Recording in immobile animals as has frequently been the practice, may, by preventing activity during waking, leave the erroneous impression that these cells are selectively active in REM sleep (Hobson *et al.*, 1974).

While most cells in the brainstem reticular formation show similar patterns of activity in waking and REM sleep, several cell groups do show specific changes in their discharge patterns in REM sleep. One such group is in the locus coeruleus complex (Fig. 7.7) (McGinty & Sakai, 1973; Hobson *et al.*, 1975; Sakai, 1980). Many of these cells become completely silent during the SWS–REM sleep transition and remain off in REM sleep. At all other times, including periods of waking movement, they are tonically active. Recently another cell group showing this activity pattern has been seen in the dorsal medullary reticular formation, in the vicinity of the nucleus of the solitary tract (Eguchi & Satoh, 1980). A third area with cells that turn off selectively in REM sleep is the serotonergic dorsal raphe nucleus (McGinty & Harper, 1976). This last cell group is located rostral to the brainstem regions shown by the transection studies to be required for REM sleep control. It therefore nicely illustrates the danger of jumping to the conclusion that because a cell group shows a unique discharge pattern in REM sleep it has a critical role in REM sleep state control. In fact a large amount of evidence now indicates that an important function of the raphe cells is to restrict PGO waves to the REM sleep and the REM sleep transition state. Destruction of this area causes continuous PGO spiking (Simon *et al.*, 1973), while pauses in raphe discharge precede PGO spikes (McGinty & Harper, 1976).

Two other cell groups have been reported to be selectively 'on' in REM sleep. One of these cell groups is located in the locus coeruleus region, adjacent to the 'REM off' cells, while the other is in the medial medullary area (Sakai, 1980). Sakai has speculated that these cells are responsible for the atonia of REM sleep, with the locus coeruleus 'REM on' cells exciting the medullary 'REM on' cells. These medullary 'REM on' cells would then inhibit spinal motoneurons producing the atonia of REM sleep. We have also recorded in these areas (Siegel *et al.*, 1979; Siegel, 1979c), but have not seen cells selectively on in REM sleep. Since such cells were reported to constitute only a small proportion of recorded cells, our failure to encounter them is most likely a sampling problem. However, there is always the possibility that the cats in the Sakai studies were

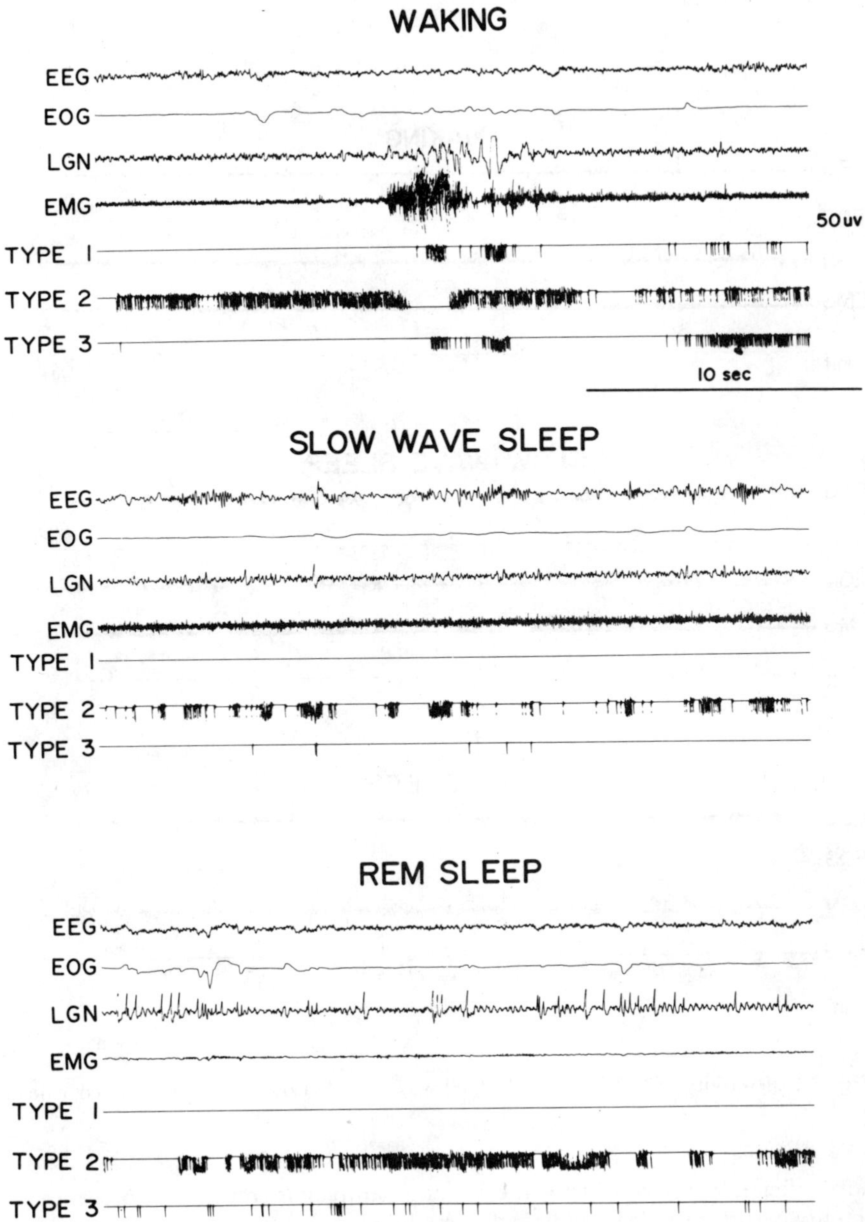

Fig. 7.6 Activity of 3 major reticular cell types seen in midbrain pontine and medullary regions during sleep cycle.

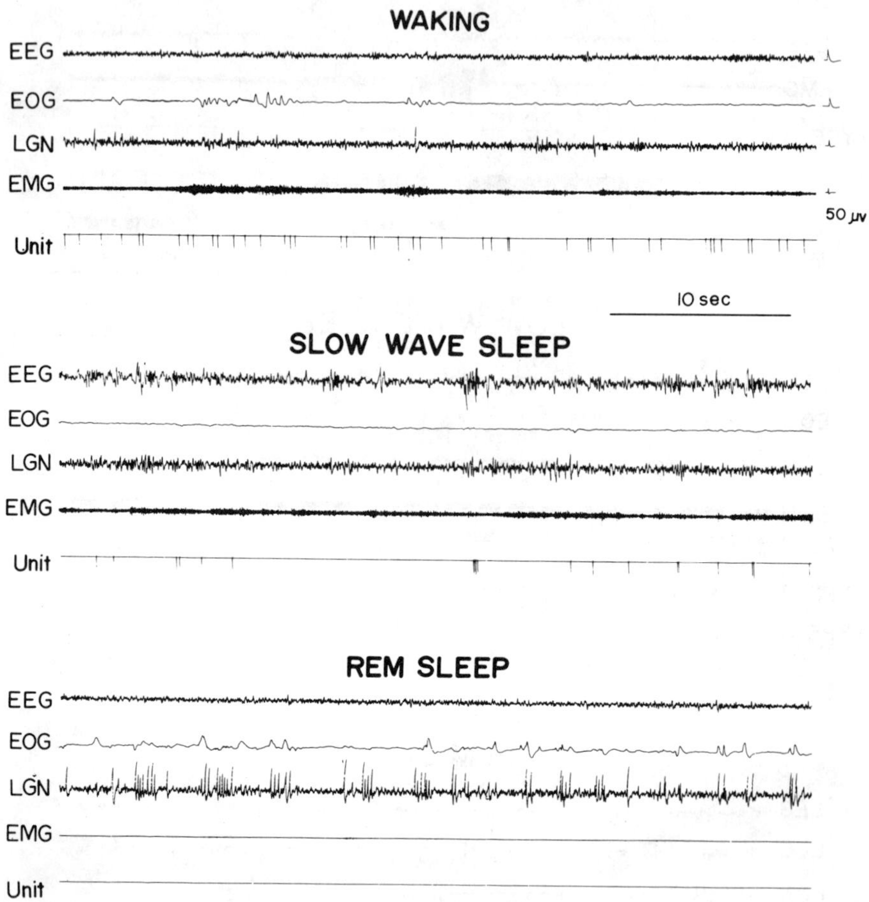

Fig. 7.7 Activity of 'REM off' cell. Cell was recorded in vicinity of locus coeruleus nucleus.

not sufficiently active during the waking samples to reveal the presence of activity in this state. It is possible that medullary inhibition of motor tone is not mediated by cells that selectively turn on in this state. Instead it may result from the synchronous discharge of medullary inhibitory cells that can also show waking activity (Siegel *et al.*, 1979).

7.4 Conclusion

While a considerable amount is known about the brain regions involved in generating REM sleep, it is not yet possible to advance a simple model of how this state is generated. Clearly, transection studies demonstrate that the pontomedullary brainstem contains systems sufficient to generate the REM sleep state. Transections behind the pons demonstrate that neither the pons nor the medulla alone contains mechanisms sufficient to generate REM sleep. The REM sleep state requires the coordinated activity of *both* regions. Further, we know that it is possible to dissociate certain aspects of REM sleep from the normally unified state. It is possible to have PGO activity without REM sleep, REM sleep without atonia and ultradian rhythmicity without REM sleep. Unit activity studies highlight several different neuronal groups which may participate in REM sleep generation. The central problem is to determine which cell groups are responsible for each of the many phenomena of REM sleep and for their coordination and timing. Is there a single medullary cell group responsible for such coordination, perhaps also being responsible for the waking basic rest–activity cycle? If so, where in this region is this group located? How does it recruit activity in cell groups responsible for each of the REM sleep phenomena? How is the timing of REM sleep controlled? Why does activity in the basic rest–activity cycle generator trigger arousal in waking and REM sleep during sleep? These questions are the focus of continuing research.

References

ADEY, W. R., BORS, E. and PORTER, R. W. (1968). EEG sleep patterns after high cervical lesions in man. *Arch. Neurol.*, **19**, 377–383.

AMATRUDA, T. T., BLACK, D. A., MCKENNA, T. M., MCCARLEY, R. W. and HOBSON, J. S. (1975). Sleep cycle control and cholinergic mechanisms; differential effects of carbachol injections at pontine brain stem sites. *Brain Res.*, **28**, 501–515.

BERMAN, A. L. (1968). *The Brain Stem of the Cat*, Madison, Wis: University of Wisconsin Press, 175 pp.

EGUCHI, K. and SATOH, T. (1980). Convergence of sleep-wakefulness subsystems onto single neurons in the region of cat's solitary tract nucleus. *Arch. Ital. Biol.*, **118**, 331–345.

GADEA-CIRIA, M. (1976). Tele-encephalic versus cerebellar control upon ponto-geniculo-occipital waves during paradoxical sleep in the cat. *Experientia*, **32**, 889–890.

HENDRICKS, J. C., MORRISON, A. R. and MANN, G. L. (1980). Behavior during paradoxical sleep differs with lesion site. *Sleep Research*, **9**, 31.

HOBSON, J. A., MCCARLEY, R. W., PIVIK, T. and FREEDMAN, R. (1974). Selective firing by cat pontine brain stem neurons in desynchronized sleep. *J. Neurophysiol.*, **37**, 497–511.

HOBSON, J. A., MCCARLEY, R. W. and WYZINSKI, P. W. (1975). Sleep cycle oscillation: reciprocal discharge by two brainstem neuronal groups. *Science*, **189**, 55–58.

HUTTENLOCHER, P. R. (1961). Evoked and spontaneous activity in single units of medial brain stem during natural sleep and waking. *J. Neurophysiol.*, **24**, 451–468.

JOUVET, M. (1962). Recherches sur les structures nerveuses et les mechanismes responsables des différentes phases du sommeil physiologique. *Arch. Ital. Biol.*, **100**, 125–206.

JOUVET, M. and DELORME, F. (1965). Locus coeruleus et sommeil paradoxal. *C.R. Soc. Biol.*, **159**, 895–899.

KLEITMAN, N. (1963). *Sleep and Wakefulness*, Chicago: University of Chicago Press, 552 pp.

KRIPKE, D. (1972). An ultradian biologic rhythm associated with perceptual deprivation and REM sleep. *Psychosom. Med.*, **34**, 221–234.

LAURENT, J. R., CESPUGLIO, R. and JOUVET, M. (1974). Delimitation des voies ascendants de l'activate ponto-geniculo-occipitale chez le chat. *Brain Res.*, **65**, 29–52.

LAVIE, P., LORD, J. W. and FRANK, R. A. (1974). Basic rest-activity cycle in the perception of the spiral after-effect: a sensitive detector of a basic biological rhythm. *Behav. Biol.*, **11**, 373–379.

MCGINTY, D. J. and HARPER, R. M. (1976). Dorsal raphe neurons: depression of firing during sleep in cats. *Brain Res.*, **101**, 569–575.

MCGINTY, D. J., LONDON, M. S., BAKER, T. L., STEVENSON, M., HOPPENBROUWERS, T., HARPER, R. M., STERMAN, M. B. and HODGMAN, J. (1979). Sleep apnea in normal kittens. *Sleep*, **1**, 393–421.

MCGINTY, D. and SAKAI, K. (1973). Unit activity in the dorsal pontine reticular formation in the cat. *Sleep Research*, **2**, 33.

MITLER, M. and DEMENT, W. (1974). Cataplectic-like behavior in cats after microinjection of carbachol in the pontine reticular formation. *Brain Res.*, **68**, 335–343.

ORR, W. C. and HOFFMAN, H. J. (1974). A 90-min cardiac biorhythm: methodology and data analysis using modified periodogram and complex demodulation. *IEEE Trans. on Biomed. Eng.*, **21**, 130–143.

PERENIN, M. T., MAEDA, T. and JEANNEROD, M. (1972). Are vestibular nuclei responsible for rapid eye movements of paradoxical sleep? *Brain Res.*, **43**, 617–621.

POMPEIANO, O. and MORRISON, A. R. (1965). Vestibular influences during sleep. I. Abolition of the rapid eye movements of desynchronized sleep following vestibular lesions. *Arch. Ital. Biol.*, **103**, 569–595.

SAKAI, K. (1980). Some anatomical and physiological properties of ponto-mesencephalic tegmental neurons with special reference to the PGO waves and postural atonia during paradoxical sleep in the cat. In: J. A. HOBSON and M. A. BRAZIER (Eds.), *The Reticular Formation Revisited*, New York: Raven Press, pp. 427–447.

SASTRE, J. P., SAKAI, K. and JOUVET, M. (1979). Persistance du sommeil paradoxal chez le chat après destruction de l'aire gigantocellulaire du tegmentum pontique par l'acide kainique. *C.R. Acad. Sci.*, **D**, 959–964.

SIEGEL, J. M. (1979a). Behavioral functions of the reticular formation. *Brain Res. Rev.*, **1**, 69–105.

SIEGEL, J. M. (1979b). Behavioral relations of medullary reticular formation cells. *Exp. Neurol.*, **65**, 691–698.

SIEGEL, J. M. (1979c). Unit activity in the reticular formation and REM sleep. In: R. DRUCKER-COLIN, M. SHKUROVICH and M. B. STERMAN (eds.), *The Functions of Sleep*. New York: Academic Press, pp. 37–71.

SIEGEL, J. M. and MCGINTY, D. J. (1976). Brainstem neurons without spontaneous unit discharge. *Science*, **193**, 240–242.

SIEGEL, J. M. and MCGINTY, D. J. (1977). Pontine reticular formation neurons: relationship of discharge to motor activity. *Science*, **196**, 678–680.

SIEGEL, J. M., MCGINTY, D. J. and BREEDLOVE, S. M. (1977). Sleep and waking activity of pontine gigantocellular field neurons. *Exp. Neurol.*, **56**, 553–573.

SIEGEL, J. M. NIENHUIS, R., TOMASZEWSKI, K. and WHEELER, R. (1981). Behavioral states after brainstem transection at the medullary level. *Soc. Neurosci. Abstr.*, **7**, 233.

SIEGEL, J. M., WHEELER, R. L., and MCGINTY, D. J. (1979). Activity of medullary reticular formation neurons in the unrestrained cat during waking and sleep. *Brain Res.*, **179**, 49–60.

SIMON, R. P., GERSHON, M. D. and BROOKS, D. C. (1973). The role of the raphe nuclei in the regulation of ponto-geniculo-occipital wave activity. *Brain Res.*, **58**, 313–330.
VILLABLANCA, J. (1966). Behavioral and polygraphic study of 'sleep' and 'wakefulness' in chronic decerebrate cats. *Electroenceph. Clin. Neurophysiol.*, **21**, 562–577.

CHAPTER 8

Pharmacological Approaches to Sleep Regulation

Alexander A. Borbély

8.1 Introduction

Two different approaches can be taken to study the pharmacology of sleep regulation (Table 8.1). In the first approach, drugs constitute the independent variable, while sleep and its substates form the dependent variable. This category includes experiments in which a hypnotic drug is administered in humans to study its effectiveness, or studies where an experimental compound is used in animals to investigate neurochemical aspects of sleep regulation. In the second approach, sleep represents the independent variable, and neurochemical brain constituents the dependent variable. In this type of experiments, sleep is sampled either during specific phases of its spontaneous occurrence or after experimental manipulation, and sleep-related neurochemical changes are studied. The focus may be either on the investigation of specific brain constituents known to be of functional importance (e.g. neurotransmitters), or on the search of unknown molecules ('sleep factors') which may play a key role in sleep regulation. A common, general aim of all pharmacological approaches to sleep is to gain insight into the chemical processes underlying sleep regulation and thus to establish a more rational basis for the therapy of sleep disorders.

On the whole, the developments of the pharmacotherapy of insomnia may be considered a 'success story' (Fig. 8.1). Chloralhydrate and paraldehyde, the

Table 8.1 Two Approaches to the Pharmacology and Neurochemistry of Sleep

	Independent variable	Dependent variable
1	Pharmacological or neurochemical compound used in therapy (e.g. hypnotic) or in experimental pharmacology (e.g. PCPA; 'sleep factor')	Sleep and its substates
2	Sleep: sampling in different substates or after experimental manipulations (e.g. sleep deprivation, electrical sleep induction)	Neurochemical brain constituents: search for changes of known constituents (e.g. transmitters, benzodiazepine binding) or search for identity of unknown constituents ('sleep factor')

first truly hypnotic therapeutic agents, were succeeded at the beginning of the present century by the more potent barbiturates which rapidly aquired a dominating position among the hypnotics. Their considerable abuse potential and their toxicity after overdose must be regarded as serious shortcomings of this class. In the last two decades, the barbiturates were substituted by the benzodiazepines which have a higher hypnotic potency and a larger margin of safety. However, the successful development of this new class of hypnotics should not detract from the fact that progress was largely a result of serendipity and trial-and-error procedures, and not a consequence of rigorous scientific deduction on the basis of facts and hypotheses.

The study of neurochemical mechanisms of sleep was stimulated in the 1960s by the discovery of specific neurotransmitter systems in the brain, and by the combined application of new morphological, electrophysiological and biochemical methods. The use of drugs as tools for influencing the metabolism of specific transmitters (e.g. p-chlorophenylalanine, an inhibitor of tryptophan hydroxylase) contributed to the formulation of an explicit neurochemical theory of sleep regulation (Jouvet, 1972). However, insights into the neurobiological processes have not yet led to innovations in the pharmacotherapy of insomnia. The amino acid tryptophan, the precursor of serotonin, is one of the few compounds which on the basis of neurochemical considerations have been tested for their hypnotic effect. However, its sleep-promoting action is limited and its efficacy in sleep disturbances controversial (Nicholson & Stone, 1979; Linnoila *et al.*, 1980). Recently, receptors of neurotransmitters, neuromodulators and hormones have received increasing attention as structures whose plasticity could play a central role in functional aspects of the brain. The

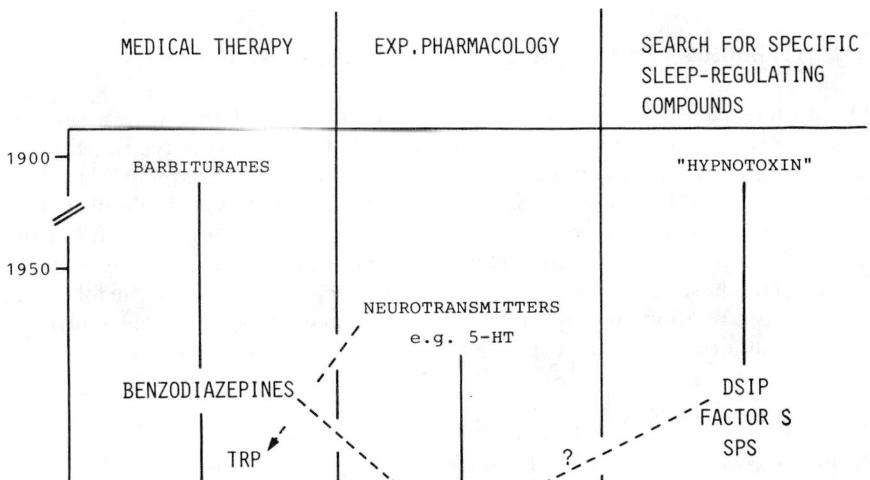

Fig. 8.1 Diagram representing three lines of development in the pharmacological approach to sleep.

discovery of specific cerebral binding sites for benzodiazepines (Möhler & Okada, 1977; Squires & Braestrup, 1977) is particularly interesting since it may provide the basis for understanding the mode of action of the most widely used class of hypnotics.

The search for specific sleep factors was undertaken mainly by groups working outside the main currents of neurobiological research. Piéron's (1913) original hypothesis that a 'hypnotoxin' accumulates during waking time and is inactivated during sleep, was re-examined in rigorous experiments by Pappenheimer and co-workers and later by Uchizono and co-workers. Monnier and Schoenenberger isolated the nonapeptide Delta Sleep Inducing Peptide (DSIP) from animals in which sleep had been induced by electrical brain stimulation. Recently attempts were made to investigate the distribution of this peptide in the organism and to study its functional aspects (Kastin *et al.*, 1980). Endogenous sleep-promoting agents will be discussed in more detail in Section 8.3.7.

The three lines of research shown in Fig. 8.1 have evolved to a large part independently from one other, and do not exhibit many cross-connections. It will be important for genuine progress in the field that on the one hand pharmacotherapy benefits from a more tangible 'spin-off' from experimental pharmacology and neurochemistry, and that on the other hand the mode of action of hypnotics and their relations to sleep regulation are better understood.

The present chapter on pharmacological approaches to sleep regulation highlights and illustrates salient problems, but does not provide an extensive or balanced review on the subject. For ample documentation the reader is referred to reviews by Kay *et al.* (1976), Gillin *et al.* (1978), Oswald (1978) and Mendelson (1980).

8.2 Hypnotics and Sleep Regulation: Studies in Man

Often pharmacological sleep studies in humans are undertaken to assess the efficacy of hypnotics. While polygraphic techniques are usually restricted to the sleep laboratory, questionnaires and self-rating scales are frequently used for the evaluation of the sleep parameters in a clinical setting or under home conditions. These procedures are generally adequate for documenting the effects and after-effects of a sleep remedy. However, it is more difficult to relate changes recorded by these procedures to physiological sleep regulation. In the following sections, two methods are presented which may facilitate a functional analysis of pharmacological effects on sleep.

8.2.1 Motor Activity Recording

Night-time motor activity has been used as a measure of the effect of hypnotics on sleep (e.g. Hinton, 1961; 1963; Oswald *et al.*, 1963; Gaillard *et al.*, 1973). We have recently applied a new activity-recording technique for monitoring the action of hypnotics outside the laboratory (Borbély *et al.*, 1981b; Mattmann *et al.*, 1982). Motor activity is measured with a wrist-worn solid-state activity monitor, a modified version of a device described by Colburn *et al.* (1976). Arm-movements are converted into electric signals by a piezo-electric transducer. The integrated signals for successive 7.5-min periods are stored in the memory of the device and read out into a computer at 5-day intervals. The method has proved to be sensitive enough to record the reduction of night-time motor activity following the administration of hypnotics to healthy volunteers (Mattmann *et al.*, 1982). When the value of the placebo night was defined as the 100% reference level (62% of the 7.5-min periods during bedtime exhibiting suprathreshold activity values), the benzodiazepine hypnotics triazolam (0.25; 0.5; 1.0 mg), nitrazepam (10 mg) and flunitrazepam (2 mg) reduced activity time by 10–30%. All but the lowest dose of triazolam reached the level of statistical significance. Fig. 8.2 illustrates the sedative effect of nitrazepam. The reduction of night-time motor activity was paralleled by the decrease in the number and duration of wake periods as estimated by the subject (Mattmann *et al.*, 1982). The unobtrusiveness of the device allows us to obtain activity data over long time periods from subjects living under their usual life conditions. Our first attempts to monitor insomniac patients and to record the effect of pharmacotherapy are promising (Borbély *et al.*, 1981b: Fig. 9).

Hypnotics are expected to promote sleep at night-time, but their effect should not persist beyond waking. Due to the long elimination half-life of several currently used hypnotics (Breimer, 1977; Mendelson, 1980, p. 49) or of their active metabolites, day-time residual effects may give rise to hangover and impaired performance (Mendelson, 1980). We used the wrist-worn activity monitor to document residual effects by recording spontaneous activity on the day following a drug night (Fig. 8.3). With the exception of the lowest dose of triazolam (0.25 mg), mean daytime activity was reduced by all hypnotics tested. Significant sedation was found for triazolam 0.5 mg and flunitrazepam 2 mg. The subjects were rated by observers as significantly more tired during the day following the flunitrazepam night than after the placebo night (Mattmann *et al.*, 1982). Another group reported a reduction of spontaneous daytime activity after flurazepam 30 mg (Crowley & Hydinger-McDonald,

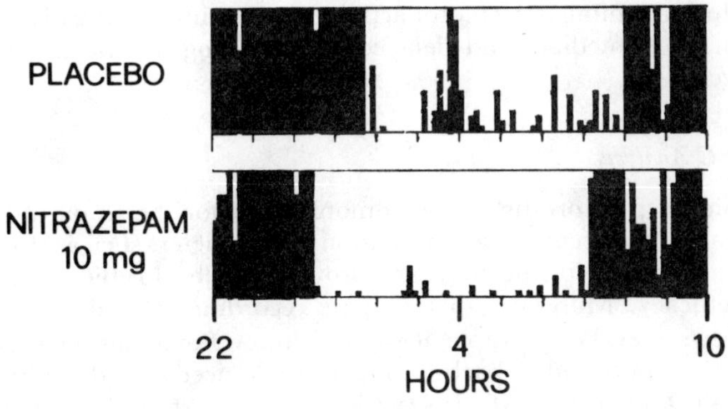

Fig. 8.2 Effect of a hypnotic on motor activity during sleep in a human subject. The plots represent activity records of successive 7.5-min intervals expressed in arbitrary units. Broad black areas represent high activity during waking. Nitrazepam 10 mg taken before bedtime causes a marked reduction in night-time activity in comparison to the placebo night. (Modified from A. A. Borbély (1981) in F. Obál and G. Benedek (Eds.), *Advances in Physiological Science*, Vol. 18, Environmental Physiology.)

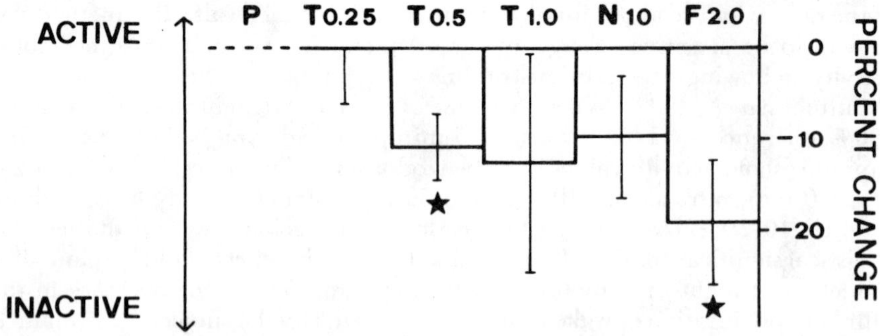

Fig. 8.3 Motor activity 10–16 h after hypnotic intake. Residual effect of various hypnotics on spontaneous daytime motor activity. The bars represent mean values with SEM of the percent change of motor activity relative to placebo (P). T: triazolam; N: nitrazepam; F: flunitrazepam. Doses are given in mg. Significant differences from placebo are indicated by asterisk ($p < 0.05$; 2-sided Wilcoxon paired signed rank test). (Reproduced from P. Mattmann *et al.* (1982), *Arzneim.-Forsch/Drug Res.*, **32**, 461–465, by permission.)

1979). In our study, the performance in the digit cancellation test in the morning was impaired following the flunitrazepam night, but not after the other hypnotics. It would be therefore premature to conclude that a reduction in spontaneous activity is a sign for a performance deficit. In the second post-drug night after triazolam 0.5 mg, sleep was characterized by a significant increase in both motor activity and self-rated restlessness. 'Rebound insomnia' has been reported after discontinuation of several other benzodiazepine hypnotics after they had been administered for several days (see Mattmann *et al.*, 1982, for references). Such delayed effects on sleep indicate that hypnotics may induce a disbalance in the long-term regulation of sleep.

In conclusion, ambulatory motor activity monitoring is a sensitive procedure for measuring immediate and delayed pharmacological effects on the rest-activity cycle.

8.2.2 EEG Analysis

Polygraphic sleep recordings are commonly used for the study of hypnotics, since they allow the accurate determination of parameters such as sleep latency, sleep duration and sleep efficiency, and provide thereby an objective measure of hypnotic efficacy. Moreover, polygraphic recordings reveal drug effects on specific sleep stages. For example, it has been known for almost two decades that REM sleep is suppressed by barbiturates and enhanced after discontinuation of these drugs (Oswald *et al.*, 1963; Oswald & Priest, 1965). Subsequent studies showed that also the slow wave sleep (SWS) fraction of non-REM sleep (Stages 3 and 4) was suppressed by barbiturate and benzodiazepine hypnotics (see Kay *et al.*, 1976; Institute of Medicine Report, Technical Supplement, 1979). The assessment of the functional significance of these observations is difficult. On the one side, changes in the distribution of sleep stages may reflect the influence of hypnotic drugs on sleep regulation, and may thus provide insights into their mode of action on sleep processes. For example, the REM sleep rebound following drug withdrawal indicates that hypnotics induce a genuine REM sleep deficit which gives rise to a compensatory response. Yet, a more basic interpretation of the effect is hampered by our ignorance of the functional significance of the various sleep stages. On the other side, one can argue that the major difficulties lie in the sleep scoring criteria which had been established on the basis of physiological sleep records (Rechtschaffen & Kales, 1968), and which may be inadequate for classifying the sleep EEG under pharmacological conditions. Changes in the distribution of the conventionally scored sleep stages may yield therefore an incomplete picture of drug effects. Such considerations led us to supplement the usual methods of sleep scoring by the spectral analysis of the EEG signal.

Fig. 8.4 shows the application of the technique to a pharmacological problem. The sleep stages scored according to the criteria of Rechtschaffen and Kales (1968) are plotted on the top. It is evident that flunitrazepam did not induce prominent changes in the sleep stage pattern. The power density records of the EEG are plotted below the sleep stages for successive frequency bands between 0.25 and 25 Hz. Vertical lines indicate the limits of non-REM–REM sleep cycles which were defined according to the criteria of Feinberg and Floyd (1979). The two initial peaks in the delta range (0–5 Hz) in the left and middle plots correspond to SWS (Stages 3 and 4). The initial peak in the 11–14 Hz band of the baseline night represents rapid alpha activity during waking, whereas high values in the 11–17 Hz range during Stage 2 reflect spindle activity.

Flunitrazepam (2 mg) induced dramatic changes in power density which consisted principally in (1) a reduction of the delta activity between 1 and 5 Hz during SWS; (2) an enhancement of the 9–14 Hz band during non-REM sleep (particularly during SWS); and (3) the appearance of prominent high-frequency peaks (14–25 Hz) during REM sleep. The reduction of delta activity and the REM sleep-related increase in high-frequency activity persisted clearly into the subsequent night starting 24 h after flunitrazepam administration. A study conducted in eight subjects confirmed that all three types of changes seen in the drug record of Fig. 8.4 were still present in the following night (Borbély *et al.*, *Eur. J. Pharmacol.* (1983) in press). The benzodiazepine hypnotics flurazepam (30 mg) and triazolam (0.5 mg) induced similar EEG effects.

The results show that all-night, spectral analysis of the EEG is an exceedingly sensitive method for demonstrating effects and after-effects of hypnotics which are not apparent from the sleep stage pattern. The question then arises whether the technique is limited to the descriptive level of EEG analysis. or if it may also provide insights into the functional aspects of sleep regulation.

We have recently used spectral analysis to investigate the regulatory responses of sleep after a 40.5-h waking period (Borbély *et al.*, 1981a). The most prominent effect of sleep deprivation (SD) consisted in the enhancement of low-frequency EEG activity (Fig. 8.5, right), an effect that was still detectable in the second recovery night. These changes corresponded in part to the increase in SWS. However, since the rise in spectral power density was present also within individual sleep stages (SWS; Stage 4, Stage 2, REM sleep), it was obvious that the sleep stage distribution did not adequately reflect the effects of SD.

The results of the SD study in conjunction with previous reports in the literature indicated that the low-frequency EEG activity may represent the intensity of a sleep process whose level is determined by the prior waking time. The

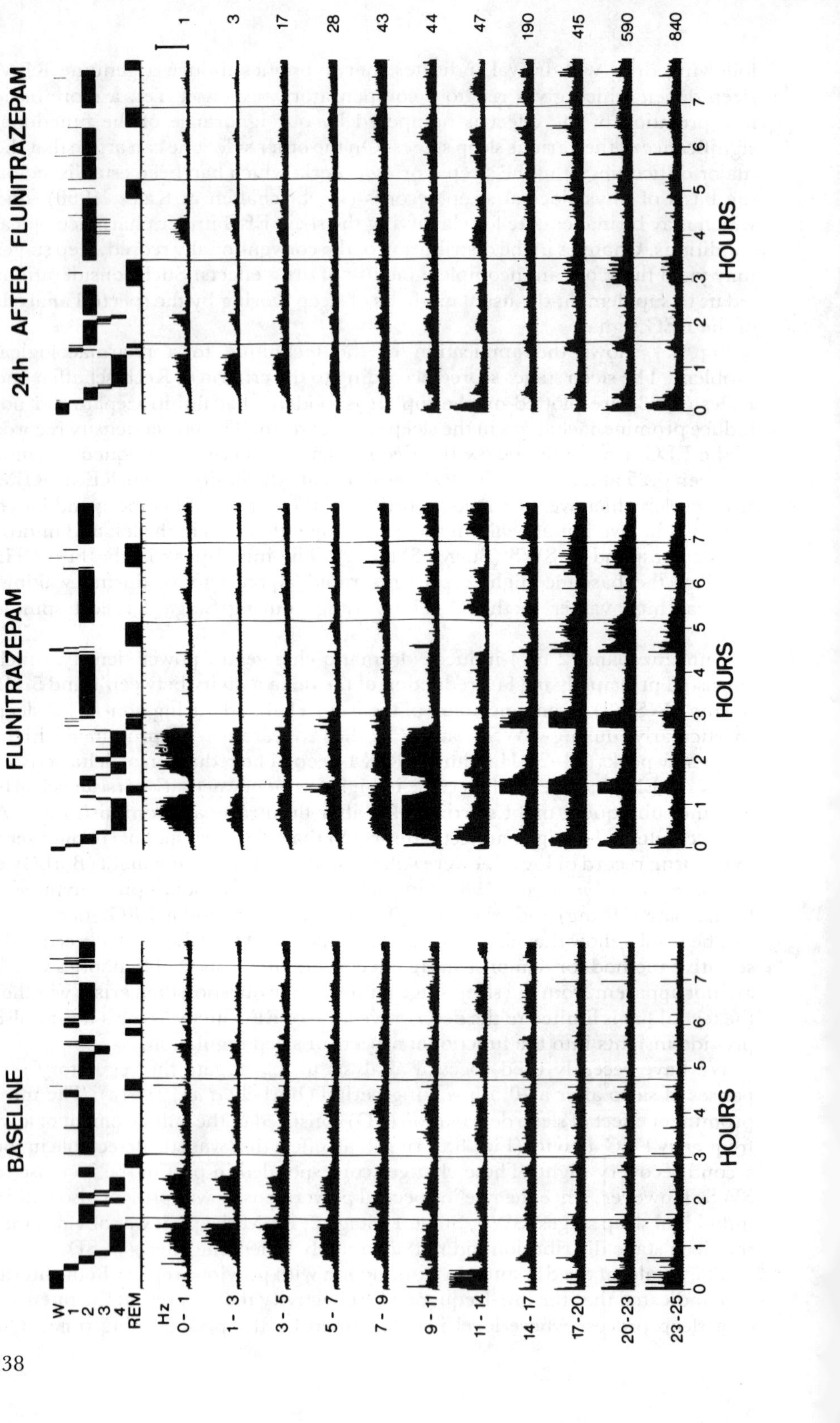
BASELINE
FLUNITRAZEPAM
24h AFTER FLUNITRAZEPAM
W
1
2
3
4
REM
Hz
0 - 1
1 - 3
3 - 5
5 - 7
7 - 9
9 - 11
11 - 14
14 - 17
17 - 20
20 - 23
23 - 25
1
3
17
28
43
44
47
190
415
590
840
0 1 2 3 4 5 6 7
HOURS

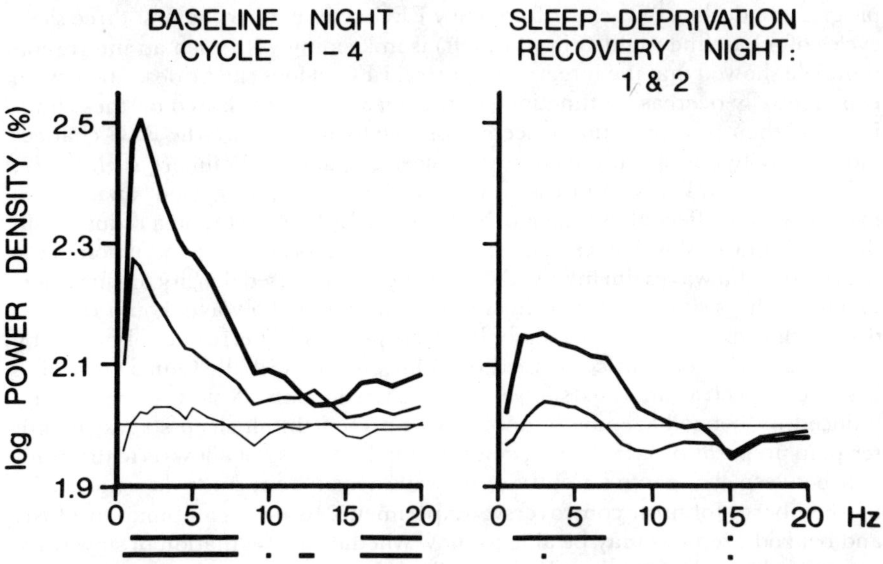

Fig. 8.5 EEG power density during baseline night (left) and two recovery nights after 40.5 h sleep deprivation (right) in man. The curves connect mean values ($n = 8$) of relative EEG power density computed for 0.5 Hz bins between 0.25 and 5.0 Hz, and for 1 Hz bins betweeen 5.25 and 25.0 Hz. In the *left panel*, values for non-REM–REM sleep cycles 1, 2 and 3 are indicated by curves of decreasing thickness. For each subject the value for sleep cycle 4 has been defined as 100% for each frequency band (horizontal line). Values of the preceding cycles are expressed relative to the corresponding values of cycle 4. In the *right panel*, the mean values of two baseline nights were defined as 100%. The curves representing recovery night 1 (thick line) and 2 (thin line) are expressed relative to the corresponding baseline values. Lines below the abscissa indicate significant differences between frequency bands ($P < 0.05$; 2-sided Wilcoxon paired signed rank test). Left panel: upper lines indicate significant differences between cycle 1 and 2, lower lines between cycle 2 and 3. Right panel: upper lines indicate difference between baseline and recovery night 1; lower lines between baseline and recovery night 2. (Modified from A. A. Borbély *et al.* (1981), *Electroenceph. Clin. Neurophys.*, **51**, 483–493.)

Fig. 8.4 Effect of flunitrazepam 2 mg on the sleep stages and EEG power density in man. The records were obtained from a young, adult healthy subject for a baseline night, a drug night and a post-drug night. Sleep scores are indicated on the top (W: waking; 1–4: stages of non-REM sleep; REM: REM sleep). Power density bands are plotted for various frequency bands (indicated on left side) for successive 1-min epochs. (Lower limit of each frequency band is 0.25 Hz higher than indicated.) The scale factors indicated on the right side were adjusted to equalize the area of the plots (see Borbély *et al.*, 1981a). Vertical lines delimit non-REM–REM sleep cycles. Note the massive changes in power density in the drug night and the residual effects in the subsequent night which are not apparent from the sleep score distribution (Borbély, Loepfe, Mattmann, Fellmann, Gerne, Strauch, Lehmann, unpublished data).

progressive decline of the low-frequency EEG activity over the first three sleep cycles of a baseline night (Fig. 8.5, left) is in keeping with such an interpretation. We showed that the integrated spectral EEG values can be described by an exponentially decreasing function (Borbély *et al.*, 1981a). Based on these findings and their interpretation it seems possible to analyse also the EEG changes induced by hypnotics in the context of sleep regulation. Feinberg *et al.* (1977, 1979) have explicitly addressed this problem. Using period analysis to investigate the effect of flurazepam on the sleep EEG, they found a reduction in the amplitude of slow waves. They reported, however, that the reduction in the density of delta waves during SWS is offset by an increased density during Stage 2. The authors suggested that this redistribution of delta waves could reflect a drug-induced slowing of a metabolic sleep process. The results obtained by Feinberg *et al.* were not confirmed by Johnson *et al.* (1979). Our own studies based on spectral analysis showed that the reduction of slow wave activity induced by benzodiazepine hypnotics was present in all sleep stages (manuscript in preparation). However, since the method does not allow us to discriminate between changes in amplitude and wave density, our study does not clarify the Feinberg–Johnson controversy. Experiments using a combination of SD and benzodiazepines may be able to show whether the regulation of slow wave activity is basically impaired by benzodiazepines.

8.3 Experimental Pharmacology and Sleep Regulation: Studies in Animals

8.3.1 Sleep Regulation in the Rat

It is well known that the two substates of sleep, non-REM sleep and REM sleep, can be discriminated on the basis of electrophysiological criteria in various mammalian species. It has been only recently recognized that the daily sleep pattern in animals and humans also shows invariant features which may reflect homologies in sleep regulation (Borbély, 1981).

Fig. 8.6 shows the distribution of the vigilance states of the rat over a period of 24 h. Under 12 h light–12 h dark conditions the rat spends close to 80% of the light phase in sleep, and approximately 80% of the dark phase in waking. This dichotomy in the daily distribution of sleep corresponds largely to the circadian rest–activity rhythm. However, by subjecting non-REM sleep to an EEG frequency analysis, prominent trends are revealed within the daily sleep and waking phases (Fig. 8.6, middle panel). Non-REM sleep in which slow waves predominate (low percentiles of zero crossing distribution; dark areas in Fig. 8.6), occurs mainly in the first part of the light phase and decreases progressively in the subsequent hours. Conversely, the non-REM sleep fraction with a high predominant EEG frequency (zero-crossing band of 70–100%) occupies a gradually increasing part of sleep. These trends were confirmed by spectral analysis of the EEG (Borbély & Neuhaus, 1979; Borbély,

Fig. 8.6 Daily distribution of sleep states in the rat. The curves connect hourly mean values from 14 animals and a total of 23 days. Interrupted vertical line and bar on top abscissa delimit the dark phase. Top: total sleep (TS) and REM sleep (REM). Middle: non-REM sleep subdivided into zero-crossing (ZCR) bands according to the percentiles (inset) of ZCR values (see Borbély *et al.*, 1981c) and expressed as percent of recording

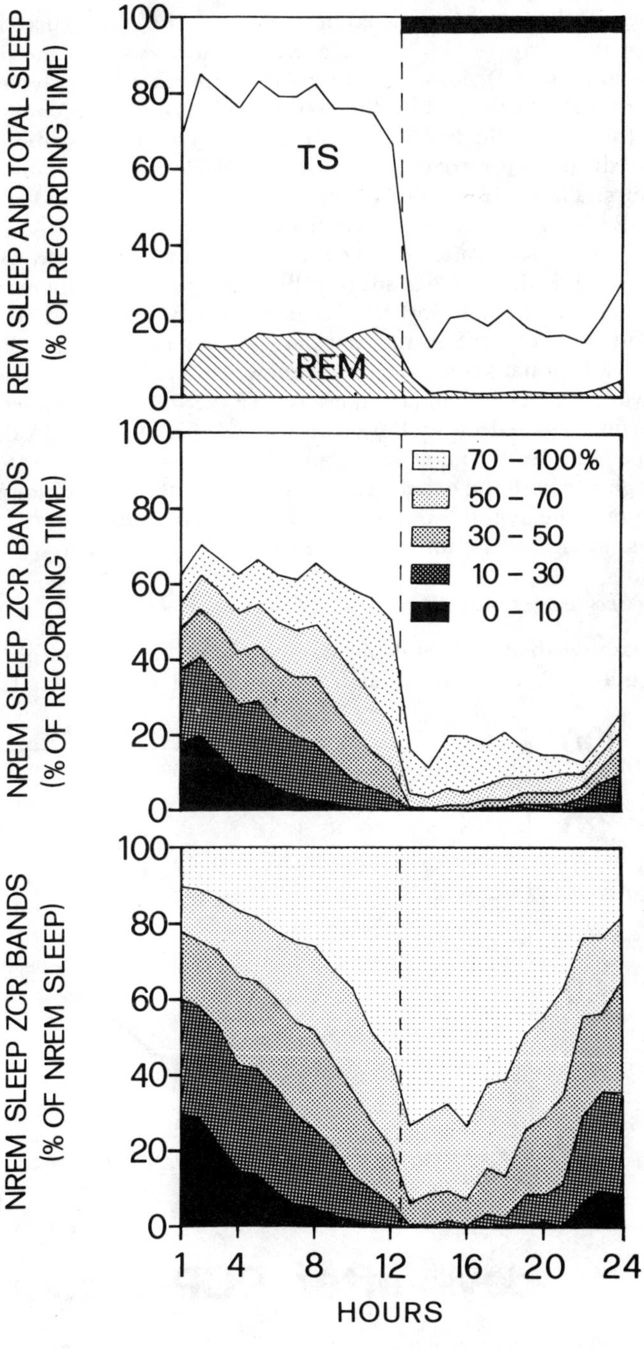

time. Areas of increasing darkness represent decreasing predominant EEG frequency. Bottom: non-REM sleep subdivided into ZCR bands and expressed as percent of total non-REM sleep, (Reproduced from A. A. Borbély *et al.* (1981), *Behav. Brain Res.*, **2**, 1–22, by permission.)

Hanagasioglu & Tobler, in preparation). Owing to the low occurrence of non-REM sleep, the zero-crossing bands are not readily seen in the dark phase (Fig. 8.6, middle panel). However, by plotting the values relative to the total amount of non-REM sleep (Fig. 8.6, bottom panel), it is apparent that slow wave sleep (defined as the lowest 30% of the zero-crossing distribution) is at a minimum at the beginning of the dark phase and increases gradually in the subsequent hours. These observations suggested to us that the proportion of SWS within non-REM sleep is a function of prior waking time. The hypothesis was supported by sleep deprivation (SD) experiments in which the slow wave sleep fraction of non-REM sleep was specifically increased after prolonged waking (Borbély & Neuhaus, 1979; Borbély, Hanagasioglu & Tobler, in preparation). The predominance of SWS in the first part of the daily sleep period has been reported also for humans (e.g. Webb & Agnew, 1971) and monkey (Reite *et al.*, 1965; Crowley *et al.*, 1972), and the increase of SWS following SD was observed in humans (first detailed study: Berger & Oswald, 1962), dog (Takahashi *et al.*, 1978), cat (Ursin, 1971) and rabbit (Pappenheimer *et al.*, 1975).

Taken together with the experiments discussed in the preceding section, the findings support the hypothesis that slow wave activity reflects the intensity of a sleep process in various mammalian species.

8.3.2 The Spontaneous Sleep–Wake Cycle after Serotonin Depletion

The 'monoamine theory' is still the most explicit neurochemical hypothesis of sleep regulation. Its conceptual framework and experimental basis was

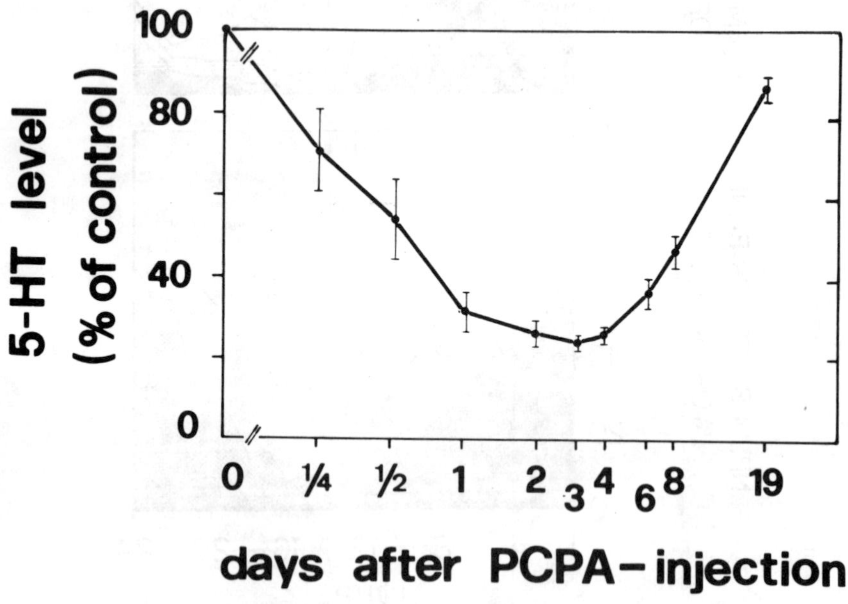

Fig. 8.7 Serotonin concentration in rat forebrain determined at various timepoints after injection of p-chlorophenylalanine (PCPA; 300 mg/kg i.p.). The points represent mean values with SEM and are expressed as a percentage of control values from non-treated animals. Note the logarithmic time scale. (Modified from P. Steigrad *et al.* (1978), *Arch. Pharmacol.* **305**, 143–148.)

established to a large degree by Michel Jouvet and his school (Jouvet, 1972, 1977). The theory was based on the discovery of ascending monoamine containing neuronal systems with cell bodies located in the brainstem. An ingenious combination of physiological and pharmacological approaches led to the hypothesis that serotonergic neurons are responsible for non-REM sleep and for the priming of REM sleep, while catecholaminergic and cholinergic systems are involved in the executive mechanisms of REM sleep as well as in the maintenance of tonic arousal (Jouvet, 1977). Our own recent data obtained in the rat will be presented to illustrate and discuss several major arguments of the hypothesis relating to the serotonin system.

Parachlorophenylalanine (PCPA) was one of the first compounds that has been used as a tool for manipulating selectively the cerebral metabolism of a transmitter. By inhibiting tryptophan hydroxylase, PCPA causes a long-lasting reduction in the concentration of brain serotonin (5HT) (Fig. 8.7), while exerting only a minor and short-lasting effect on catecholamines (Koe & Weissmann, 1966; Miller *et al.*, 1970). The reduction of brain 5HT was shown to be paralleled by insomnia in the cat (Delorme *et al.*, 1966; Koella *et al.*, 1968). Sleep could be temporarily restored by administering the 5HT precursor 5-hydroxytryptophan (5HTP) which causes a transient rise in cerebral 5HT (Mouret *et al.*, 1967; Koella *et al.*, 1968). Insomnia could be also produced by lesions of the raphe nuclei, a result predicted by the 'serotonin hypothesis' (see Jouvet, 1972, 1977, for reviews). However, in recent years the general validity of the hypothesis was questioned on several grounds. The critical arguments included inconsistent effects of PCPA (Rechtschaffen *et al.*, 1973) and 5, 7-dihydroxytryptamine (a 5HT neurotoxin) on sleep in the rat (Ross *et al.*, 1976), and the recovery of sleep during chronic administration of PCPA in the cat (Dement *et al.*, 1972; see also Steigrad *et al.*, 1978, for similar findings in the rat).

We investigated the effect of a single injection of PCPA (300 mg/kg i.p.) on the vigilance states of the unrestrained rat by continuous telemetric recordings during six post-injection days (Fig. 8.8). In the hours immediately following drug injection, the SWS fraction of non REM sleep was enhanced, while REM sleep and motor activity were reduced (Borbély *et al.*, 1981c). During the dark phase starting 12 h after drug injection in which the 5HT level decreased from 60% to 40% of control (Fig. 8.7), total sleep time was increased. This initial phase of sedation was followed by a phase of partial insomnia which was most prominent in the light phase of the day following PCPA injection (Fig. 8.8: PCPA + 1 d). Although all sleep states were significantly reduced, REM sleep and SWS were proportionately more decreased than non-REM sleep. Total sleep time was still significantly shortened in the light phase of the second post-drug day (PCPA + 2 d), but did not differ from the control level on subsequent days.

The low level of cerebral 5HT 24 h after PCPA administration could be raised within 1 h from 38% to 61% of control by injecting tryptophan (Trp; 150 mg/kg i.p.) (Borbély *et al.*, 1981c). When Trp was administered 28 h after PCPA, SWS and REMS were temporarily enhanced (Fig. 8.9), while motor activity was reduced. No effect was seen when the same dose of Trp was administered to untreated animals. Our results are consistent with the findings by Laguzzi and Adrien (1980) who described the effect of large doses of PCPA on sleep in the rat and showed that the insomnia could be reversed by 5HTP.

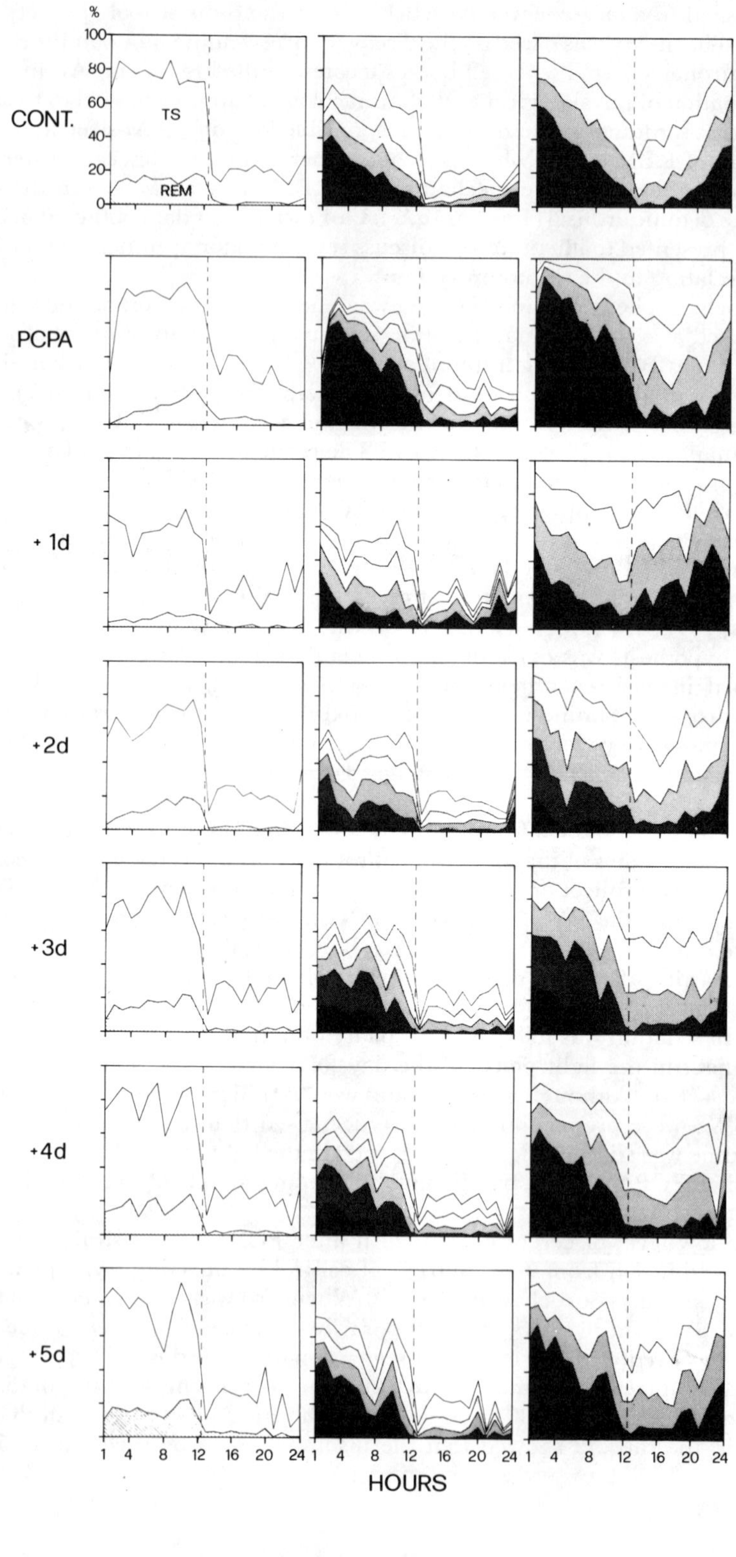

%
100
80
60
40
20
0
CONT.
TS
REM
PCPA
+ 1d
+2d
+3d
+4d
+5d
1 4 8 12 16 20 24
HOURS

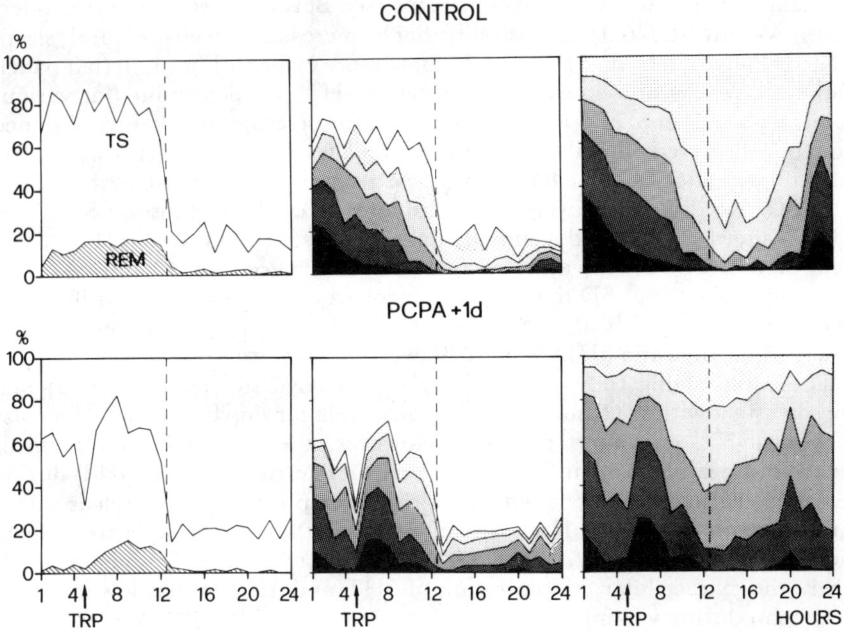

Fig. 8.9 Effect of L-tryptophan (150 mg/kg i.p.; TRP, arrow) on sleep states in PCPA- pretreated rats (PCPA + 1d corresponding to day starting 24 h after PCPA administration). Column of panels correspond to those in Fig. 8.8. (Reproduced from A. A. Borbély *et al.* (1981), *Behav. Brain Res.*, **2**, 1–22, by permission.)

However, the mechanisms involved in the antagonism of PCPA insomnia by 5HT precursors may be more complex than previously thought. There was a marked delay between the systemic or intraventricular administration of 5HTP or Trp, and the increase in sleep (Laguzzi & Adrien, 1980; Petitjean *et al.*, 1980; Borbély *et al.*, 1981c), indicating that the reappearance of sleep may depend on an unknown intervening process.

8.3.3 Brain Serotonin as a Dependent Variable

The 'serotonin hypothesis' of sleep is based to a large part on experiments in which manipulations of the 5HT system affected sleep. However, if 5HT does play a key role in sleep regulation, changes in its turnover should accompany the physiological sleep–wake cycle. The few studies that have addressed this

---

Fig. 8.8 Effect of p-chlorophenylalanine (PCPA; 300 mg/kg i.p.) on the daily distribution of sleep states in the rat. The curves represent hourly mean values. Interrupted vertical lines delimit light and dark phase. Top panels: control day (mean of 2 days per animal). Subsequent rows of panels: day of PCPA administration (injection before hour 1) and successive 5 days (+ 1d to + 5d). Left column of panels: total sleep (TS) and REM sleep (REM) (% of recording time). Middle column: non-REM sleep with zero-crossing bands (% of recording time; see legend of Fig. 8.6). Right column: non-REM sleep with zero-crossing bands (% of total non-REM sleep). (Reproduced from A. A. Borbély *et al.* (1981), *Behav. Brain Res.*, **2**, 1–22, by permission.)

problem, remain as a whole inconclusive (see Borbély *et al.*, 1980, for references). We investigated the possibility that by increasing 'sleep pressure', sleep-related changes in brain 5HT may become more evident. Fig. 8.10 (left panel) shows the results of a study in which brain 5HT was determined at various points after a 24-h SD period and compared to corresponding values obtained from non-deprived animals. The cerebral 5HT level did not differ from control immediately after SD or 1 h later, but was significantly increased 2 h and 6 h after SD. No differences were seen 12 h after SD. The increase in SWS and REMS after SD exhibited a similar timecourse as the 5HT values (Fig. 8.10, right panel). The mean values of 5-hydroxyindole acetic acid (5HIAA) were generally higher after SD than in the control group, but significant differences were present only 1 h after SD (Borbély *et al.*, 1980). No differences were observed for the ratio 5HIAA/5HT between the two groups.

The results of this study confirm those reported by Tsuchiya *et al.* (1969), and are consistent with the assumption of a causal relationship between the increase in brain 5HT and sleep rebound. However, the subcellular mechanisms involved are difficult to infer from the data. The rise in brain 5HT during recovery sleep could reflect a reduction in the synaptic transmitter release. This interpretation is supported by experiments using the cortical superfusion technique (Puizillout *et al.*, 1979) or the voltammetric technique (Cespuglio, 1981) where the extracellular concentration of 5HT and 5HIAA was lower during sleep than during waking.

Recent progress in neurobiology makes it necessary to revise earlier concepts on the functions of the serotonergic system. Among the new results that are

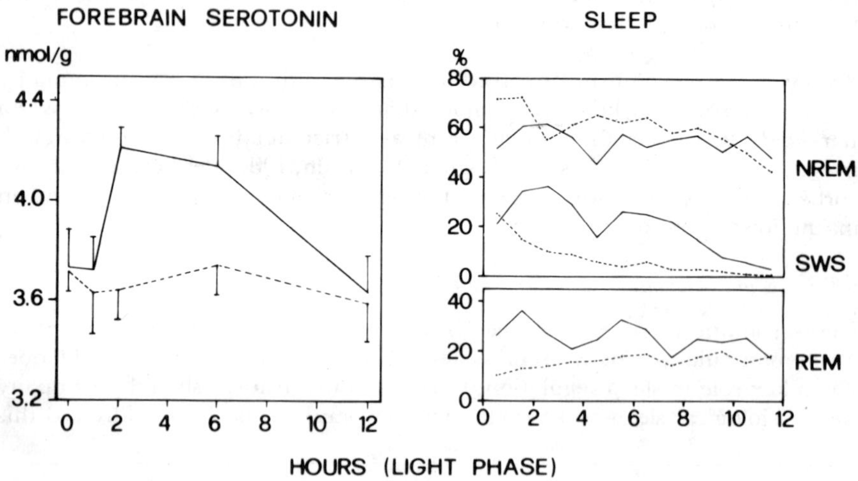

Fig. 8.10 Concentration of forebrain serotonin (left) and distribution of sleep states (right) in rats recovering from 24-h sleep deprivation (SD: solid line) and in a control group (interrupted lines). The curves represent mean values (with SEM indicated in left panel). Significant differences of serotonin between SD group and control group at 2 h ($p < 0.001$) and 6 h ($p < 0.05$; 2-sided t-test). Serotonin is expressed as nmol/g tissue wet weight, sleep as percent of recording time. Hours after 24-h SD are indicated on the abscissa, 0 h corresponding to light onset. (Reproduced from A. A. Borbély *et al.* (1980), *Behav. Brain Res.*, **1**, 205–210, by permission.)

particularly relevant for sleep regulation is the observation that classical transmitters may coexist with biologically active peptides in the same neuron (e.g. 5HT and Substance P in raphe neurons), a discovery that adds a new dimension to the problem of the functional role of neurotransmitters in general (Hökfelt *et al.*, 1980). New efforts at a synthesis will have to take into account these developments.

8.3.4 Sleep Regulation after Serotonin Depletion

In the following study, the focus is on the physiological sleep regulating mechanisms and not on the neurochemical processes involved.

The effect of 5HT-depleting compounds was usually studied in animals exhibiting spontaneously occurring sleep. However, insomnia under such an experimental paradigm cannot be attributed to the impairment of specific sleep-regulating mechanisms, since non-specific pharmacological effects may also interfere with sleep. We studied sleep regulation in 5HT deficient rats by combining the administration of PCPA with sleep deprivation (Tobler & Borbély, 1982). Fig. 8.11 shows the main results. While the sleep-inhibiting and REM sleep-reducing effects of PCPA were not antagonized by the combined treatment, delta activity in non-REM sleep was massively enhanced. The result indicates that SWS regulating mechanisms are still functional in 5HT-deficient animals. Moreover, typical effects of SD such as regular cycles of

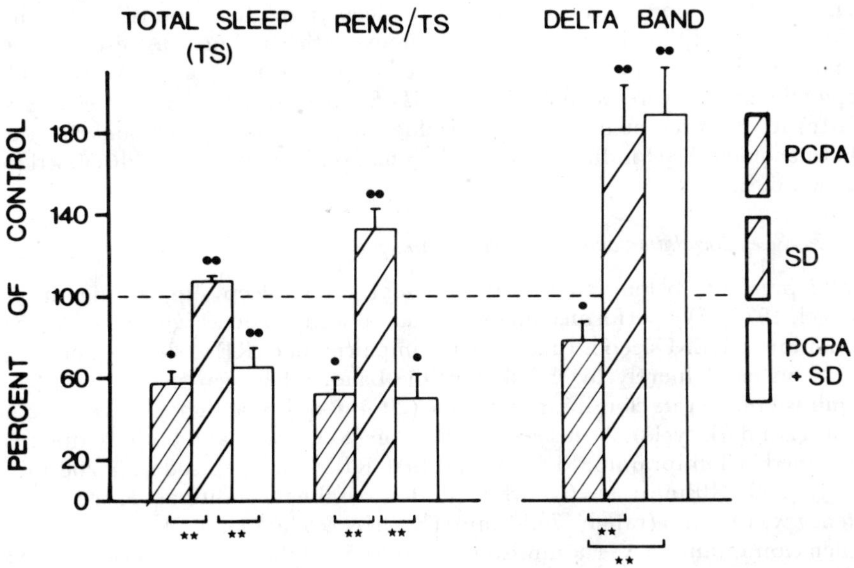

Fig. 8.11 Effect of treatment with PCPA (300 mg/kg i.p.), sleep deprivation (SD) and the combined treatment (PCPA + SD) on sleep in the rat. Mean values with SEM expressed as percent of control day (100%). The power density of the delta band (1.25—4.0Hz) is expressed relative to nonREMS. Dots indicate significant differences from control, asterisks significant differences between the values indicated by brackets (° and * : $p<0.05$; °° and ** : $p<0.01$; Wilcoxon paired and unpaired signed rank test, 2-sided). (Modified from I. Tobler and A. A. Borbély (1982), *Sleep*, **5**, 145–153.)

Table 8.2 Effect of Clomipramine, Sleep Deprivation (SD) and the Combined Treatment with Clomipramine and SD on Sleep in the Rat (mean values; $n = 6$)

	Control	Clomipramine	SD	Clomipramine & SD
Total sleep (%)				
light phase	76.2	77.7	80.3	85.4*
dark phase	20.0	31.4*	35.9*	38.6*
REM sleep (%)				
light phase	14.9	9.4*	21.0*	17.7
dark phase	2.7	6.9*	6.6*	8.9*

* $p < 0.05$; from control (Wilcoxon paired signed-rank test, two-sided).

synchronized and desynchronized EEG, and REM sleep rebound in one animal, suggested that the depression of REM sleep after the combined treatment may have been a consequence of the shortened total sleep time rather than a sign for the impairment of REM sleep regulation. The results of this study are consistent with the notion that a general hyper-responsiveness, rather than the disruption of the regulation of sleep states, is responsible for the insomnia in 5HT-deficient animals. Moreover, the findings suggest that the striking early recovery of normal rest and sleep patterns at a time when 5HT depletion is still severe (Dement *et al.*, 1972; Steigrad *et al.*, 1978; Borbély *et al.*, 1981c) may represent in part a physiological compensatory response to the pharmacological SD induced by PCPA. This issue will be further discussed in Section 8.4.

8.3.5 Sleep Regulation and the Effect of Antidepressants

Antidepressants belong to the most potent REM sleep suppressing drugs (Vogel, 1975). We performed an experimental study to investigate whether the inhibition of REM sleep is caused by the impairment of REM sleep generating mechanisms or merely by the shift in the balance between sleep states. We administered to rats clomipramine alone (20 mg/kg i.p. at light onset of a 12 h light–12 h dark cycle), 24-h sleep deprivation (SD) alone, and both treatments combined. Clomipramine delayed the first REM sleep episode for 288 min (range 250–340 min; $n = 6$), while under baseline conditions REM sleep latency was 42 min (range 27–98 min) (Borbély & Hagmann, in preparation). When clomipramine was administered at the end of the 24-h SD period, REM sleep latency was 65 min (range 19–125 min) which was significantly less than after clomipramine alone ($p < 0.05$; 2-sided Wilcoxon paired signed-rank test), and not significantly different from baseline. The values recorded for the entire 12-h light phase also showed that the REM sleep suppressing action of clomipramine was antagonized by SD (Table 8.2). Non-REM sleep as well as its SWS fraction (defined as the lowest 30% of the zero-crossing values) were enhanced in the light phase after clomipramine alone (112% and 155% of control) and SD and clomipramine (110% and 159% of control) (all $p < 0.05$).

The results of this study show that physiological REM sleep regulating mechanisms are still functional at a time when REM sleep is suppressed by a tricyclic antidepressant.

8.3.6 *Benzodiazepine Binding as a Dependent Variable*

The discovery of specific benzodiazepine binding sites in the brain of animals raises the possibility that these structures are in some way involved in the regulation of sleep, and that benzodiazepine hypnotics exert their effects via physiological mechanisms. There is preliminary evidence that benzodiazepine binding is altered as a function of the sleep–wake cycle. Thus Poddar *et al.* (1980) reported that (^{3}H) diazepam binding to a hamster cerebral membrane preparation was decreased in the presence of supernatant obtained from awake animals, but not from sleeping animals. Moreover the inhibition of binding decreased as a function of sleeping time. Scatchard analysis suggested that affinity, but not the number of binding sites, was changed. Mendelson *et al.* (1982) reported that supernatant from rat brain homogenates obtained after a 24-h sleep deprivation period caused significantly less inhibition of (^{3}H) diazepam binding to rat brain than the supernatant (the liquid phase remaining after centrifugation of the tissue sample) obtained from control animals. Both studies indicate that in normally awake animals a brain constituent inhibits benzodiazepine binding.

The inhibitory factor does not appear to be present in the membrane fraction of the brain, since without the supernatant, no difference was seen between sleeping and waking animals (Poddar *et al.*, 1980). On the other hand, a clear circadian rhythm of (^{3}H) diazepam binding to the rat forebrain membrane fraction has been documented which is little affected by sleep deprivation (Wirz-Justice *et al.*, 1981). The circadian rhythm in binding was caused by variations in the number of binding sites, while the affinity for the ligand remained stable. Taken together, the results suggest the possibility that the affinity of cerebral benzodiazepine binding sites is modified by a sleep-dependent factor, while their number undergoes circadian variations which are largely independent of the sleep-wake cycle.

In conclusion, new insights may be gained into the mode of action of benzodiazepines by combining EEG studies in which sleep is the dependent variable, with neurochemical investigations in which sleep constitutes the independent variable.

8.3.7 *The Search for Endogenous 'Sleep Factors'*

The search for endogenous sleep-promoting compounds is essentially an 'agnostic' approach since it does not originate from any contemporary hypothesis on the role of specific neurochemical processes or systems in sleep regulation. In this type of study, sleep constitutes initially the independent variable whose manipulations in the donor animal is designed to enhance the level of a sleep-promoting agent in the extracellular fluid space. However, since the sleep-enhancing activity can be tested only in intact recipient animals, sleep is by necessity also the dependent variable (Table 8.1). The stringent criteria of this experimental approach allow therefore a more rigorous study of the chemical aspects of sleep regulation than most other procedures, and provide therefore the opportunity for the discovery of new fundamental mechanisms. On the other side, the lack of explicit neurochemical hypotheses entails certain risks. One of them derives from the fact that no physiological process that is comparable to sleep in terms of generality and complexity, has been shown to be regulated by a single neurochemical compound. It is possible that a variety of constituents participate interactively in the regulation of sleep and waking, and that the search for a single regulatory agent is futile. Success will be the most convincing argument to dispel such doubts.

The search for endogenous sleep-promoting agents is based on the assumption that the level of a 'hypnotoxin' (Piéron, 1913) builds up during waking time and is responsible for the subsequent sleep. In the approach taken by Pappenheimer *et al.* and by Uchizono *et al.*, sleep deprivation was the main method for obtaining 'sleep factor' containing material from donor animals. In contrast, Monnier *et al.* induced sleep artificially by electric stimulation in the thalamus. The results of the two approaches will be briefly summarized and discussed.

In their first experiments, Pappenheimer *et al.* extracted CSF from sleep-deprived goats, and investigated the presence of a sleep-enhancing factor by infusing the CSF or its fractions into the cerebral ventricle of rats. The recipient rats exhibited a reduction in motor activity and an increase in sleep (Fencl *et al.*, 1971). The active principle was designated as Factor S (for sleep). The authors also showed that the CSF level of Factor S increased progressively during the 48-h period of sleep deprivation. In later experiments, Factor S was extracted, partially purified and concentrated from the brain of goats, sheep, rabbits and slaughterhouse cattle (Pappenheimer *et al.*, 1975; Krueger *et al.*, 1978). Although its sleep-enhancing action had been demontrated also in the rat and cat, rabbits were used in recent routine assays. The sleep-promoting effect of Factor S is characterized by a gradual enhancement of the percentage of SWS and a concomitant increase in the amplitude of EEG delta waves, changes that reach their maximum 2 h after intraventricular infusion, and last for 5–10 h. The sleep and EEG changes correspond closely to those seen after SD. Recently, Factor S has been isolated and purified from human urine (Krueger *et al.*, 1980). The factor is a glycopeptide which is effective at an intraventricular dose of 5 pmol/kg (Krueger *et al.*, 1982).

Uchizono *et al.* studied a brain extract from sleep-deprived rat (Nagasaki *et al.*, 1974; Uchizono *et al.*, 1978; Inoué *et al.*, 1982). When administered to recipient rats by intraperitoneal route, a long-lasting reduction of motor activity as well as an increase in sleep time and EEG delta activity was observed. A dose-effect relationship was demonstrated in the mouse (Nagasaki *et al.*, 1980). The group is presently working on the purification of the Sleep Promoting Substance (SPS) which seems to resemble Factor S in various respects.

The experiments started by Monnier *et al.* in the 1960s culminated in the identification of the Delta Sleep Inducing Peptide (DSIP) (Schoenenberger *et al.*, 1978). The authors reported that synthetic DSIP also rapidly induces sleep (within minutes following the intraventricular administration in the rabbit) which is characterized by the predominance of slow wave activity in the EEG. The typical effective dose was 30 nmol/kg for intravenous administration, and 6 nmol/kg for intraventricular injection. Increasing the dose above the optimal level resulted in a reduction or abolition of sleep-inducing activity. The sleep-promoting action of DSIP was reported also for the cat (Polc *et al.*, 1978) and rat (Kafi *et al.*, 1979). However, in contrast to the initial experiments in the rabbit, the main effect in the cat consisted in an increase of REM sleep, and not in the enhancement of SWS. In neither of the two studies was a dose-effect relationship observed. A slight sleep-promoting effect of DSIP has been reported in preliminary human studies (Schneider-Helmert *et al.*, 1981a, b). On the other hand, various groups failed to observe consistent effects of DSIP on sleep and motor activity (Krueger *et al.*, 1980; Mendelson *et al.*, 1980; Tobler & Borbély, 1980). The presence of high levels of DSIP-like material outside the brain is intriguing (Kastin *et al.*, 1978, 1980). Moreover, DSIP in conjunction with amphetamine was reported to affect thermoregulation (Yehuda *et al.*, 1980). It is possible that the thalamic stimulation in the rabbit which led to the identification of the peptide not only induced sleep, but also had further, unspecified biological effects. Presently, convincing evidence that DSIP is centrally involved in sleep regulation is still lacking, and the biological functions of the peptide are unclear.

Research of endogenous factors promoting REM sleep are at a very preliminary stage and will be only briefly mentioned. Brainstem perfusion studies in the cat indicated that an increase in the protein content of the perfusate occurs during REM sleep, and that antibodies against these proteins suppress this sleep state (Drucker-Colin *et al.*, 1980a, b). In another study, CSF obtained from REM sleep deprived donor cats was reported to restore sleep in PCPA-pretreated recipient animals (Sallanon *et al.*, 1981). The results suggest the possibility that specific REM sleep regulating compounds exist in the brain.

8.4 Outline of a Two-Process Model and Some Pharmacological Implications

It has been recently proposed that two separate processes underlie sleep regulation (Borbély, 1980, 1981, 1982a, b; Borbély *et al.*, 1981d; Daan & Beersma, 1983): a sleep-dependent process (process S), and a sleep-independent process (process C). The level of process S is assumed to increase during waking and to decrease during sleep. EEG slow wave activity is considered to be a correlate of this process, since in animals and humans its level at sleep onset is a function of prior waking time, and since it declines during sleep (see Sections 8.2.2 and 8.3). Process C reflects mainly the circadian variation of sleep propensity which is largely independent of the occurrence of sleep, since it persists even during prolonged sleep deprivation (Akerstedt & Fröberg, 1977). In humans, circadian sleep propensity is at a maximum in the early morning hours, and at a minimum in the late afternoon. In animals, process C is closely related to the circadian rest–activity rhythm. While sleep deprivation has a profound effect on the rat's sleep states (Section 8.3), it leaves the period and phase of the free-running rest–activity rhythm unaffected (Borbély, 1982a: Fig. 3). Process C appears therefore to correspond to a rather rigidly programmed rhythm controlled by a circadian oscillator which is practically independent of sleep and waking. Since a circadian rest–activity rhythm is present also in simple organisms that do not exhibit electrographic signs of sleep, it may constitute a phylogenetic precursor of sleep. We have argued that sleep-related aspects of sleep regulation (process S) may have evolved later (Borbély & Neuhaus, 1979; Borbély, 1980). By providing an intensity dimension to the sleep process, they may have increased the adaptive capability of the organism to environmental challenges that require a resting period outside the circadian rest phase.

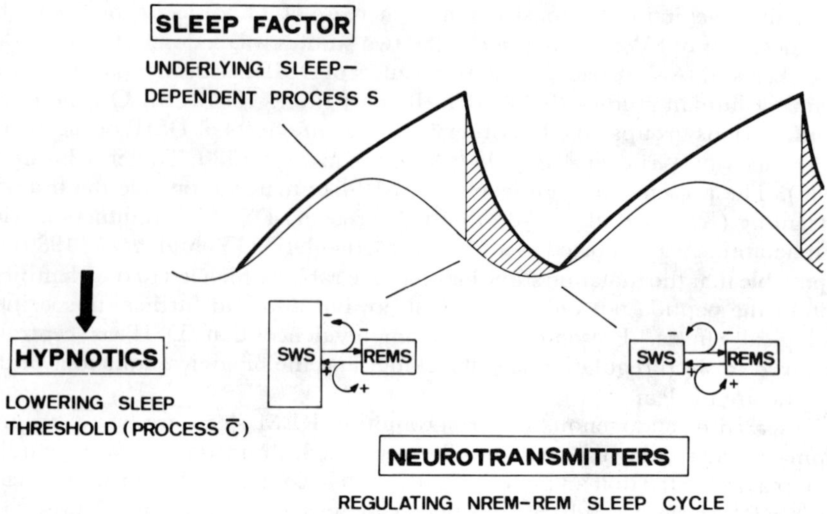

Fig. 8.12 Two-process model of sleep regulation and possible action of neurochemical and pharmacological agents. The level of process S increases during waking and declines exponentially during sleep. Curve $\overline{C}$ (the negative function of process C) exhibits a circadian rhythm. Sleep propensity during waking and sleep (hatched area) is represented by the difference between S and $\overline{C}$. The two diagrams below the curve indicate the reciprocal interaction between SWS and REM sleep.

In the model, sleep propensity during waking, and sleep intensity during sleep, is represented by the sum of the two processes. In Fig. 8.12 the negative function of process C ($\overline{C}$) has been plotted to represent the sum of the processes as the difference between two curves. Curve $\overline{C}$ may be regarded as a 'sleep threshold' which is highest when the circadian sleep propensity is lowest (in the late afternoon in humans).

While the level of EEG slow wave activity was used to simulate the time course of process S (Borbély, 1981, 1982a, b; Daan & Beersma, 1983), REM sleep was not incorporated in the original version of the model. In contrast to SWS, the daily distribution of REM sleep is strongly determined by circadian variables (Webb & Agnew, 1971). Nevertheless, since REM sleep deprivation gives rise to a compensatory increase of this sleep state, also a sleep-dependent aspect of REM sleep regulation is clearly present. There seem to be differences, however, between the regulatory characteristics of the two sleep states. Thus while SWS appears to be finely regulated around a reference level, a REM sleep deficit has to exceed a certain threshold for the regulatory mechanisms to become activated (see Borbély & Neuhaus, 1979). The following discussion will be focused on the interaction between the two sleep states.

Sleep is characterized by the cyclic alternation of non-REM sleep and REM sleep. Based on their neurophysiological studies of brainstem mechanisms underlying the sleep cycles, McCarley & Hobson (1975) proposed a reciprocal interaction between REM sleep enhancing and REM sleep inhibiting neuronal populations. They applied the Lotka-Volterra equations to simulate this interaction. The reciprocal interaction model has been extended to account for the non-REM–REM sleep cycle in the framework of the present model. Here only the main arguments will be briefly summarized, and a more detailed discussion will be provided elsewhere (Borbély, 1982b).

Since under ordinary sleep–wake conditions, REM sleep propensity is largely determined by circadian variables, it could have been indicated in Fig. 8.12 as the difference between a horizontal line and curve C. According to this model, the maximum of REM sleep propensity would coincide with the maximum of circadian sleep propensity. The data obtained from human subjects living in an environment without time cues are consistent with this prediction (Czeisler *et al.*, 1980: Figs 5, 6). SWS propensity which in the model is represented by the level of process S, shows quite a different time-course. It exhibits a maximum at sleep onset and then declines gradually throughout the sleep period. Since the reciprocal interaction between the two sleep processes is assumed to be influenced by their respective level, the interaction is a function of both sleep time and circadian phase. Thus in the beginning of a typical sleep period, the balance between the two processes is strongly in favor of SWS (Fig. 8.12: large SWS box), whereas towards the end of sleep it becomes more equally distributed (Fig. 8.12: small SWS box). This type of interaction can account for the observation that in human sleep the REM sleep fraction of a sleep cycle increases throughout the sleep period. A progressive increase of the REM sleep fraction of total sleep in the course of the daily sleep phase has been also documented for the rat (Borbély & Neuhaus, 1978).

The present model was originally conceived to simulate physiological aspects of sleep regulation (effects of sleep deprivation, sleep patterns under time-free conditions, etc.). In the following, its possible relevance for pharmacological and neurochemical aspects will be examined. While at this stage the propositions are bound to be highly speculative, they may serve as a working hypothesis for the analysis of drug effects in the framework of sleep regulation.

Of all sleep processes the non-REM–REM sleep cycle lends itself most readily to an examination of neurochemical mechanisms and the involvement of neurotransmitters. The McCarley–Hobson model rests on the interaction of two cell groups: the large pontine neurons in the giganto tegmental field (FTG) which exhibit maximum activity during REM sleep, and smaller neurons located in the raphe nuclei and in the locus coeruleus which show minimum activity during REM sleep (Amatruda *et al.*, 1975; Hobson *et al.*, 1975). While the former cells are cholinergic and cholinoceptive, the latter are monoaminergic. The topical application of minute amounts of transmitter agonists or antagonists can shift the balance between the interacting cell groups and produce dramatic effects on the sleep cycle. Thus a spectacular enhancement of a REM sleep-like state was produced by the local administration of the cholinergic agonist carbachol or the β-adrenergic antagonist propranolol (Amatruda *et al.*, 1975; Silberman *et al.*, 1980; Vivaldi *et al.*, 1980). Results from human studies are also consistent with the hypothesis that the sleep cycle is regulated by the interaction of cholinergic and monoaminergic processes. Thus while a REM sleep promoting action of the cholinergic compounds physostigmine and arecoline was apparent from the shortening of REM sleep latency when these drugs were administered intravenously during sleep, the opposite effect was observed for the cholinergic blocking agent scopolamine (Sitaram *et al.*, 1976, 1978). The prominent REM sleep suppressing effect of antidepressant drugs could be explained by the same mechanism, since by inhibiting transmitter re-uptake, these compounds activate the monoaminergic system, and at the same time exert often also anticholinergic effects.

While the time-course of process S (Fig. 8.12) has been derived from EEG criteria, it may equally reflect a neurochemical process. Factor S and the Sleep Promoting Substance (SPS) are potential humoral correlates of process S, since their level apparently increases during waking and declines during sleep (see Section 8.3.7). Moreover, there is evidence that the level of Factor S in CSF increases as a function of waking time (Fencl *et al.*, 1971) and that a dose-effect relationship is obtained for SPS (Nagasaki *et al.*, 1980). However, all these results must be regarded as tentative until the identity of the compounds is conclusively established and their effects confirmed in different laboratories. In contrast to process S, there is no evidence for a possible neurochemical correlate of process C.

In Fig. 8.12, the sleep-inducing effect of hypnotics has been attributed to the lowering of the level of curve $\overline{C}$. According to the present model, this curve not only represents the circadian variation in the sleep threshold, but also may reflect short-term changes which lie in the order of seconds or minutes (Borbély, 1982a). Process C may be seen therefore as the target of external and internal arousing stimuli which may readily inhibit sleep or reduce sleep propensity. Conversely, sleep-promoting conditions (e.g. the absence of environmental stimuli; repetitive stimuli or monotonous tasks; warm ambient temperature; satiety, etc.) may lower the sleep threshold and enhance sleep propensity. Thus, superimposed on its circadian rhythm, process C may undergo short-term modifications by a variety of different extrinsic and intrinsic stimuli. According to this hypothesis, hypnotic and stimulant drugs favour or inhibit sleep by changing the level of this process. It is an interesting aspect of this proposition that the drugs are supposed to affect a relatively non-specific process of sleep regulation which is not dependent on prior sleep or waking. Hypnotics could be considered as 'sleeping aids' which, like a darkened and quiet room, favour the transition from waking to sleep. However, on the basis of the EEG studies of benzodiazepines (Fig. 8.4) this is unlikely to be the whole story as these drugs exert also selective effects on the electrographic aspects of non-REM sleep and REM sleep. The possibility that the affinity of cerebral benzodiazepine receptors is affected by sleep itself has been pointed out before (Section 8.3.6). The mode of action of hypnotics indicated in Fig. 8.12 must be therefore regarded as highly tentative.

It is interesting to re-examine the action of PCPA in the light of the model. As has been mentioned in Section 8.3.2, PCPA leaves the daily pattern of sleep states in the rat largely unchanged (Fig. 8.8), and does not abolish the SWS maximum after light onset. Moreover, the compensatory increase of SWS after sleep deprivation can be demonstrated at the time of maximum insomnia (Fig. 8.11). Therefore, if slow wave activity constitutes an indicator of process S, PCPA does not appear to have a major effect on this process. On the other hand, serotonin depletion may elevate the sleep threshold by an action on process C. This would lead to a shortening of sleep time due to the easy disruption of sleep episodes by extrinsic and intrinsic stimuli. In fact, the effect of PCPA has been described as consisting in a general hyper-responsiveness of the animal which is manifested not only by a reduction of sleep and an enhancement of daytime motor activity (Borbély *et al.*, 1973), but also by the increased reactivity to neutral and noxious stimuli, and the enhancement of sexual activity and aggressivity (see Messing *et al.*, 1978, for a review). The present interpretation of the mode of action of PCPA is basically in agreement with the views of Trulson and Jacobs (1979) and Ursin (1980). It illustrates the possibility that drugs may affect sleep by relatively non-specific physiological mechanisms while acting on highly specific neurochemical processes.

The functional significance of the two processes postulated in the present model may not be limited to sleep regulation, but may extend to other areas. This assumption is based mainly on the observation that not only are sleep disorders frequent concomitants of psychopathology, but also pathological conditions can be favourably influenced by manipulating sleep. While this theme is briefly mentioned here in view of its general and pharmacological implications, it is discussed in detail elsewhere (Borbély & Wirz-Justice, 1982). Sleep in endogenous depression is characterized by a short REM sleep latency, a long sleep latency, a tendency for fragmentation and early morning awakening (Gillin *et al.*, 1979). Surprisingly, depressive symptomatology can be temporarily alleviated by sleep deprivation (see Rudolf *et al.*, 1977, for a review). We have indicated how both the pathognomic changes in the sleep pattern and the therapeutic effect of sleep deprivation can be explained in the framework of the two-process model by assuming a deficiency in process S (Borbély *et al.*, 1981d; Borbély & Wirz-Justice, 1982) or an increase in the level of threshold $\overline{C}$. It is relevant for the present pharmacological discussion, that an antidepressant effect has been reported also after a prolonged, selective REM sleep deprivation (Vogel *et al.*, 1975, 1980). Vogel (1975) has drawn attention to the fact that antidepressant drugs produce a most prominent suppression of REM sleep, and proposed that this effect might be causally related to their therapeutic effect. This hypothesis can be also accommodated in the framework of the two-process model.

In summary, selective physiological and pharmacological effects on sleep regulation could be relevant for the understanding and treatment of affective disorders.

8.5 Concluding Remarks

Pharmacological studies of sleep are still too much confined to a descriptive level of analysis. For example, the effect of benzodiazepines and other hypnotics on sleep is well documented, but their mode of action, and the functional significance of the altered sleep stages remain obscure. The neurophysiological and neurochemical investigation of central nervous mechanisms involved in sleep regulation has given rise to appealing hypotheses, but it has failed so far to pave the way for new, effective sleep remedies. More tangible results may be expected from focusing explicitly on the regulatory aspects of sleep. The search for endogenous sleep-promoting compounds is a prime example for an approach which starts out from physiological sleep regulation and aims at physiological sleep induction. Possibly, a similar two-way relationship will be established a posteriori between sleep and the benzodiazepines whose hypnotic action is being widely exploited, but whose possible role in physiological sleep regulation is still largely unexplored.

Historically, pharmacology has long been a sub-discipline of physiology. The explosive growth of the analytic and synthetic potential of chemistry has attracted pharmacology into its sphere of influence, and has caused at the same time an unwholesome estrangement from physiology. The recent discovery, that the benzodiazepines and opiates exert their action via specific brain receptors and possibly mimic the effect of endogenous ligands, has stimulated efforts to analyse their action within the framework of physiological regulatory processes. It is to be hoped that these developments will accelerate a *rapprochement* between the two disciplines.

8.6 Summary

Two developments have renewed the interest in pharmacological approaches to sleep regulation: (1) the widespread use of benzodiazepine hypnotics as drugs of choice in the treatment of insomnia coupled with the limited understanding of their mechanisms of action; and (2) the possibility of recording drug-induced intra-sleep changes with polygraphic techniques in an increasing number of laboratories coupled with the ignorance about their functional significance. The use of more sensitive techniques of measurement and analysis in experiments which explore the regulatory aspects of sleep, may contribute to progress in the field.

The effect of hypnotics on movement activity at night can be easily recorded by an ambulatory activity monitor. The method is sensitive enough to document residual sedative effects on the day following drug intake and a rebound insomnia on a subsequent night. EEG techniques offer the possibility of investigating drug effects on the various sleep states. However, progress may have been hampered by the too strict adherence to sleep scoring procedures that do not adequately reflect the changes. All-night spectral analysis of the sleep EEG reveals effects of sleep deprivation as well as immediate and residual effects of hypnotics which are not apparent from the sleep stage distribution. Slow wave activity may be particularly important as an indicator of the intensity of a sleep process whose level depends on prior waking time in humans and animals. Sleep deprivation was applied to study the regulatory sleep response in rats treated with a serotonin synthesis inhibitor or with an antidepressant drug. The compensatory increase in SWS and REM sleep indicated that the pharmacological manipulation induced merely a shift in the balance between the vigilance states rather than disrupting the sleep regulating mechanisms.

A model of sleep regulation is proposed in which sleep propensity results from the combined action of a sleep-dependent process (process S) and a sleep-independent process which is largely controlled by a circadian oscillator (process C). The action of neurochemical and pharmacological compounds is discussed in the framework of the model.

Acknowledgements

I wish to thank Dr Irene Tobler for her comments on the manuscript, Ms Karin Schwarz for preparing the figures and Ms Rita Steiger for typing. The experimental work presented in this article was supported by grants from the Swiss National Science Foundation.

References

AKERSTEDT, T. and FRÖBERG, G. E. (1977). Psychophysiological circadian rhythms in women during 72 h of sleep deprivation. *Waking and Sleeping*, **1**. 387–394.

AMATRUDA, T. T., BLACK, D. A., MCKENNA, T. M. MCCARLEY, R. W. and HOBSON, J. A. (1975). Sleep cycle control and cholinergic mechanisms: differential effects of carbachol injections at pontine brain stem sites. *Brain Research*, **98**, 501–515.

BERGER, R. J. and OSWALD, I. (1962). Effects of sleep deprivation on behaviour, subsequent sleep, and dreaming. *J. Ment. Sci.*, **108**, 457–465.

BORBÉLY, A. A. (1980). Sleep: circadian rhythm versus recovery process. In: M. KOUKKOU, D. LEHMANN and J. ANGST (Eds.), *Functional States of the Brain: Their Determinants*, Amsterdam: Elsevier, pp. 151–161.

BORBÉLY, A. A. (1981). The sleep process: circadian and homeostatic aspects. In: F. OBÁL and G. BENEDEK (Eds.), *Adv. Physiol. Sci*, Vol. 18, *Environmental Physiology*, Oxford: Pergamon Press, pp. 85–91.

BORBÉLY, A. A. (1982a). Sleep regulation: circadian rhythm and homeostasis. In: D. GANTEN and D. PFAFF (Eds.), *Sleep: Clinical and experimental aspects. Current Topics in Neuroendocrinology*, Vol. 1, Berlin: Springer Verlag, pp. 83–103.

BORBÉLY, A. A. (1982b). A two-process model of sleep regulation, *Human Neurobiology*, **1**, 195–204.

BORBÉLY, A. A. and NEUHAUS, H. U. (1978). Daily pattern of sleep, motor activity and feeding in the rat: effects of regular and gradually extended photoperiods. *J. Comp. Physiol.*, **124**, 1–14.

BORBÉLY, A. A. and NEUHAUS, H. U. (1979). Sleep-deprivation: effects on sleep and EEG in the rat. *J. Comp. Physiol.*, **133**, 71–87.

BORBÉLY, A. A., STEIGRAD, P. and TOBLER, I. (1980). Effect of sleep deprivation on brain serotonin in the rat. *Behav. Brain Res.*, **1**, 205–210.

BORBÉLY, A. A., BAUMANN, F., BRANDEIS, D., STRAUCH, I. and LEHMANN, D. (1981a). Sleep deprivation: effect on sleep stages and EEG power density in man. *Electroenceph. Clin. Neurophys.*, **51**, 483–493.

BORBÉLY, A. A., NEUHAUS, H. U., MATTMANN, P. and WASER, P. G. (1981b). Langzeitregistrierung der Bewegungsaktivität: Anwendungen in Forschung und Klinik. *Schweiz med. Wschr.*, **111**, 730–736.

BORBÉLY, A. A., NEUHAUS, H. U. and TOBLER, I. (1981c). Effect of p-chlorophenylalanine and tryptophan on sleep, EEG and motor activity in the rat. *Behav. Brain Res.*, **2**, 1–22.

BORBÉLY, A. A., TOBLER, I. and WIRZ-JUSTICE, A. (1981d). Circadian and sleep-dependent processes in sleep regulation: outline of a model and implications for depression. *Sleep Research*, **10**, 19.

BORBÉLY, A. A., HUSTON, J. P. and WASER, P. G. (1973). Physiological and behavioral effects of parachlorophenylalanine in the rat. *Psychopharmacologia* (Berlin), **31**, 131–142.

BORBÉLY, A. A. and WIRZ-JUSTICE, A. (1982). Sleep, sleep deprivation and depression: a hypothesis derived from a model of sleep regulation. *Human Neurobiology*, **1**, 205–210.

BREIMER, D. D. (1977). Clinical pharmacokinetics of hypnotics. *Clin. Pharmacokinet.*, **2**, 93–109.

CESPUGLIO, R. (1981.) Les phénomènes phasiques du cycle veille-sommeil chez le chat, le rat et la souris. Leur contrôle par le système du raphé. Doctoral dissertation, University of Lyon, France.

COLBURN, T. R., SMITH, B. M., GUARINI, J. J. and SIMMONS, N. N. (1976). An ambulatory activity monitor with solid state memory. *Biomedical Sciences Instrumentation Symposium*, ISA BM 76322, pp. 117–122.

CROWLEY, T. J., KRIPKE, D. F., HALBERG, F., PEGRAM, G. V. and SCHILDKRAUT,

J. J. (1972). Circadian rhythms of Macaca mulatta: sleep, EEG, body and eye movement, and temperature. *Primates*, **13**, 149–168.

CROWLEY, T. J. and HYDINGER-MCDONALD, M. (1979). Bedtime Flurazepam and the human circadian rhythm of spontaneous motility. *Psychopharmacology*, **62**, 157–161.

CZEISLER, C. A., ZIMMERMAN, J. C., RONDA, J. M., MOORE-EDE, M. C. and WEITZMAN, E. D. (1980). Timing of REM sleep is coupled to the circadian rhythm of body temperature in man. *Sleep*, **2**, 329–346.

DAAN, S. and BEERSMA, D. (1983). Circadian gating of human sleep and wakefulness. In: M. C. MOORE-EDE (Ed.), *Mathematical Modeling of Circadian Systems*, Raven Press, in press.

DELORME, F., FROMENT, J. L. and JOUVET, M. (1966). Suppression du sommeil par la p.chlorométhamphétamine et la p.chlorophénylalanine. *C.R. Soc. Biol.* (Paris), **160**, 2347–2351.

DEMENT, W. C., MITLER, M. M. and HENRIKSEN, S. J. (1972). Sleep changes during chronic administration of parachlorophenylalanine. *Rev. Canad. Biol.*, **31**, 239–246.

DRUCKER-COLIN, R., DE GOMEZ-PUYOU, M. T., DEL CARMEN GUTIÉRREZ, M. and DREYFUS-CORTÉS, G. (1980a). Immunological approach to the study of neurohumoral sleep factors: effects on REM sleep of antibodies to brain stem proteins. *Experimental Neurology*, **69**, 563–575.

DRUCKER-COLIN, R., DEL CARMEN GUIÉRREZ, M. and BERNAL-PEDRAZA, J. G. (1980b). Polypeptide regulation of REM sleep. *Front Hormone Res.*, **6**, 138–155.

FEINBERG, I. and FLOYD, T. C. (1979). Systematic trends across the night in human sleep cycles. *Psychophysiology*, **16**, 283–291.

FEINBERG, I. FEIN, G., WALKER, J. M., PRICE, L. J., FLOYD, T. C. and MARCH, J. D. (1977). Flurazepam effects on slow-wave sleep: Stage 4 suppressed but number of delta waves constant. *Science*, **198**, 847–848.

FEINBERG, I. FEIN, G., WALKER, J. M., PRICE, L. J., FLOYD T. C. and MARCH, J. D. (1979). Flurazepam effects on sleep EEG. *Arch. Gen. Psychiatry*, **36**, 95–102.

FENCL, V., KOSKI, G. and PAPPENHEIMER, J. R. (1971). Factors in cerebrospinal fluid from goats that affect sleep and activity in rats. *J. Physiol.* (London), **216**, 565–589.

GAILLARD, J. M., SCHULZ, P. and TISSOT, R. (1973). Effects of three benzodiazepines (Nitrazepam, Flunitrazepam and Bromazepam) on sleep of normal subjects, studied with an automatic sleep scoring system. *Pharmakopsychiat.*, **6**, 207–217.

GILLIN, J. C., MENDELSON, W. B., SITARAM, N. and WYATT, R. J. (1978). The neuropharmacology of sleep and wakefulness, *Ann. Rev. Pharmacol. Toxicol.*, **18**, 563–79.

GILLIN, J. C., DUNCAN, W., PETTIGREW, K. D., FRANKEL, B. L. and SNYDER, F. (1979). Successful separation of depressed, normal, and insomniac subjects by EEG sleep data. *Arch. Gen. Psychiatry*, **36**, 85–90.

HINTON, J. M. (1961). The actions of amilobarbitone sodium, butobarbitone and quinalbarbitone sodium upon insomnia and nocturnal restlessness compared in psychiatric patients. *Brit. J. Pharmacol.*, **16**, 82–89.

HOBSON, J. A., MCCARLEY, R. W. and WYZINSKI, P. W. (1975). Sleep cycle oscillation: reciprocal discharge by two brainstem neuronal groups. *Science*, **189**, 55–58.

HÖKFELT, T., JOHANSSON, O., LJUNGDAHL, A., LUNDBERG, J. M. and SCHULTZBERG, M. (1980). Peptidergic neurones. *Nature*, **284**, 515–521.

INOUÉ, S., UCHIZONO, K. and NAGASAKI, H. (1982). Endogenous sleep-promoting factors. *Trends Neurosci.* **5**, 218–220.

INSTITUTE OF MEDICINE (1979). Sleeping pills, insomnia, and medical practise. National Academy of Sciences, Washington DC.

JOHNSON, L. C., SEALES, D. M., NAITOH, P., CHURCH, W. M. and SINCLAIR, M. (1979). The effects of flurazepam hydrochloride on brain electrical activity during sleep. *Electroenceph. Clin. Neurophys.*, **47**, 309–321.

JOUVET, M. (1972). The role of monoamines and acetylcholine-containing neurons in the regulation of the sleep-waking cycle. *Ergebn. Physiol.*, **64**, 166–307.

JOUVET, M. (1977). Neuropharmacology of the sleep-waking cycle. In: S. D. IVERSEN, L. L. IVERSEN and S. H. SNYDER (Eds.), *Handbook of Psychopharmacology*, Vol. 8, New York: Plenum, pp. 233–293.

KAFI, S., MONNIER, M. and GAILLARD, J. M. (1979). The delta-sleep inducing peptide (DSIP) increases duration of sleep in rats. *Neuroscience Letters*, **13**, 169–172.

KASTIN, A. J., NISSEN, Ch., SCHALLY, A. V. and COY, D. H. (1978). Radioimmunoassay of DSIP-like material in rat brain. *Brain Research Bulletin*, **3**, 691–695.

KASTIN, A. J., OLSON, G. A., SCHALLY, A. V. and COY, D. H. (1980). DSIP — more than a sleep peptide? *Trends in Neurosciences*, **3**, 163–165.

KAY, D. C., BLACKBURN, A. B., BUCKINGHAM, J. A. and KARACAN, I. (1976). Human pharmacology of sleep. In: R. L. WILLIAMS and I. KARACAN (Eds.), *Pharmacology of sleep*, New York: Wiley, pp. 83–210.

KOE, B. K. and WEISSMAN, A. (1966). P-chlorophenylalanine: a specific depletor of brain serotonin. *J. Pharmacol. exp. Ther.*, **154**, 499–516.

KOELLA, W. P., FELDSTEIN, A. and CZICMAN, J. S. (1968). The effect of para-chlorophenylalanine on the sleep of cats. *Electroenceph. Clin. Neurophys.*, **25**, 481–490.

KRUEGER, J. M., PAPPENHEIMER, J. R. and KARNOVSKY, M. L. (1978). Sleep-promoting factor S: purification and properties. *Proc. Nat. Acad. Sci.* (USA), **75**, 5235–5238.

KRUEGER, J. M., BACSIK, J. and GARCIA-ARRARAS, J. (1980). Sleep-promoting material from human urine and its relation to factor S from brain. *Am. J. Physiol.*, **238** (Endocrinol. Metab. 1): E116–E123.

KRUEGER, J. M., PAPPENHEIMER, J. R. and KARNOVSKY, M. L. (1982). The composition of sleep-promoting factor isolated from human urine. *J. Biol. Chem.*, **257**, 1664–1669.

LAGUZZI, R. F. and ADRIEN, J. (1980). Inversion de l'insomnie produite par la parachlorophenylalanine chez le rat. *Arch. Ital. Biol.*, **118**, 109–123.

LINNOILA, M., VIUKARI, M., NUMMINEN, A. and AUVINEN, J. (1980). Efficacy and side effects of chloral hydrate and tryptophan as sleeping aids in psychogeriatric patients. *Int. Pharmacopsychiat.* **15** 124–128.

MATTMANN, P., LOEPFE, M., SCHEITLIN, T., SCHMIDLIN, D., GERNE, M., STRAUCH, I., LEHMANN, D. and BORBÉLY, A. A. (1982). Day-time residual effects of motor activity after three benzodiazepine hypnotics. *Arzneim.-Forsch/Drug Res.*, **32**, 461–465.

MENDELSON, W. B. (1980). *The use and misuse of sleeping pills*. New York: Plenum.

MENDELSON, W. B., GILLIN, J. C. and WYATT, R. J. (1980). Studies with the delta sleep-inducing peptide in the rat. *Sleep Research*, **9**, 55.

MENDELSON, W. B., GILLIN, J. C. and WYATT, R. J. (1982). The search for circulating sleep-promoting factors. In: H. YOSHIDA, Y. HAGIHARA and S. EBASHI (Eds.), *CNS Pharmacology — Neuropeptides*. Advances in pharmacology and therapeutics II, Vol. 1. Oxford: Pergamon Press, pp. 227–240.

MESSING, R. B., PETTIBONE, D. J., KAUFMAN, N. and LYTLE, L. D. (1978). Behavioral effects of serotonin neurotoxins: an overview. *Annals N. Y. Acad. Sci.*, **305**, 480–496.

MCCARLEY, R. W. and HOBSON, J. A. (1975). Neuronal excitability modulation over the sleep cycle: a structural and mathematical model. *Science*, **189**, 58–60.

MILLER, F. P., COX, R. H. jun., SNODGRASS, W. R. and MAICKEL, R. P. (1970). Comparative effects of p-chlorophenylalanine, p-chloroamphetamine and p-chloro-N-methylamphetamine on rat brain norepinephrine, serotonin and 5-hydroxyindole-3-acetic acid. *Biochem. Pharmacol.*, **19**, 435–442.

MÖHLER, H. and OKADA, T. (1977). Benzodiazepine receptor: demonstration in the central nervous system. *Science*, **198**, 849–851.

NAGASAKI, H., IRIKI, M., INOUÉ, S. and UCHIZONO, K. (1974). The presence of sleep-promoting material in the brain of sleep-deprived rats. *Proc. Jpn. Acad.*, **50**, 241–247.

NAGASAKI, H., KITAHAMA, K., VALATX, J-L. and JOUVET, M. (1980). Sleep-promoting effect of the sleep-promoting substance (SPS) and delta sleep-inducing peptide (DSIP) in the mouse. *Brain Research*, **192**, 276–280.

NICHOLSON, A. N. and STONE, B. M. (1979). L-Tryptophan and sleep in healthy man. *Electroenceph. Clin. Neurophys.*, **47**, 539–545.

OSWALD, I., BERGER, R. J., JARAMILLO, R. A., KEDDIE, K. M. G., OLLEY, P. C. and PLUNKETT, G. B. (1963). Melancholia and barbiturates: a controlled EEG, body and eye movement study of sleep. *Brit. J. Psychiat.*, **109**, 66–78.

OSWALD, I. and PRIEST, R. G. (1965). Five weeks to escape the sleeping-pill habit. *Brit. med. J.*, **2**, 1093–1095.

OSWALD, I. (1978). Drug research and human sleep. In: E. JUCKER (Ed.), *Progress in Drug Research*, Vol. 22, Basel: Birkháuser, pp. 356–372.

PAPPENHEIMER, J. R., KOSKI, G., FENCL, V., KARNOVSKY, M. L. and KRUEGER, J. (1975). Extraction of sleep-promoting factor S from cerebrospinal fluid and from brains of sleep-deprived animals. *J. Neurophysiol.* **38**, 1299–1311.

PETITJEAN, F., BUDA, C., JANIN, M., SALLANON, M. and JOUVET, M. (1980). Neurophysiologie — L'insomnie provoquée par la p-chloropheénylalanine chez le chat. Sa réversibilité par l'injection intraventriculaire d'indolamines. *C.R. Acad. Sc.* (Paris), **291**, 1063–1066.

PIÉRON, H. (1913). *Le probème physiologique du sommeil*. Paris: Masson.

PODDAR, M. K., URQUHART, D. and SINHA, A. K. (1980). Diazepam binding in brain after sleep and wakefulness. *Brain Research*, **193**, 519–528.

POLC, P., SCHNEEBERGER, J. and HAEFELY, W. (1978). Effect of the delta sleep inducing peptide (DSIP) on the sleep-wakefulness cycle of cats. *Neuroscience Letters*, **9**, 33–36.

PUIZILLOUT, J. J., GAUDIN-CHAZAL, G., DASZUTA, A., SEYFRITZ, N. and TERNAUX, J. P. (1979). Release of endogenous serotonin from 'encéphale isolé' cats. II — Correlations with raphe neuronal activity and sleep and wakefulness. *J. Physiol.* (Paris), **75**, 531–537.

RECHTSCHAFFEN, A. and KALES, A. (Eds.) (1968). *A Manual of standardized terminology, techniques and scoring system for sleep stages of human subjects*. National Institutes of Health, Publication **204**, US Govt Printing Office, Washington, DC.

REITE, M. L., RHODES, J. M., KAVAN, E. and ADEY, W. R. (1965). Normal sleep patterns in macaque monkey. *Arch. Neurol.* **12**, 133–144.

ROSS, C. A., TRULSON, M. E. and JACOBS, B. L. (1976). Depletion of brain serotonin following intraventricular 5, 7-dihydroxytryptamine fails to disrupt sleep in the rat. *Brain Research*, **114**, 517–523.

RUDOLF, G. A. E., SCHILGEN, B. and TOLLE, R. (1977). Antidepressive Behandlung mittels Schlafentzug. *Nervenarzt*, **48**, 1–11.

SALLANON, M., BUDA, C., JANIN, M. and JOUVET, M. (1981). L'insomnie provoquée par la p-chlorophénylalanine chez le chat. Sa réversibilité par l'injection intraventriculaire de liquide céphalorachidien prélevé chez des chats privés de sommeil paradoxal. *C.R. Acad. Sc.* (Paris), **292**, 113–117.

SCHNEIDER-HELMERT, D., GRAF, M. and SCHOENENBERGER, G. A. (1981a). Synthetic delta-sleep-inducing peptide improves sleep in insomniacs. *Lancet*, **1**, 1256.

SCHNEIDER-HELMERT, D., GNIRSS, F., MONNIER, M., SCHENKER, J. and SCHOENENBERGER, G. A. (1981b). Acute and delayed effects of DSIP (delta sleep-inducing peptide) on human sleep behavior. *Intern. J. of Clin. Pharmac. Therapy and Toxicology*, **19**, 341–345.

SCHOENENBERGER, G. A., MAIER, P. F., TOBLER, H. J., WILSON, K. and MONNIER, M. (1978). The delta EEG (sleep)-inducing peptide (DSIP). XI. Amino-acid analysis, sequence, synthesis and activity of the nonapeptide. *Pflügers Arch.* **376**; 119–129.

SILBERMAN, E. K., VIVALDI, E., GARFIELD, J., MCCARLEY, R. W. and HOBSON, J. A. (1980). Carbachol triggering of desynchronized sleep phenomena: enhancement via small volume infusions. *Brain Research*, **191**, 215–224.

Sitaram, N., Wyatt, R. J., Dawson, S. and Gillin, J. C. (1976). REM sleep induction by physostigmine infusion during sleep. *Science*, **191**, 1281–1283.

Sitaram, N., Moore, A. M. and Gillin, J. C. (1978). Experimental acceleration and slowing of REM sleep ultradian rhythm by cholinergic agonist and antagonist. *Nature*, **274**, 490–492.

Squires, R. F. and Braestrup, C. (1977). Benzodiazepine receptors in rat brain. *Nature*, **266**, 732–734.

Steigrad, P., Tobler, I., Waser, P. G. and Borbély, A. A. (1978). Effect of p-chlorophenylalanine on cerebral serotonin binding, serotonin concentration and motor activity in the rat. *Arch. Pharmacol.*, **305**, 143–148.

Takahashi, Y., Ebihara, S., Nakamura, Y. and Takahashi, K. (1978). Temporal distribution of delta wave sleep and REM sleep during recovery sleep after 12-h forced wakefulness in dogs: similarity to human sleep. *Neurosci. Lett.*, **10**, 329–334.

Tobler, I. and Borbély, A. A. (1982). Sleep regulation after reduction of brain serotonin: effect of p-chlorophenylalanine combined with sleep-deprivation in the rat. *Sleep*, **5**, 145–153.

Trulson, M. E. and Jacobs, B. L. (1979). Raphe unit activity in freely moving cats: correlation with level of behavioral arousal. *Brain Research*, **163**, 135–150.

Tsuchiya, K., Toru, M. and Kobayashi, T. (1969). Sleep deprivation: changes of monoamines and acetylcholine in rat brain. *Life Sci.*, **8**, 867–873.

Uchizono, K., Higashi, A., Iriki, M., Nagasaki, H., Ishikawa, M., Komoda, Y., Inoué, S. and Honda, K. (1978). Sleep-promoting fractions obtained from the brain-stem of sleep-deprived rats. In: M. Ito, K. Kubota, N. Tsukahara and K. Yagi (Eds.), *Integrative Control Functions of the Brain*, Vol. 1, Amsterdam: Elsevier, pp. 392-396.

Ursin, R. (1971). Differential effect of sleep deprivation on the two slow wave sleep stages in the cat. *Acta. Physiol. Scand.* **83**, 352–361.

Ursin, R. (1980). Does para-chlorophenylalanine produce disturbed waking, disturbed sleep or activation by ponto-geniculo-occipital waves in cats? *Waking and Sleeping*, **4**, 211–221.

Vivaldi, E., McCarley, R. W. and Hobson, J. A. (1980). Evocation of desynchronized sleep signs by chemical microstimulation of the pontine brain stem. In: J. A. Hobson and M. A. B. Brazier (Eds.), *The Reticular Formation Revisited*, New York: Raven Press, pp. 513–529.

Vogel, G. W. (1975). A review of REM sleep deprivation. *Arch. Gen. Psychiatry*, **32**, 749–761.

Vogel, G. W., Thurmond, A., Gibbons, P., Sloan, K., Boyd, M. and Walker, M. (1975). REM sleep reduction effects on depression syndromes. *Arch. Gen. Psychiatry*, **32**, 765–777.

Vogel, G. W., Vogel, F., McAbee, R. S. and Thurmond, A. J. (1980). Improvement of depression by REM sleep deprivation. New findings and a theory. *Arch. Gen. Psychiatry*, **37**, 247–253.

Webb, W.B. and Agnew, H. W. jun. (1971). Stage 4 sleep: influence of time course variables. *Science*, **174**, 1354–1356.

Wirz-Justice, A., Tobler, I., Kafka, M. S., Naber, D., Marangos, P. J., Borbély, A. A. and Wehr, T. A. (1981). Sleep deprivation: effects on circadian rhythms of rat brain neurotransmitter receptors. *Psychiatry Research*, **5**, 67–76.

Yehuda, S., Kastin, A. J. and Coy, D. H. (1980). Thermoregulatory and locomotor effects of DSIP: paradoxical interaction with d-amphetamine. *Pharmacology Biochemistry and Behavior*, **13** 895–900.

CHAPTER 9

Mammalian Sleep Function with Particular Reference to Man

J. A. Horne

9.1 Introduction and Summary of Main Proposals

The putative functions for mammalian sleep range from a non-restorative 'non-behaviour' occupying unproductive hours, providing safety and conserving energy, to an essential and special restitutive process. There is a tendency for such proposals to be seen to be: (1) mutually exclusive, (2) equally applicable across the mammalia. The standpoint adopted here will be that mammalian sleep serves both these functions. However, for various mammalian groups sleep will contain different and interacting proportions of these functions. That sleep which provides some form of essential restitutive function will be referred to as 'obligatory sleep' and the non-restitutive form will be referred to as 'facultative sleep', being more able to be extended or reduced, according to environmental constraints. The prescription for the amounts of this obligatory and facultative sleep within any given species will depend upon several factors, which include phylogeny, ontogeny, body size, brain development and safety.

Facultative sleep, which is seen here to be largely governed by a circadian oscillator, switches in during the normal sleep period and lifts during the normal waking period. This lifting seems apparent even if sleep is not taken. Obligatory sleep is seen to be largely oriented towards cerebral restitution and plays an increasing role in sleep as the phylogenetic scale of cerebral advancement is ascended. Such development also appears to bring a greater propensity for relaxed (advanced) wakefulness. Obligatory sleep need accumulates with wakefulness and perhaps with waking cerebral metabolic load. Both facultative and obligatory sleep mechanisms may work in parallel at sleep onset, but there will be a faster decline in the obligatory mechanism, leaving the facultative sleep to continue. In less cerebrally advanced mammals this decline may be even more rapid. Human Stages 3 and 4 sleep, together with the temporally associated REM and Stage 2 sleep may fit an obligatory sleep model, with the remainder of sleep (wherein much of REM sleep lies) fitting a facultative sleep model (see Fig. 9.1).

Body restitution (not necessarily brain restitution) seems to be influenced mostly by food intake, increasing with food absorption and declining with fasting. Hence in mammals such as humans, where sleep is generally a fasting state, sleep is a condition of reduced body restitution. Less cerebrally advanced mammals such as insectivores and rodents tend to be almost constantly physically active, and display little of the relaxed wakefulness found in the more

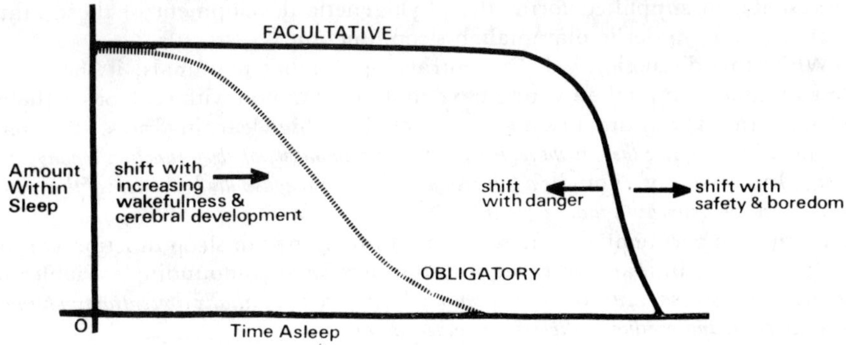

Fig. 9.1 Hypothesized trends during sleep for obligatory and facultative sleep mechanisms, and the major influences seen to affect these trends. See text for details.

advanced mammals. So for the less advanced mammals, sleep (which may be largely composed of facultative sleep) could be the main immobilizer where a resting metabolic rate is obtained, and where needless physical energy expenditure is prevented. The fall in metabolism during the sleep of rodents seems large when compared with the normal metabolism of wakefulness (comprising mostly of physical activity). However, for the more advanced mammal this fall is small, as the normal waking metabolism mostly reflects a more relaxed condition. This suggests that for these mammals the energy conservation value of sleep, particularly facultative sleep, is not so substantial. Facultative sleep in those cerebrally advanced mammals sleeping under relatively safe conditions may still be of considerable importance as it may be the main means for occupying the period of darkness. For example, in mammals very reliant upon colour vision (which needs good light) night-time would be tedious without sleep. Humans, the obvious example, can extend sleep easily and even learn to shorten sleep. This flexibility would seem to be with the latter (facultative) sleep cycles. Fig. 9.2

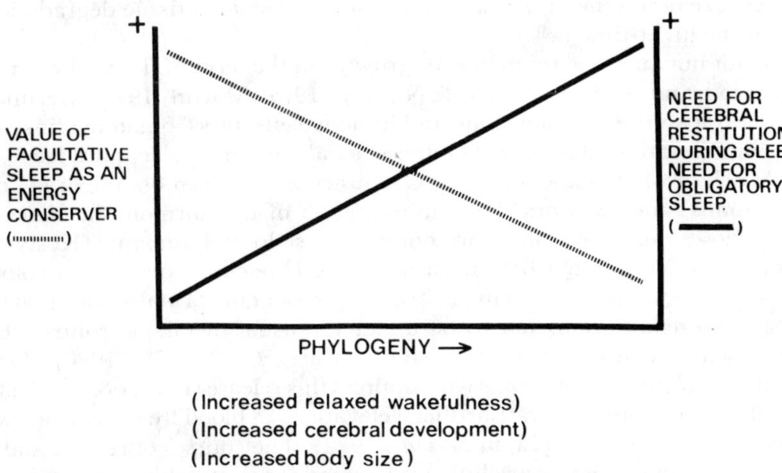

Fig. 9.2 A simplified representation of the interactions between the main variables hypothesized to influence mammalian sleep function. See text for details.

represents, in simplified form, the phylogenetic development of these main factors seen to underlie mammalian sleep function.

While this discussion will concentrate upon adult mammals, it should be noted that as mammalian young have more in common with each other (helplessness, rapid body and brain growth, relatively high learning rates, etc.) than do the adult forms, *there is more likely to be a commonality of sleep function amongst the young*. Interestingly, though, *adult humans being neotenous may have more of their sleep function in common with that of the infant primate*.

Because experimental studies relating to mammalian sleep function can be carried out on humans with the minimum of such confounding variables as behavioural stress, and so on, *the ensuing discussion will initially concentrate on human sleep function and gradually diversify to other mammals*.

9.2 Human Sleep and Body Restitution

9.2.1 The Sleep-Related Growth Hormone Release

One of the major findings appearing to support the restitutive hypothesis for sleep function is that certain hormones, which amongst their various activities have anabolic actions, display a heightened release during human sleep, and prominent within this group is human growth hormone (hGH). The substantial sleep-hGH output is mostly associated with Stages 3 and 4 sleep (collectively called slow wave sleep — SWS; but not to be confused with this same term which is used, unfortunately, for animal sleep as a synonym for non-REM sleep in its entirety). However, the significance of the sleep-hGH release for this restitution starts to become obscure when one notes that other hormones integral to anabolism, such as insulin, display no sleep-related release (Jefferson, 1980). As will be seen, there are several other findings which have been taken as signs of this restitution, which on further analysis turn out to be misleading in this respect. In fact it is beginning to appear that for the majority of tissues, excluding the brain, sleep may well be a state of tissue degradation, owing to the night-time fast.

For adult humans, the reference to 'growth' in the term hGH is now generally seen to be misleading (Kostyo & Nutting, 1974; Martin, 1977; Merimee, 1979). The actions of this hormone and its active effectors (somatomedins) are many, and their roles during wakefulness, let alone during sleep, are far from clear. Much of what is known about GH function has been obtained: (1) not from humans, and (2) from the administration of the hormone in pharmacological doses, and not from more normal physiological amounts (Kostyo & Nutting, 1974; Merimee, 1979). In sleep, the hGH release is unrelated to blood levels of glucose, amino acids, fatty acids, etc., present in normal amounts at the time, and therefore seems not to be under the usual metabolic control, but under obscure neurogenic mechanisms (Parker *et al.*, 1972, 1980). Only induced high blood glucose levels will suppress this release (Parker & Rossman, 1971), although more moderate artificial elevations in blood free fatty acids will be effective in this respect (Lipman *et al.*, 1972). The courses of release and of action of the somatomedins are little understood for sleep, although for one of them, somatomedin C, sleep onset brings a fall in the serum level, which remains low during sleep (Minuto *et al.*, 1981).

Mammalian GH seems to have a major effect as a sparer of amino acid breakdown, and as a mobilizer of fats. When the body's carbohydrate reserves start becoming depleted, amino acids and fats can be used as alternative energy sources. However, GH protects amino acids in this respect and encourages the utilization of fats for energy. This hormone *permits*, but not necessarily stimulates, increases in protein synthesis if the levels of amino acids (the protein building blocks) available to the cell are sufficiently high which, as will be seen, does not appear to be the case in human sleep. As noted already, insulin, a hormone promoting the cellular uptake of amino acids and a stimulus to protein synthesis (Jefferson, 1980), *does not show any enhanced release during sleep*; such an enhancement usually closely follows food intake. The sleep-hGH release might be linked with the human's usual night-time fast, sparing amino acids from degradation, although such a link is not yet clear.

Only a few other primates have been assessed for a sleep-related GH release. Whilst the rhesus monkey and baboon display SWS, it now appears that despite earlier claims, GH release in the former animal is not linked to sleep or to SWS (Quabbe *et al.*, 1981). For the latter, there are only limited data available claiming this release (Parker *et al.*, 1972a), and these are now disputed by Quabbe *et al.* (1981). In the normal sleep of the rat, cat and dog, there is no such release (Quabbe, 1977; Parker *et al.*, 1981), but it can be found in the recovery sleep of dogs following total sleep deprivation (cf. Takahashi, 1979). It seems therefore that the sleep-GH release is a rare event amongst mammals, of unknown purpose. Any claims that this release is of a restitutive nature must take into consideration the animal findings and whether, for example, in the absence of any clear sleep-GH release, their sleep is non-restitutive.

9.2.2 *Protein Turnover During Sleep*

Tissue protein is in a continuous state of turnover. That is, breaking down into the constituent amino acids, which are either deaminated (oxidized) or reused together with exogenous amino-acids from recent food intake, for further protein synthesis. In accordance with the literature, protein turnover will be described here, in terms of synthesis, breakdown and oxidation. If an excess of 'wear and tear' were present during wakefulness, presumably the rate of synthesis would be exceeded by the rate of breakdown, leading to a decrease in the protein content of cells. Sleep, it has been proposed (Adam & Oswald, 1977; Adam, 1980), redresses this imbalance, allowing synthesis to proceed at a high rate, faster than that of breakdown and oxidation, leading to 'repair' and a net increase in tissue protein. However, this viewpoint, that human sleep is a state of enhanced tissue growth, can be disputed on several accounts, with the main criticism stemming from the substantive review on protein metabolism by Waterlow *et al.* (1978).

These authors concluded that the main stimulus to protein synthesis and to an increase in the protein content of cells was food absorption. Hence, because of the human's night-time fast, often lasting 12 h from evening meal to breakfast, it could be predicted that protein synthesis during sleep would be low. Until recently, no investigation has assessed protein turnover during human awake and sleep periods. Two reports (Garlick *et al.*, 1980; Clugston & Garlick, 1982), one a preliminary finding of the other have thrown light on this area by describing trends in whole-body protein turnover for 24 h, using a $1^{14}C$ leucine infusion technique. Although this method may have some drawbacks, these are not major (Waterlow *et al.*, 1978; Garlick *et al.*, 1981), and the method would seem to be valid. An interesting debate on this point can be seen elsewhere (Adam & Oswald, 1981; Garlick *et al.*, 1981).

Group data were presented in 12-h epochs, 08.00–20.00 and 20.00–08.00, with the latter period mostly consisting of sleep. Approximately hourly time-course data relating to synthesis, breakdown and oxidation of protein were given throughout the 24 h for one subject, whose trends were typical of the group. Although sleep EEGs were not taken at night, subjects appeared to sleep satisfactorily. Ten obese but otherwise healthy subjects, and five lean subjects were used. During the 12-h daytime period all subjects were given normal food to eat, at one hourly intervals throughout, while during the night-time period there was a complete fast. From the summary of the findings in Table 9.1, it can be seen that both subject groups showed very similar responses in protein turnover, with feeding leading to increases in the protein content of tissue (i.e. increased synthesis and decreased breakdown), but with increased oxidation of amino acids owing to their elevated availability through absorption. Fasting caused the reverse to happen to all these indices, with synthesis falling by about 27% and breakdown rising by about 35%. The more detailed hourly data showed that these changes began about 1–2 in after the last meal, levelling out to more stable values after about a further 4–5 h, (at around 02.00), for the rest of the night (i.e. sleep). Re-feeding, not wakefulness, re-established the daytime levels. Oxidation showed a substantial 50–60% fall from feeding to fasting, with the hourly data revealing a more rapid decline over the first 4 h of fasting (prior to sleep), then also levelling off for the rest of the night.

One possible criticism on the relevance of these findings to the restitutional hypothesis may come from the unusual feeding regimen employed, given that subjects were normally meal feeders rather than 'nibblers'. Whilst this may have had some effect upon absorption characteristics and protein turnover during the daytime, the value of this study to sleep research lies in what happened during the fasting state; most people normally cease eating between 20.00 and 08.00.

These findings relate to the body as a whole, and it has been pointed out by

Table 9.1

Summary of findings from Clugston & Garlick (1982). Mean and s.d. of rates of protein turnover during feeding, 08.00–20.00, and fasting (including sleep), 20.00–08.00, in 10 obese and 5 lean subjects. Note that during fasting, synthesis is exceeded by breakdown, indicating protein loss. See text for further details.

		mmol leucine/h		
		Synthesis	Breakdown	Oxidation
Obese	Fed	6.07 (0.75)	3.98 (0.82)	2.37 (0.37)
	Fasted	4.45 (0.79)**	5.40 (0.93)*	0.95 (0.21)**
Lean	Fed	5.70 (1.24)	3.82 (0.95)	2.19 (0.38)
	Fasted	4.15 (0.77)*	5.11 (0.78)*	0.96 (0.18)*

* $P \leq 0.01$.
** $P \leq 0.001$.

Garlick *et al.* (1981) that it is possible for certain tissues, perhaps the brain, to have shown opposite trends during sleep, with other tissues displaying even greater protein losses. However, the course of brain protein turnover during sleep is not known.

The reduction in amino acid oxidation during sleep was substantial, indicating amino acid conservation. This, together with the significant reduction in the utilization of protein as energy, suggests some form of active amino acid conservation, although, as noted already, it is not known whether hGH had any role to play here. The main point made by this research group was to emphasize the importance of food intake, with protein content of tissue rising after feeding and falling during fasting. Indeed, as predicted, the night-time fast (the obvious consequence of sleep), not sleep itself, seemed to be the prime cause of the protein turnover changes.

A preliminary report (Clugston & Garlick, 1981) of a further study by this group also failed to show any significant increases in protein synthesis during the sleep period, and also demonstrated the importance of protein intake for tissue protein synthesis. Adaptation to a low-energy, protein-free diet given for 12 h in the daytime, with nil food intake at night-time, led to the abolition of any day–night changes in protein turnover. Both levels were typical of those found at night-time under the previous experimental conditions.

It has been suggested by Adam & Oswald (1977, 1981) and Adam (1980) that amino acids from recent dietary intake could be stored during wakefulness, perhaps by the expansion of the free amino acid pool, for restitutive purposes during sleep. However, calculations by Garlick *et al.* (1981) and Clugston & Garlick (1982) now show that this is very unlikely, and that the bulk of recently absorbed amino acids are either oxidized or converted to protein with very little delay.

Laboratory rodent studies appear to show that under ad lib feeding, protein synthesis is higher during the light hours (the putative sleep period) than in the dark hours (although most of these studies give no indication about actual sleep and waking patterns). These studies are described elsewhere (Adam & Oswald, 1977; Adam, 1980). Although such findings appear contrary to those of human studies, the investigations are limited in that they have not measured adequately the specific activity of the free amino acids at the sites of protein synthesis, and neither did they control for food intake (Garlick, personal communication). Also, assessment of protein synthesis was made only once or twice; the trend over time in amino acid activity must be measured before a clear picture can be established. Consequently, very *little is known from the animal data about protein turnover, particularly the rates in protein breakdown and in amino acid oxidation. Without data on breakdown it cannot be assumed that there is an increase in tissue protein (restitution) during sleep*. The elevated synthesis, if this were correct, may simply reflect an increased protein turnover, with breakdown also heightened, leading to no net increase or even a decrease in tissue protein. Such a situation seems to be apparent from the findings by Rebolledo and Gagliardino (1971), where C^{14} leucine incorporation into mouse diaphragm was assessed. Whilst protein synthesis seemed greater in the light period, the total protein content of this tissue was highest at the end of the dark period.

Laboratory rodents, being 'nibblers', have different feeding styles from those of present-day humans who are 'meal feeders'. Consequently, as feeding seems to be so important in determining protein turnover rates, these rates will display qualitative differences from rodent to humans. The rodent does not fast during its sleep period, but wakes up frequently and nibbles food; about one-third of the daily food intake is eaten at this time. A recent study by Wannemacher and Dinterman (1980) meal fed rats and, like the study of Garlick *et al.* (1980, 1981), assessed all three phases of protein turnover. Again it was found that the major stimulus to protein synthesis was food intake, particularly dietary protein.

Finally, it should be noted that prolonged physical activity may attenuate and/or delay food absorption until a resting state is achieved. In an animal spending much of wakefulness in physical activity, sleep may (by default) be the main permissor (not stimulus) of increased body restitution. Rodents and insectivores in the wild are continually active during wakefulness. They display little relaxed wakefulness, or what Kleitman (1963) called 'advanced (contemplative) wakefulness', which appears to be a reflection of cerebral advancement. *Sleep is probably the only mechanism which brings prolonged inactivity to these animals*. However, in a caged or otherwise restricted rodent, of course, such a caveat may not be so applicable.

9.2.3 Cellular Energy Charge and Energy Cost of Protein Synthesis

According to Atkinson (1977), increases in tissue protein (anabolism) are positively correlated with the cellular energy charge (EC), which is the ratio of ATP + 1/2 ADP to the total cellular adenylate pool. It has been proposed by Adam & Oswald (1977) and Adam (1980) that during sleep EC rises, leading to an increase in anabolism (i.e. increased restitution). However, *a high EC does not cause such an increase, only promotes it*, given adequate levels of intra-cellular amino acid substrate. Because of the probability that in sleep these levels are reduced owing to the fast, and that cells cannot store amino acids to any extent without converting them to protein, it is unlikely that EC changes during sleep would affect protein turnover. There are some data available, only from animal studies, on EC changes from waking to sleep. However, none of these studies assessed protein turnover. The few reports available have concentrated on brain tissue. Two (Van den Noort & Brine, 1970; Reich *et al.*, 1972) found very small EC increases in the sleeping brain, with one (Reich *et al.*, 1972) observing that acclimatization of the animal to the laboratory setting reduced this increase to insignificance. The third investigation (Durie *et al.*, 1978) found large increases in EC from waking to sleep in both brain and muscle. However, the waking EC levels given by this study seem lower than the usual norm (Chapman *et al.*, 1971) and it would seem from the data that rather than EC being increased during sleep, EC has been depressed somehow during wakefulness. Also, it should be noted that caution should be exercised in relating the EC levels from these laboratory studies to possible changes in protein synthesis rates. It has been pointed out (Veech, 1980) that the EC of mitochondria containing tissue, such as brain and muscle, does not fully reflect the free-ADP concentrations within the cytoplasm, as this chemical is found in different cellular compartments, which have been combined together in all of the studies described. Such a pooling cannot give a valid 'cellular ADP level'.

In humans, *EC levels are very high during wakefulness*, almost at maximum, even after exercise (Harris *et al.*, 1974). From the hypothetical graphs given by Atkinson (1977) linking EC with protein synthesis rates, such levels would permit very high protein synthesis rates.

While the energy cost of protein synthesis is difficult to assess, it certainly makes a significant contribution to the overall resting metabolic rate (RMR). Although Waterlow *et al.* (1978) have estimated that mammalian protein synthesis makes up about 17% of RMR, this covers only the formation of peptide bonds. The true figure is likely to be much higher (Young *et al.*, 1975) if all the associated processes such as amino acid transport to the cell are taken into account. The correlation between growth (net protein increase) and RMR has been given as 0.9 (Webster, 1980), although the data forming this correlation are from sources outside sleep research. With these factors in mind, it would seem unlikely that the approximately 10% drop which occurs in RMR from relaxed wakefulness to sleep in humans (Brebbia & Altschuler, 1965; Webb & Heistand, 1975) could embody a significant increase in the net content of protein within tissues. However, this argument applies to the body as a whole, and it is possible that some tissues (e.g. the cerebrum) could be in a state of net protein increase. Whilst protein breakdown would liberate some energy which could be 'reused' for protein synthesis without affecting RMR, the significant drop in sleep RMR still militates against high protein synthesis rates during human sleep. It could be countered, though, that sleep brings extra postural relaxation compared with pre-sleep levels of lying relaxed. Hence energy could be 'diverted' so to speak from maintaining muscular tonus, to an increase in protein synthesis during sleep, with little net change to RMR. However, whilst it is clear that head and neck muscles can display a profound drop during (REM) sleep, there is as yet little evidence to show that there is a significant drop in the tonus of other muscles from this relaxed wakefulness to sleep.

9.2.4 Mitosis

Another index of body restitution has been seen to be rate of mitosis. For at least some human tissues, the circadian peak in mitosis appears within the usual sleep period (Scheving, 1959; Fisher, 1968). Although such findings appear to support a restitutional hypothesis for human sleep function, it has been pointed out by Scheving (1959) that *these peaks are not sleep dependent*, as they are present in the absence of sleep, (and therefore unrelated to the sleep-hGH release). In humans these peaks seem to be influenced by corticosteroid and adrenaline levels, being inversely related to the output of these hormones. As the circadian rhythms of these hormones are not sleep dependent (Weitzman, 1976; Parker *et al.*, 1980), it would seem that these peaks are also not sleep dependent. The extent to which these peaks may be related to feeding patterns are not really known, although it would seem that as food intake may promote the growth of individual cells, subsequent cell division may also be so influenced. This appears to be the case in a recent study by Halberg and Nelson (1978), where alteration of feeding schedules, but not of light–dark schedules in laboratory rodents, was reflected in shifts in mitotic peaks. Although under normal feeding schedules sleep is the state of increased mitosis in rodents (Clark & Korst, 1969; Halberg & Barnum, 1961), the association between these events appears to be indirect.

Physical activity seems to attenuate mitosis (cf. Fisher, 1968), and it should be remembered that in the case of rodents and insectivores, which display little relaxed wakefulness in the wild, sleep may simply facilitate these mitotic peaks. Finally, an important point which must be noted with respect to the significance of the mitotic peaks for sleep function, is that *nothing is known of the rate of cell death at these times*. Hence these peaks may simply reflect a higher rate of cell turnover, with no net increases in tissue cell numbers; there could even be a decrease. However, of course, such a turnover of cells could still be interpreted as 'restorative' in the broad sense, but not necessarily as a sign of growth.

9.2.5 Exercise and Sleep

The topic of exercise and sleep has been seen to be of relevance to our understanding of the function of human sleep. If sleep were a state of enhanced body restitution, overcoming the physical wear and tear of waking activity, then exercise would be expected to lead to a further enhancement of this restitution during subsequent sleep, and consequently may affect this sleep. This leads to the supposition that the types of sleep showing changes following exercise may be related to these processes. However, it has just been argued that the evidence now points to human sleep being a state of decreased body restitution. This together with the fact that no exercise and sleep study has actually measured any body restitutive process during the recovery sleep, lead to the conclusion that there is *no support for any interpretation that the sleep EEG changes which do occur following exercise are signs of enhanced body restitution*. As already noted, SWS has been assumed to be particularly oriented towards body restitution mainly because of the association between this sleep and the sleep-related hGH release. So of all the types of sleep which could change following exercise, the findings that it appears to be SWS which shows the most significant effects (an increase) fit in with the original expectations. But because SWS is unlikely to be a state of elevated body restitution under normal circumstances, there are no grounds for expecting SWS increases following exercise to be signs of a further enhancement to this restitution.

As already noted in the previous section, it is quite possible for certain restitutive functions, such as mitosis, which are normally relatively active during wakefulness, to be suppressed during exercise, perhaps leading to a rebound effect at night-time *with or without sleep*. Although this could happen at the time of increased SWS, these two events would obviously not be causally related. Exercise does heighten tissue protein breakdown and oxidation, and the ensuing rest is accompanied by increases in net amounts of tissue protein, given adequate feeding (Molé & Johnson, 1971; Rennie *et al.*, 1980), and of course this increase may intrude into sleep. Interestingly though, this heightened protein oxidation and breakdown may not be a sign of increased 'wear and tear' in muscle, as Rennie *et al.* suggest that muscle is not the source of this catabolism, but more likely it is the viscera. Here tissue protein is probably being used to provide energy (via gluconeogenesis) for muscle contraction, and consequently it is the viscera rather than muscle which is the major site of tissue growth and repair following exercise.

Respiratory recovery processes may intrude into sleep, and this is indicated by the findings of Hauri (1968) and Walker *et al.* (1978), where elevations in heart-rate and related measures were observed during recovery sleep. These findings are also important in that the sleep EEG was unaffected, again indicating that the EEG is not sensitive to changes in somatic functioning; a factor casting further doubt on the validity of the EEG as an index of body restitution. Even in the single case of a significant increase in the sleep hGH output following exercise (Adamson *et al.*, 1974), SWS was not significantly affected.

There are findings of substantial SWS increases following increased daytime exercise in fit (trained) subjects (e.g. Shapiro *et al.*, 1975; Griffin & Trinder, 1978), although there are also nil findings in this respect (Walker *et al.*, 1978). The relatively large body of evidence from studies employing unfit (untrained) subjects points to exercise having little effect upon SWS or other forms of subsequent sleep (see review by Horne, 1981). Even careful analysis of the delta EEG activity in Stage 2 sleep revealed no substantive changes (Horne & Porter, 1976). These contrasting findings may well pose problems for any body restitutional proposals for SWS, as it could be argued that untrained subjects would experience as much, if not more, muscle wear and tear during exercise than would trained subjects. Horne (1981) concluded that the reason for these SWS differences between the two groups may relate to the greater exercise endurance in fit subjects and consequently the greater the likelihood of a higher and more sustained thermal load upon both body and brain. Support for this proposal has come recently from a study by Horne and Staff (1982) of fit subjects, which passively increased core temperature to a similar level to that of a high intensity exercise condition, for a period of 1.5 h during the afternoon. Both conditions produced similar SWS increases during the subsequent night-time sleep. These findings were interpreted in terms either of a torpor-like response stimulated by rapid dehydration, along the lines proposed for other mammals by Walker and Berger (1980) (see Section 9.6.2), or due to increased cerebral metabolism through body heating, and perhaps an increased need for some form of cerebral restitution. For reasons just described, both these interpretations centred on the brain and not on the body.

9.2.6 *Effects of Total Sleep Deprivation on Body Functioning*

Further evidence doubting a body restitutional role for at least human sleep, comes from the *large numbers of nil findings on the physiological effects of total sleep deprivation*, although as will be seen in Section 9.3, there are clear signs of CNS impairment. It should be noted, however, that most sleep deprivation studies have been oriented towards a stress perspective, believing reasonably that this condition would be a potent stressor. Hence, while there are many reports on such putative measures of stress as, corticosteroid output and cardiovascular functioning, there are little data on measures relating to body restitution, for example, protein metabolism.

A recent review by Horne (1978) of the sleep deprivation literature reported that:

(a) Out of the nine studies assessing urinary corticosteroid output over 24–205 h of continuous wakefulness, none reported any significant changes. Although two subsequent investigations have reported increases (Palmblad *et al.*, 1976; Francescioni *et al.*, 1978), both also involved military battle simulation.
(b) Out of the five reports measuring one or more of blood sedimentation rate, haematocrit, glucose, free fatty acids, none found any significant change.
(c) Of the ten studies monitoring urinary catecholamine levels, only one reported a significant increase. Subsequently, Palmblad *et al.* (1976) also found an increase.

(d) Heart-rate increased in three studies, decreased in five, and showed no change in nine.
(e) Systolic blood pressure decreased in three studies and remained unchanged in nine.

Most of these measures retained their circadian rhythm during sleep deprivation, and this topic has been reviewed by Akerstedt (1980).

From data available on measures which could give some guidance to body restitution, there seem to be no adverse effects of sleep deprivation. If this deprivation were to impair muscle tissue restitution, then the physiological ability to do physical work (physical work capacity) would be impaired. Only two studies (Brodan *et al.*, 1969; Harris & O'Hanlon, 1972) have examined this index, both measuring daily for either 72 h or 120 h total deprivation. Neither found any work capacity decrement. Recent findings by Martin (1981) have shown that apparent reductions in exercise endurance during sleep deprivation are due to failing psychological motivation, rather than to physiological factors. It is remarkable how well subjects can endure sustained exercise, given the motivation. For example, 92 h of near-continuous football playing in five subjects resulted in only minor physical effects (Reilly & Walsh, 1981). Although there was obvious but not serious behavioural impairment, there were apparently no adverse sequelae.

Two studies (Luby *et al.*, 1960, 1962) coming from the same laboratory, but using different subject groups, assessed blood adenylate activities over 123 or 220 h total sleep deprivation. 'Emergency responses' were claimed with ADP levels during both studies. However, both claims were based on only one observation half-way through each study, with ADP activity returning to normal levels on the second (last) measurement taken at the end of each vigil. Of the seven studies cited by Horne (1978), reporting on creatinine excretion (a rough guide to energy utilization) during sleep deprivation, only one (Luby *et al.*, 1960) found a significant change over 48 h of deprivation. However, the changes were well within the normal range. Of the three studies assessing urinary nitrogen levels (a crude guide to amino acid/protein metabolism), two found no changes, and one (Scrimshaw *et al.*, 1966) reported a significant but small fall (6%) on the first day of deprivation and a similar rise on the second day. These changes were also well within the biological norm.

A recent investigation by Vondura *et al.* (1981) on the effects of 120-h deprivation upon the activity of certain enzymes in skeletal muscle, sampled by biopsy at the end of deprivation, reported several significant changes when these data were compared with prior baseline values. Also, there was a significant rise in serum lactate. However, there was no control group, and details of exercise levels, method of deprivation, and of diet, were not given.

There remain several body systems where the response to total sleep deprivation is unknown, and so the picture is far from complete in this respect. For example, it is commonly believed that sleep loss heightens susceptibility to infection, and although two investigations (Palmblad *et al.*, 1976, 1979) have demonstrated that 72 h of sleep deprivation produces statistically significant (but not biologically significant) changes to certain aspects of the immune-response system, the changes could not be interpreted as being 'adverse', but simply as changes of unknown consequence. Of course, if any physiological system were to have seriously malfunctioned during those studies assessing corticosteroid output, then this output should have increased, which as noted does not appear to have been the case.

It is clear that there has been confusion with the interpretation of the few findings of statistical significance from several of these total sleep deprivation studies, and this has not necessarily been by the authors themselves. *Even though a physiological change may have been statistically significant, little can be made of the finding if the level does not fall outside the resting normal range.* Conversely, the data can be outside this biological range on pre-sleep deprivation baseline days (for example, through apprehension) and show a statistically significant change back to the norm during deprivation. Another problem of interpretation of findings which may have been compounded by a statistical rather than a clinical approach to these studies, is that there are clear individual differences in physiological response styles. Hence, averaging group data may convert these valuable data into 'noise', in the hunt for a common denominator. Clearly there is a need not only for a statistical approach which takes cognizance of the biological norms for the parameter under observation, but also a more clinical analysis which attempts to integrate the various physiological, as well as psychological changes within an individual.

One of the major stimuli to the elevation of corticosteroid output is psychological stress (Bush, 1962). Apprehension (not sleep loss alone) has been identified as the cause in the one recent sleep deprivation study (Francesconi *et al.*, 1978) to report a substantial rise in this output. However, it would seem that because of the absence of such corticosteroid changes in the other studies, sleep deprivation does not appear to be very stressing psychologically, even though it is tiring. This is one indication of several suggesting that humans could survive adequately with less sleep, and is a subject which will be covered in detail in Section 9.3. It must be remembered, though, that most sleep deprivation studies have carefully selected mentally stable subjects, and have encouraged a sanguine approach by their subjects to sleep deprivation. Furthermore, subjects are usually well looked after, and apart from lack of sleep, have most of their needs catered for very adequately. So sleep deprivation may be much more stressful in less 'stable' individuals, and under 'real world' conditions. However, whether or not 'body restitution' would suffer to any great extent is an unknown quantity, although, from the conclusions so far, it seems that with the sleep-deprived subject given some rest and sufficient food, this would be unlikely.

9.3 Brain Restitution and Sleep

Postural muscle can reduce its activity and relax to a similar extent during wakefulness as in sleep, but the equivalent situation does not apply to the human cerebral cortex. Even with a subject lying awake with the eyes closed in a sound-damped room, the EEG reveals that the cortex is still active, and in a state of quiet readiness, still attending to the environment. A significant degree of shut-down from the processing of sensory input, perhaps allowing for rest and recovery, *only seems to occur during sleep*, and as will be seen, probably more so during SWS. For muscle, the greater state of rest after exercise, the more efficient and rapid the recovery. A similar situation may occur with the cerebrum, as sleep may be the means for the most efficient and rapid recovery.

The cerebrum has been identified, here, as the part of the brain which is in most need of sleep, perhaps for recovery of and changes in plastic processes. Such a hypothesis is, of course, not new, and dates back to Jackson (1884). Moruzzi (1966, 1972) has endorsed this need for 'off-line' recovery, and pointed out that from the neurophysiological data it seems that the midbrain and brainstem structures never really rest. These structures appear to undergo 'on-line' restitution, even though sleep control mechanisms are mostly located within them.

9.3.1 CNS Effects of Sleep Deprivation

Total sleep deprivation soon brings psychological performance decrements, behavioural irritability and suspiciousness, some enhancement of paroxysmal EEG activity, but few other neurological effects (Wilkinson, 1965; Naitoh, 1976; Horne, 1978). While these changes indicate some form of CNS impairment and a need for the brain to sleep rather than to rest, it will be seen that the extent of these changes are not so extensive as one might expect if humans needed all of 8 h of sleep per day for brain restitution.

Wilkinson (1965) has pointed out that the psychological performance tests which are most vulnerable to sleep deprivation are not those which might be construed as 'cerebrally demanding', such as IQ tests and other complex decision-making tasks like 'battle games', but simple low-interest long-duration tasks, such as 1 h of auditory vigilance. One might expect the former tasks to be the first to show the effects of sleep deprivation, if sleep deprivation soon brought on impairment to cerebral restitution. However, these tasks being inherently interesting induce compensatory effort, and performance can be maintained at almost normal levels up to 64 h of deprivation (Wilkinson, 1964), indicating a 'cerebral capacity' to perform well under limited sleep deprivation. On the other hand, complex tasks which are uninteresting are soon vulnerable to sleep deprivation. Usual performance levels at the simpler tasks can also be maintained up to 2–3 days of deprivation by giving some form of reward or other incentive for doing well. Of course, with increasing deprivation the ability to sustain this compensatory effort declines and performance at whatever type of task will eventually drop.

The implication of these findings for the understanding of sleep function for the human cerebral cortex are complex. For example, the cerebrum may have the capacity to perform well because cortical cells do not need much off-line restitution (i.e. sleep), and/or there is much redundancy within the cortex, enabling 'reserves' to be called upon. The clear circadian rhythm of sleepiness which is apparent during sleep deprivation (Williams *et al.*, 1959; Froberg *et al.*, 1975; Akerstedt, 1980) is most interesting in this respect. Subjects have the greatest difficulty in remaining awake during the usual sleep period, and consequently exhibit their daily worst performance levels at this time. The lifting of much of this tiredness in the latter part of the day, with improved performance but without any sleep, suggests that *a significant degree of performance impairment is not due to a lack of cerebral restitution, but may be due to some form of 'non-restorative' sleep drive (cf. Murray, 1966) which switches in at night-time but lifts in the daytime*. This interpretation would also account for the changes in performance over sleep deprivation with respect to complex and interesting tasks, versus simple and uninteresting tasks. That is, the extra effort induced by the former tasks combats the non-restorative sleepiness, and not the inherent cerebral capacity to perform. The latter is more resilient to sleep loss, as only a portion of sleep may be necessary for cerebral restitution. The possible purposes of the sleep drive will be discussed later (Section 9.4).

Sleep deprivation has obvious effects on behaviour. Apart from tiredness, there is irritability, suspiciousness and speech slurring which soon become evident; mild forms of paranoia are not uncommon (Morris *et al.*, 1960, Berger & Oswald, 1962). Time disorientation and visual mis-preceptions such as 'spiders on the wall' are usually encountered at least once after 1–2 nights sleep deprivation, although seldom for more than a few occasions. Full-blown hallucinations are rare, and for examples were apparently not encountered on two of the longest sleep deprivation studies of 265 h (Gulevich *et al.*, 1966) and 205 h (Pasnau *et al.*, 1968). The neurological abnormalities in these two studies were relatively minor (Ross, 1966), amounting to some hand tremor, nystagmus, ptosis and hyperaesthesia. In these and other studies the waking EEG simply reflects tiredness, with a loss of alpha activity and increased theta (Rodin *et al.*, 1962; Johnson *et al.*, 1965; Naitoh *et al.*, 1969), except in the case of subjects with a history of epilepsy. Here, one night of sleep deprivation appears to bring paroxysmal (wave and spike) activity in about 25% of these subjects (Pratt *et al.*, 1968; Geller *et al.*, 1969).

The significance of these behavioural and perceptual findings for human sleep function is unclear. They could be due to some form of conflict behaviour between a sleep drive and the need to stay awake, along the lines described by Murray (1966), and/or some form of lack of cerebral restitution. The neurological tests employed during sleep deprivation have been very limited and have not assessed cerebral functoning, although the EEG is doing this to some extent. All that can be said of these findings is that they do not point to serious cerebral malfunction. Probably the only way to begin to understand the significance of sleep for cerebral functioning in cerebrally advanced mammals will be through sophisticated, as yet undeveloped neurochemical techniques allowing *in vivo* measurements of protein turnover and other restitutive changes inside neurones and glia, and to establish whether these changes are solely confined to sleep.

9.3.2 Neurophysiological and Neurochemical Evidence for Brain Restitution

Cerebral neural firing rates are not that much reduced in sleep when compared with those of waking levels, and may even be higher during REM sleep. Although the sleep EEG of SWS and REM sleep would suggest low and high firing respectively, such an assumption cannot necessarily be made. What does differ between these states is the pattern and organization of firing rates (cf. Hobson & McCarley, 1971; Schlag, 1974; Cruetzfelt, 1975; Webb, 1976). Unfortunately, these changes tell us little about cerebral restitution during sleep.

One of the most recent and detailed studies of single unit activity in the cerebrum during both sleep and wakefulness was by Livingstone and Hubel (1981), studying primary cortical cells in the cat. Transition from sleep to wakefulness brought reduced but smoother levels of spontaneous firing rates with enhanced evoked reponses, indicating an increased signal to noise ratio. Non-REM sleep seemed to have a dampening effect on the evoked activity, particularly in the deeper cortical layers (layers 5 and 6). 2-Deoxyglucose measurements (a guide to neural energy metabolism) showed similar levels for both non-REM sleep and wakefulness within the upper layers, but substantial reductions during non-REM sleep for these deeper layers. The significance of the apparent shut-down of these latter layers is unknown, and the authors pointed out that it seemed to represent an insulation of the animal from the sensory environment, either to permit uninterrupted sleep and/or to allow some form of recovery and regeneration (p. 561). Livingstone and Hubel pointed out that although during wakefulness many cerebral neurones seem to be relatively inactive and in a form of resting state, they are in a condition of 'quiet readiness' and slaves of incoming sensory input. In sleep there seemed to be some form of shut-down allowing freedom from this constraining condition. Although, instead, they are 'at the mercy of events related to the still all-too-mysterious slow waves' (p. 560).

In view of the similarities between the cat and man in the structure of their cerebral cortices, it is likely that similar findings with layers 5 and 6 would be apparent during human non-REM sleep. During SWS, the cerebrum is certainly in a peculiar state of unresponsiveness, as for example Sato *et al.* (1975) reported in a study of photic stimulation during sleep, that during SWS the cerebrum seems to be functionally disconnected from subcortical mechanisms, a condition unlike that to be found during REM sleep and other non-REM sleep stages.

From the restitutive perspective little can be gleaned from the limited data available on the neurochemical changes during sleep. Although there are reports that protein synthesis increases in the brain during sleep, nothing is known of the rate of protein breakdown. So this increase cannot yet be assumed to be signs of increased nerve growth or of the laying down of 'memory proteins'. Findings of increased amounts of extracellular protein during sleep can easily be wrongly interpreted. For example, a series of well-executed studies by Drucker-Colin (summarized by Drucker-Colin, 1981) has shown that during REM sleep in the cat there is a significant increase of extra-cellular proteins in samples perfused from the midbrain reticular formation. This has led others to speculate that REM sleep has a special role in the formation of proteins, particularly those relating to long-term memory. However, these samples were neither taken from the cerebrum, where long-term memory is believed to be located, nor taken from within cells, where presumptive memory proteins are more likely to be located. Hence, the real functional significance of his findings remains unknown.

Several studies have shown that drugs which inhibit protein synthesis (usually antibiotics — for example, anisomycin and chloramphenicol) also reduce REM sleep but not non-REM sleep, and again this evidence is often taken as further sign of a specific link between REM sleep and brain restitution or memory consolidation. At the dosages often given, these drugs can produce adverse reactions (such as diarrhoea) which may be distressing to the animals. Information on their vetinary status is seldom given. REM sleep is a 'fragile' state (cf. Hartmann, 1973) and is more prone to disruption than is non-REM sleep. Hence REM sleep reductions with these drugs may at least in part be due to an artefact of the method (e.g. substitution of wakefulness for REM sleep because of the latter's fragility), rather than to any central inhibition of protein synthesis. Any concomitant long-term memory disruptions may also have this underlying cause (i.e. due to arousal and behavioural distress). Certain anti-tumour drugs such as 'vincristine' have also been employed in high doses. They are cytotoxic, of course, and apart from inhibiting protein synthesis have a host of systemic effects.

Sterne and Morgane (1977) have shown that injections of bovine growth hormone in rats will increase REM sleep, and again this could be interpreted as signs of increased protein synthesis in the brain, and of REM sleep being linked with brain restitution. However, the authors pointed out that these findings, as well as those from the drug studies just described, could be due to changes in REM sleep triggering mechanisms, without affecting any underlying function of REM sleep (e.g. protein synthesis facilitation). Sterne and Morgane proposed that these two factors could be teased out by observing whether or not there was any subsequent REM sleep rebound. A nil rebound would indicate that it was the triggering mechanism that was being affected, and a positive rebound would imply it was the underlying function.

There seem to be qualitative changes in RNA turnover in neurones during sleep, but these changes are dependent upon the neurone type, and the overall significance of these changes for protein synthesis, etc. are not really known. One of the most recent studies in this area was by Giuditta *et al.* (1980a, b). The content of radioactively labelled RNA within large nuclei (of neuronal and astroglial origin) taken from the rabbit cerebral cortex was found to increase with increasing EEG synchrony (presumably increasing sleep 'depth'), indicating that this labelling was lowest during REM sleep. While a significant but smaller trend in the opposite direction was found with cytoplasmic (ribosomal) RNA, no changes of either sort were observed for cells with small nuclei (of oligodendroglial origin). The only conclusions that can be drawn from these findings for a brain restitution perspective is that RNA changes of unknown significance do occur in sleep and the quality and quantity of these changes vary with the type of neural tissue examined. The situation is further complicated by the review of brain RNA and protein synthesis by Dunn and Rees (1977) who pointed out that for various reasons, it is almost impossible to relate changes in the labelling of RNA to changes in RNA synthesis, let alone try and draw conclusions for protein synthesis.

9.4 Obligatory Sleep

The theme running through this section is that *only a part of mammalian sleep seems to be obligatory*, perhaps serving some form of essential cerebral restitution, and that *the remainder of sleep is 'facultative', being able to accommodate such restitution if necessary*. In essence, facultative sleep is a more flexible form of sleep, designed to keep the organism asleep for a sleep length which is optimal for purposes of energy conservation, keeping the organism out of harm's way, or simply relieving boredom. This facultative sleep is well engrained into the sleep habit, although it is amenable to change. It could represent *some form of basic (non-restorative) sleep drive*, which shows a distinct circadian rhythm. The need to sleep at *the beginning of the usual sleep period may well be brought about by both obligative (restitutive) and facultative mechanisms running concurrently*. However, it seems that the former lifts more rapidly during the usual sleep period, leaving the facultative mechanism to carry on. In humans, Stages 3 and 4 sleep (particularly the latter), that is delta activity, and the first few sleep cycles in which this is contained, together with the accompanying non-REM and REM sleep, may well represent this obligatory sleep. Much of our nightly REM and non-REM sleep occurs in later cycles, and it will be proposed that these forms of non-REM and REM sleep may be largely facultative. It should be noted that the terms obligatory sleep and facultative sleep have been used by Parmeggiani *et al.*, (1969) and Ruckesbuch (1972a, 1977).

9.4.1 Recovery Sleep Following Sleep Deprivation

The psychological performance impairments and behavioural changes produced by sleep deprivation are largely reversed after only 1–3 nights of recovery sleep, even in the longest deprivation studies (Pasnau *et al.*, 1968; Johnson *et al.*, 1965). Whilst it appears that much of the lost sleep is never regained, there are substantial qualitative changes in this recovery sleep whereby, over the first few recovery nights, most of the lost Stage 4 sleep is reclaimed, but less so for the lost REM sleep. On the other hand, as far as can be ascertained from the limited number of recovery nights recorded, all of the lost Stages 1 and 2 seem to be lost for good. For example, in the 265-h deprivation study (Gulevich *et al.*, 1966) the single subject was allowed to sleep ad lib on each of the first 3 recovery nights, which were recorded. From Table 9.2 summarizing these data, it can be seen that on the first night, sleep was double the usual length, with Stage 4 and REM sleep being about 3–4 times greater than for baseline values. Over the 3 nights, a total of 68% and 53% of the lost Stages 4 and REM sleep were regained respectively. Recovery of these two types of sleep was clearly incomplete by the end of the third night, and extrapolation of the data would suggest that there was more Stage 4 sleep than REM sleep to come over the next few nights. In all, only

Table 9.2 Recovery Sleep

Characteristics following 11 nights total sleep deprivation. From Gulevich *et al.* (1966). (1 subject) Note that recovery was incomplete by recovery 3. (TST = total sleep time)

	Sleep stages (min)				
	2	3	4	REM	TST
Baseline*	205	42	23	65	390
Total lost	2255	462	253	715	4290
Recovery sleep nights: amount in excess of baseline					
Recovery 1	192	91	90	171	490
Recovery 2	53	67	44	123	235
Revovery 3	19	56	37	87	153
Total	264	214	171	381	878
% regained	12%	46%	68%	53%	20%

* Average of 6 and 10 week post-sleep deprivation follow-up nights.

Table 9.3

Recovery sleep characteristics following 8 nights total sleep deprivation. From Kales *et al.* (1970). Total sleep time data unavailable owing to 12, 9 and 9 h limitations to recovery sleep.

	Sleep stages (min)			
	2	3	4	REM
Baseline	265	63	38	104
Amount lost	2120	504	304	832
Recovery sleep nights: amount excess of baseline				
Recovery 1	– 76	37	126	154
Recovery 2	– 114	24	70	81
Recovery 3	– 39	23	42	39
Total	– 229	84	238	274
% regained	– 11%	17%	78%	33%

about 20% of the total sleep lost seemed to have been regained over these first 3 nights.

The 205-h deprivation study (Kales *et al.*, 1970) also reported on the first 3 recovery nights, but here, the sleep was restricted to 12, 9 and 9 h over these nights. From Table 9.3, also summarizing the data, it can be seen that over the 3 nights 70% of the lost Stage 4 sleep was regained, and there was obviously more to come. Only 33% of the lost REM sleep was reclaimed, although again, there was more to come. *Both these studies indicate a greater pressure for the return of lost Stage 4 sleep than for the return of the lost REM sleep*. Indeed, further REM sleep may have been reclaimed moe gradually over many subsequent recovery nights, but the key point to be made here is that for both studies, *psychological performance and behaviour seemed to be back to normal levels by the fourth recovery day, despite any REM sleep deficiency*.

Shorter-term sleep deprivation investigations of 1–2 nights duration (Berger *et al.*, 1971; Williams *et al.*, 1964; Horne, 1976; Benoit *et al.*, 1980; Borbély *et al.*, 1981) show similar Stage 4 and REM sleep rebound characteristics, with the emphasis on an almost complete Stage 4 reclaim, and about a 30% return of the entire sleep loss.

9.4.2 Partial Sleep Deprivation and Chronic Sleep Reduction

Clearly, humans can oversleep by 90 min or so, simply by going back to sleep after the usual morning awakening (Verdone, 1968; Aserinsky, 1969, 1973; Webb & Agnew, 1975; Feinberg *et al.*, 1980). Although it has been argued that humans may be chronically sleep deprived (Webb & Agnew, 1975), there is little other evidence to support such an hypothesis, and it is more likely that this extra sleep is probably superfluous type of facultative sleep. Further evidence favouring this latter hypothesis will be discussed in Section 9.4.3. Because the EEG quality of this sleep is similar to that of the last 1–2 sleep cycles of our usual night's sleep, it is possible that these cycles may also be superfluous from a restitutional standpoint. Although short-term partial sleep deprivation studies indicate that these two cycles are necessary to prevent daytime sleepiness, it will be seen that what might be called 'cerebral capacity' is not impaired, and it is proposed that this sleepiness is due to some residual facultative effect from the already mentioned non-restorative facultative sleep drive.

One of the most elaborate of these short-term studies (Wilkinson, 1968) reduced sleep to 0, 1, 2, 3, or 5 h per night form 7.5 h per night, for 2 consecutive nights. The author applied a signal detection theory analysis to vigilance data, and described the courses of d′ and β (Swets *et al.*, 1961). d′, which can be considered to be a form of measure of the inherent functioning capacity of the cerebrum (as opposed to a subject's motivation or 'willingness' to perform, which is reflected in β) did not display an appreciable decline on the first night until sleep was down to about 3 h per night, and then fell substantially. On the second night there was a more evident decline in d′ from 7 h to 3 h of sleep per night. This decline became much more severe on further sleep reduction. On the other hand, β dropped rapidly (less willingness) from 7.5 h to 3 h sleep per night and then improved, indicating an increase in compensatory effort trying to overcome the failing d′. This trend in β was similar for both deprivation nights. While no sleep EEG records were taken, the author noted that the severe decline in d′ from 3 to zero hours sleep per night coincided with the part of sleep containing the majority of Stage 4 sleep. He speculated that provided that the usual amount of Stage 4 sleep is obtained, there will only be a limited reduction in cerebral capacity to perform, although willingness and motivation to perform will be affected. This is one of the earliest reports indicating that Stage 4 sleep may be some form of obligatory sleep, necessary to overcome a decline in cerebral capacity.

Further indications of some sort of optionality in at least the last two usual sleep cycles comes from two longer-term investigations of chronic sleep reduction (Johnson & Macleod, 1973; Friedman *et al.*, 1977). Both came from the same laboratory and used similar designs. A total of ten subjects systematically reduced their sleep length by 0.5 h every three weeks, from an initial 7.5–8 h sleep per day, until they could go no further. Problems of difficulty in arising and daytime sleepiness began to appear when sleep was down to about 6 h, and most subjects gave up at the 5 h point. There were no significant performance impairments up to this point. However, practice effects could not be fully assessed as there was no control group undergoing regular performance assessment without sleep reduction. Hence, any performance detriment due to sleep loss may have been offset by an improvement due to practice. Nevertheless, probably the most significant finding from both studies was that a 10 month to 1 year follow-up, showed that the subjects *had maintained 1–2.5 h sleep reductions without any adverse effects such as daytime sleepiness or difficulty in arising*. Another shorter-term partial sleep deprivation study (Webb & Agnew, 1974) required subjects to reduce their sleep to 5.5 h per day, from their usual 7.5–8 h per day, and maintain this regimen for 60 days. Few psychological performance deficits were found, but again, as no control group was used, the findings may have been confounded by practice effects.

All three of these longer-term partial sleep deprivation studies provided data on the quality of the restricted sleep, and all indicated that sleep had become shortened rather than condensed. That is, subjects responded by *demonstrating a*

Table 9.4 Sleep Stage Minutes under Gradual Sleep Reduction

Note that proportions of REM and Stage 3 sleep remain constant, but Stage 4 increases. From Mullaney *et al.* (1977).

Sleep length (h)	Stage 3	Stage 4	Stages 3 + 4	REM sleep
8	34	48	82	115
7½	36	45	81	112
7	38	42	80	101
6½	39	58	97	101
6	36	54	90	90
5½	30	56	86	82
5	30	51	81	81
4½	27	35	62	67
Follow-up (6 h)	36	58	94	90

loss of the latter part of sleep rather than pro rata reductions in all of the sleep stages. For example, from Table 9.4, adapted from Mullaney *et al.* (1977) (which is the sister paper to Friedman *et al.*) it can be seen that the absolute level of Stage 4 sleep was unaffected, but REM sleep was reduced. In relative terms, Stage 4 sleep increased and REM sleep remained about the same, and it should be noted that these findings also applied to the later follow-up sleep.

9.4.3 Extension of Sleep

Flexibility of sleep length makes sense if one considers humans before the advent of artificial lighting. In the UK the ratio of daily hours of light to dark goes from 16:8 to 8:16 from summer to winter. Given that we are visually oriented animals, requiring reasonably good light to interact with the environment, the ability to change sleep length by a few hours over the year may well have helped overcome boredom of the long hours of winter darkness and have kept us out of harm's way. Relaxation and lack of stimulation in the daytime also promotes sleep, and it would seem that such (facultative) sleep can also act as a time-filler, contrasting with the more obligatory form of sleep already described.

As already noted, sleep can be extended relatively easily by asking subjects to return to sleep upon their normal awakening. Similarly, subjects not used to taking daytime naps can usually nap quite easily (Evans *et al.*, 1977). Karacan *et al.* (1970) reported that naps taken in the morning contained a preponderance of REM sleep and little SWS (an observation confirmed by Agnew & Webb, 1973; Moses *et al.*, 1973; Hume & Mills, 1975; Akerstedt & Gillberg, 1981), whereas afternoon naps contained more SWS and less REM sleep. Although subjects had taken extra sleep during the day, there was no shortening of the subsequent night's total sleep time, again suggesting, like the findings from the extended sleep studies, that this extra nap sleep was in many respects superfluous.

Karacan *et al.* also observed important qualitative changes in the subsequent sleep. Whilst the extra REM sleep of both the morning and afternoon naps *resulted in no pro rata reductions in the following night's REM sleep, there were such reductions for SWS.* Similar findings were also reported by Whitehead *et al.* (1969). Consequently, the ability of REM sleep to be extended and the role of this extra REM sleep, need to be explained by proponents of hypotheses specifically identifying REM sleep as the type of sleep oriented towards brain restitution.

The daily amount of SWS cannot be extended by taking extra sleep; quite the reverse in fact, as this sleep is positively correlated with the length of prior wakefulness (Webb & Agnew, 1971). If sleep is substituted for part of this wakefulness, SWS is often reduced. A positive relationship between wakefulness and SWS is, of course, indicated in the recovery sleep data following total sleep deprivation. REM sleep, on the other hand, shows the opposite temporal trends to SWS by not being related to the length of prior wakefulness, but being positively correlated to the length of sleep (Agnew & Webb, 1973). A strong circadian rhythm in REM sleep has been observed, with SWS showing only slight circadian trends (Berger *et al.*, 1971; Moses *et al.*, 1975; Hume & Mills, 1975; Zulley, 1980; Czeisler *et al.*, 1980; Akerstedt & Gillberg, 1981) and this will be described in the next section.

All of the extended sleep studies (Aserinsky, 1969, 1973; Verdone, 1968, Feinberg *et al.*, 1980) reported that the extended sleep contained mostly Stage 2 sleep, little SWS, and about 25–30% REM sleep. The EEG of this superfluous REM sleep as well as that of the last 1–2 usual sleep cycles, appears similar to the REM sleep EEG found during much of a usual night's sleep. Detailed spectral analyses of the usual nightly succession of REM cycles by Borbély *et al.* (1981) has only revealed some decrease in total power density in the delta range from the first to the second REM cycle; beyond this latter cycle there was no obvious further trend. Finally, both Aserinsky (1969) and Feinberg *et al.* (1980) noted a steady increase in eye movement density during REM sleep periods up to about 7 h of sleep, and Aserinsky considered this density as an index of sleep satiety. Both groups also reported that the duration of REM sleep periods decreased during extended sleep, but the frequency of REM cycling increased.

9.4.4 Circadian Rhythm of Sleep Propensity

The propensity for sleep is not necessarily governed by the amount of prior wakefulness (although this is the case for SWS) but follows a distinct circadian rhythm. A large and systematic study into the relationships between total sleep time, temperature phase and REM sleep preponderance has recently been completed by Czeisler *et al.* (1980). Twelve subjects lived under free-running conditions for 16–189 days. The major finding concerned the relationship between temperture phase and sleep length. When self-selected bedtimes were near the temperature cycle minimum, the average sleep duration was about 7.8 h, whereas if a subject chose to retire at the temperature cycle maximum, sleep length averaged 14.4 h. This relationship persisted even when the chosen bedtime followed more than 20 h of prior wakefulness. No significant correlation was observed between sleep duration and length of prior wakefulness (provided that subjects had been awake for at least 14 h previously).

Circadian peaks of tiredness corresponded with the temperature troughs, and not surprisingly, the greatest likelihood of going to bed. It should be remembered that similar circadian rhythms of tiredness have been reported by several total sleep deprivation studies (Section 9.2.1). Czeisler *et al.* noted that the propensity for REM sleep was greatest about 4 h after the temperature cycle trough and lowest about 6 h after the temperature maximum. Stage 4 sleep exhibited little by way of a circadian rhythm, but as expected, was positively correlated with the length of prior wakefulness. Czeisler *et al.* concluded that there was a clear relationship between the circadian rhythms of REM sleep and body temperature and that both can oscillate together at a period different from that of the sleep–wake cycle itself. Most (86%) spontaneous endings of sleep occurred on the upturn of the temperature cycle, and it would appear that this may be a trigger for wakening. Hence, if bedtime occurs after this point, the duration of sleep continues until this point is reached again. Similar conclusions about the relationship between the temperature cycle and REM sleep were made by Zulley (1980).

If the findings by Czeisler *et al.* can be translated into non-free-running clock times, and circadian temperature peak and trough times are assumed to be about 19.00 and 05.00 respectively, then the propensity to display the most and least amounts of REM sleep will be at about 09.00 and 01.00 respectively. These estimates are supported by the nap sleep study of Moses *et al.* (1975), the split sleep investigation by Hume and Mills (1978), and more recently by the 'displaced sleep' experiment by Akerstedt and Gillberg (1981). Here, six subjects had their sleep shifted to different times of the day under a time-free (but not necessarily free-running) environment. Sleep was allowed to end spontaneously. As expected, the likelihood to wake coincided with the circadian peak of least tiredness. The authors noted that as time awake increased from 23.00 to 11.00, sleep length, accumulated REM sleep and self-reported sleepiness actually decreased. They suggested some sort of barrier to sleep at about noon. No matter what the sleep length, SWS seemed to be completed well before the end of sleep, and was mostly related to the length of prior wakefulness.

If sleep were wholly restitutive, then it is very difficult to see what restitutional purpose would be served by the extended sleep which can occur at more unusual times of the day. This sleep must simply be facultative and, in many respects, superfluous. Again, the near absence of SWS in this extended sleep and the apparent dependence of SWS upon length of prior wakefulness suggest that this form of sleep, and presumably its associated non-REM and REM sleep, are of some necessity, perhaps for brain restitution. In contrast, the preponderance of REM sleep at a time of day (late morning) when a (restitutional?) need for sleep seems least necessary, suggests that this type of REM sleep may even be some form of substitute for wakefulness. Hence, we may now begin to view REM sleep as possibly of two types, 'restitutive' (obligatory) and 'non-restitutive' (facultative). Possibly, the two may be differentiated by the amount of delta activity they contain, with the former containing more than the latter.

9.4.5 *Naturally Long and Short Human Sleepers*

Total sleep time amongst healthy sleepers follows a normal distribution within any age group. For example, in young adults the mean and standard deviation are about 7.5 and 1 h respectively. Webb and Agnew (1970) reported on the sleep stage characteristic of long (8.5 h and above) and short (6.5 h and below)

Table 9.5 Sleep Stage Characteristics of Long and Short Sleepers
From Webb & Agnew (1970).

	Minutes		
	Long (8½ h +)	Short (6½ h −)	Control
Stages 0 + 1 + 2	317	182	241
3	22	18	29
4	72	81	81
REM	155	96	101
Total	566	377	452

good sleepers, and it can be seen from a summary of the authors' data in Table 9.5 that the amounts of SWS in both groups was about the same. The differences lay in the amounts of REM sleep and other non-REM sleep stages. A later study by Webb and Friel (1971) on 9.5 h and above versus 5.5 h and below sleepers, produced similar findings with regard to these sleep stages, and reported that the two groups did not differ on a battery of personality, scholastic and medical measures. However, in the earlier study, short sleepers seemed to be more hypomanic. Johns *et al.* (1974) reported that short sleepers rated higher on the MMPI hysteria scale, and Hicks and Pellegrini (1977) found their short sleepers to be more anxious. The most recent study of such sleepers was by Benoit *et al.* (1980). Short and long sleepers had mean sleep times of 5 h and 9 h respectively, and again, the sleep stage differences between the two groups were similar to those reported by Webb and Agnew (1970). In particular, REM and Stage 2 sleep differed between the two groups by a factor of two.

Interestingly, Benoit *et al.* (1980) also a sleep deprived the two groups for 36 h. While the average sleep length of the short sleepers was significantly lengthened, this was not so for the long sleepers. SWS increased to a similar extent in the two groups, with REM sleep also increasing (by 30%) in the short sleepers, but not in the long sleepers. This study also confirmed the findings, already described, of a negative relationship between body temperature slope and the durations of total sleep and REM sleep. It might seem as though *the long sleepers had more facultative sleep in their usual sleep than did short sleepers*, and that this has the capacity to take up any extra obligatory sleep need.

Individuals naturally sleeping less than 3–4 standard deviations below the norm (e.g. less than 3.5 h sleep in the case of middle-aged adults) will be very rare. No non-sleepers have ever been found, although a few particularly short, natural, non-insomniac sleepers have been reported. Jones and Oswald (1966) found two male subjects, aged 30 and 54, who averaged 164 min sleep per day between them, and Stuss and Broughton (1978) described one 57-year-old man who slept on average 97 min per day. All three subjects had similar absolute amounts of SWS, which occupied about 50% of total sleep, and although in relative terms this was about three times the age-related norm, it was normal in absolute terms. They exhibited little absolute and relative amounts of REM sleep, ranging from an average of 14% for the subjects of Jones and Oswald to 6% for the other subject. What is of particular importance with all three subjects is that the absolute and relative amounts of REM sleep, Stage 2 and SWS were akin to what would be expected from *similar lengths of sleep taken from usual sleep onset* in age-related normal sleepers. One might speculate, therefore, that these very short sleepers are down to their obligatory minimum of sleep and have little facultative sleep.

A third report by Meddis *et al.* (1973), of a 70-year-old woman, found very variable amounts (0–204 min) of night-time sleep over a six-day study period. Average data revealed 67 min sleep per night with absolute SWS levels similar to that of the age-related norm. The amount of REM sleep was similar (10 min) to that found in the first sleep cycle of the norm. Although the authors noted that her daily temperature peak was at night, with the trough during the day, the possibility that her sleep–wake rhythm was also 180° out of phase was not discussed. This may have affected the findings as sleep-EEG records were taken only at night-time.

Jones and Oswald described the behaviour of their subjects as vigorous but not hypomanic, but no personality measures were performed. Stuss and Broughton, on the other hand, in assessing the personalities of six very short sleepers (1.5–4 h per day) (one of whom had the sleep EEGs taken) reported that MMPI scores indicated four subjects to have tendencies for hypomania and repression, but nevertheless seemed well adjusted. No personality tests were given to Meddis *et al.*'s subject, although she was described as despising inactivity and kept busy. (My own observation of her later indicated that she was very active, continually fidgeting and talking, and seemingly unable to cease activity.) Overall then, these very short sleepers seem to be very active, if not hypomanic. Hence the question arises whether this activity and the short sleep are related, and if so is one factor causing the other or are they both the result of some common cause? Unfortunately, little further information is available to resolve these questions. Nevertheless, it would seem that notwithstanding their limited sleep *these subjects lead healthy and relatively normal lives*. They have no obvious cognitive deficits, particularly of memory (despite their little REM sleep), or seem to suffer any problems of physical health which could be ascribed to a 'lack of body restitution'. Of course, it could be argued that what sleep they do have is of superior restitutive quality than that of normal sleepers, and while the relatively large amounts of SWS suggest that this may be so, it must be remembered that the SWS obtained by these people only seems to be equivalent to the first part of sleep in age-related normal sleepers.

9.4.5 *Selective Deprivation of SWS and REM Sleep*

Because of the putative need for SWS, particularly of Stage 4 sleep, it might be expected that Stage 4 sleep deprivation would have a more adverse effect than the deprivation of all other forms of sleep, including REM sleep. However, it has been postulated, here, that REM sleep associated with SWS cycles may be of significant restitutive benefit, and both REM sleep and SWS may well work in harmony in this respect. So to deprive selectively one or other of these sleep states would adversely affect the integrity of any restitutive processes during obligatory sleep. It is not therefore surprising that all of the few studies which have compared the psychological performance effects of both forms of sleep deprivation have reported no significant difference in the amounts of performance decrement between the two conditions (Agnew *et al.*, 1967; Lubin *et al.*, 1974; Johnson *et al.*, 1974).

While there have been so few studies of Stage 4 or SWS deprivation, there have been numerous investigations into REM sleep deprivation (RSD) alone, with most using rodents. RSD has been total or near total in all these studies and, for example, they have not just reduced the amount of REM sleep in the latter part of sleep. Such data would have been of particular interest to the present viewpoint as the functions of obligatory and facultative REM sleep are presumed to differ.

The most detailed and recent review of the effects of RSD has been by McGrath and Cohen (1978). For both human and rodent studies, the literature was categorized under (1) type of experimental design (pre-RSD, post-RSD, and mixed), and (2) the degree of task complexity (prepared vs unprepared). This latter division was instituted primarily because of the proposal by Greenberg and Pearlman (1974) that REM sleep is not funtionally oriented to the consolidation of the learning of habitual responses closely linked with survival, but is necessary for the consolidation of learning which involves the assimilation of unusual material. In this respect, 'prepared tasks' were interpreted by McGrath and Cohen to mean that the organism has a built-in readiness to perceive, store and relate to the tasks, such that successful adjustments to the tasks are made quickly and tend to persist longer (p. 26). 'Unprepared tasks' implies less biological preparedness, and learning more typical of the laboratory condition.

With rodent studies, McGrath and Cohen concluded that prior-RSD (RSD followed by training and testing) produced similar performance decrements for both RSD and 'stress control' conditions with both types of task. On the other hand, subsequent RSD (training followed by RSD and testing) and mixed RSD do generally result in a greater decremental effect of RSD, particularly with unprepared tasks. With humans, and for prepared tasks, it appeared that for both prior and post-RSD conditions (there being no 'mixed' studies), RSD had no greater effect than equivalent amounts of non-REM sleep deprivation, although there seems to be a significantly greater decrement with RSD for unprepared tasks. Finally, while intense daytime learning does seem to increase REM sleep as well as non-REM sleep in rodents, McGrath and Cohen concluded that this is not so for humans.

Overall, the literature on REM sleep and learning does suggest that REM sleep may be involved in the consolidation of complex learning. However there are several methodological problems associated with rodent studies and generally, it is not known to what extent these findings are specific to RSD alone, rather than to a more intense form of sleep deprivation. As will be seen in Section 9.5.4, there are reasons unrelated to a learning consolidation hypothesis for REM sleep, that these findings may indeed be specific to REM sleep. Much of the learning impairment attributed to RSD could, for example, be an artefact of an apparent arousing effect of RSD (to be described). Hence, application of an inverted 'U' model of arousal and performance (Yerkes & Dodson, 1908; Hebb, 1955) would predict that increased arousal would lead to a decline in learning performance, which would be more severe for complex and unprepared tasks; a situation similar to that found with RSD.

Finally, another factor which has to be taken into account when one considers any specific role REM sleep may have with the consolidation of learning, concerns the drop in REM sleep during the early ontogeny of all mammals. In humans, for example, the daily amounts of REM sleep fall progressively and substantially by about 320 min per 24 h in the age period from 1 week to 4 years, compared with only a 90-min drop in non-REM sleep (Williams *et al.*, 1974). This age span encompasses a period of considerable learning, which would presumably invoke a great need for learning and memory consolidation. If all of REM sleep was functionally oriented towards these processes, *then such a drop would not be expected*. It would seem therefore that whilst some REM sleep may well be associated with this consolidation, a significant proportion of REM sleep is not for this purpose.

9.4.6 Obligatory and Facultative Sleep in Other Mammals

The concept of obligatory and facultative sleep has been applied to the sleep of other mammals (Parmeggiani *et al.*, 1969, 1980; Ruckesbusch, 1972a, 1975, 1977). Farm animals sleep about 30% more in the safe confines of a stable than in the open field, and Ruckesbusch (1972a) referred to this extra sleep as 'luxury sleep'. A cross-species statistical survey by Allison and Cicchetti (1976) correlated several sleep variables with safety factors, and reported a significant positive correlation between sleep safety and usual sleep length. Interestingly, although both REM and non-REM sleep were less in the vulnerable sleepers, a significantly greater reduction was apparent in REM sleep; findings again suggesting a degree of redundancy in REM sleep.

Parmeggiani *et al.* (1969, 1980), Parmeggiani and Sabbatini (1972) performed studies on cats sleeping in a cold environment. One of the significant effects (see also Section 9.5.3) was a reduction in total sleep time mostly at the expense of REM sleep; the colder the environment, the less sleep. Recovery sleep in a thermoneutral environment showed no REM sleep rebound until the amount of prior REM sleep deprivation exceeded about 40–50%. The authors referred to the non-rebound REM sleep as 'facultative' with the remainder being 'obligate'. They were amongst the first to use these terms within the context of sleep. Interestingly, findings similar to these have also been observed with man sleeping in the cold (Buguet *et al.*, 1979). A 20% reduction in REM sleep over 16 nights resulted in no subsequent REM sleep rebound.

All mammals sleep, despite some earlier claims to the contrary. If sleep were entirely facultative, or non-restitutional, *mammals living under very adverse sleeping conditions would be expected to forego sleep entirely*. Kristal and Noonan (1979) observed in a non-EEG study of sleep in the giraffe that this animal lies down for periods of between 3 and 75 min, 3–8 times a night. While most of this time is spent awake, chewing cud and with the neck vertical, part of the time is taken up by sleep, with what was assumed to be non-REM sleep (neck 'S' shaped, no cud chewing and with open but unfocused eyes) lasting 5–30 min, followed by short periods of putative REM sleep (head and neck rotated on to the flank in a 'sleeping swan' position, with eyes closed) lasting for 1–10 min. Sleep totalled about 2 h per night, but this is clearly a particularly vulnerable state in such an ungainly animal, which for example, takes 10 or so seconds to stand up. Presumably the advantage of sleep in this mammal outweighs the disadvantage, and it would be reasonable to conclude that its sleep is at an obligatory minimum, with little facultative sleep. The giraffe is quite able to display long periods of relaxed wakefulness at night-time. So if there were no essential need for sleep, evolution would presumably have extended this relaxed wakefulness by a further 2 h or so, and have eliminated sleep entirely.

Further evidence for an essential need of some sleep comes from studies of sleep in the dolphin. Pilleri (1979) reported that the blind Indus dolphin (Platanista indi), which lives in turbid and muddy estuarine waters, has to keep constantly on the move or else risk injury on rocks, etc. While no EEG assessments were performed, the author was able to monitor sound emissions from these animals and claimed that these ceased only during sleep. Sleep periods lasted for only about 90 s at a time, but were very frequent, summating to about 7 h a day. This animal must sleep under one of the most hazardous of circumstances, and again it is argued here, that if sleep were entirely inessential, evolution would have removed it, as it has done to this animal's sight. Instead, evolution has altered the scheduling of sleep in a remarkable way.

Even more intriguing is the sleep in both the bottlenose dolphin (Tursiops truncatus) and the Black Sea porpoise (Phocoena phocoena), reported on by Mukhametov *et al.* (1977) and Mukhametov & Polyakova (1981) respectively. Electrocorticograms (ECoGs) were performed on free-swimming animals. During wakefulness there is typical bilateral synchrony of the ECoG, however, in the sleep period the animals sleep with one hemisphere at a time, with the other remaining awake. This condition lasts for about 1 h and is followed by 1 h of wakefulness in both hemispheres, with bilateral ECoG symmetry. Then follows 1 h of unilateral sleep in the other hemisphere. This 3-h cycle is repeated throughout the night. Of considerable importance were the claims by both groups of authors that both species had no apparent REM sleep, in terms of ECoG, of eye movements, or, as Kovalzon (1977) reported, of no temperature changes in the desynchronized ECoG hemisphere. Clearly, there have been sophisticated developments to the neural pathways controlling sleep in these animals, as demonstrated by the remarkable unilateral isolation of a sleeping hemisphere. Here is an advanced state of sleep evolution, and it is *difficult to conceive why such a further development should occur if (some) sleep was not essential.* Body movements do not cease during these animals' sleep, and so it would seem that sleep offers little by way of energy conservation. However, this development may be a response for maintaining respiratory ventilation, as drug-induced bilateral ECoG synchrony produces partial apnoea (Mukhametov & Polyakova, 1981). Nevertheless, the point is that sleep has been modified and retained, and the cortical isolation suggests a need for the cerebrum itself to sleep.

Hypotheses claiming that mammalian sleep has no restorative benefit, (particularly for the brain) and that sleep is an adaptive non-behaviour simply to occupy unproductive hours (Webb, 1976), or a redundant instinct (Meddis, 1977), may have difficulty in explaining the sleep characteristics of dolphins, if not of the giraffe. Any rebuttal that the sleep of these animals simply reflects behavioural adaptation to an optimal level, is inadequate *unless the question of the behavioural advantages of the remaining sleep in these advanced mammals is addressed further.* For reasons already described in Sections 9.2.1–9.2.6, it is likely that these mammals obtain as much, if not more, body restitution during wakefulness than in sleep, particularly as they are able to demonstrate prolonged periods of relatively relaxed wakefulness. On the other hand, like humans they have advanced cerebral cortices (i.e. having substantial cerebral convolutions), and this is the most likely target organ for sleep function. As already described in Section 9.3.2, owing to the lack of available technology, there is to date no substantive evidence of neurochemical changes within the brain which can be claimed to be restitutive and solely confined to sleep. Consequently, proposals eschewing a brain restitutive role for sleep, based on the absence of positive findings, seem premature if not dogmatic.

9.5 The Functional Significance of Other REM Sleep Epiphenomena

9.5.1 Brain Metabolism

While obligatory REM sleep may well have some restorative role for the brain, probably interacting with SWS and/or delta activity in this respect, it has been argued in Section 9.4 that a significant amount of REM sleep is surplus to this requirement. The various neurophysiological phenomena which accompany REM sleep, taken by many investigators as support for a restitutive role, *occur as soon as REM sleep commences, regardless of when in sleep the REM period occurs*. As these phenomena appear both in what has been identified as obligatory and facultative REM sleep, their significance for any restitutive aspects of REM sleep might now seem obscure, and perhaps can be viewed as 'epiphenomena', along the lines described by Moruzzi (1966, 1972).

Increases in neural firing rates during REM sleep provide little guidance to REM sleep function. For example, these increases are more evident in brainstem and midbrain structures rather than in the cerebrum, where restitution is believed to be more necessary. High firing rates may well militate against efficient restitution, for similar reasons already described with muscle (Section 9.3), that is, inactivity not activity promotes recovery. Although certain cortical neurones fire more rapidly during REM sleep, others reduce their firing rate (Evarts, 1961). As already noted in Section 9.3.2, what is clear is that it is the pattern and organization of firing which changes during this sleep, not so much the rate. Non-REM sleep has its own distinct firing patterns, and like those of REM sleep, these provide little help for the understanding of sleep function.

Brain metabolism does seem to increase during REM sleep, to much greater levels than those found in either non-REM sleep or in relaxed wakefulness. Although there is a paucity of direct measurement during sleep (cf. Seisjo, 1978) there is a highly significant positive correlation between EEG frequency and cerebral oxygen uptake ($CMRO_2$) in humans during waking states (cf. Ingvar *et al.*, 1979), indicating that $CMRO_2$ will be raised in REM sleep compared with that of non-REM sleep. There have been several studies of brain blood flow (BBF) during sleep in both animals and humans, and without doubt, BBF rises substantially during REM sleep, and this finding has been taken as a sign of increased $CMRO_2$. However, as will be seen, this BBF increase appears to be well in excess of any raised $CMRO_2$ requirement.

Greater BBF increases during REM sleep have been found in the brainstem and midbrain than in the cerebrum, in both the cat (Reivich *et al.*, 1968) and humans (Sakai *et al.*, 1979), and this seems to be correlated with the differential neural firing rates. Both Seylaz *et al.* (1971) and Townsend *et al.* (1973) were among the first to consider that the REM sleep BBF increases were in excess of metabolic requirements, being under neural rather than metabolic control. For example, the increases were instantaneous on REM sleep onset and did not show the gradual increase expected through metabolic causes. One of the most detailed and recent studies on humans (Sakai *et al.*, 1979) reported that in both brainstem and cortical regions there was a progressive drop in BBF (totalling about 25%) from relaxed wakefulness, through Stages 1 and 2 sleep, to SWS. On the other hand, in both brain regions, REM sleep was accompanied by a 50% BBF increase from relaxed wakefulness levels. However, the reduced cerebral vasodilatory response to increased arterial blood pCO_2 levels during REM sleep suggested to the authors that, indeed, this particular BBF increase was largely under some central rather than metabolic control; the reason for this is unknown. Perhaps the one obvious conclusion which can be drawn from these BBF studies is that *during SWS the cerebrum seems to be in a greater state of rest than during REM sleep*.

There is an increase in brain temperature during REM sleep in several mammalian species, although, this is *not very evident in the monkey (Reite & Pegram, 1968), nor probably in humans*. Such increases have also been taken as signs of brain restitution, but this is almost certainly an erroneous conclusion (cf. Horne, 1977). These increases are particularly evident in mammals which utilize panting as the main (thermolytic) mechanism for disposing of waste heat from the body (e.g. the cat, dog and many even-toed ungulates). A carotid rete is located in the cavernous sinus of the nose, and blood travelling up the carotid artery is shunted through the rete where it is cooled, via a counter-current system, by the latent heat of water evaporation from the nasal mucosa. The first major organ encountered by the cooled blood is the brain. During REM sleep in these animals their thermolytic system becomes inoperative (cf. Hayward & Baker, 1969). This is probably due to the drying up of the nasal mucosa (which is particularly evident in REM sleep of the cow — Toutain & Ruckesbusch, 1972) and to the suppression of the panting response (which has been well documented for the cat — Parmeggiani & Sabbatini, 1972; Parmeggiani *et al.*, 1977). Consequently, heat clearance from the brain is reduced and the brain heats up.

Thermolytic organs in other animals, including humans, also become less effective during REM sleep, and in those animals where the brain is near to such an organ, brain temperature seems to increase for the same reasons as before. For example, the horns of certain even-toed ungulates act as minor thermolytic organs by virtue of their rich peripheral vascular supply. During REM sleep this blood flow is substantially reduced (Taylor, 1960), and a similar effect has been observed in the major thermolytic organ of the rabbit, the ear capillaries (Baker & Hayward, 1967). In humans, sweating during REM sleep is curtailed (Shapiro *et al.*, 1974; Henane *et al.*, 1977; Haskell *et al.*, 1981), although as noted, this seems to have little effect upon brain temperature. All these changes during REM sleep have been considered by some to be signs that REM sleep is a primitive thermoregulatory (poikilothermic) state, but it will be seen in Section 9.6.3 that this may not be quite the case.

9.5.2 REM Sleep Deprivation (RSD) and Arousal

There are numerous reports indicating that in rodents RSD produces a state of heightened cerebral excitability. For example, RSD reduced seizure thresholds have been reported by Cohen & Dement (1965), Cohen *et al.* (1970), Handwerker & Fishbein (1975), Hartmann *et al.* (1968), Owen & Bliss (1970) and enhanced recovery functions inevoked cortical potentials reported by Dewson *et al.* (1967), Satinoff *et al.* (1971). RSD diminishes fear in rats (Hicks & Moore, 1979), and it also seems to enhance drive motivated behaviour such as, intracranial self-stimulation (Cohen *et al.*, 1972; Steiner & Ellman, 1972), eating during the usual sleeping period (Elomaa & Johanasson, 1980a), aggressiveness (Hicks *et al.*, 1979; Mollenhour *et al.*, 1977; Morden *et al.*, 1968; Sloan, 1972), and exploratory or locomotor behaviour (Albert *et al.*, 1970; Elomaa & Johansson, 1980b; Hicks & Adams, 1976; Hicks & Moore, 1979; Moore *et al.*, 1979). In summary, the above effects of RSD seem to produce *enhanced drive-related behaviours, and increased arousal.*

In rodents, the enhancement of drive-related and stereotyped behaviours by RSD may well be a direct effect of REM sleep loss, indicating that this form of sleep may modulate drive-related behaviour, allowing a greater degree of behavioural plasticity. Such a hypothesis for REM sleep function has been postulated recently by Vogel (1979). Alternatively, these behaviours may be due indirectly to RSD via some form of stress, as they are very similar to those behaviour patterns elicited by stress alone. For example, in a non-sleep oriented review of stress behaviour in rodents, Antelman and Caggiula (1980) include amongst various stressors, frustration, confinement and isolation; all of which may be particularly pertinent to the usual RSD 'pedestal' procedure. This method is generally assumed to be 'stressful', because additional 'stress control conditions' are almost invariably employed. However, several reviewers have argued that such controls are inadequate (Plummer *et al.*, 1974; Vogel, 1975; Albert, 1975; Karnovsky & Reich, 1977; Ellman *et al.*, 1978). For example, in general terms, the control pedestal is larger, and so the animal is less confined, less frustrated, falls into the surrounding water less often and gets fewer sleep interruptions. Methodological problems prevent a non-REM sleep deprivation condition for rodents, and so it is not clear whether the behavioural effects of RSD are specific to RSD alone.

Increased stereotype may also have implications for Jouvet's (1978, 1980) 'genetic programming' hypothesis for REM sleep function, where it is proposed that REM sleep facilitates the transcription of genetic material associated with innate behaviour patterns. Any modification to these programmes would be accomplished in REM sleep. He has postulated that chronic RSD will inhibit the modification of these programmes by learning, and that a given behaviour pattern found in RSD treated animals will show a greater between-animal similarity (i.e. a greater degree of stereotyped behaviour) than for behaviour observed between animals not REM sleep deprived. However, the stress produced by RSD may also cause stereotype through the mechanisms just described, unrelated to Jouvet's hypothesis, and so give artificial support to his hypothesis.

The real significance for REM sleep function of the increases in stress, cerebral excitability and stereotyped behaviour which are apparent with RSD are not really known. Even Vogel's (1979) hypothesis provides only a part explanation and, for example, needs to be integrated with his well-known proposals that RSD is an effective method for treating depression (Vogel, 1975; Vogel *et al.*,

1980). All these effects may be the result of some common neurochemical change. But in turn these changes may well be an effect of a deeper cause and function of REM sleep.

Because of their more primitive cerebrum, rodents may require less REM sleep for cerebral restitutive purposes, if this is a function of (obligatory) REM sleep. Hence, for them much of this sleep may be facultative. If the arousal effects of RSD are indeed specific to REM sleep, it could be postulated that one function of facultative REM sleep is to reduce arousal, that is, promote sleep for the purposes of energy conservation, and so on. This suggestion has already been made with respect to human facultative REM sleep (Section 9.4.3), but more for the purposes of occupying the dark hours rather than for energy conservation.

In humans there have been relatively few studies on the effects of RSD on behaviour or on arousal. Although effects may be apparent, they appear not so marked as in the case of rodents. Increased appetite and aggression have been recorded by Dement (1965) and Sampson (1966), heightened sexual interest observed by Zarcone *et al.*, (1974) and elevated cortical excitability, as reflected in evoked cortical, potential changes, shown by Kopell *et al.* (1972).

Obviously, deprivation of both REM and non-REM sleep stages brings tiredness in humans, and from an uni-dimensional arousal perspective it would be erroneous to state that RSD simply brings arousal. However, arousal has more than one parameter; for example, Thayer (1979) has proposed a two dimensional model having two scales representing 'energy-sleep' and 'tension-placidity'. Such an approach can explain certain well-known arousal paradoxes, such as that displayed by the insomniac who is both tired and anxious. So to put these dimensions into the RSD and arousal perspective, it is possible that in humans at least, RSD may produce tension, but the inherent sleep deprivation causes sleepiness. However, in the absence of data from human RSD studies concerning details of these two dimensions, as well as the lack of data on psychophysiological measures of arousal during RSD, further speculation along these particular lines must be curtailed. Clearly, apart from a need for such studies, an examination needs to be made on the effects of RSD in the last 2–3 REM sleep periods within the usual human sleep period. Such deprivation of putative facultative REM sleep may have quite a different effect to that of total RSD, whereby the effects of obligatory RSD may even counter to some extent those of facultative RSD.

9.5.3 REM Sleep: A Primitive Form of Sleep?

It is tempting to draw parallels between the ontogeny of sleep and its phylogeny, but although Haeckel's (1866) theory of recapitulation (whereby ontogeny recapitulates phylogeny) can still be used for guidelines in various fields of biology, it has serious shortcomings (cf. de Beer, 1958). REM sleep is particularly evident very early on in mammalian ontogeny. However, there is as yet no clear evidence that it is present in reptiles or in more primitive animals, or for that matter in egg-laying mammals, although it is evident in birds (suggesting parallel evolution of REM sleep rather than evolution from a common ancestor). Nevertheless, REM sleep is often classed as 'primitive'. Such a viewpoint is endorsed by Jouvet (1961), but for different reasons. Because

REM sleep is primarily a hind brain (archibrain) phenomenon, he has referred to this sleep as 'archisleep'.

Non-REM sleep seems not so readily evident at the time of the first ontogenetic appearance of REM sleep, and in many respect it seems to be a later development. On the other hand, there is some recent evidence that certain aspects of non-REM sleep may be present in reptiles. Two studies of young caimans kept under environmental temperatures close to that of the natural habitat reported high voltage slow wave EEG activity similar to that of mammalian non-REM sleep (Warner & Huggins, 1978; Meglasson & Huggins, 1979). Although REM sleep is usually more preponderant in the young of birds and mammals, it was not evident in these young alligators. However, reptiles do display high voltage spikes during inactivity, and Walker and Berger (1980) have suggested that these may be analogues or homologues of pontine-geniculate-occipital (PGO) spikes of REM sleep. Consistent with this interpretation they claim, is evidence that EEG spiking activity in the tortoise is possibly generated by the optic lobe (Walker & Berger, 1973). Although Flanigan *et al.* (1973) originally suggested that reptilian EEG spikes were similar to PGO spikes, Flanigan (1974) subsequently argued that they were analogues of mammalian and avian slow waves. More recently, Hartse (1980) has reported that certain of the sub-cortical activities accompanying non-REM sleep in mammals, particularly the limbic spike (not to be confused with the PGO spike), are also found in reptiles. Furthermore, experimental manipulations which influenced this activity in mammals seemed to have similar effects with reptiles. So although the extent to which reptiles may or may not have REM and non-REM sleep is still a matter for debate, evidence favouring their having REM sleep is indeed limited.

The question of whether REM sleep is present in the monotremes is still unresolved as, so far, investigators have studied only adult animals (e.g. Allison *et al.*, 1972), and particularly, have not manipulated the environmental temperature. It must be remembered that REM sleep is not only preponderant in the young of mammals, but also enhanced during sleep under conditions of thermoneutrality (e.g. Szymusiak & Satinoff, 1981).

Findings proposed to support the primitiveness of REM sleep have come from various studies of thermoregulation, where it has been claimed that this sleep is poikilothermic, that is, a reversion to the reptilian thermoregulatory state (e.g. Parmeggiani & Sabbatini, 1972; Parmeggiani *et al.*, 1977; Heller & Glotzbatch, 1977; Walker & Berger, 1980). Although thermoregulation appears to become relatively unresponsive to changes in environmental temperature with, for example, impairments to shivering and panting (cf. Parmeggiani, 1980) (see Section 9.5.1), Horne (1977) has pointed out that REM sleep is probably not quite such a primitive thermoregulatory state. For example, if the usual definition of poikilothermy is taken to be limited thermogenesis and the inability to maintain a stable body temperature under varying environment temperatures, then such a difinition has only limited application to REM sleep, as there are no clear indications that either of these conditions is evident. Humans can display long periods of REM sleep, hence thermal inertia can be overcome to some extent. Here, body core temperature does not show any significant fall in a cold environment, and heat production (0_2 uptake) does not decline (cf. Haskell *et al.*, 1981). Also it must be remembered, that in humans REM sleep is preponderant at a time of the night when body temperature is rising (see Section 9.4.4), with little change in heat production (Dallosso *et al.*, 1982); an efficient state of affairs which would be unlikely to occur if REM sleep were truly poikilothermic.

While Parmeggiani *et al.* (1969, 1977) have reported a body temperature fall during REM sleep in cats sleeping at environmental temperatures below 0 °C, the measurement site was subcutaneous in the relatively hairless inguinal region; core temperature was not taken. Recent work on the Tasmanian Devil (Sarcophilus harrisii) by Nicol and Maskrey (1980) has found no core temperature fall during REM sleep in the cold, although it must be remembered that these mammals do have a relatively short REM period (similar to that of the cat), and that thermal inertia may have confounded the outcome.

An interesting finding by Walker *et al.* (1979) was the progressive diminution of REM sleep with increasing torpor, and although this was attributed to the hypothesis that REM sleep is a poikilothermic state, where body temperature cannot be satisfactorily stabilized etc., it could be argued that if REM sleep were poikilothermic, *this sleep could have been usefully adapted during evolution, for the purposes of promoting torpor*. Horne (1977, 1978) has proposed that REM sleep may be oriented towards energy (heat) conservation, rather than towards poikilothermy, whereby body temperature can be kept at an optimal level close to that of wakefulness, by reducing heat loss. If this were to be the case, then any need for sleep to progress into torpor would have to exclude REM sleep. That is, rather than REM sleep being unable to regulate a systematic drop in body temperature and stabilizing this at a low level, owing to its hypothesized poikilothermic nature, the alternative explanation from the present viewpoint is that REM sleep is incompatible with torpor as it is a form of sleep designed to maintain temperature at near waking levels.

Horne has postulated that the model taken for thermoregulatory changes during REM sleep should not be that of the reptilian condition, but that of early mammalian ontogeny. In the case of humans, for example, this would be up to the neonatal stage. The human newborn has a heterothermic-cum-homeothermic state of temperature control, maintained mostly by mechanisms effecting the reduction of heat loss, rather than by the heightening of shivering thermogenesis (cf. Smith, 1959); the latter method is poorly developed, as is active thermolysis (sweating). Non-shivering thermogenesis (brown adipose tissue — BAT thermogenesis) is a more primitive form of mammalian heat production and BAT deposits are well developed in the neonate, although this tissue seems to be largely absent in the adult. As REM sleep may be primarily a foetal state (to be described) carried into adulthood, it is possible that *during REM sleep in the adult, thermoregulation, as well as other homeostatic control mechanisms, revert to a foetal mode of control*. It should be noted that in the neonate, the level of these control mechanisms during REM sleep appears to be the same as those for other sleeping and waking conditions.

REM sleep is at its most abundant in the mammalian foetus, occupying most of sleep. As has been well demonstrated in the classical study by Jouvet-Mounnier *et al.* (1970), ontogenetic development of the CNS seems to be inversely related to the amount of REM sleep. These investigators reported that REM sleep occupied about 90% of sleep in the neonatal rat and cat, which are both born in an immature state of CNS development. On the other hand, the guinea-pig, which is born in a more mature state presents only about 15% of sleep as REM sleep. In its earlier foetal development, the guinea-pig displays much more REM sleep, comparable with that of the neonatal rat and cat.

REM sleep is the first of the two major sleep states (REM and non-REM sleep) to appear in the developing mammalian foetus (Astic, 1973). In humans, REM sleep is evident at six months post-conception, before recognizable non-REM sleep, and occupies much of sleep. It falls to about 50% of sleep at birth, and to about 30% three months later (cf. Williams *et al.*, 1974). In human REM sleep, there seems to be little qualitative change to the EEG over this postnatal period or thereafter. On the other hand, the non-REM sleep EEG undergoes a considerable change, particularly from birth to 3–6 months of age, probably reflecting changes in cerebral development (Dittrichova, 1969; Metcalf *et al.*, 1971; Sternman *et al.*, 1977; Feinberg *et al.*, 1977; Ellingson & Peters, 1980).

In essence then, *REM sleep may be a special adaptation for the foetal condition* (i.e. it is caenogenetic). De Beer (1957) pointed out that phylogenetic precedence is not necessary for caenogenetic developments, as for example, there are numerous special embryological adaptations to the mammalian lungs, liver, kidneys, thyroid and skull, which are not represented in any ancestral condition. REM sleep in the adult may be a vestige of that found in the foetus. Both obligatory and facultative REM sleep in the adult may serve similar functions to those of the foetus, with perhaps some changes, such as much more facultative REM sleep in the foetus. If REM sleep is essentially a foetal state, physiological regulatory mechanisms in adult REM sleep may revert to the foetal level of control.

The reduction of REM sleep over a short time period following birth, particularly in humans, suggests that this may be mostly with facultative REM sleep, which in certain respects may subserve wakefulness. It will be remembered that this form of REM sleep may be de-arousing in the adult, and the same may hold for foetal facultative REM sleep, i.e. the prevention of needless physical activity which would occur if the foetus spent more time awake. This may be not so much for energy conservation, but for minimizing physical discomfort to the mother. Also, as there is a relative lack of waking sensory stimulation for the foetus in the uterus, REM sleep may well substitute for this. A similar proposal to this latter suggestion has been made by Roffwarg *et al.* (1966) in their 'Ontogenetic Hypothesis'. They considered that the developing CNS needs stimulation in order to mature adequately, and that REM sleep supplies endogenous input. This 'active' hypothesis complements their second, 'passive hypothesis', where it was postulated that the immaturity of the early foetal CNS is unable to inhibit REM sleep, with later maturity reversing this condition. However, Roffwarg *et al.* do not make clear to what extent REM sleep may substitute for wakefulness. Recent evidence in support of a significant amount of REM sleep subserving wakefulness comes from Denenberg and Thoman's (1981) analysis of the sleep–wakefulness data of normal human infants. The amounts of REM sleep and quiet wakefulness reciprocated each other, and the authors proposed that the former subsumed the latter, with both acting to stimulate the CNS.

Although Sterman (1979) has stressed that REM sleep cycling may hold the key to REM sleep function, there are few details of this possible significance. The present review has avoided the topic of REM sleep cycling, as it is felt that this characteristic of REM sleep may well be another epiphenomenon. All biological phenomena display rhythmicity and it is to be expected that the architecture of sleep would do the same. Sleep might be of greater interest in this respect if it did not demonstrate cyclicity.

Exactly how SWS and obligatory REM sleep would interact for the purpose of brain restitution in both infant and adult mammals, is an unknown matter. There have been a few other hypotheses (Jackson, 1884; Laborit, 1972; Feinberg, 1974) outside the concept of obligatory and facultative sleep (of course) which have centred this restitution on non-REM sleep rather than on REM sleep (with Feinberg specifying SWS in this respect). Although Ephron and Carrington (1966) in their 'Homeostatic Hypothesis' proposed that non-REM sleep was a state of cortical deactivation, with REM sleep reversing this condition by increasing cortical tonus through 'endogenous afferentation', they only implied restitution for non-REM sleep.

Finally, while there may be changes in obligatory sleep function from infancy to adulthood, the extent of this change may be less for humans owing to his neotenous condition. Also, because of the greater anatomical and morphological similarities between adult humans and the infant primate, rather than with the adult primate, *human adult sleep function may also have more in common with that of the infant primate*. Adult humans display a relatively high proportion of REM sleep within sleep, compared with other advanced mammals, and it is tempting to suggest that this may partly reflect a neotenous continuation of the preponderance of REM sleep in the neonate.

9.6 Further Aspects of Mammalian Sleep Function

9.6.1 Overview of Main Points So Far

Although the behavioural and EEG manifestations of sleep throughout the Mammalia are similar in many respects, particularly with most exhibiting REM and non-REM sleep, these characteristics probably represent vehicles for functions which may gradually change with phylogeny. Factors which have been proposed, so far, to influence these functions are cerebral development, the propensity for relaxed wakefulness, sleep safety, and feeding habits. The interactions of these factors, which have been summarized in the Introduction and in Fig. 9.2, will prescribe the amounts of obligatory and facultative sleep. However, there are also other factors which need to be taken into consideration, especially body size and energetics in relation to energy conservation; these will now be discussed in more detail.

As already noted, those mammals not able to display much physically relaxed wakefulness (Kleitman's 'advanced', contemplative wakefulness) are typically the insectivores and rodents, for whom sleep could well play a significant energy conservation role through immobilization. However, the laboratory rodent may not be typical of the Rodentia in this respect, owing to its being bred and reared in a restricted and unstimulating environment. Wild rodents are very active during wakefulness (this is very evident from 'wild-life' films). Even following several weeks in captivity, such activity is very noticeable (Pearson, 1947). Not only do insectivores and rodents display less cerebral development by having a smooth cerebral cortex and relatively little grey matter, but also *they are usually small in size*. Consequently, because of their relatively and absolutely higher metabolic rate, generally (disregarding differences in food availability and the protein-energy content of food) they will need to eat more per kg of body weight than in the case of larger mammals, and hence may need to spend more of wakefulness in search of food. The extent to which relaxed wakefulness was facilitated in the larger mammals by (1) what could be loosely described as more spare time through a lesser need for feeding activity, and/or (2) to advanced cerebral development which allowed relaxed waking activities, are not really known. It is likely, though, that these two events acted to mutual advantage.

However, it should be remembered that an increasingly advanced cerebrum may have had other effects upon sleep need. On the one hand it may have permitted a *transfer of physical inactivity from sleep to wakefulness*, reducing the energy conservation role for sleep. On the other hand, if cerebral restitution necessitates sleep, which may well be the case, cerebral advancement would have brought an *increasing need for this form of restorative (obligatory) sleep*. This obligatory sleep may only necessitate a few hours a day even in advanced mammals, with any remaining sleep being facultative and governed largely by some form of circadian modulated non-restorative sleep drive. In the less cerebrally advanced mammal, facultative sleep may occupy the great majority of sleep for enforcing immobility and conserving energy, but because of the propensity for relaxed wakefulness in advanced mammals, facultative sleep may have become more of an occupier of time for relieving boredom, particularly during darkness. Rodents and insectivores would still *need some sleep for cerebral restitution*, and it is important to note that Borbély and Neuhaus (1981) have found in the rodent a 'deeper' form of non-REM sleep which predominates during the first part of each sleep period. While this type of sleep is less apparent than the more obvious SWS of humans, it may represent obligatory sleep.

Also, it must be remembered that *increasing body size permits an increasing tolerance to foodstuffs with a low nutrient content*, and has allowed the evolution of large herbivores, especially ruminants. Such a diet reduces ranging and has led to much of wakefulness being spent in stereotyped feeding behaviour (cf. Eisenberg, 1981). So, for example, the rate of novel stimulation for the CNS is relatively low. Such a situation may have contributed to the low encephalization quotients of these mammals (Jerison, 1973), compared with those of carnivores the same size and having contrasting behavioural styles. Consequently, there may have been a *reduced need for brain restitution during the sleep of these herbivores*. This, coupled with their sedentary life-styles, suggesting a lessened need for sleep as an immobilizer and energy conserver, *may account for why these mammals seem to take relatively little sleep*.

In the rodent, sleep could be a state of body restitution simply because this animal nibbles food and sleeps intermittently throughout the 24-h period, although more sleep and less eating occur during the sleep (daylight) period (cf. Borbély, 1978). However, the extent to which the level of this restitution compares with that of wakefulness has not yet been clearly established. Sleep is bound to follow eating closely in these animals, owing to their polyphasic daily sleeping habit, and coincide with food absorption; more so during the light period. Furthermore, the relatively high degree of physical activity during wakefulness in these animals may reduce and/or delay food absorption and any potential increase in tissue protein content.

9.6.2 Energy Conservation and Sleep — General Principles

The cross-species analysis by Zepelin and Rechtschaffen (1974) which looked for significant correlations between sleep and constitutional variables, has provided sleep research with invaluable information, acting as a stimulus for further thought on sleep function. However, even the more substantial findings, for example a correlation of 0.64 between total sleep time and metabolism, leave most of the variance unaccounted for, even though these findings may well support a hypothesis that sleep is an energy conserver. Such correlations can all too easily lead to ubiquitous and perhaps naïve conclusions about mammalian sleep function, as there are several confounding variables (which Zepelin & Rechtschaffen acknowledge).

There is a differential energy saving effect of immobility depending upon body size. Before describing this factor further, it should be remembered that because of obvious methodological problems, no mammal apart from humans has had its metabolism assessed during objectively determined waking and sleeping states (i.e. as measured by the EEG or ECoG) under *free and natural environmental circumstances*. Although there have been a few detailed studies of 24-h trends in 0_2 consumption in wild rodents and insectivores (one of the most notable being by Pearson, 1947), animals are (1) confined to a cage, and (2) are given ad lib access to food. These animals naturally spend most of wakefulness foraging for food, but unfortunately this activity is prevented in the laboratory. Hence, *the metabolic data are not a true reflection of those which might be found for animals in the wild state.*

Nevertheless, there are laboratory data from which inferences might be drawn, particularly on the energy cost of differing physical activity levels in a variety of species. From these, estimates can be made of the energy saving attainable by being inactive, and in the case of animals showing little relaxed wakefulness, what the energy saving of sleep might be. The energy cost of movement, particularly running, is inversely proportional to body weight, with the smaller the mammal the greater the cost, not only over a given distance, but also per unit time of movement at the mammal's average movement speed (cf. Taylor *et al.*, 1970). For example, in a mouse, the difference between its average running speed (running occupies much of its wakefulness) and immobility is about 5 calories per gram of body weight per hour, but for an 18 kg dog this difference is about 2 $cal/g^{-1}/h^{-1}$. Hence, in *general terms* the mouse has to consume more of the environment's food in being active than does a dog. While a dog demonstrates much relaxed wakefulness and can conserve energy while being awake, the enforced immobility of sleep in the mouse will act as a considerable energy saver, not only because of this animal's relative lack of relaxed wakefulness, but also *because of the further saving through its smallness.*

There is also a third, more indirect, form of energy saving produced by sleep in these small mammals, which could well be the most significant in this respect. Sleep will usually confine these mammals *to a well-insulated nest and encourage huddling together*, both of which will result in substantive reductions in heat loss, and in energy expenditure. Pearson (1947) has clearly shown (Fig. 9.3) that at 26 °C (which is about 4 °C below thermoneutrality 0_2 consumption of four mice huddled together is approximately one-half of the summated 0_2 expenditures of the animals sleeping alone. The more individuals in a huddle, the greater this saving. However, Pearson observed that the propensity to huddle is reduced at

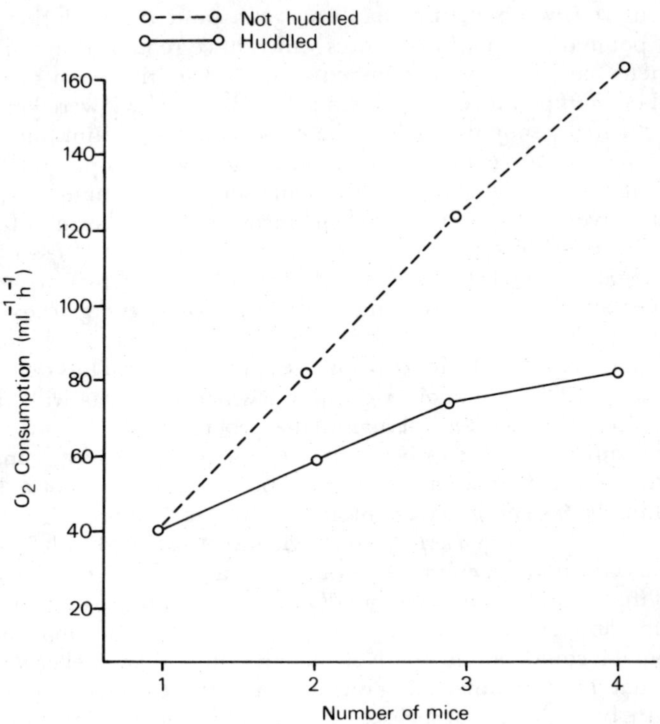

Fig. 9.3 Oxygen consumption of mice measured singly compared with that of huddling together. All measurements at an environmental temperature of 26 °C. (Reproduced from O. Pearson (1947), *Ecology*, **28**, 127–145, © 1947, The Ecological Society of America. Reprinted by permission.)

thermoneutrality, presumably owing to the possibility of over-heating.

The energy saving of sleep over relaxed wakefulness is indeed small in the case of larger (cerebrally advanced) mammals. In the cow and sheep, oxygen consumption drops from relaxed wakefulness to sleep by 10% and 13% respectively (Toutain & Webster, 1975). In humans, the main studies of metabolism during sleep (Kreider *et al.*, 1958; Kreider & Iampetro, 1959; Brebbia & Altschuler, 1965; Webb & Hiestand, 1975; Haskell *et al.*, 1981; Goll & Shapiro, 1981) indicate a drop in 0_2 consumption of about 10% from relaxed wakefulness levels (within or around the sleep period) to sleep. Although these findings are confounded by the circadian rhythm in that metabolism is lower during the usual sleeping period, regardless of whether the individual is asleep or awake. Also, of course, in man, sleep in the usual period is mostly post-absorptive (e.g. protein turnover and the energy demands of protein synthesis and related activities will be reduced), unlike that of much of the waking period. Hence, any comparison of the 0_2 consumption between sleep in the usual sleep period and relaxed waking levels taken earlier in the day may show a greater difference between these two conditions than is the real case.

The type of energetics displayed by a mammal and whether it has a nocturnal or diurnal lifestyle must also be taken into consideration when trying to relate energy conservation with sleep length across species. Crompton *et al.* (1978), in their recent review on mammalian energetics and the evolution of homeothermy, pointed out that insectivores which have remained in the nocturnal environment have in general retained a more primitive form of energetics, whereby body temperature is regulated at 25–30 °C, with lowered metabolism. Other nocturnal mammals, such as the echidna and opossum, have acquired typically mammalian energetics, maintaining body temperature at about 30–35 °C and fitting Kleiber's (1961) equation. These mammals, although nocturnal, have evolved from diurnal ancestors. Both forms of nocturnal mammal have much lower body temperatures than that (37–40 °C) of the typical diurnal mammals. So in general terms, because of the warmer environment of the day, sleeping by day may present less of an energy (heat) loss than sleeping by night, irrespective of the type of energetics. In the case of the nocturnal mammal with the more primitive energetics, heat loss during sleep in the day may well be nominal; a condition which contrasts with that of the nocturnal sleeper having typical mammalian energetics.

Another confounding factor between sleep quality and energy conservation, is the degree to which an animal utilizes torpor during sleep. For at least some small mammals, the energy saving of sleep may even be more substantial *if sleep is allowed to develop into a mild torpor*, which will be accentuated with food deprivation and/or a drop in the environmental temperature. Heller *et al.* (1978) have estimated that in an environment of 0 °C a 100 g mammal can, by lowering its body temperature by 2 °C during sleep, survive 5 days without food; a day longer than if it could remain relatively inactive but awake. Heller *et al.* go on to point out that, by the animal going into a shallow torpor and dropping the body temperature by 10 °C, it can survive 7 days, and by hibernating and regulating its body temperature at 7 °C it can survive 65 days. In many respects, as Heller *et al.* suggest, all three states, sleep, torpor and hibernation are extensions of each other, along an energy saving continuum.

Berger (1975), Walker *et al.* (1979), and Walker and Berger (1980) proposed in a series of review and experimental articles that non-REM sleep (in allowing an apparently regulated fall in body temperature) is specially oriented towards energy conservation, evolved to offset the high costs of endothermy. Supportive evidence comes from (1) the strong correlation between non-REM sleep amounts and metabolic rate (Zepelin & Rechtschaffen, 1975), (2) the parallel ontogenetic developments of non-REM sleep and thermoregulation, and (3) the absence of non-REM sleep in poikilotherms. Although, Walker and Berger admit that there is dispute over this latter point in that non-REM sleep may be present in reptiles (see Section 9.5.3). The most powerful finding favouring Walker and Berger's hypothesis comes from Glotzbatch and Heller (1976), who reported a regulated decrease in body temperature during non-REM sleep in the ground squirrel. This could, of course, be a reversion to a more primitive form of energetics of the type described by Crompton *et al.* (1980). It is likely though, that this hypothesis is more appropriate to smaller mammals rather than to larger mammals, as the ability of the latter to reduce body temperature during non-REM sleep seems more limited, mostly because of their lessened relative heat loss and greater thermal inertia. As noted, for humans, the real extent to which sleep per se (especially non-REM sleep) permits a metabolic fall, is still not clear.

Sleep safety, it will be remembered, interacts with any role sleep may have for energy conservation and, for example, mammals sleeping under hazardous circumstances will have little facultative sleep. However, both the safe and vulnerable sleeper within a mammalian order may have similar amounts of obligatory sleep.

A final point which must be kept in mind when considering the role sleep may have for energy conservation, is that one must not just consider this conservation from the point of energy expenditure of an individual organism, but *also in terms of the conservation of food resources*, and consequently, the maximization of numbers of individuals of a given species within a given environment. Sleep quality and quantity for mammals living in their natural habitat are set at finely adjusted levels which mediate between the constraints set by the optimal daily time necessary for foraging and feeding, and the minimal protein-energy requirement necessary for the animal to survive and reproduce successfully.

References

ADAM, K. (1980). Sleep as a restorative process and a theory to explain why. *Progress in Brain Research*, **53**, 289–306.

ADAM, K. and OSWALD, I. (1977). Sleep is for tissue restoration. *Journal of the Royal College of Physicians*, **11**, 376–388.

ADAM, K. and OSWALD, I. (1981). Diurnal pattern of protein metabolism in man: some doubts. *American Journal of Clinical Nutrition*, **34**, 1624–1626.

ADAMSON, L., HUNTER, W. M., OGUNREMI, O. O., OSWALD, I. and PERCY-ROBB, I. W. (1974). Growth hormone increase during sleep after daytime exercise. *Journal of Endocrinology*, **62**, 473–478.

AGNEW, H. W. and WEBB, W. B. (1973). The influence of time course variables on REM sleep. *Bulletin of the Psychonomic Society*, **3**, 131–133.

AGNEW, H. W., WEBB, W. B. and WILLIAMS, R. L. (1967). Comparison of stage 4 and 1-REM sleep deprivation. *Perceptual and Motor Skills*, **24**, 851–858.

AKERSTEDT, T. (1980). Altered sleep/wake patterns and circadian rhythms. *Acta Physiologica Scandinavia*, Suppl. **469**.

AKERSTEDT, T. and GILLBERG, M. (1981). The circadian variation of experimentally displaced sleep. *Sleep*, **4**, 159–170.

ALBERT, I. (1975). REM sleep deprivation. *Biological Psychiatry*, **10**, 341–351.

ALBERT, I., CICALA, G. and SIEGEL, J. (1970). The behavioural effect of REM sleep deprivation in rats. *Psychophysiology*, **6**, 550–555.

ALLISON, T. and CICCHETTI, D. V. (1976). Sleep in mammals: ecological and constitutional correlates. *Science*, **194**, 732–734.

ALLISON, T., VAN TWYVER, H. and GOFF, W. R. (1972). Electrophysiological studies of the echidna (Tachyglossus aculeatus). *Archives of Italian Biology*, **110**, 145–184.

ANTELMAN, S. M. and CAGGIULA, A. R. (1980). Stress-induced behaviour: chemotherapy without drugs. In: S. M. DAVIDSON and R. J. DAVIDSON (Eds.), *Psychobiology of Consiousness*, New York: Plenum Press, 65–104.

ASERINSKY, E. (1969). The maximal capacity for sleep: rapid eye movement density as an index of sleep satiety. *Biological Psychiatry*, **1**, 147–159.

ASERINSKY, E. (1973). Relationship of REM density to the prior accumulation of sleep and wakefulness. *Psychophysiology*, **10**, 545–558.

ASTIC, L. (1973). Ontongenese des états de vigilance chez le foetus de cobaye, *Electroencephalography and Clinical Neurophysiology*, **22**, 54–64.

ATKINSON, D. E. (1977). *Cellular Energy Metabolism and its Regulation*, New York: Academic Press.

BAKER, M. A. and HAYWARD, J. N. (1967). Autonomic basis for the rise in brain temperature during paradoxical sleep. *Science*, **157**, 1586–1588.

BENOIT, O., FORET, J., BOUARD, G., MERLE, B., LANDAU, J. and MARC, M. E. (1980). Habitual sleep length and patterns of recovery sleep after 24 hours and 36 hours sleep deprivation. *Electroencephalography and Clinical Neurophysiology*, **50**, 477–485.

BERGER, R. J. (1975). Bioenergetic functions of sleep and activity rhythms and their possible relevance to ageing. *Federation Proceedings*, **34**, 97–102.

BERGER, R. J. and OSWALD, I. (1962). Effects of sleep deprivation on behaviour, subsequent sleep, and dreaming. *Journal of Mental Science*, **108**, 457–465.

BERGER, R. J., WALKER, J. M., SCOTT, T. D., MAGNUSON, L. J., and POLLACK, S. L. (1971). Diurnal and nocturnal sleep stage patterns following sleep deprivation. *Psychonomic Science*, **23**, 273–275.

BORBÉLY, A. A. (1978). Effects of light on sleep and activity rhythms. *Progress in Neurobiology*, **10**, 1–31.

BORBÉLY, A. A., BAUMANN, F., BRANDEIS, D., STRAUCH, I., and LEHMANN, D. (1981). Sleep deprivation: effect on sleep stages and EEG power density in man. *Electroencephalography and Clinical Neurophysiology*, **51**, 483–493.

BORBÉLY, A. A. and NEUHAUS, H. U. (1979). Sleep deprivation: effects on sleep and EEG in the rat. *Journal of Comparative and Physiological Psychology*, **133**, 71–87.

BREBBIA, D. R. and ALTSHULER, K. Z. (1965). Oxygen consumption rate and electroencephalographic stage of sleep. *Science*, **150**, 1621–1623.

BRODAN, V., VOSTECHOVSKY, M., KUHN, M., and CEPELAK, J. (1969). Changes of mental and physical performance in sleep deprived healthy volunteers. *Activitas Nervosa Superior*, **11**, 175–181.

BUGUET, A. G. C., ROUSSEL, B. H. E., WATSON, W. J. and RADOMSKI, M. W. (1979). Cold-induced diminution of paradoxical sleep in man. *Electroencephalography and Clinical Neurophysiology*, **46**, 29–32.

BUSH, I. E. (1962). Chemical and biological factors in the activity of adrenocortical steroids, *Pharmacological Reviews*, **14**, 317–428.

CHAPMAN, A. G., FALL, L. and ATKINSON, D. E. (1971). Adenylate energy charge in Escherichia coli during growth and starvation. *Journal of Bacteriology*, **108**, 1072–1086.

CLARK, R. H. and KORST, D. R. (1969). Circadian periodicity of bone marrow mitotic activity and reticulocyte counts in rats and mice. *Science*, **166**, 236–237.

CLUGSTON, G. A. and GARLICK, P. J. (1981). Diurnal patterns of protein turnover in obese subjects given a protein-free diet. *Proceedings of the Nutrition Society*, **40**.

CLUGSTON, G. A. and GARLICK, P. J. (1982). The response of protein and energy metabolism to food intake in lean and obese man. *Human Nutrition: Clinical Nutrition*, **36C**, 57–70.

COHEN, H. B. and DEMENT, W. C. (1965). Sleep: changes in threshold of electroconvulsive shock in rats after deprivation of 'paradoxical' phase. *Science*, **150**, 1318–1319.

COHEN, H. B., EDELMAN, A. and BOWEN, R. (1972). Sleep and self stimulation in the rat. *Sleep Research*, **1**, 158.

COHEN, H. B., THOMAS, J. and DEMENT, W. C. (1970). Sleep styles, REM deprivation and electroconvulsive threshold in the cat. *Brain Research*, **19**, 317–321.

CROMPTON, A. W., TAYLOR, C. R. and JAGGER, J. A. (1978). Evolution of homeothermy in mammals. *Nature*, **272**, 333–336.

CREUTZFELDT, O. D. (1975). Neurophysiological correlates of different functional states of the brain. In: D. H. INGVAR and N. A. LASSEN (Eds.), *Brain Work*, Copenhagen: Munksgaard, 21–46.

CZEISLER, C. A., WEITZMAN, E. D., MOORE-EDE. M. C., ZIMMERMAN, J. C. and KRAUER, R. S. (1980). Human sleep: its duration and organisation depends on its circadian phase. *Science*, **210**, 1264–1267.

DALLOSSO, H., MURGATROYD, P. R. and JAMES, W. P. T. (1982). Feeding frequency and energy balance in adult males. *Human Nutrition: Clinical Nutrition*, **36C**, 25–39.

DE BEER, G. (1958). *Embryos and Ancestors*, Oxford: Oxford University Press.

DEMENT, W. C. (1965). Recent studies on the biological role of REM sleep. *American Journal Psychiatry*, **122**, 404–408.
DEMENT, W. C. (1973). Commentary. *In*: W. B. WEBB (Ed.), *Sleep: an Active Process*. Illinois: Scott, Foresman pp. 48–58.
DENNENBERG, V. H. and THOMAN, E. B. (1981). Evidence for a functional role for active (REM) sleep in infancy. *Sleep*, **4**, 185–192.
DEWSON, J. H., DEMENT, W. C., WAGENER, T. E. and NOBEL, K. (1967). Rapid eye movement sleep deprivation: a central neural change during wakefulness. *Science*, **156**, 403–406.
DITTRICHOVA, J. (1969). Development of sleep in infancy. *In*: R. J. ROBINSON (Ed.), *Brain and Early Behaviour*, New York: Academic Press, 193–204.
DRUCKER-COLIN, R. P. (1981). Neuroproteins, brain excitability and REM sleep. In: W. FISHBEIN (Ed.), *Sleep, Dreams and Memory*, New York: MTP Press, pp. 73–94.
DUNN, A. J. and REES, H. D. (1977). Brain RNA and protein synthesis during training: the interpretation of changes of precursor incorporation. In: R. R. DRUCKER-COLIN and J. L. MCGAUGH (Eds.), *Neurobiology of Sleep and Memory*, New York: Academic Press, pp. 33–56.
DURIE, D. J. B., ADAM, K., OSWALD, I. and FLYNN, I. W. (1978). Sleep: cellular energy charge and protein synthetic capability. *IRCS Medical Science*, **6**, 351.
EISENBERG, J. F. (1981). *The Mammalian Radiations*. London: Athlone Press.
ELLINGSON, R. J. and PETERS, J. F. (1980). Development of EEG and daytime sleep patterns in normal full-term infants during the first 3 months of life: longitudinal observations. *Electroencephalography and Clinical Neurophysiology*, **49**, 112–124.
ELLMAN, S. J., SPIELMAN, A. J., LUCK, D., STEINER, S. S. and HALPERIN, R. (1978). REM deprivation: a review. In: A. M. ARKIN, J. S. ANTROBUS and S. J. ELLMAN (Eds.), *The Mind in Sleep*, New Jersey: Lawrence Erlbaum, pp. 419–457.
ELOMAA, E. and JOHANSSON, G. G. (1980a). Daily rhythm of locomotor activity is dropped during REM sleep deprivation in the rat. *Physiology and Behaviour*, **24**, 327–330.
ELOMAA, E. and JOHANSSON, G. G. (1980b). REM stage of sleep participates in the generation of the nocturnal meal patterns of the rat, *Physiology and Behaviour*, **24**, 331–336.
EPHRON, H. S. and CARRINGTON, P. (1966). Rapid eye movement sleep and cortical homeostasis. *Psychological Review*, **73**, 500–526.
EVANS, F. J., COOK, M. P., COHEN, H. D., ORNE, E. C. and ORNE, M. T. (1977). Appetitive and replacement naps: EEG and behaviour. *Science*, **197**, 687–689.
EVARTS, E. V. (1961). Effects of sleep and waking on activity of single units in the unrestrained cat. In: G. E. W. WOLSTENHOLME and M. O'CONNOR (Eds.), *The Nature of Sleep*, London: Churchill.
FEINBERG, I. (1974). Changes in sleep cycle patterns with age. *Journal of Psychiatric Research*, **10**, 283–306.
FEINBERG, I., FEIN, G. and FLOYD, T. C. (1980). EEG patterns during and following extended sleep in young adults. *Electroencephalography and Clinical Neurophysiology*, **50**, 467–476.
FEINBERG, I., HIBI, S. and CARLSON, V. R. (1977). Changes in EEG amplitude during sleep with age. In: K. NANDY and I. SHERWIN (Eds.) *The Aging Brain and Senile Dementia*. New York: Plenum Press, pp. 85–98.
FISHER, L. B. (1968). The diurnal mitotic rhythm in the human epidermis. *British Journal of Dermatology*, **80**, 75–80.
FLANIGAN, W. F. (1974). Sleep and wakefulness in chelonian reptiles, II The red-footed tortoise. *Archives of Italian Biology*, **112**, 253–277.
FLANIGAN, W. F., WILCOX, R. H. and RECHTSCHAFFEN, A. (1973). The EEG and behavioural continuum of the crocodilian, Caiman sclerops. *Electroencephalography and Clinical Neurophysiology*, **34**, 521–538.
FRANCESCIONI, R. P., STOKES, J. W., BANDERET, L. E. and KOWAL, D. M. (1978).

Sustained operations and sleep deprivation: effects on indices of stress. *Aviation, Space and Environmental Medicine*, **49**, 1271–1274.
FROBERG, J., KARLSSON, C-G., LEVI, L. and LIDBERG, L. (1975). Circadian rhythms of catecholomine excretion, shooting range preference and self-ratings of fatigue during sleep deprivation. *Biological Psychology*, **2**, 175–188.
FRIEDMAN, J., GLOBUS, G., HUNTLEY, A., MULLANEY, D., NAITOH, P. and JOHNSON, L. (1977). Performance and mood during and after gradual sleep reduction. *Psychophysiology*, **14**, 245–250.
GARLICK, P. J., CLUGSTON, G. A., SWICK, R. W. and WATERLOW, J. C. (1980). Diurnal pattern of protein and energy metabolism in man. *American Journal of Clinical Nutrition*, **33**, 1983–1986.
GARLICK, P. J., CLUGSTON, P. J., WATERLOW. J. C. and SWICK, R. W. (1981). Diurnal pattern of protein and energy metabolism in Man: a defense. *American Journal of Clinical Nutrition*, **34**, 1626–1628.
GELLER, M. R., GOURDJI, N., CHRISTOFF, N. and FOX, E. (1969). The effects of sleep deprivation on the EEGs of epileptic children. *Developmental Medicine and Child Neurology*, **11**, 771–776.
GIUDITTA, A., RUTIGLIANO, B., and VITALE-NEUGEBAUER, A. (1980a). Influence of synchronised sleep on the biosynthesis of RNA in neuronal and mixed fractions isolated from rabbit cerebral cortex. *Journal of Neurochemistry*, **35**, 1267–1272.
GIUDITTA, A., RUTIGLIANO, B., and VITALE-NEUGEBAUER, A. (1980b). Influence of synchronised sleep on the biosynthesis of RNA in two nuclear classes isolated from rabbit cerebral cortex. *Journal of Neurochemistry*, **35**, 1259–1266.
GLOTZBACH, S. F. and HELLER, H. C. (1976). Central nervous regulation of body temperature during sleep. *Science*, **194**, 537–539.
GOLL, C. C. and SHAPIRO, C. M. (1981). Oxygen consumption during sleep. *Journal of Physiology*, **313**, 35p–36p.
GREENBERG, R. and PEARLMAN, C. A. (1974). Cutting the REM nerve: an approach to the adaptive role of REM sleep. *Perspectives in Biology and Medicine*, **17**, 513–521.
GRIFFIN. S. J. and TRINDER, J. (1978). Physical Fitness, exercise and human sleep, *Psychophysiology*, **15**, 447–450.
GULEVICH, G., DEMENT, W. and JOHNSON L. C. (1966). Psychiatric and EEG observations on a case of prolonged (264 hours) wakefulness. *Archives of General Psychiatry*, **15**, 29–36.
HAECKEL, E. (1866). *Generell Morphologie der Organismen*, Berlin.
HALBERG, F. and BARNUM, C. P. (1961). Continuous light or darkness and circadian periodic mitosis and metabolism in C and D8 Mice. *American Journal of Physiology*, **201**, 227–230.
HALBERG, F. and NELSON, W. (1978). Chronobiologic optimization of aging. In: H. V. SAMIS and S. CAPOBIANCO (Eds.), *Aging and Biological Rhythms*, New York: Plenum, pp. 5–56.
HANDWERKER, M. J. and FISHBEIN, W. (1975). Neural excitability after paradoxical sleep deprivation: a replication and further examination. *Physiological Psychology*, **3**, 137–140.
HARTMANN, E. (1973). *The Functions of Sleep*, New Haven: Yale University Press.
HARTMANN, E., MARCUS, J. and LEINOFF, A. (1968). The sleep-dream cycle and convulsive threshold. *Psychonomic Science*, **13**, 141–142.
HARRIS, R. C., HULTMAN, E. and NORDESJO, L-O. (1974). Glycogen, glycolytic intermediates and high energy phosphates determined in biopsy samples of quadriceps muscle of man at rest. *Scandinavian Journal Clinical Laboratory Investigation*, **33**, 109–120.
HARRIS, W. and O'HANLON, J. F. (1972). A study of recovery functions in man. US Army Technical Memorandum 10–72, Aberdeen Research and Development Center, Maryland.

HARTSE, K. M. (1980). The limbic spike: an electrophysiological correlate of sleep in mammals and reptiles. *Sleep Research*, **9**, 30.

HASKELL, E. H., PALCA, J. W., WALKER, J. M., BERGER, R. J. and HELLER, H. C. (1981). Metabolism and thermoregulation during stages of sleep in humans exposed to heat and cold. *Journal of Applied Physiology: Respiration, Environmental and Exercise Physiology*, **51**, 948–954.

HAURI, P. (1968). Effects of evening activity on early night sleep. *Psychophysiology*, **4**, 267–277.

HAYWARD, J. M. and BAKER, M. A. (1969). A comparative study of the role of the cerebral arterial blood in the regulation of brain temperature in five mammals. *Brain Research*, **16**, 417–440.

HEBB, D. O. (1955). Drives and the CNS. *Psychological Review*, **62**, 243–254.

HELLER, H. C. and GLOTZBATCH, S. F. (1977). Thermoregulation during sleep and hibernation. *Environmental Physiology II International Review of Physiology* **15**, 147–188.

HELLER. H. C., WALKER, J. M., FLORANT, G. L., GLOTZBACH, S. F. and BERGER, R. J. (1978). Sleep and hibernation: electrophysiological and thermoregulatory homologies. In: L. Wang and J. W. Hudson (Eds.), *Strategies in Cold: Natural Thermogenesis and Torpidity*, New York: Academic Press, pp. 225–265.

HENANE, R., BUGUET, A., ROUSSEL, B., and BITTEL, J. (1977). Variations in evaporation and body temperatures during sleep in man. *Journal of Applied Physiology*, **42**, 50–55.

HICKS, R. A. and ADAMS, G. (1976). REM sleep deprivation and exploration in young rats, *Psychological Reports*, **38**, 1154.

HICKS, R. A., MOORE, J. D., HAYES, C., PHILLIPS, N. and HAWKINS, J. (1979). REM sleep deprivation increases aggressiveness in male rats. *Physiology and Behaviour*, **22**, 1097–1100.

HICKS, R. A. and MOORE, J. D. (1979). REM sleep deprivation diminishes fear in rats. *Physiology and Behaviour*, **22**, 689–692.

HICKS, R. A. and PELLEGRINI, R. J. (1977). Anxiety levels of short and long sleepers. *Psychological Reports*, **41**, 569–570.

HICKS, R. A., PETTY, B., OKUDA, A. and THOMSON, D. (1979). Effects of REM sleep deprivation and age on locomotion activity in rats. *Psychological Record*, **29**, 355–360.

HOBSON, J. A. and MCCARLEY, R. W. (1971). Cortical unit activity in sleep and waking. *Electroencephalography and Clinical Neurophysiology*, **30**, 97–112.

HORNE, J. A. (1976). Recovery sleep following different visual conditions during total sleep deprivation in man. *Biological Psychology*, **4**, 107–118.

HORNE, J. A. (1977). Factors relating to energy conservation during sleep in mammals, *Physiological Psychology*, **5**, 403–408.

HORNE, J. A. (1978a). A review of the biological effects of total sleep deprivation in man. *Biological Psychology*, **7**, 55–102.

HORNE, J. A. (1978b). Dreaming sleep in man: a reappraisal. *Perspectives in Biology and Medicine*, **21**, 591–601.

HORNE, J. A. (1981). The effects of exercise upon sleep: a critical review. *Biological Psychology*, **12**, 241–290.

HORNE, J. A. and PORTER, J. M. (1976). Time of day effects with standardised exercise upon subsequent sleep. *Electroencephalography and Clinical Neurophysiology*, **40**, 178–184.

HORNE, J. A. and STAFF, L. H. E. (1983). Exercise and sleep: body heating effects, *Sleep*, **6**, 52–63.

HUME, K. I. and MILLS, J. N. (1977). Rhythms of REM and slow wave sleep in subjects living or abnormal time schedules, *Waking and Sleeping*, **3**, 291–296.

INGVAR, D. H., ROSEN, I. and JOHANNESSON, G. (1979). EEG related to cerebral metabolism and blood flow. *Pharmakopsychiatry*, **12**, 200–209.

JACKSON, J. H. (1884). Evolution and dissolution of the nervous system. In: J. TAYLOR, (Ed.), *Selected Writings of John Hughlings Jackson* (1958), London: Staples, pp. 45–75.

JEFFERSON, L. S. (1980). Role of insulin in the regulation of protein synthesis, *Diabetes*, **29**, 487–496.

JERISON, H. J. (1973). *Evolution of Brain and Intelligence*, New York: Academic Press.

JOHNS, M. W., BRUCE, D. W. and MASTERSON, J. P. (1974). Psychological correlates of sleep habits reported by healthy young adults. *British Journal of Medical Psychology*, **47**, 181–187.

JOHNSON, L. C. and MACLEOD, W. L. (1973). Sleep and awake behaviour during gradual sleep reduction. *Perceptual Motor Skills*, **36**, 87–97.

JOHNSON, L. C., NAITOH, P., MOSES, J. M. and LUBIN, A. (1974). Interaction of REM deprivation and stage 4 deprivation with total sleep loss: experiment 2. *Psychophysiology*, **11**, 147–159.

JOHNSON, L. C., SLYE, E. S. and DEMENT, W. C. (1965). Electroencephalographic and autonomic activity during and after prolonged sleep deprivation. *Psychosomatic Medicine*, **27**, 415–423.

JONES, H. S. and OSWALD, I. (1968). Two cases of healthy insomnia. *Electroencephalography and Clinical Neurophysiology*, **24**, 378–380.

JOUVET, M. (1961). Telencephalic and rhombencephalic sleep in the cat. In: G. WOLSTENHOLME and M. O'CONNOR (Eds.), *CIBA Foundation Symposium on the Nature of Sleep*, Boston: Little, Brown.

JOUVET, M. (1978). Does a genetic programming of the brain occur during paradoxical sleep? In: P. A. Buser and A. Rougel-Buser (Eds.), *Cerebral Correlates of Conscious Experience*, Amsterdam: Elsevier.

JOUVET, M. (1980). Paradoxical sleep and the nature–nurture controversy. *Progress in Brain Research*, **53**, 331–346.

JOUVET-MOUNIER, D., ASTIC, L. and LACOTE, D. (1970). Ontogenesis of the states of sleep in the rat, cat and guinea pig during the first postnatal month. *Developmental Psychobiology*, **2**, 391–399.

KALES, A., TAN, T-L., KOLLAR, E. J., NAITOH, P., PRESTON, T. A. and MALMSTROM, E. J. (1970). Sleep patterns following 205 h of sleep deprivation. *Psychosomatic Medicine*, **32**, 189–200.

KARACAN, I., WILLIAMS, R. L., FINLEY, W. W. and HURSCH, C. J. (1970). The effects of naps on nocturnal sleep: influence on the need for stage 1-REM and stage 4 sleep. *Biological Psychiatry*, **2**, 391–399.

KARNOVSKY, M. L. and REICH, P. (1977). Biochemistry of sleep. *Advances in Neurochemistry*, **2**. 213–275.

KLEIBER, M. (1961). *The Fire of Life: An Introduction to Animal Energetics*, New York: Wiley.

KLEITMAN, M. (1963). *Sleep and Wakefulness*, Chicago: Chicago University Press.

KOPEL, B. S., ZARCONE, V., DE LA PENA, A. and DEMENT, W. C. (1972). Changes in selective attention as measured by the visual averaged evoked potential following REM deprivation in man. *Electroencephalography and Clinical Neurophysiology*, **32**, 322–325.

KOSTYO, J. L. and NUTTING, D. F. (1974). Growth hormone and protein metabolism. In: *American Physiological Society Handbook of Physiology*, **7, (IV)** 187–210.

KOVALZON, V. M. (1977). Brain temperature variations and ECoG in free-swimming bottlenosed dolphin. In: W. P. KOELLA, (Ed.), *Sleep 1976*, Basel: Karger, pp. 239–241.

KREIDER, M. B., BUSKIRK, E. R. and BASS, D. E. (1958). Oxygen consumption and body temperatures during the night. *Journal of Applied Physiology*, **12**, 361–366.

KREIDER, M. B. and IAMPETRO, P. F. (1959). Oxygen consumption and body temperatures during sleep in cold environments. *Journal of Applied Physiology*, **14**, 765–767.

KRISTAL, M. B. and NOONAN, M. (1979). Note on sleep in captive giraffes (Giraffa camelopardalis reticulata) *South African Journal of Zoology*, **14**, 108.

LABORIT, H. (1972). Correlations between protein and serotonin synthesis during

various activities of the central nervous system. *Research Communications in Chemical Pathology and Pharmacology*, **3**, 51–81.
LIPMAN, R. L., TAYLOR, A. L., SCHENK, A. and MINTZ, D. H. (1972). Inhibition of sleep related growth hormone release by elevated free fatty acids. *Journal of Clinical Endocrinology and Metabolism*. **36**, 592–594.
LIVINGSTONE, M. S. and HUBEL, D. H. (1981). Effects of sleep and arousal on the processing of visual information in the cat. *Nature*, **291**, 554–561.
LUBIN, A., MOSES, J., JOHNSON, L. C. and NAITOH, P. (1974). The recuperative effects of REM Sleep and Stage 4 sleep on human performance after complete sleep loss: experiment 1. *Psychophysiology*, **11**, 133–146.
LUBY, E. D., FROHMAN, C. E., GRISELL, J. L., LENZO, J. E. and GOTTLIEB, J. S. (1960). Sleep deprivation: effects upon behaviour, thinking, motor performance and biological energy transfer system. *Psychosomatic Medicine*, **22**, 182–192.
LUBY, E. D., GRISELL, J. L., FROHMAN, C. E., LEES, H., COHEN, B. D. and GOTTLIEB, J. S. (1962). Biochemical, psychological and behavioural responses to sleep deprivation. *Annals of the New York Academy of Science*, **96**, 71–79.
MARTIN, B. J. (1981). Effect of sleep deprivation on tolerance of prolonged exercise. *European Journal of Applied Physiology*, **47**, 345–354.
MARTIN, C. R. (1976). *Textbook of Endocrine Physiology*, Baltimore: Williams & Wilkins.
MCGRATH, M. J. and COHEN, D. B. (1975). REM Sleep facilitation of adaptive waking behaviour: a review of the literature. *Psychological Bulletin*, **85**, 24–57.
MEDDIS, R. (1977). *The Sleep Instinct*, London: Routledge & Kegan Paul.
MEDDIS, R., PEARSON, A. J. D. and LANGFORD, G. (1973). An extreme case of healthy insomnia. *Electroencephalography and Clinical Neurophysiology*, **35**, 391–394.
MEGLASSON, M. D. and HUGGINS S. E. (1979). Sleep in a crocodilian, Caiman sclerops. *Comparative Biochemistry and Physiology*, **63A**, 561–567.
MERIMEE, T. J. (1979). Growth hormone secretion and action. In: L. J. DEGROOT *et al.* (Eds.), *Endocrinology*, *Vol. 1*, New York: Grune and Stratton, pp. 123–132.
METCALF, D. R., MONDALE, J. and BUTLER, F. K. (1971). Ontogenesis of spontaneous K complexes. *Psychophysiology*, **8**, 340–347.
MINUTO, F., UNDERWOOD, L. E., GRIMALDI, P., FURLANFO, R. W., VAN WYK, J. J. and GIORDANO, G. (1981). Decreased serum somatomedin C concentrations during sleep: temporal relationship to the nocturnal surges of growth hormone and prolactin. *Journal of Clinical Endocrinology and Metabolism*, **52**, 399–403.
MOLE, P. A. and JOHNSON, R. E. (1971). Disclosure by dietary modification of an exercise-induced protein catabolism in Man. *Journal of Applied Physiology*, **31**, 185–190.
MOLLENHOUR, M. N., VOORHEES, J. W., DAVIS, S. F. (1977). Sleepy and hostile: the effects of REM sleep deprivation on shock-elicited aggression. *Animal Learning and behaviour*, **5**, 148–152.
MORDEN, B., CONNER, R., MITCHELL, G., DEMENT, W. C. and LEVINE, S. (1968). Effects of REM sleep deprivation upon shock induced fighting. *Physiology and Behaviour*, **3**, 425–428.
MOORE, J. D., HAYES, C. and HICKS, R. A. (1979). REM sleep deprivation increases preference for novelty in rats. *Physiology and Behaviour*, **23**, 975–976.
MORRIS, G. O., WILLIAMS, H. L. and LUBIN, A. (1960). Misperception and disorientation during sleep deprivation. *AMA Archives of General Psychiatry*, **2**, 247–254.
MORUZZI, G. (1966). The functional significance of sleep with particular regard to the brain mechanisms underlying consciousness. In J. C. ECCLESS (Ed.), *Brain and Conscious Experience*, Berlin: Springer-Verlag. pp. 345–388.
MORUZZI, G. (1972). The sleep-waking cycle. *Reviews of Physiology*, **64**, 1–165.
MOSES, J. M., HORD, D. J., LUBIN, A., JOHNSON, L. C. and NAITOH, P. (1975). Dynamics of nap sleep during a 40 hour period. *Electroencephalography and Clinical Neurophysiology*, **39**, 627–636.
MUKHAMETOV, L. M. and POLYAKOVA, I. G. (1981). EEG investigation of the sleep in

porpoises (Phocoena phocoena) *Journal of Higher Nervous Activity SSR (Russ)* **31**, 333–339.
MUKHAMETOV, L. M., SUPIN, A. Y. and POLYAKOVA, I. G. (1977). Interhemispheric asymmetry of the electroencephalographic sleep patterns in dolphins, *Brain Research*, **134**, 581–584.
MULLANEY, D. J., JOHNSON, L. C., NAITOH P., FRIEDMAN, J. K., and GLOBUS G. G. (1977). Sleep during and after gradual sleep reduction. *Psychophysiology*, **14**, 237–244.
MURRAY, E. J. (1966). *Sleep Dreams and Arousal*, New York: Appleton-Century-Crofts.
NAITOH, P. (1976). Sleep deprivation. *Waking and Sleeping*, **1**, 53–60.
NAITOH, P., KALES, A., KOLLAR, E. J., SMITH, J. C. and JACOBSON, A., (1969). Electro-encephalographic activity after prolonged sleep loss. *Electroencephalography and Clinical Neurophysiology*, **27**, 2–11.
NICOL, S. C. and MASKREY, M. (1980). Thermoregulation, respiration and sleep in the Tasmanian Devil (Sarcophilus harrisii). *Journal of Comparative Physiology*, **140**, 241–248.
OWEN, M. and BLISS, E. (1970). Sleep loss and cortical excitability. *American Journal of Physiology*, **218**, 171–173.
PALMBLAD, J., CANTELL, K., STRANDER, H., FROBERG, J., KARLSSON, C-G., LEVI, L., GRANSTROM, M. and UNGER, P. (1976). Stressor exposure and immunological response in man: interferon-producing capacity and phagocytosis. *Journal of Psychosomatic Research*, **20**, 193–199.
PALMBLAD, J., PETRINI, B., WASSERMAN, J. and AKERSTEDT, T. (1979). Lymphocyte and granulocyte reactions during sleep deprivation. *Psychosomatic Medicine*, **41**, 373–378.
PARKER, D. C. and ROSSMAN, L. G. (1971). Human growth hormone release in sleep: non-suppression by acute hyperglycaemia. *Journal of Clinical Endocrinology*, **32**, 65–69.
PARKER, D. C., ROSSMAN, L. G., KRIPKE, D. F., HERSHMAN, J. M., GIBSON, W., DAVIS, D., WILSON, K., and PEKARY, E. (1980). Endocrine rhythms across sleep-wake cycles in normal young men under basal state conditions. In: J. OREM, and C. D. BARNES (Eds.), *Physiology in Sleep*, New York: Academic Press, pp. 145–179.
PARKER, D. C., ROSSMAN, L. G. and VAN DER LAAN, E. F. (1972). Persistence of rhythmic growth hormone release during sleep in fasted and non-isoçalorically fed normal subjects. *Metabolism*, **21**, 241–252.
PARKER, D. L., MORISHIMA, M., KOERKER, D. J., GALE, C. C. and GOODNER, C. J. (1972). Pilot study of growth hormone release in the sleep of the chair — adapted baboon: potential as a modal of human sleep release. *Endocrinology*, **91**, 1462–1467.
PARMEGGIANI, P. L. (1980). Temperature regulation during sleep: a study in homeostasis. In: J. OREM and C. D. BARNES (Eds.), *Physiology in Sleep*, New York: Academic Press, pp. 97–143.
PARMEGGIANI, P. L., CIANCI, T., CALASSO, M., ZAMBONI, G. and PEREZ, E. (1980). Quantitative analysis of short-term deprivation and recovery of desynchronised sleep in cats. *Electroencephalography and Clinical Neurophysiology*, **50**, 293–302.
PARMEGGIANI, P. L., RABINI, C. and CATTALINI, M. (1969). Sleep phases at low environmental temperature. *Archives of Science and Biology*, **53**, 277–290.
PARMEGGIANI, P. L. and SABBATINI, L. (1972). Electromyographic aspects of postural, respiratory and thermoregulatory mechanisms in sleeping cats. *Electroencephalography and Clinical Neurophysiology*, **33**, 1–13.
PARMEGGIANI, P. L., ZAMBONI, G., CIANCI, T. and CALASSO, M. (1977). Absence of thermoregulatory vasomotor responses during fast wave sleep in cats. *Electroencephalography and Clinical Neurophysiology*, **42**, 372–380.
PASNAN, R. O., NAITOH, P., STIER, S. and KOLLAR, E. J. (1968). The psychological effects of 205 hours of sleep deprivation. *Archives of General Psychiatry*, **18**, 496–508.
PEARSON, O. (1947). The rate of metabolism of some small mammals. *Ecology*, **28**, 127–145.
PILLERI, G. (1979). The blind Indus dolphin (Platanista Indi) *Endeavour*, **3**, 48–56.

PLUMMER, S., MATTHEWS, L., TUCKER, M. and COOK, T. (1974). The water tank technique: avoidance conditioning as a function of water level and pedestal size. *Physiology and Behaviour*, **12**, 285–288.

PRATT, K. L., MATTSON, R. H., WEIKERS, N. J. and WILLIAMS, R. (1968). EEG activation of epileptics following sleep deprivation: a prospective study of 114 cases. *Electroencephalography and Clinical Neurophysiology*, **24**, 11–14.

QUABBE, H-J. (1977). Chronobiology of growth hormone secretion. *Chronobiologia*, **4**, 217–246.

QUABBE, H-J, GREGOR, M., BUM KE-VOGT, C., ECKHOF, A. and WITT. I. (1981). Twenty-four hour pattern of growth hormone secretion in the rhesus monkey: studies including alterations of the sleep/wake and sleep stage cycles. *Endocrinology*, **109**, 513–522.

REBOLLEDO, O. R. and GAGLIARDINO, J. J. (1971). Circadian variations of the protein metabolism in musle. *Journal of Interdisciplinary Cycle Research*, **2**, 101–108.

REICH, P., GEYER, S. J. and KARNOVSKY, M. L. (1972). Metabolism of brain during sleep and wakefulness. *Journal of Neurochemistry*, **19**, 487–497.

REILLY, T. and WALSH, T. J. (1981). Physiological, psychological and performance measures during an endurance record for a 5-a-side soccer play. *British Journal of Sports Medicine*, **15**, 122–128.

REITE, M. L. and PEGRAM, G. V. (1968). Cortical temperature during paradoxical sleep in the monkey. *Electroencephalography and Clinical Neurophysiology*, **25**, 36–41.

REIVICH, M., ISAACS, G., EVARTS, E. and KETY, S. (1968). The effect of slow wave sleep and REM sleep on regional cerebral blood flow in cats. *Journal of Neurochemistry*, **15**, 301–306.

RENNIE, M. J., EDWARDS, R. H. T. DAVIES, C. T. M., KRYWAWYCH, S., HALLIDAY, D., WATERLOW, J. C. and MILLWARD, D. J. (1980). Protein and amino acid turnover during and after exercise. *Biochemical Society Transactions*, **8**, 499–501.

RODIN, E. A., LUBY, E. D. and GOTTLEIB, J. S. (1962). The EEG during prolonged experimental sleep deprivation. *Electroencephalography and Clinical Neurophysiology*, **14**, 544–551.

ROFFWARG, H. P., MUZIO, J. N. and DEMENT, W. C. (1966). Ontongenetic development of the human sleep-dream cycle. *Science*, **152**, 604–609.

ROSS, J. J. (1966). Neurological findings after prolonged sleep deprivation. *Archives of Neurology*, **12**, 399–403.

RUCKEBUSCH, Y. (1972). The relevance of drowsiness in the circadian cycle of farm animals. *Animal Behaviour*, **20**, 637–643.

RUCKEBUSCH, Y. (1972). Development of sleep and wakefulness in the foetal lamb. *Electroencephalography and Clinical Neurophysiology*, **32**, 119–128.

RUCKEBUSCH, Y. (1975). The hypnogram as an index of adaptation of farm animals to changes in their environment. *Applied Animal Ethology*, **2**, 3–18.

RUCKEBUSCH, Y. (1977). Sleep and the environment. In: W. P. KOELLA, (Ed.), *Sleep 1976*, Basel: Karger, pp. 152–169.

SAKAI, F., MEYER, J. S., KARACAN, I., DERMAN, S., YAMAMOTO, M. (1979). Normal human sleep: regional cerebral haemodynamics. *Annals of Neurology*, **7**, 471–478.

SAMSON, H. (1966). Psychological effects of deprivation of dreaming sleep. *Journal of Nervous and Mental Diseases*, **143**, 305–317.

SATINOFF, E., DRUCKER-COLIN, R. R. and HERNANDEZ-PEON, R. (1971). Paelocortical excitability and sensory filtering during REM sleep deprivation. *Physiology and Behaviour*, **7**, 103–106.

SATO, S., DREIFUSS, F. E. and PENRY, J. K. (1975). Photic sensitivity of children with absence seizures in slow wave sleep. *Electroencephalography and Clinical Neurophysiology*, **39**, 479–489.

SCHEVING, L. E. (1959). Mitotic rhythm in the human epidermis. *Anatomical Record*, **135**, 7–20.

SCHLAG, J. (1974). Reticular influences on thalamo-cortical activity. In: A. REMOND

(Ed.), *Handbook of Electroencephalography and Clinical Neurophysiology* (Vol. 2, part C), Amsterdam: Elsevier, pp. 119–135.
SCRIMSHAW, N. S., HABICHT, J. P., PELLET, P., PICHE, M. L. and CHOLAKOS, B. (1966). Effects of sleep deprivation and reversal of diurnal activity on protein metabolism of young men. *American Journal of Clinical Nutrition*, **19**, 313–318.
SEYLAZ, J., MAMO, H., GOAS, J. Y. and HOUDART, R. (1971). Human cerebral blood flow regulation and physiological sleep. In: R. W. RUSSEL (Ed.), *Brain and Blood Flow*, London: Pitman, pp. 143–149.
SHAPIRO C. M., GRIESEL, R. D., BARTEL, P. R. and JOOSTE, P. L. (1975). Sleep patterns after graded exercise. *Journal of Applied Physiology*, **2**, 187–190.
SHAPIRO, C. M., MOORE, A. T., MITCHELL, D. and YODAIKEN, M. L. (1974). How well does man thermoregulate during sleep? *Experientia*, **30**, 1279–1281.
SIESJO, B. K. (1978), *Brain Energy Metabolism*, New York: Wiley.
SLOAN, M. A. (1972). The effects of deprivation of REM sleep on maze learning and aggression in the albino rat. *Journal of Psychiatric Research*, **9**, 101–111.
SMITH, C. A. (1959). *The Physiology of the Newborn Infant*, Springfield, Ill: C. C. Thomas.
STERN, W. C. and MORGANE, P. J. (1977). Sleep and memory: effects of growth hormone on sleep brain neurochemistry and behaviour. In: R. R. DRUCKER-COLIN and J. L. MCGAUGH (Eds.), *Neurobiology of Sleep and Memory*, New York: Academic Press, 373–400.
STEINER, S. S. and ELLMAN, S. J. (1972). Relation between REM sleep and intracranial self-stimulation. *Science*, **177**, 1122–1124.
STERMAN, M. B. (1979). Ontogeny of sleep: implications for function. In: R. DRUCKER-COLIN, M. SHKUROVICH and M. B. STERMAN (Eds.), *The Functions of Sleep*, New York: Academic Press.
STERMAN, M. B., HARPER, R. M., HAVENS, B., HOPPENBROUWERS, T., MCGINTY, D. J. and HODGMAN, J. E. (1977). Quantitative analysis of infant EEG development during quiet sleep. *Electroencephalography and Clinical Electroencephalography*, **43**, 371–385.
STUSS, D. and BROUGHTON, R. (1978). Extreme short sleep: personality problems and a case of sleep requirement. *Waking and Sleeping*, **2**, 101–105.
SWETS, J. A., TANNER, W. P. and BIRDSALL, T. G. (1961). Decision processes in perception. *Psychological Review*, **68**, 301–340.
SZYMUSIAK, R. and SATINOFF, E. (1981). Maximal REM sleep time defines a narrower thermoneutral zone than does minimal metabolic rate. *Physiology and Behaviour*, **26**, 687–690.
TAKAHASHI, Y. (1979). Growth hormone secretion related to the sleep and waking rhythms. In: R. DRUCKER-COLIN *et al.* (Eds.), *The Functions of Sleep*, New York: Academic Press, pp. 113–145.
TAYLOR, C. R. (1966). The vascularity and possible thermregulatory function of the horns in goats. *Physiology and Zoology*, **39**, 127–139.
TAYLOR, C. R., SCHMIDT-NIELSEN, K. and RAAB, J. L. (1970). Scaling of the energetic cost of running to body size in Mammals. *American Journal of Physiology*, **219**, 1104–1107.
THAYER, R. E. (1978). Towards a psychological theory of multidimensional activation (arousal), *Motivation and Emotion*, **2**, 1–34.
TOUTAIN, P-L. and RUCKESBUSCH, Y. (1972). Secretions nasolabiales au cours du sommeil paradoxal chez les bovins. *C.R. Academie de Science* (Paris), **274**, 2519–2522.
TOUTAIN, P-L. and WEBSTER, A. J. (1975). Equilibre energetique au cours du sommeil chez les ruminants. *C.R. Academic des Science* (Paris), **281**, 1605–1608.
TOWNSEND, R. E., PRINZ, P. N. and OBRIST, W. D. (1973). Human cerebral blood flow during sleep and waking. *Journal of Applied Physiology*, **35**, 620–625.
VAN DEN NOORT, S. and BRINE, K. (1970). Effect of sleep on brain labile phosphates and metabolic rate. *American Journal of Physiology*, **218**, 1434–1439.

VEECH, R. L. (1980). Freeze-blowing of brain and the interpretation of the meaning of certain metabolite levels. In: J. V. PASSONNEAU, *et al.* (Eds.), *Cerebral Metabolism and Neural Function*, Baltimore: Williams & Wilkins, pp. 34–41.

VERDONE, P. (1908). Sleep satiation: extended sleep in normal subjects. *Electroencephalography and Clinical Neurophysiology*, **24**, 417–423.

VOGEL, G. W. (1975). A review of REM sleep deprivation. *Archives of General Psychiatry*, **32**, 749–761.

VOGEL, G. W. (1979). A motivational function of REM sleep. In: R. DRUCKER-COLIN, M. SHKUROVICH and M. B. STERNMAN (Eds.), *The Functions of Sleep*, New York: Academic Press.

VOGEL, G., VOGEL, F., MCABEE, R. A. and THURMOND, A. J. (1980). Improvement of depression by REM sleep deprivation. *Archives of General Psychiatry*, **37**, 247–253.

VONDURA, K., BRODAN, V., BASS, A., KUHN, E., TEISINGER, J., ANDEL, M. and VESELKOVA, A. (1981). Effects of sleep deprivation on the activity of selected metabolic enzymes in skeletal muscle. *European Journal of Applied Physiology*, **47**, 41–46.

WALKER, J. M. and BERGER, R. J. (1973). A polygraphic study of the tortoise (Testudo denticulata): absence of electrophysiological signs of REM sleep. *Brain and Behavioural Evolution*, **8**, 453–467.

WALKER, J. M. and BERGER, R. J. (1980). Sleep as an adaptation for energy conservation functionally related to hibernation and shallow torpor, *Progress in Brain Research*, **53**, 255–278.

WALKER, J. M., FLOYD, T. C., FEIN, G., CAVNESS, C., LUALHATI, R. and FEINBERG, I. (1978). Effects of exercise on sleep. *Journal of Applied Physiology*, **44**, 945–951.

WALKER, J. M., GARBER, A., BERGER, R. J. and HELLER, H. C. (1979). Sleep and estivation (shallow torpor): continuous process of energy conservation. *Science*, **204**, 1098–1100.

WANNEMACHER, R. W. and DINTERMAN, R. E. (1980). Diurnal response in endogenous amino acid oxidation of meal-fed rats. *Biochemical Journal*, **190**, 663–671.

WARNER, B. F. and HUGGINS, S. E. (1978). An electroencephalographic study of sleep in young caimans in a colony. *Comparative Biochemistry and Physiology*, **59A**, 139–144.

WATERLOW, J. C., GARLICK, P. J. and MILLWARD, D. J. (1978). *Protein Turnover in Mammalian Tissues and in the Whole Body*, Amsterdam: Elsevier.

WEBB, A. C. (1976). The effects of changing levels of arousal on the spontaneous activity of cortical neurones. 1. Sleep and Wakefulness. *Proceedings of the Royal Society, London, B*, **194**, 225–237.

WEBB, P. and HIESTAND, M. (1975). Sleep metabolism and age, *Journal of Applied Physiology*, **38**, 257–262.

WEBB, W. B. (1975). *Sleep, the Gentle Tyrant*, Englewood Cliffs, NJ: Prentice Hall.

WEBB, W. B. and AGNEW, H. W. (1970). Sleep stage characteristics of long and short sleepers, *Science*, **168**, 146–147.

WEBB, W. B. and AGNEW. H. W. (1971). Stage 4 sleep: influence of time-course variables. *Science*, **174**, 1354–1356.

WEBB, W. B. and AGNEW, H. W. (1974). The effects of a chronic limitation of sleep length. *Psychophysiology*, **11**, 265–274.

WEBB, W. B. and AGNEW, H. W. (1975). Are we chronically sleep deprived? *Bulletin of the Psychonomic Society*, **6**, 47–48.

WEBB, W. B. and FRIEL, J. (1971). Sleep stage and personality characteristics of 'natural' long and short sleepers. *Science*, **171**, 587–588.

WEBSTER, A. J. F. (1980). The energetic efficiency of growth. *Livestock Production Science*, **7**, 243–252.

WEITZMAN, E. D. (1976). Circadian rhythms and episodic hormone secretion in man. *Annual Review of Medicine*, **27**, 225–243.

WHITEHEAD, W. E., ROBINSON, T. M., WINCOR, M. Z. and RECHTSCHAFFEN, A. (1969). The accumulation of REM sleep need during sleep and wakefulness. *Communications in Behavioural Biology*, **4**, 195–201.

WILKINSON, R. T. (1964). Effects of up to 60 hours sleep deprivation on different types of worm. *Ergonomics*, **7**, 175–186.

WILKINSON R. T. (1965). Sleep deprivation. In: O. G. EDHOLM and A. L. BACHARACH (Eds.), *Physiology of Survival*, London: Academic Press.

WILKINSON, R. T. (1968). Sleep deprivation: performance tests for partial and selective sleep deprivation. In: L. E. ABT and B. F. RIESS (Eds.), *Progress in Clinical Psychology: Dreams and Dreaming*, London: Grune & Stratton, pp. 28–43.

WILLIAMS, H. L., HAMMACK, J. T., DALY, R. L., DEMENT, W. C. and LUBIN, A. (1964). Responses to auditory stimulation, sleep loss and the EEG stages of sleep. *Electroencephalography and Clinical Neurophysiology*, **16**, 269–279.

WILLIAMS, H. L., LUBIN, A. and GOODNOW, J. J. (1959). Impaired performance with acute sleep loss. *Psychological Monographs*, **73**, 1–26.

WILLIAMS, R. L., KARACAN, I. and HURSCH, C. J. (1974). *Electroencephalography (EEG) of Human Sleep: Clinical Application*, New York: Wiley.

YERKES, R. M. and DODSON, J. D. (1908). The relation of strength of stimulus to rapidity of habit formation. *Journal of Comparative and Neurological Psychology*, **18**, 459–482.

YOUNG, V. R., STEFFEE, W. P., PENCHARIZ, P. B., WINTERER, J. G. and SCRIMSHAW, N. S. (1975). Total human body protein synthesis in relation to protein requirements at various ages. *Nature* (London), **253**, 192–194.

ZARCONE, V., DE LA PENA, A. and DEMENT, W. C. (1974). Heightened sexual interest and sleep disturbance. *Perceptual and Motor Skills*, **39**, 1135–1141.

ZEPELIN, H. and RECHTSCHAFFEN, A. (1974). Mammalian sleep, longevity and energy metabolism. *Brain and Behavioural Evolution*, **10**, 425–470.

ZULLEY, J. (1980). Distribution of REM sleep in entrained 24 hour and free-running sleep-wake cycles, *Sleep*, **2**, 377–390.

CHAPTER 10

Cognitive Processes During Sleep: Evolutionary Aspects

David Foulkes

Soon after the discovery of REM sleep, and of its correlation with vivid dreaming in the adult human (Aserinsky & Kleitman, 1953), Dement (1958) reported that the REM stage also could be observed in the sleep of cats. Subsequent research (summarized e.g. by Allison & Van Twyver, 1970) has established that most mammals have clearly identifiable periods of REM ('paradoxical') sleep. Brief episodes of REM sleep also have been observed in chickens and pigeons (Klein *et al.*, 1964).

That humans share REM sleep with a variety of related species naturally enough raises the question as to whether they also share the experiencing of dreams with some or all of these species. Leaving aside, for the moment, how this question might be addressed observationally, one can see how its answer might be of great value to the struggling science of human dreams. Should the experiencing of dreams be shared by other species than our own, dream psychology would have a greatly expanded sphere of potentially pertinent observation and experimentation, as well as the opportunity to make the sorts of comparative observations that have illuminated our understanding of so many other physiological processes and behavioural phenomena. Conversely, should dreaming prove to remain an essentially human prerogative, it might then be the case that a number of possible conceptualizations of dreaming and of dream function (specifically those based on subhuman evolutionary considerations) would be less tenable and that our attention would be redirected to specifically human phenomena in whose study the riddles of dreaming more appropriately could be resolved.

But one cannot, of course, hope for answers with wide-ranging implications of these sorts unless the question of dream experiencing in other species actually can be investigated in any meaningful way. In this chapter, I shall present two subhuman experimental models of human dreaming, and one human observational model of subhuman dreaming. I want to use the discussion of these models to show that the question of dreaming in other species may not be so refractory to reasonable analysis as it is sometimes imagined to be. I will also argue that the resolution of this question suggested by presently available evidence has significant implications for how we can best conceptualize and study human dreams.

First, however, I want to provide a context of observations of dreaming in the adult human. These observations will provide an appropriate empirical base from which to launch a more speculative foray into the nocturnal mental life of other species. What, in brief, do we really know about *our own* dreams?

10.1 Dreaming in the Adult Human: Descriptive Data

After early childhood, the proportion of total sleep time that humans spend in REM sleep stabilizes at somewhere between 22% and 28% (Williams *et al.*, 1974). This REM sleep generally occurs in discrete periods of 5–45 min duration, each period terminating an approximately 90-min sleep cycle whose earlier constituent is EEG slow wave and/or spindle sleep unaccompanied by rapid eye movement. The first REM period of the night generally is the shortest, and occurs only after an hour or more of non-REM (NREM) sleep. Following the first REM period, NREM sleep recurs, to be terminated by a second REM period. A normal night's sleep may include 4–6 discrete REM periods, whose lengths generally increase as the night progresses.

The likelihood that reasonably well-motivated and articulate subjects will remember a dream following experimental interruptions of REM sleep is very high. Over 80% of REM awakenings produce dream reports (Dement, 1965), and, with some subjects, the figure is likely to be close to 100%.

It was believed at first (e.g. Dement & Kleitman, 1957) that NREM sleep is unaccompanied by significant mental activity, but later research suggested that dreamlike mentation can accompany NREM sleep as well as REM sleep. At the initial onset of sleep, fairly vivid NREM dream episodes occur for many persons at a rate at least equalling that of REM dreaming (e.g. Foulkes & Vogel, 1965). On awakenings from succeeding periods of NREM sleep, the quantity and dreamlike quality of subjects' mentation reports is somewhat less than at sleep onset, but these NREM reports still clearly refute any hypothesis of an exclusive association of dreaming with the REM stage (e.g. Foulkes, 1962). Thus, although REM sleep is most frequently associated with vivid dream recollections, REM sleep does not appear to be a *necessary* condition of experiencing dreams in the adult human.

In addressing the question of animals' dreams, I will focus on REM-sleep dreaming, for it is in REM sleep that human dreaming seems to be both most well developed in form and most obligatory in occurrence. Is REM sleep a *sufficient* condition of experiencing dreams? If so, most mammals must dream, for they possess REM sleep, as it ordinarily has been defined (Rechtschaffen & Kales, 1968).

While my focus is on REM sleep, it may prove useful to consider briefly some of the differences often observed between NREM reports and REM reports in adult humans, for these differences have been influential in shaping researchers' notions of what is so distinctive about REM dreaming. In trying to decide whether NREM reports were really 'dream' reports (as opposed to reports of 'thoughts' or other forms of experience and/or mentation), researchers were forced to attend to those properties of full-blown (i.e. REM) dream experience that might be considered hallmarks of 'dreaming'. Consensus generally is reached on the following characteristics of fully developed dreams.

First, the manifest form of the dream experience is generally imaginal, rather than imageless and/or verbal. Some NREM reports seem 'undreamlike', because, in them, subjects claim merely to have been thinking verbally or in some other abstract, non-imaginal way.

Second, in the manifest dream experience there is a constructive rearrangement of one's past experiences and thoughts according to principles somewhat foreign to waking thought. Some NREM reports seem undreamlike in that they seem merely to be relatively unreconstructed memories of events in the subject's life history or in that they seem to portray situations or contents of literal or immediate interest to the subject. They are either the sort of thing one already has thought of or experienced in wakefulness or the sort of thing one might well think or experience in the waking state.

Third, the manifest dream is a narrative. The dream's reordering of our memories and knowledge is far from a random one. Dream images generally cohere sequentially as sensible parts of an overall dream story. The dream is not a succession of unrelated images nor an isolated single image which leads nowhere else. By these criteria, some NREM reports are defective cases of well-developed dreaming.

Fourth, the manifest dream is a hallucination. While dreaming a dream, we ordinarily do not question the truth of what we are experiencing. So long as we are dreaming the dream, its story-line is our reality, and our sole reality (Rechtschaffen, 1978). We do not bring our critical judgement or our history of waking reality testing to bear on what we see and hear. We do not tell ourselves that this is all nonsense or that this cannot be. We believe. By the hallucination criterion, some NREM and sleep-onset reports are not fully dreamlike.

What do these four hallmarks of the adult human's REM dreams suggest about the possibility that subhuman mammals experience dreams during their REM sleep? The first and fourth characteristics might be viewed as favouring that possibility: dreaming is an unreflective, automatic process of a sort that might not depend on the possession of language or of abstract thought; it occurs in a 'primitive language' of perceptual experience. However, the second and third characteristics listed above challenge both this interpretation of human dreaming and the possibility that dreaming is experienced by other species. Our dreaming is not a 'replay' of our perceptual experience, but an active symbolic reorganization of our discrete memories and our more general knowledge. The very same imaginal character of the dream that neurophysiologists are wont to see as indexing the primitiveness of dreaming suggests to the student of human cognition (and to the human neuropsychologist) that dreaming is a symbolic, rather than a perceptual process. Linking the phylogeny of dreaming to the development of symbolic processes must place greatly more restrictive limits on subhuman dreaming than does the linkage of dreaming to effective waking sensorimotor processing. Moreover, the *kind* of symbolic reorganization we experience in our dreams, namely the synthesis of internally consistent story-lines, suggests that dreaming requires not merely symbolism but also the capability of deploying high-level operations upon symbols in the service of integrative narrative schemata. By this criterion, dreaming in the full-blown adult sense must be viewed as an implausibility not only for most if not all subhuman organisms but also for human beings before the age (5–7) at which children's thought becomes 'operational' (Flavell, 1963).

10.2 Dreaming in the Adult Human: Functional Considerations

Of theories of human dreaming there seemingly is no end, no view that someone, somewhere, has not espoused. Betraying their origins in clinical psychiatry, many of these theories have remained remarkably insensitive to what empirical observations have been made about dreams, particularly to observations made in recent years about REM dreaming. It is, for example, a feature of most of these theories that they propose that dreaming serves some essential function in overt adaptation to the external world and/or in the creation or maintenance of the internal programming that permits such adaptation. However, there is very little satisfactory evidence that human REM dreaming serves any demonstrable function. It boggles the mind to think that something as pervasive as human REM dreaming (in which we may spend the equivalent of five full years of our lifetimes) has no function, and yet reliable evidence of any such function has yet to appear (Kramer, 1981).

REM deprivation in the adult human does not seem to 'drive' dreaming to other states, either in sleep (Arkin *et al.*, 1978) or in wakefulness (Vogel, 1975). Thus REM-sleep deprivation can be considered to be REM-dream deprivation. Yet such deprivation has no deleterious effect on 'mental health', and no consistent or reliable effect on external adaptation, memory, or cognitive organization in normal human subjects (Vogel, 1975; Ellman *et al.*, 1978).

Besides this major evidential problem with the hypothesis that REM dreaming serves some vital adaptive function, there is also a substantial methodological problem in ever determining the functions of REM dreaming. If, by function, we mean 'effect', then, because we generally have reliable control neither of REM dreaming *per se* nor of particular kinds of dream imagery (Griffin & Foulkes, 1977), it is impossible to know the effects either of dreaming or of particular kinds of dreams. In the face, at the human level, of these evidential difficulties, of methodological problems in achieving dream control and/or REM deprivation, and of ethical constraints on experimental manipulation, many investigators have turned to animal models to determine REM-sleep functions.

In these models, the REM-deprived subhuman subject is compared to a non-deprived control animal on some learning or memory task or in the manifestation of some drive-regulated behaviour (see e.g. reviews by McGrath & Cohen, 1978; Ellman *et al.*, 1978). Results for the body of this research are only somewhat more promising than those for the human studies which the subhuman research is meant to supplement or replace. However, as a model for determining the function of *dreaming*, the subhuman REM-deprivation study is appropriate only to the extent that one believes (1) that the subhuman organism generally experiences REM dreams and (2) that this dreaming is being suppressed by the concomitant suppression of REM sleep. It is, to the contrary, quite possible that the subhuman REM-deprivation paradigm at best speaks only to the functions of REM sleep and not at all to those of dreaming.

Indeed, given the nature of the human dream as I have reviewed it above on the one hand, and the nature of the neural mediation of REM sleep (e.g. Jouvet, 1962; Hobson & McCarley, 1977) on the other hand, there is reason to believe that little is to be learned about the functions of the human dream from the study of the REM-deprived or REM-observed rat or cat. The nervous structures which seem to be involved in the most elementary manifestations of REM sleep are primitive ones in the brain stem. The narrative complexity and ingenuity of the adult human dream argue for the critical engagement of central nervous system (CNS) functions of an altogether different and higher order. We have no solid justification for believing that these latter functions are even present in, for example, the cat.

If one *were* to believe in the appropriateness of studying dream function via the observation or manipulation of REM sleep in the cat (e.g. Hobson & McCarley, 1977), one would have to guess, from reports of enhanced drive-state activity (e.g. sexuality, aggression) and of interference with certain kinds of information-processing and information-retention following subhuman REM deprivation, that the dream serves to regulate primitive drive states and to facilitate certain elementary forms of behavioural adaptation. There is much room for doubt, however, in making that kind of extrapolation, for, as we have seen, at the human level there is scant evidence in its favour. If the dream serves such relatively primitive functions as can be mimicked in the animal model, it surely is strange that they cannot readily be demonstrated in human REM-deprivation studies.

In sum, human research does not immediately suggest any particular function for dream generation or dream experiencing, nor that dreams play any sort of critical role in phylogenetically primitive forms of behavioural regulation or information processing. Subhuman animal models suggest that some adaptive significance may attach to REM sleep itself, but the relevance of these models to the function of *dreams* is questionable, both on empirical and on theoretical grounds. At a minimum, to use effectively observations or manipulations of subhuman REM sleep to address questions of dream function, it would be desirable to show that the subhuman species in question actually generates and experiences dreams. The questions remain, 'Do animals really dream during their REM sleep?' and 'How could we *show* that they do so?'

10.3 Animal Models of Human REM Dreaming

Allison and Van Twyver (1970) were 'willing to conclude that imagery occurs during paradoxical sleep in animals' (p. 65). They specifically mention two sorts of evidence indicative of 'dream life in animals' (ibid.). First, they cite data from an unpublished dissertation by Vaughan (1963). Vaughan trained rhesus monkeys in wakefulness to press a lever in the presence of experimenter-generated visual stimuli. Later, the monkeys were reported to have spontaneously lever-pressed during REM sleep, as if they were responding to the imagery of their dreams. Second, Allison and Van Twyver refer to early observations by Jouvet, recently organized in a systematic way by Sastre and Jouvet (1979). Jouvet reported that, when the brainstem structure responsible for their muscular atonia during REM sleep was lesioned, cats exhibited various overt behaviours during REM sleep, as if they were responding to hallucinatory imagery and/or acting out a dream.

Because the Vaughan study and Jouvet's observations remain the most convincing experimental demonstrations of animal dreaming, they deserve our close attention. Have these investigators in fact been able to circumvent the inability of other species to tell us in words whether or not they dream? Have they found reliable, non-verbal indicators of the presence and contents of dream consciousness during REM sleep in subhuman organisms?

Vaughan. Luce (1965; Luce & Siegel, 1966) was largely responsible for calling wider attention to Vaughan's (1963) study. She reported that:

> Until recently nobody had ever taught an animal to report 'seeing things' in sleep, but this has now been done by Dr. Charles J. Vaughan of the University of Pittsburgh with rhesus monkeys . . . (1965, p. 85)

In brief, Vaughan's (1963) experimental design was as follows. He adapted each monkey to spending long periods of time in a restraining chair inside a closed phone booth. Facing the monkey was an illuminated projection screen on which visual patterns of varying degrees of complexity could be displayed. The monkey was taught to press a lever in the presence of projected stimuli in order to avoid foot shocks. After a period in which rates of lever pressing could be assessed in the absence of the projected stimuli, the monkey was fitted with contact lenses that eliminated patterned visual stimulation. The lenses were worn continuously for 74–96 h. The intent here was to see if the animals would signal autogenous visual imagery by bar-pressing during this extended period of 'sensory deprivation.' Vaughan's major finding was that what bar-pressing did occur during this period of visual monotony generally was initiated from sleep accompanied by eye movements. He argued that 'the animals were dreaming when responding began, and the responding was to dream images' (p. 144). Luce accepted and popularized Vaughan's interpretation of his findings.

There are, however, many reasons to doubt Vaughan's hypothesis that his monkeys were signalling their experience of visual dream imagery. Not the least among them is that the replications and extensions of Vaughan's study which Luce (1965, pp. 85–86) so confidently anticipated never have materialized. The Vaughan study stands quite alone in its promise that animals can be trained to tell us if they 'see things' during REM sleep. (Indeed, it is quite difficult even to programme human subjects to signal dream imagery during sleep (Brown & Cartwright, 1979).) But Vaughan's hypothesis also is suspect merely on the basis of the data which he himself described. Indeed, a more detailed analysis of Vaughan's work begins to suggest some of the reasons why it never has been repeated by others.

Here are some of the internal evidential problems weakening the force of Vaughan's interpretation of his own findings. (1) There was no physiological recording of brain-wave or eye-movement activity to verify that Vaughan's animals were in fact asleep, or in REM sleep, when they signalled during the period of visual monotony. The necessity of such recording seems especially critical in a study in which the animals were reported to have behaved queerly. While wearing lenses, Vaughan's monkeys were described variously as: 'virtually motionless for hours'; 'virtually comatose during the first 27 hours'; and showing 'increasingly erratic behavior' (Vaughan, 1963, pp. 86, 93, 103).

(2) The patterning of bursts of responding during visual monotony — these bursts generally occurred many hours apart and themselves lasted for up to 5.25 h — bears no resemblance to the patterning of REM sleep in the monkey under other conditions (Weitzman *et al.*, 1965). It also bears no resemblance to any experimentally induced alteration of REM sleep ever documented elsewhere.

(3) There are a substantial number of difficulties attaching to Vaughan's interpretation that his animals' bar presses during visual monotony meant 'I

see imagery'. Specifically: (a) in the training phase of the study (i.e. before the application of the contact lenses), when Vaughan's animals gave the best evidence that their bar-pressing was somehow related to the presence of visual experience, bar-pressing was *not* observed during 'sleep' periods; (b) the appearance of responding during 'sleep' in the visual-monotony phase of the experiment, then, may well have been a non-specific response to the condition of visual deprivation, and Vaughan had no control animals (untrained at the specific task of signalling visual displays by lever-pressing, but also observed during visual monotony) to rule out this possibility; (c) the conditions of the experiment — the highly restricted environment and the animals' extensive shock-avoidance training with one particular response favoured by that environment, namely lever-pressing — may well have made that response an obvious choice for signalling or trying to reduce distress; (d) there is no doubt but that, even before the insertion of the lenses in both eyes of the experimental animals, the experimental situation was highly stressful: two of Vaughan's six animals could not be tested under visual monotony because 'experimental neurosis' or 'agitation' during training precluded their acquisition of bar-pressing in the presence of the experimenter's visual displays; (e) at best, Vaughan's procedures could not have taught his animals to signal visual experience but only visual-displays-on-the-screen — other visual experiences during training were not made discriminitive stimuli for lever-pressing; (f) during training itself, most animals could be trained to lever-press at the onset of the visual displays, but did not cease lever-pressing at their offset — that is, even during training, lever-pressing did not reliably index the sort of visual experience under experimental control; (g) no animal responded as well after visual monotony as during training to the experimental displays, suggesting that whatever degree of stimulus control Vaughan obtained of the lever-press response during training may not have been sustained, or may have been altered, during the monotony condition.

Based on her understanding of Vaughan's results, Luce went on to suggest that:

> Perhaps a next step — training monkeys to respond to particular images or to smells, for instance — may allow us to find out *what* a monkey dreams about (1965, p. 86, emphasis added).

Vaughan's experiment was, in fact, initiated with the intent of having his monkeys signal what kind of visual experience they had had. Three classes of stimuli (dots of light, simple shapes and complex scenes) were meant to be paired with their own specific levers; the left lever, for example, was to be pushed in the presence of the complex scenes. Neither of the two animals run under these conditions could be taught reliably to signal what kind of slide had been displayed. It was on the basis of their failure, in Vaughan's training conditions, to be able to signal *what* had been seen that these two animals, and the other animals in the study, then were trained at the simpler (but more ambiguous) response of the single lever-press, the supposed index *that* something had been seen.

Thus, a careful reading of Vaughan's study dashes one's casual optimism about the feasibility of quickly training subhuman primates to 'tell' us either what sorts of imagery they experience during REM sleep or even whether or not they in fact experience any such imagery. In such a reading one begins to appreciate why Vaughan's study did not lead to further programmatic research on either the 'dream-reporting' or the waking 'introspection' of subhumans. And, Vaughan's results themselves clearly are far too equivocal to be viewed as offering any consequential evidence of subhuman dreaming.

Jouvet. Bilateral lesioning in the brainstem (in the area of the medial portion of the nucleus locus coeruleus [LC] alpha) suppresses the muscular atonia otherwise characteristic of REM sleep in the cat. In other words, REM sleep is no longer accompanied by a continuous motoric inhibition. Jouvet has documented that the cat released from such inhibition engages, *during* REM sleep, in a variety of stereotyped behaviours. Sastre and Jouvet (1979) have reported that these behaviours include predatory attack (most frequently observed), rage, flight, grooming and exploration. They call these responses 'oneiric' behaviours, implying that they are related to dreams.

How could they be so related? One interpretation might be that, since the LC-lesioned cat can act out its dreams, we see 'externalized' a dream process that ordinarily is more effectively constrained as purely 'mental'. Cohen (1979), after having viewed a film of the 'oneiric' behaviour of Jouvet's cats, has reported his 'compelling' impression that Jouvet's cats must actually have been dreaming. But, wisely I think, he also suggests that one should not rely solely on such captivating impressions in evaluating Jouvet's data.

There are several substantial problems in viewing the behaviour of the LC-lesioned cat as either part of its typical dream process or as a disinhibited behavioural response to its typical dream imagery. First, there are the general difficulties one has in interpreting any lesion data and the specific difficulties attaching to the interpretation of the effects of any brainstem lesion. In the former regard, one cannot be sure that the behaviour of an experimentally scrambled CNS is comparable to that of a normal one; in the latter regard, brainstem lesions generally carry in their wake considerable disruption of the regulation of waking behaviour (and this was the case for Sastre and Jouvet's cats), and one has, therefore, even less confidence than in the case of circumscribed cortical lesions that one is observing a nervous system in which, except for the state or behaviours of experimental interest, all other factors are assuming their normal functional roles. In fact, Morrison and associates (Morrison *et al.*, 1980) have shown that Jouvet's lesions lead to a similar release of locomotor activity during wakefulness as during REM sleep, and plausibly argue that this shows that the REM phenomenon cannot be interpreted simply as 'a release of normal oneiric behaviour'.

Second, there are particular problems in accepting the hypothesis that behaviour during sleep invariably indexes symbolic processes during sleep. Until the advent of modern electrophysiological investigations of sleep, for instance, it often was believed that sleep walkers are acting out their dreams. But it is now known that somnambulism generally is *not* initiated from REM sleep and that somnambulists aroused during their walking episodes generally *cannot* provide a dream account consistent with their pre-arousal behaviours. Most often, they claim not to have been dreaming at all (Jacobson *et al.*, 1965). During sleep there can be a considerable dissociation of behavioural acts — which may simply have been disinhibited — and symbolic processes. Thus, while one might be justified in describing the LC-lesioned cat's comportment during REM sleep as 'REM behaviour', it requires a considerable leap of faith to accept it as 'dream behaviour.'

Third, were the Sastre-Jouvet tabulation of oneiric behaviour to have any strong implications for the understanding of human dream processes, it would seem to be that dreaming is devoted to the exercise of instinctive behaviour, or, as Jouvet (1980) has put it more recently, to the reinforcement of 'genetic programming' and its integration with 'epigenetic stimulation'. In formal terms, this animal model would seem to suggest dream-process mechanisms not unlike those of Freud's (1900) theory, in which the dream is instigated by primitive drive stimuli. In its specific content, however, this animal model would be quite different from Freud's theory. For Freud, the almost invariable instigator of the dream would be a sexual instinct, while Sastre and Jouvet never observed sexual behaviour during the REM sleep of the LC-lesioned cat.

What, then, *would* be the implications for human dream content of the Sastre–Jouvet model? At the level of these authors' *general theoretical position*, the implications are far from clear. Precisely what separates us from lower evolutionary forms is the relative absence in our case of the kinds of pre-programmed behavioural routines readily observed in the cat. Moreover, as Freud acknowledged, and as any careful observer of human dreams would have to attest, our dreams do *not* consist simply of the exercise of primitive drive-related behaviours. While, in the Freudian view, our dream imagery may (but need not, and often does not) *directly refer to* elementary drive states, it rarely, if ever, consists of the vicarious *enactment* of some fixed pattern of drive expression. As Freud would have it, our dreams *are* not our instincts. They are, instead, our mind's attempts to *manage* our instincts. From an evolutionary perspective, what distinguishes us from the cat is the elaboration of a flexible mental-symbolic system that permits our dreams vast latitudes of indirection in the management of elementary systems of adaptation, if indeed we can be said to have such systems at all in the way that the cat does.

In what sense, then, even if cats *do* dream, and even if the Sastre–Jouvet observations *do* offer testimony to the content of their dreams, could the LC-lesioned cat offer a useful model of human dreaming? It bears emphasis, moreover, that even Freud's model of the dream, in which the role of genetic programming is attenuated *vis-à-vis* Jouvet's, is seriously questioned by many empirical students of dreaming. The instinctive biology of Freud's dream model rests more on Freud's own theoretical preoccupations than upon any parsimonious reading of the dream evidence (Foulkes, 1978). What must concern us is not the convergence of a Sastre–Jouvet dream model with an archaic and heavily discredited *theory* of dreaming, but its usefulness in understanding the *facts* of human dreaming, as we now know them.

At the level of Sastre and Jouvet's *specific observations*, the implication for human dream content might be that one would expect a high incidence of primitive drive-related behaviours, such as aggressive displays, in human dreams. Ontogenetically, one would expect such displays to be most visible in the dreams of young children, whose ability symbolically to manage or distort the dreams' sources in mechanisms underlying genetically programmed behaviour would be least well developed. Recent observations of the ontogeny of REM dream reporting (Foulkes, 1982), to be detailed in the next section of this chapter, refute this expectation. They also, not so coincidentally, offer a strong refutation of the like-minded Freudian model of the dream as an affectively or instinctively driven process. What is critically absent in both the Sastre–Jouvet model and in Freudian theory is recognition of what a dream *is* — a *symbolic reorganization of knowledge*.

As the child data will demonstrate, the requisite for the experiencing of dreams seems to be a certain level of symbolic ability. One cannot assume, from the fact that organisms (whether cats or human infants) manifest certain behaviours (whether instinctive behaviour sequences or diffuse emotionality) in any state (whether wakefulness or REM sleep) that their dreams therefore must portray such behaviours. The pertinent questions, both phylogenetically and ontogenetically, in asking whether or what an organism dreams are not 'Can it act?' and 'How does it act?' but 'Can it think?' and 'How does it think?'

By these criteria, stipulated by the fact that the dream is a symbolic process, claims from cat observations of *any* sort that one has a model of how or why or what we dream would have to be so modest as to be imperceptible. And, as I have tried to show, there is no good reason to believe that the particular observations of Sastre and Jouvet have potential relevance to human dreaming or that they indicate that cats dream. Let us, therefore, now take another tack in our consideration of subhuman dreaming, one which adequately recognizes dreaming as the symbolic act that it is, and asks, first, 'What are the cognitive prerequisites of dreaming?' and then, 'What evidence is there that these prerequisites exist in other species besides our own?' (cf. Bates, 1979).

10.4 A Human Model of Dream Phylogeny

Longitudinal observations of REM dream reports (Foulkes, 1982) are consistent with the following pattern of the early ontogenesis of dreaming in the human. In the *pre-operational* or early-symbolic (ages 2–5) period of cognitive development, dream activity is not continuous during REM sleep, and what dreaming does occur consists of isolated static images rather than of kinematic dream narratives. The content of these images generally does not symbolically recreate the social circumstances of the child's waking world but is strongly influenced by dreamer body states such as fatigue, hunger, and thirst. However, self characters as such are absent, and self-concerns most generally are ascribed manifestly to animal characters which seem to stand in for the self.

These various features of pre-operational children's dreams are consistent with children's concurrent cognitive-symbolic performance in wakefulness. Specifically: pre-operational children cannot recreate visual movement in their mental imagery (Piaget & Inhelder, 1966; Kerr *et al.*, 1980); their thinking is episodic, distractible, and liable to be centred on momentary circumstances or states of the self (Flavell, 1963); and pre-operational children are deficient in their awareness of, and in their ability symbolically to recreate themselves as objects and their behaviour as activites (Piaget, 1974; this suggests, of course, an immediate problem in interpreting the LC-lesioned cat's REM behaviour as its enactment of a dream role). Also supporting the hypothesis that the unfolding of dreams is related to cognitive-symbolic ability is the absence of affect in children's earliest REM reports, for, while pre-operational children surely can and do 'behave' emotionally, they generally are quite deficient in their knowledge of feelings and in their ability symbolically to recreate feelings (Shantz, 1975).

It is only in the *transition to operational* thinking (ages 5–7) that children begin to experience dreams with rudimentary narrative sequencing supported by kinematic visual imagery. Also consistent with qualitative changes in waking cognition, dreams now begin effectively to recreate the outlines of the social world outside the child's own skin. However, the experiencing of dreams is considerably less than continuous during REM sleep, and the effective deployment of a self character and the presence of affective accompaniment still are largely lacking in dream scenarios.

The early *concrete operational* (ages 7–9) child, on the other hand, is able to generate and experience REM dreams that formally are very much like those of adults. Dreaming is relatively continuous during REM sleep, and its narrative organization is increasingly complex. There now is a self-character who is capable of various forms of 'participation' in the dream scenario. Feelings (mostly pleasant ones) and thoughts can be generated as imagery accompaniments, although most dreams are hedonically neutral and unreflective. Animal characters assume a decreasingly important and increasingly realistic role in the elaboration of dream stories.

All of these achievements also reflect changes in waking cognitive development: in a way that is not true of the pre-operational child, the concrete-operational child gives evidence of systematized thinking, of versatile mental operations, and of incipient comprehension of an inner-psychological plane of human experience. Neither the development of REM dreaming nor its dependence on waking cognitive maturation ceases in the early operational period (see Foulkes, 1982, Chapters 6–8). However, for purposes of modelling dream phylogeny, this is as far as we need to carry the developmental scenario suggested by children's REM-report data.

It bears reiteration that it is children's REM *reporting* which suggests the sequence described above for the *generation* and *experiencing* of REM dreams. It is possible, therefore, that the developmental changes observed in REM reports do not index developmental changes in dreaming itself. Perhaps, as children become older, they simply are better able to describe a dream process which is relatively constant developmentally. Since our access to children's dreamlife is limited to children's verbal reports, this hypothesis of report, but not of dream, changes cannot definitively be refuted. It can, however, be shown to be implausible.

Theoretically, the hypothesis assumes dreaming to be the sole exception to the principle that adult-level cognitive achievement has a substantial history. No other adult-level human symbolic skill emerges full-blown in early childhood. It seems unparsimonious to assume that children, who otherwise behave as children (including in their descriptive behaviour regarding their dream experiences), are uniquely able to behave as adults when they dream.

My argument here rests on the presupposition that dreaming is a cognitive-symbolic act, rather than a perceptual one. Is there any evidence in favour of this argument? The independence of visual imagination and visual perception can be demonstrated in several ways. Neuropsychological evidence indicates 'that visual imagery is mediated by neural mechanisms that are distinct from the mechanisms of true visual experience' (Gazzaniga & LeDoux, 1978, p. 123). Phenomenologically, late-adventitiously blinded persons may sustain the capability of visual imagination, despite an absence of visual perception (Kirtley, 1975), and some persons with specific cognitive deficits cannot generate kinematic waking mental imagery or dream in visual imagery although they have had a standard history of visual experience and retain the ability to perceive visually their waking world (Kerr *et al.*, 1978; Kerr & Foulkes, 1981). Thus, although both neurophysiologists and behaviourists (e.g. Skinner, 1963) would have us believe in the position of the British empiricists that images are weak copies of 'sensory' sensations, there is, in fact, now substantial reason to doubt this position. Images are cognitive-symbolic constructions, depending on cognitive-symbolic skill. Having seen the world is not a sufficient condition of being able to imagine it visually; one also needs the cognitive operations that permit the symbolic reconstruction of the perceptual act (Piaget & Inhelder, 1966).

The hypothesis that dream-report changes in early childhood are report changes rather than dream ones also encounters a considerable number of direct evidential problems. Although children's reports of known and constant visual stimuli do improve with age, so too does their ability to construct complex narrative representations (Foulkes, 1982). It seems at least as likely that it is *what* is being reported, as *how* it is being reported, that mediates dream-report development. The most consistent cognitive correlates of REM report rate in childhood are visuospatial skills, rather than verbal ones. Such skills presumably have less to do with the ability to describe dreams than with the ability to generate them. Finally, the case of two young adolescents who had normal verbal and memory skills for their age but who had a specific deficit in visuospatial analytic ability (as indexed by block-design and embedded-figure tests) is instructive: these boys reported REM dreams so infrequently (on 1 of 30 awakenings at ages 13–15) as to cast considerable doubt as to whether in fact they REM-dreamed (Foulkes, 1979). These boys had no known visual-perceptual deficits, and they experienced the tonic and phasic physiological aspects of REM sleep. But, with a specific *cognitive* deficit, they seemed not to dream, or not to dream at all well *vis-à-vis* peers of comparable age, physical maturation, *and* verbal/memorial skill.

I conclude from the foregoing lines of evidence that the changing frequency and nature of children's overt reports of REM dreams *do* have something to tell us about the frequency and nature of children's private dream experience. What they have to say is this: dreaming is, in fact, a process whose very presence depends on the capacity for symbolic thought, and whose pervasiveness and nature during REM sleep depend upon the availability and versatility of an organism's mental representations and operations. On this account, dreaming conforms to the cognitive-developmental analysis Piaget has provided for other forms of thinking. Specific implications are that, in the absence of representational or symbolic thought, there can be no mental experience at all during sleep, and that 'dreaming', as we ordinarily understand it, depends upon at least the partial achievement of concrete-operational reasoning. These implications, in turn, have substantial entailments both for deciding whether it is plausible to imagine that subhuman organisms in general dream and for addressing the question of dreaming with relevant empirical observations in the case of any particular subhuman species. The question of an animal's dreaming is indissolubly tied to that of an animal's cognition more generally.

10.5 Subhumans as Thinkers — and Dreamers

The most prominent recent studies of higher cognitive processes in subhumans have been various attempts to teach apes visual or gestural 'languages' (e.g. Gardner & Gardner, 1969; Premack, 1971). Certainly it is these studies that have given rise to the most spectacular claims of experimentally demonstrated communalities in cognition between subhumans and humans. Thus it will be useful to determine what these studies — the 'best' subhuman evidence, coming from both the most cognitively eligible of species and the most exhaustively trained and observed of individual subhuman subjects — in fact suggest about the potentialities of subhuman thinking — and dreaming.

As of this writing (late 1981), the bubble has burst regarding the often extravagant claims made in the past decade or so to the effect that apes can be taught to behave linguistically, in the human sense (Gardner, 1980). One significant concern of researchers on subhuman language has been to demonstrate that chimpanzees or gorillas can be taught syntax, specifically, to generate lawful novel 'sentences' comprised of gestures or visual 'symbols' with discrete semantic reference. Despite early claims of sentence production by apes, it now appears that no satisfactory demonstration exists that apes combine gestures or 'lexical objects' in a fashion mimicking the combinatorial aspects of human language (Premack, 1976; Terrace *et al.*, 1979). Indeed, a second wave of revisionism now casts doubt on whether 'linguistic' apes generally even have acquired reference in the human sense, that is, on whether their use of gestures or lexical objects has, in fact, been symbolically mediated.

Savage-Rumbaugh (Savage-Rumbaugh *et al.*, 1980a; Savage-Rumbaugh *et al.*, 1980b) has spearheaded this second challenge to the major purported demonstrations of language in the ape. Based on more recent testing, for example, she and her associates now doubt that their own well-known chimpanzee model of language use, 'Lana', was behaving symbolically in her deployment of 'lexigrams' (distinctive keys on a console keyboard). This doubt is reinforced by demonstrations, both in computer simulation (Thompson & Church, 1980) and in experiments with birds (Epstein *et al.*, 1980) that the performance of 'linguistic' apes can be duplicated in conditioned-response models not requiring the assumption of symbolic mediation. Thus, it is now less than clear that the most famous demonstrations of chimpanzee and gorilla 'language acquisition' even have involved rudimentary symbol formation.

A symbol, in Savage-Rumbaugh's sense (Savage-Rumbaugh *et al.*, 1980a), can stand for an object in the physical absence of that object. The contrast is with what McNeill (1979) calls 'indexical signs', which 'refer to' an object, but which are under the control of the physical presence of that object. 'Symbolic signs', on the other hand, refer to conceptual structures, and function independently of objects denoted by concepts. Savage-Rumbaugh wants to distinguish between those gestures or manipulations of lexical objects that only superficially resemble word usage, and those gestures or manipulations of lexical objects that imply 'understanding' (or 'representational intelligence': McNeill, 1979) in the post-sensorimotor human sense. She suggests that most or all of the accomplishments of the most famous linguistic apes have not, in fact, rested upon genuine semantic comprehension.

Thus, the study of ape language seems to be returning to the point from which it might well have started, the study of ape intelligence, and of the presence in subhumans of the *cognitive bases* of human linguistic ability. Of those prominent in the first wave of the study of ape language, only Premack (1976) has conceptualized the problem in this manner. He sought to show that his chimpanzee, 'Sarah', organized her knowledge of her world in representational forms much like those of human knowledge (e.g. that she thought of state transformations in terms of 'causality'). In further tests, he sought to demonstrate that Sarah conserved quantity across transformations in shape, much as concrete-operational children do (Woodruff *et al.*, 1978), and that she 'understood' problem situations on a human model (Premack & Woodruff, 1978). In view of Savage-Rumbaugh's findings, these specific claims must be viewed as somewhat questionable (see e.g. Savage-Rumbaugh & Rumbaugh, 1979), but clearly the thrust of Premack's programme is appropriate: determine the degree to which the processes of ape and human intelligence are comparable, rather than (or as well as) whether apes can be shaped into performances that mimic human linguistic accomplishment.

Savage-Rumbaugh *et al.* (Savage-Rumbaugh *et al.*, 1980b) trained three chimpanzees (including Lana) to label (i.e. select the appropriate lexigram) three inedible objects as 'tools' and three edible objects as 'food'. Later they presented the names (i.e. lexigrams previously paired singly with their appropriate referents) of various additional foods and tools to the chimpanzees, and 'requested' that these be appropriately labelled as foods or tools. To solve this problem, the researchers reasoned, the chimpanzee would have to possess symbolism: specifically, the name would have to evoke a representation of the object, since the names in test never had, themselves, been paired with categorical labels, and the object-representation would then have to be matched with a functional-categorical representation. Two of the chimpanzees (but not Lana) correctly labelled these new names on their first presentations. These results were used to argue that the two chimpanzees who were successful evidenced a 'representational symbolic function' and that Lana's failure suggests that her earlier 'linguistic' performances were achieved without 'either semantic comprehension or representational symbolic ability' (p. 924).

The Savage-Rumbaugh *et al.* observations, then, indicate a far more restricted interpretation of ape language-learning performances than one might have hazarded ten years ago. On the other hand, they also suggest that, suitably trained at sufficient length, apes can manifest the sort of symbolic representation on which both language and dreaming must, at least in part, depend.

In evaluating the current status of research on ape language and/or on the cognitive skills on which language rests, one faces the inevitable problem of catching in a fixed frame the rapidly moving current of any research field. Specifically, there is the risk of depending too much upon the most recent events in that current, of relying too heavily upon the most recent research study in an area in which it seems to be the fate of each of today's firm conclusions that it appears highly questionable tomorrow. None the less, I think that the last decade or so of research on ape cognition does suggest several tentative conclusions to the question as to whether apes, our closest 'cognitive cousins' and our best bets for animal dreaming could, in fact, be plausibly considered as REM dreamers.

First, when careful attention is given the question of its symbolic mediation, ape 'language' seems less like the language of operational or pre-operational children and implicates far more rudimentary cognitive talent than earlier reports would have suggested. More direct approaches suggest that, at least under certain training conditions, apes have some potential for functioning symbolically, in a Piagetian sense, although this potential was not well enlisted in typical attempts to teach artificial languages to them. The extent of this potential is as yet not well known, but current evidence justifies caution in assuming that it is sufficiently great to support such complex symbolic constructive-combinatorial acts as language or dreaming, as we understand these phenomena at the adult human level.

Second, the demonstration of symbolic potentiality is not the same as that of symbolic actuality. Apes do not *spontaneously* develop a symbolic-communicative system of the flexibility and complexity of our verbal language. By the same token, one may doubt that, spontaneously, they have a REM symbolic-expressive system of the flexibility and complexity of most human dreaming. There remains the possibility that apes might be *trained* to develop the cognitive representations and operations requisite to dreaming, but there is good reason to believe that any such training programme would have to be so massive and so pervasive as to render its graduates highly unrepresentative of their own species. The great lengths to which researchers have had deliberately to structure ape environments to produce even superficial analogues of elementary forms of human language suggest that comparable dream-training exercises, whose success only could be verified by concomitant development of genuine linguistic skill, must for now be consigned to the realm of science fiction.

Third, even where apes can be demonstrated to be teachable in symbolic or pseudo-symbolic performance, at whatever degree of effort, it does not seem to be the case that they show a predilection to spontaneous production or deployment of symbolic or proto-symbolic behaviour outside of highly restrictive contexts related to those of the acquisition of such behaviour. One gets no sense of the enthusiastic symbol-seeking and symbolic generalization that routinely characterizes child language-learners. Because dreaming, far more than language, would seem to depend on spontaneous rather than on evironmentally elicited or environmentally supported production motives, there is even more reason to doubt that chimpanzees and gorillas spontaneously dream than that they spontaneously use symbolic language for social communication. Moreover, even human ontogenetic evidence on REM dreaming (previous section of this chapter), and on spoken language acquisition (e.g. Foss & Hakes, 1978), suggest that dreaming is the more difficult production skill for preoperational children to master. And, in focusing on the fact that dream generation is a *production* skill depending upon *spontaneous* deployment, we can review the history of recent attempts to teach apes language feeling only the most meagre encouragement for the hypothesis that apes dream.

10.6 Ontogeny Again: Consciousness

Dreaming is *consciously experienced* symbolic activity occurring in the human during sleep, most saliently perhaps during REM sleep. Heretofore, our focus in thinking about the possibility that other species dream has been on whether they possess the symbolic skills requisite to dream generation. One might, however, equally well ask if they can experience consciousness. If not, it scarcely seems imaginable that they can 'dream'. I have postponed consideration of this question until now for the obvious reason that it is more difficult to conceive of evidence that might answer it. None the less, it is a question about which it can be fun, and perhaps even instructive, to speculate.

The problem of defining consciousness never has been satisfactorily resolved by those who have had good reason to try to do so, be they philosophers, psychologists or biologists. We adult humans all 'know' what 'consciousness is', but we experience hopeless confusion in trying to explicate that knowledge so that we can consider, rationally and/or empirically, if others 'experience it' as we do. Do subhuman species experience consciousness in our sense? In any sense? In what sense?

Griffin (1976) has recently attempted to marshal evidence from studies of animal behaviour in favour of evolutionary continuity in 'mental experience', which he defines as thought 'about objects and events that are remote in time and space from the immediate flux of sensations' (p. 5), and in 'awareness', which he defines as 'the whole set of interrelated mental images of the flow of events'. As we have seen, even in higher primates it is hard to come by much evidence that would seem to fit Griffin's first definition, which seems to reduce to the question of symbolic behaviour, in Savage-Rumbaugh's sense. And, as Griffin attempts to apply his definition of awareness, it unsurprisingly slips off into the obscurities suggested by its own verbalisms. What precisely is 'mental imagery' or 'internal imagery'? How, if at all, can it be reliably indexed? Is the possession of spatial orientation, for example, as Griffin seems to think, adequate to indicate 'some sort of internal imagery' (p. 14)? What 'sort'? The confusions of Griffin's broadside for 'animal awareness' amply illustrate the phylogenetic thicket which other, less bold but perhaps more wise, students of consciousness strenuously have avoided.

Interestingly, although Griffin espouses applying the theories of human cognitive psychology to subhuman species, he does not use any evidence from cognitive *developmental* psychology. That is, he does not consider how human ontogeny might bear on the phylogeny of consciousness. Nor does he seriously reflect upon the implications of current accounts of adult-human cognitive processing (as recently discussed, for instance, by Shallice, 1978) for his question of animal awareness. In wholly or largely ignoring the literatures of these two areas, Griffin has, in my judgement, cut himself off from precisely those sources of greatest potential relevance to answering his question. Perhaps not so coincidentally, these sources point to a far different answer from Griffin's confident assertion of interspecies similarities in consciousness/awareness.

When we use the term 'consciousness', we ordinarily imply the existence of something more than sheer responsiveness to external stimulation. That we can displace a house-fly by rapidly moving our hand towards it seldom gives rise to an attribution of full consciousness to that insect. Our kind of consciousness requires something more than responsiveness to stimulation. The question is, what is that 'something more'?

One conventional philosophical account (e.g. Dennett, 1969) would reduce awareness in our sense to the capacity for verbalization. While the fly is aware ('aware_2') of our hand in the sense that its current behaviour is influenced by our hand, we alone can be aware ('aware_1') of that exchange in the sense that it provides input to processes capable of generating verbalizations that are (in some sense) descriptive of it. Even our awareness_1 of stimuli demonstrably influencing our behaviour can be and frequently is quite limited (Nisbett & Wilson, 1977).

While this account is by no means unhelpful, it may place too much stress on verbalization, at least on overt vocalization. Those with a congenital inability to produce motor speech acts (anarthria) do not seem to lack linguistic comprehension nor to be less than fully human in their capacity for consciousness (Lenneberg, 1962; Fourcin, 1975.) From the perspective of contemporary cognitive psychology, one might better define $awareness_1$ (our awareness) in terms of the more general phenomenon of multiple information processing, and of a capability to metaprocess, i.e. to $process_1$ the fact that we are $processing_2$ some self-environment exchange such as shooing a fly (Battista, 1978). Inherent in this multiple processing is some division of internal self-reference: we are aware that we are shooing a fly.

In this sense, our consciousness implies a certain level of complexity in symbolic functioning. It is doubtful that the neonatal human possesses it, or that the cat possesses it. Indeed, in the sense of being able to metaprocess our own acts with any degree of accuracy, Piaget (1974) has demonstrated that human self-consciousness develops according to a timetable much like that for other human symbolic achievements. Consciousness, in our sense, is not a biological 'given' for any creature with a central nervous system; it is, rather, a symbolic construction dependent on the potential a central nervous system develops for self-referential metaprocessing and on whether or not we are in fact employing that potential at any particular moment in time. It seems highly unlikely that most of us employ that potential to its full extent most of the time (Jaynes, 1976; Rechtschaffen, 1975), or that the metaphor of a continuous 'stream of consciousness' (James, 1892) adequately fits our deployment of our potential for multiple, self-referential cognitive processing. Ontogenetically, the best evidence suggests that the symbolic processing on which human consciousness must depend does not appear until well into the second year of life (Inhelder *et al.*, 1972).

If dream experiencing depends on consciousness, ontogenetic evidence on self-consciousness does not suggest an earlier appearance of dreaming than does ontogenetic evidence on waking symbolism, for self-consciousness itself depends on symbolism. In fact there is reason to believe, from dream phenomenology (Rechtschaffen, 1978), that REM sleep is an environment that places more restrictive limits on our utilization of multiple self-referential processing than does wakefulness. Specifically, our capability to become aware, during REM sleep, *that* we are dreaming is much inferior to our capability of becoming aware, while we are thinking in wakefulness, *that* we are thinking. And, as we have seen, accurate self-reconstructions are remarkably slow in developing in children's REM dreams (Foulkes, 1982). Thus, one would have to imagine that the conditions of REM sleep are even less favourable than those of wakefulness for the demonstration in subhuman species of those forms of symbolism and mental processing on which consciousness depends.

There are several senses, then, in which the philosophical account that only language users can be (humanly) conscious seems substantially correct, if somewhat imprecise: (1) The cognitive bases of language are likely similar to the cognitive bases of consciousness; (2) As Trevarthan (Lenneberg, 1974) has suggested, social language must depend on children's development of a consciousness of the self as actor in relation to particular characterizations of events and persons outside that self — a 'sense of intersubjectivity', in which one has things to communicate to other actors not dissimilar to one's self (see also Bates, 1979); (3) Human neuropsychological observation (LeDoux *et al.*, 1979) suggests that the surgically isolated human right brain hemisphere shows genuine self-consciousness only to the degree that it retains substantial language function.

LeDoux *et al.* go on to argue that, since the right-hemisphere performance of split-brain patients without substantial right-lateralization of language function does *not* suggest independent right-hemisphere consciousness, and since the behaviour of most subhuman species does not suggest cognitive aptitude superior to that evidenced by these patients' right-hemisphere-mediated performance, then it is unlikely that other species share consciousness, in our sense. These authors view self-consciousness as a verbal interpretation that can be supplied for sensorimotor acts, and see human uniqueness lying in our 'ability to verbalize and in so doing create a personal sense of reality and conscious unity out of the multiple mental systems present' (p. 550).

By linguistic criteria, as we have seen, the prospects for subhuman consciousness, even in other primates, seem gloomy indeed. But it would be wise not altogether to foreclose that possibility for the great apes. Gallup (1970, 1977) observed that chimpanzees (but not monkeys) responded to mirror reflections as if they were self-representations, rather than 'other' organisms. This demonstration (I [here] see me [there]) seems to suggest that higher subhuman primates may be capable of the kind of multiple, self-referential cognition on which consciousness depends. At the same time, it casts further doubt on whether the subprimate organisms most fervently advanced as dream candidates (cats, dogs) even possess the kind of consciousness necessary for dreaming. Interestingly enough, studies cited by Gallup (1977) suggest that children do not show mirror self-recognition until their approach to their second birthday.

At best, Gallup's observations suggest that chimpanzees might be able to dream. It is worth mentioning, however, another possible impediment to their actually doing so. As Premack (1975) has observed, chimpanzees do not:

> construct copies of existing or imaginary figures by any device — drawing, assembling pieces of existing material, or otherwise. In this apparent failure to reproduce or transform parts of the visual world, the ape differs from man no less profoundly than it does in the case of language. (p. 228)

This production deficit, even more germane to the dream question than the linguistic one, reminds us that sufficient conditions of dream experiencing include not only possession of adequate symbolic representations but also possession of and proclivity to employ operations that work on such representations to produce the creative imagery of dream experience.

Gallup's observations provide a convenient bridge for our return to the human dream, its nature and its possible functions. Fraiberg and Adelson (1975) have reported that blind children are defective in constructing an adequate self-representation, and have suggested that this is because they lack the opportunity to see that kind of mirror-image visual representation that best promotes a sense of the self as a totality, and as a totality that can be externalized into a world of other selves. Even under more optimal conditions, nature can be somewhat stingy in its affordance of opportunities for mirror-image self-portrayals. It is interesting to 'reflect' that, except for the most narcissistic souls among us, we probably 'see ourselves' more frequently in our dreams than in any other circumstances. Could this indicate a possible function (effect) of REM dreaming? Specifically, could visual dreaming promote (as personality theorists would have it, but for different reasons) the growth of 'self', i.e. of a continuing and well-defined representation of what's inside our skins *vis-à-vis* what's outside them?

10.7 Human Implications of the Phylogenetic/Ontogenetic Review

My review of evidence pertinent to the question of subhuman dreaming suggests that other species do not, and largely cannot, experience dreams. Human dreaming represents the joining together of certain permissive patterns of general neural activation during sleep (most saliently, REM sleep) with specific neurocognitive systems which permit the exploitation of this permissive environment for the production of consciously experienced symbolic acts. The patterns of general neural activation ('REM sleep') cannot, in and of themselves, produce dreaming and, because of the absence of the specific neurocognitive conditions of consciousness and of spontaneous and creative symbolism in all or almost all other mammalian species, the REM sleep of other mammals does not index dreaming. We dream because we can; other species don't, because they can't. This viewpoint finds supporting evidence in the ontogenesis of human dreaming, in which dreaming unfolds in synchrony not with changes in 'REM sleep' but with changes in symbolic capability (Foulkes, 1982).

Having staked out what I believe to be a reasonable answer, given our current knowledge, to the question of animals' dreaming, I would now, as promised in the introduction to this chapter, like to consider the possible implications of my answer for the problem of the functions of dreaming. Does dreaming have a function or some functions? It scarcely seems conceivable that so much symbolic activity could occur during our lifetimes, and leave no traces behind, have no effects. It seems unlikely, however, that these effects could be critical to elementary requirements of realworld adaptation or of body-state maintenance, because such requirements arise (and are met satisfactorily) long before the presumed evolutionary appearance of dreaming. Even if one focuses on *how* these requirements are met (in fixed action patterns in lower mammals vs. in increasingly flexible and environmentally programmable ways in subhuman primates), it does not seem that flexibility and programmability *per se* can be intimately linked with dreaming, for the former again predate the latter.

I would suggest, then, that it is most plausible to look for dream functions that uniquely fit the level at which dreaming itself first appears. Specifically, it seems most appropriate to think about dream functions intra-symbolically. If dreaming has any critical role to play in the larger fabric of our lives, that role must be in relation to the synchronously appearing phenomena of self-consciousness and symbolic metaprocessing.

Prehuman data and considerations, then, seem unlikely sources for measurably advancing our thinking about dream function. On the other hand, a kind of evidence that is highly pertinent, and highly suggestive as well, can be found in the particular forms of symbolism and the particular mental operations evident in our own dreams. Although it may be a given that organisms with capability of self-consciousness, of symbolic representation, and of 'operational' organization of symbolic representations will experience *some kind* of semi-continuous mental experience during sleep, it is by no means self-evident why our REM dream thinking almost invariably assumes the particular form that it does.

For example, our dream thinking is narratized. We create world-analogues, and imagine interrelated temporal sequences of activity within those world-analogues. The serial integration of consciously experienced dream content suggests that dreaming may serve some integrative function in our organization of knowledge, most specifically in our organization of knowledge susceptible to 'conscious' recall (i.e. Piaget's 'evocative', as opposed to 'recognition' memory). What sort of integration might this be? Perhaps it is both within and across different modalities of conscious memory organization, e.g. Tulving's (1972) 'episodic' and 'semantic' memory systems. Thus, although the dream typically makes at least occasional reference to actual life experiences we have had ('episodes'), it also intermingles them, and weaves them together with wholly new experiences fabricated from our general ('semantic') knowledge of what the world is like.

Our dream thinking is experienced in generally vivid sensory imagery, although its sources and very construction seem also to depend on verbal knowledge and 'inner speech' (Foulkes, 1978; Epstein & Simmons, 1983). The suggestion here is of an integration or cross-referencing of conscious memory at the level of verbal and visuo-spatial coding systems.

Our dreams generally contain both memories or knowledge that we recognize as having been very recently acquired (Freud's [1900] 'day residues') and knowledge-representations that we recognize (more dimly, perhaps) as deriving from our more distant past. There is the possibility that dreaming links recent evocative memories to more persistent ones. That the dream itself often is forgotten may simply indicate that the fact of linkage is important, while the means is not.

Increasingly through childhood (Foulkes, 1982), and most strongly in adult life, our dreams are, by the standards of waking life, unrealistic. They portray experiences unlikely to be afforded by waking life, and do so in such a convincing manner that we are not immediately able to discount or terminate their improbabilities and impossibilities. I can see at least two kinds of effect that might follow from our nocturnal participation in a theatre of the absurd. First, dreams greatly expand upon the range of experience permitted by the socialized routines of our waking lives. If socialization prepares our self-awareness for adaptive adjustment, dreaming may prepare it for adaptive innovation. Second, precisely because dreams go well beyond the limits of predictable waking experience, and in a context in which we are able to determine their falsity as such experience (i.e. by virtue of what it means to 'wake up'), they may aid in the development of reality testing. That is, dreams permit the formation of control mechanisms commensurate with the major risk inherent in our symbolic development: that we will take as literally real (i.e. part of our everyday commerce with the world) everything that we are able to conceive (cf. Applebee, 1978).

Finally, our dream thinking is heavily self-referential. The most frequent character in our dreams is a 'self' character and, freed from external control and monitoring, our dreams examine our own, intensely personal concerns, rather than those urged upon us by others or by the larger society in which we spend our waking lives. Ontogenetically, dreaming assumes its most characteristic adult form just as children's self-knowledge becomes organized in a systematic and relatively realistic way. Dreaming may be a medium through which knowledge at the level of motor memory and recognition memory becomes recoded and interrelated as conscious 'self-knowledge' (cf. Rycroft, 1979). Certainly, over time children's dreams become better and better able to portray a conscious self-representation with the behavioural, affective and cognitive properties which other observers earlier can recognize in wakefulness (Foulkes, 1982). The transfer of knowledge from motor and recognition memory to consciously retrievable memory may serve the function of permitting relatively inflexible forms of knowledge coding to be operated on by the more flexible and generalizable processes of conscious memory (Rozin, 1976; Davidson, 1980).

These are several ways of thinking about dream function that are compatible with the phylogenetic and ontogenetic conclusions drawn above. They are not meant as precise hypotheses. At present, it is perhaps sufficient merely to begin the process of reconceptualizing the problem of dream function in ways that are more appropriate to what our dreams in fact are like and to the kinds of cognitive-symbolic capabilities that must be deployed in constructing them. Empirical entailments may follow, although as I already have indicated, there are few grounds for immediate optimism about the possibility of confirming *any* theory of dream function. The particular possibilities I am suggesting do, however, have some unique implications for the more general problem.

For instance, one recurring difficulty in thinking about the function of dreams is whether dreaming actually could participate in achieving whatever functions one suspects it to have, or whether dream experiences are simply epiphenomena of other cognitive or brain processes occurring during sleep that have both the supposed effects of dreaming *and* dreaming itself as their consequences. Insofar as one proposes dream functions at a level of consciousness and conscious self-representations, it scarcely seems likely that the dream itself would not participate in the process of change.

There are significant methodological implications, as well, of the sort of position for which I am arguing. For example, behaviouristically influenced research paradigms may not be adequate to test functional hypotheses specifying variables at the level of the organization of conscious experience around a self reference. Neither lever-press nor questionnaire score will prove sufficient to determine something as subtle and complex as the way one organizes one's conscious self-representations. In principle, there must be reliable means by which such a process *can* be indexed, but it is a mark of the primitivity of our approach as psychologists to things truly human that at present we scarcely can imagine what they might be. Our continuing ignorance of dream function and our inability experimentally to demonstrate such function may well reflect the scientific inappropriateness of continuing to act as if rat and cat methods can answer significant human questions. To understand dreams, as to understand language, the phylogenetic implication of this essay is that there's no place to start but at the very top.

References

APPLEBEE, A. N. (1978). *The child's concept of story: Ages two to seventeen*. Chicago: University of Chicago Press.

ALLISON, T., and VAN TWYVER, H. (1970). The evolution of sleep. *Natural History*, **79**, 56–65.

ARKIN, A. M., ANTROBUS, J. S., ELLMAN, S. J. and FARBER, J. (1978). Sleep mentation as affected by REMP deprivation. In: A. M. ARKIN, J. S. ANTROBUS and S. J. ELLMAN (Eds.), *The mind in sleep: Psychology and psychophysiology*, Hillsdale, NJ: Lawrence Erlbaum, pp. 459–484.

ASERINSKY, E. and KLEITMAN, N. (1953). Regularly occurring periods of eye motility, and concomitant phenomena, during sleep. *Science*, **118**, 273–274.

BATES, E. (1979). *The emergence of symbols: Cognition and communication in infancy*, New York: Academic Press.

BATTISTA, J. R. (1978). The science of consciousness. In: K. S. POPE and J. L. SINGER (Eds.), *The stream of consciousness: Scientific investigations into the flow of human experience*, New York: Plenum Press, pp. 55–87.

BROWN, J. N. and CARTWRIGHT, R. D. (1979). Locating NREM dreaming through instrumental responses (review). *Sleep Research*, **8**, 352–355.

COHEN, D. B. (1979). *Sleep and dreaming: Origins, nature and functions*, Oxford: Pergamon Press.

DAVIDSON, R. J. (1980). Consciousness and information processing: a biocognitive perspective. In: J. M. DAVIDSON and R. J. DAVIDSON (Eds.), *The psychobiology of consciousness*, New York: Plenum Press, pp. 11–46.

DEMENT, W. (1958). The occurrence of low voltage, fast, electroencephalogram patterns during behavioural sleep in the cat. *Electroencephalography and Clinical Neurophysiology*, **10**, 291–296.

DEMENT, W. C. (1965). An essay on dreams. *New Directions in Psychology*, **2**, 135–257.

DEMENT, W. and KLEITMAN, N. (1957). The relation of eye movements during sleep to dream activity: An objective method for the study of dreaming. *Journal of Experimental Psychology*, **53**, 339–346.

DENNETT, D. G. (1969). *Content and consciousness*, London: Routledge & Kegan Paul.

ELLMAN, S. J., SPIELMAN, A. J., LUCK, D., STEINER, S. S. and HALPERIN, R. (1978). REM deprivation: a review. In: A. M. ARKIN, J. S. ANTROBUS and S. J. ELLMAN (Eds.), *The mind in sleep: Psychology and psychophysiology*, Hillsdale, NJ: Lawrence Erlbaum, pp. 419–457.

EPSTEIN, A. W. and SIMMONS, N. N. (1983). Aphasia with reported loss of dreaming. *American Journal of Psychiatry*, **140**, 108–109.

EPSTEIN, R., LANZA, R. P. and SKINNER, B. F. (1980). Symbolic communication between two pigeons (*Columbia livia domestica*). *Science*, **207**, 543–545.

FLAVELL, J. H. (1963). *The developmental psychology of Jean Piaget*, Princeton, NJ: D. Van Nostrand.

FOSS, D. J. and HAKES, D. T. (1978). *Psycholinguistics: An introduction to the psychology of language*, Englewood Cliffs, NJ: Prentice-Hall.

FOULKES, D. (1962). Dream reports from different stages of sleep. *Journal of Abnormal and Social Psychology*, **65**, 14–25.

FOULKES, D. (1978). *A grammar of dreams*, New York: Basic Books.

FOULKES, D. (1979). Home and laboratory dreams: four empirical studies and a conceptual reevaluation. *Sleep*, **2**, 233–251.

FOULKES, D. (1982). *Children's dreams: Longitudinal studies*, New York: John Wiley.

FOULKES, D. and VOGEL, G. (1965). Mental activity at sleep onset. *Journal of Abnormal Psychology*, **70**, 231–243.

FOURCIN, A. J. (1975). Language development in the absence of expressive speech. In: E. H. LENNEBERG and E. LENNEBERG (Eds.), *Foundations of language development: A multidisciplinary approach. Vol. 2*, Paris: UNESCO Press, pp. 263–268.

FRAIBERG, S. and ADELSON, E. (1975). Self-representation in language and play: observations of blind children. In: E. H. LENNEBERG and E. LENNEBERG (Eds.), *Foundations of language development: A multidisciplinary approach. Vol. 2*, Paris: UNESCO Press, pp. 177–192.

FREUD, S. (1955). *The interpretation of dreams*, New York: Basic Books, (orig. 1900).

GALLUP, G. G. (1970). Chimpanzees: self-recognition. *Science*, **167**, 86–87.

GALLUP, G. G. (1977). Self-recognition in primates: a comparative approach to the bidirectional properties of consciousness. *American Psychologist*, **32**, 329–338.

GARDNER, M. (1980). Monkey business. *New York Review of Books*, 20 March, pp. 3–6.

GARDNER, R. A. and GARDNER, B. T. (1969). Teaching sign language to a chimpanzee. *Science*, **165**, 664–672.

GAZZANIGA, M. S. and LEDOUX, J. E. (1978). *The integrated mind*, New York: Plenum Press.

GRIFFIN, D. R. (1976). *The question of animal awareness: Evolutionary continuity of mental experience*, New York: Rockefeller University Press.

GRIFFIN, M. L. and FOULKES, D. (1977). Deliberate pre-sleep control of dream content: an experimental study. *Perceptual and Motor Skills*, **45**, 660–662.

HOBSON, J. A. and MCCARLEY, R. W. (1977). The brain as a dream state generator: an activation-synthesis hypothesis of the dream process. *American Journal of Psychiatry*, **134**, 1335–1348.

INHELDER, B., LEZINE, I., SINCLAIR, H. and STAMBAK, M. (1972). Les débuts de la fonction symbolique. *Archives de Psychologie*, **41**, 187–243.

JACOBSON, A., KALES, A., LEHMANN, D. and ZWEIZIG, J. R. (1965). Somnambulism: All-night electroencephalographic studies. *Science*, **148**, 975–977.

JAMES, W. (1892). *Psychology (briefer course)*, New York: Henry Holt.

JAYNES, J. (1976). *The origin of consciousness in the breakdown of the bicameral mind*, Boston, Mass: Houghton Mifflin.

JOUVET, M. (1962). Recherches sur les structures nerveuses et les mécanismes responsables des différentes phases de sommeil physiologique. *Archives of Italian Biology*, **100**, 125–206.

JOUVET, M. (1980). The functions of dreaming: a neurophysiologist's point of view. Presented to Association for the Psychophysiological Study of Sleep, 27 March 1980, Mexico City.

KERR, N. H., CORBITT, R. and JURKOVIC, G. J. (1980). Mental rotation: Is it stage-related? *Journal of Mental Imagery*, **4**, 49–56.

KERR, N. H. and FOULKES, D. (1981). Right-hemispheric mediation of dream visualization: a case study. *Cortex*, **17**, 603–610.

KERR, N. H., FOULKES, D. and JURKOVIC, G. J. (1978). Reported absence of visual dream imagery in a normally sighted subject with Turner's syndrome. *Journal of Mental Imagery*, **2**, 247–264.

KIRTLEY, D. D. (1975). *The psychology of blindness*, Chicago: Nelson-Hall.

KLEIN, M., MICHEL, F. and JOUVET, M. (1964). Etude polygraphique du sommeil chez les oiseaux. *Comptes Rendus des Séances de la Société de Biologie*, **158**, 99–103.

KRAMER, M. (1981). The function of psychological dreaming: a preliminary analysis. In: W. P. KOELLA (Ed.), *Sleep 1980*, Basel: Karger, pp. 182–185.

LEDOUX, J. E., WILSON, D. H. and GAZZANIGA, M. S. (1979). Beyond commissurotomy: clues to consciousness. In: M. S. GAZZANIGA (Ed.), *Handbook of Behavioral Neurobiology, Vol. 2*, New York: Plenum Press, pp. 543–554.

LENNEBERG, E. H. (1962). Understanding language without ability to speak: a case report. *Journal of Abnormal and Social Psychology*, **65**, 419–425.

LENNEBERG, E. H. (1974). Language and brain: developmental aspects. *Neurosciences Research Program Bulletin*, **12**, 513–656.

LUCE, G. G. (1965). *Current research on sleep and dreams*, Washington, DC: US Govt Printing Office (PHS publication **1389**).

LUCE, G. G. and SIEGEL, J. (1966). *Sleep*, New York: Coward-McCann.

McGrath,, M. J. and Cohen, D. B. (1978). REM sleep facilitation of adaptive waking behavior: a review of the literature. *Psychological Bulletin*, **85**, 24–57.
McNeill, D. (1979). *The conceptual basis of language*, Hillsdale, NJ: Lawrence Erlbaum.
Morrison, A. R., Mann, G. and Hendricks, J. C. (1980). Paradoxical sleep without atonia and increased exploratory behaviour in wakefulness: effects of pontine lesions. *Sleep Research*, **9**, 36 (Abstract).
Nisbett, R. E. and Wilson, T. D. (1977). Telling more than we can know: verbal reports on mental processes. *Psychological Review*, **84**, 231–259.
Piaget, J. (1976). *The grasp of consciousness: Action and concept in the young child*, Cambridge, Mass.: Harvard University Press, (orig. 1974).
Piaget, J. and Inhelder, B. (1971). *Mental imagery in the child*. New York: Basic Books (orig. 1966).
Premack, D. (1971). Language in chimpanzee? *Science*, **172**, 808–822.
Premack, D. (1975). Putting a face together. *Science*, **188**, 228–236.
Premack, D. (1976). *Intelligence in ape and man*. Hillsdale, NJ: Lawrence Erlbaum.
Premack, D. and Woodruff, G. (1978). Chimpanzee problem-solving: a test for comprehension. *Science*, **202**, 532–535.
Rechtschaffen, A. (1975). Scientific method in the study of altered states of consciousness with illustrations from sleep and dream research. In: *Altered states of consciousness: Current views and research problems*, Washington, DC: Drug Abuse Council, pp. 135–191.
Rechtschaffen, A. (1978). The single-mindedness and isolation of dreams. *Sleep*, **1**, 97–109.
Rechtschaffen, A. and Kales, A. (Eds.) (1968). *A manual of standardized teminology, techniques and scoring system for sleep stages of human subjects*, Washington, DC: US Govt Printing Office (NIH publication **204**).
Rozin, P. (1976). The evolution of intelligence and access to the cognitive unconscious. *Progress in Psychobiology and Physiological Psychology*, **6**, 245–280.
Rycroft, C. (1979). *The innocence of dreams*, New York: Pantheon.
Sastre, J. P. and Jouvet, M. (1979). Le comportement onirique du chat. *Physiology and Behaviour*, **22**, 979–989.
Savage-Rumbaugh, E. S. and Rumbaugh, D. M. (1979). Chimpanzee problem comprehension: insufficient evidence. *Science*, **206**, 1201–1202.
Savage-Rumbaugh, E. S., Rumbaugh, D. M. and Boysen, S. (1980a). Do apes use language? *American Scientist*, **68**, 49–61.
Savage-Rumbaugh, E. S., Rumbaugh, D. M., Smith, S. T. and Lawson, J. (1980b). Reference: the linguistic essential. *Science*, **210**, 922–925.
Shallice, T. (1978). The dominant action system: an information-processing approach to consciousness. In: K. S. Pope and J. L. Singer (Eds.), *The stream of consciousness: Scientific investigations into the flow of human experience*, New York: Plenum Press, pp. 117–157.
Shantz, C. U. (1975). *The development of social cognition*, Chicago: University of Chicago Press.
Skinner, B. F. (1963). Behaviorism at fifty. *Science*, **140**, 951–958.
Terrace, H. S., Petitto, L. A., Sanders, R. J. and Bever, T. G. (1979). Can an ape create a sentence? *Science*, **206**, 891–902.
Thompson, C. R. and Church, R. M. (1980). An explanation of the language of a chimpanzee. *Science*, **208**, 313–314.
Tulving, E. (1972). Episodic and semantic memory. In. E. Tulving and W. Donaldson (Eds.), *Organization of memory*, New York: Academic Press, pp. 381–403.
Vaughan, C. J. (1963). The development and use of an operant technique to provide evidence for visual imagery in the rhesus monkey under 'sensory deprivation'. PhD dissertation, University of Pittsburgh.
Vogel, G. W. (1975). A review of REM sleep deprivation. *Archives of General Psychiatry*, **32**, 749–761.

WEITZMAN, E. D., KRIPKE, D. F., POLLACK, C. and DOMINGUEZ, J. (1965). Cyclic activity in sleep of *Macaca mulatta*. *Archives of Neurology*, **12**, 463–467.

WILLIAMS, R. L., KARACAN, I. and HURSCH, C. J. (1974). *Electroencephalography (EEG) of human sleep: Clinical applications*, New York: John Wiley.

WOODRUFF, G., PREMACK, D. and KENNEL, K. (1978). Conservation of liquid and solid quantity by the chimpanzee. *Science*, **202**, 991–994.

CHAPTER 11

Overview: Comments on General Themes and a Discussion of Sleep Pathology

Andrew Mayes

11.1 Introduction

This book comprises chapters which specifically review theories of sleep (Webb), rhythmical aspects of sleep (Hume), sleep phylogeny (Meddis), sleep ontogeny (Harper, Frostig and Taube, and Zepelin), physiological and biochemical mechanisms of quiet and active sleep control (Steriade, Siegel, and Borbély), the nature of human dreaming and its potential occurrence in non-human animals (Foulkes), and the possible functional significance of sleep (Horne). These reviews highlight the impact on thinking about sleep, made by the use of new techniques and approaches. Part of this impact has been the undermining of hypotheses advanced in the 1960s and 1970s. For example, research by Siegel and his co-workers (see Chapter 7) has cast doubt on Hobson, McCarley and Wyzinski's (1975) hypothesis that active sleep (AS) is controlled by a reciprocity of firing levels in neurons of the locus coeruleus and giganto-cellular tegmental field (FTG). It now seems that the increased firing of FTG neurons is not uniquely associated with AS onset and maintenance, but rather, more generally to movement, or at least, activity in motor neurons.

Conclusions about sleep phylogeny, ontogeny, mechanisms and functions must be tentative and may often be polemical. Nevertheless, there is a broad consensus among the contributors that AS and quiet sleep (QS) reflect basically distinct processes. (There is not, however, agreement about terminology. Some refer to REM sleep rather than AS and to slow wave sleep rather than QS. It is safest to regard AS as subsuming REM sleep and QS as subsuming slow wave sleep, in both phylogenetic and ontogenetic contexts). Levels of AS seem to be mainly controlled by a circadian clock, whereas those of slow wave sleep depend on a self-regulatory process, influenced by the duration of preceding wakefulness. These two kinds of sleep probably have different evolutionary histories and in mammals are weakly associated with each other. They appear to be controlled by distinct biochemical and physiological mechanisms and respond differently to sleep deprivation. Their early ontogenetic courses are also different as AS levels initially decline whereas slow wave sleep levels initially increase. Their later development and senescence also suggests the existence of two processes. The two kinds of sleep have been related to different types of mental activity, with AS having a special association with vivid dreaming.

Although sleep pathology is only incidentally discussed by some of the contributors it corroborates further the distinction between active and slow wave sleep processes. For example, narcolepsy may be seen as a disorder of the control mechanisms of AS. Sleep pathologies should also illuminate other aspects of sleep and as a recent taxonomy has galvanized research in this area, the next section will outline this classification and illustrate it with a few examples of sleep disorders.

11.2 Sleep Pathologies — The New Taxonomy

The nosology of sleep disorders was compiled by a special committee of the Association of Sleep Disorders Centers under the chairmanship of Howard Roffwarg (Association of Sleep Disorders Centers, 1979). The nosological classification was based on the natural clustering of clinical symptoms, including measures of EEG and autonomic activity, and did not rely on identification of hypothetical causes or tissue damage. The taxonomy is shown in Table 11.1. Its dependence on patient complaints is acknowledged and its creators regard it as 'a provisional working construct'. Its introduction is intended to encourage careful differential diagnosis, and the search for mechanisms and appropriate treatment.

Table 11.1 shows four major kinds of disorder comprising disorders of sleep initiation and maintenance (the insomnias or DIMS), disorders of excessive somnolence (the hypersomnias or DOES), disorders of the sleep–wake rhythm (circadian rhythm problems), and dysfunctions associated with sleep (the parasomnias). A recent review of disorders in these four categories is given by Weitzman (1981). It is clear that different kinds of complaint (e.g. insomnia or hypersomnia) may be associated with apparently similar causes. For example, sleep-induced respiratory impairments lead to both DIMS and DOES. Complaints of insomnia are, however, mainly associated with central apnea (cessation of breathing), which is most severe in AS, especially during REM bursts. In contrast, complaints of excessive sleep are more often linked to obstructive and sub-obstructive apneas (absence of, or reduced, airflow with respiratory effort) and mixed apnea (central and obstructive apnea). These apneas are also more severe in AS and, in some patients, may be accompanied by cardiac arrhythmias (see Weitzman, 1981, for a discussion). They also increase with age (see Chapter 5).

The respiratory impairments so apparent in AS may represent an exaggerated form of the lability of this state. Several contributors have discussed the reduced thermoregulatory responses which are associated with it in mammals (see chapters by Meddis and Horne). The loss of thermoregulatory control in AS contrasts with its continued presence in quiet sleep. It also seems that normal mechanisms of respiratory control are markedly changed in AS. Thus, ventilation during AS is less responsive to increases in arterial carbon dioxide and other metabolic inputs, and respiratory control is not influenced by vagal mediation (see Orr, 1982, for a discussion). Parmeggiani (1979) has suggested these changes in AS may be caused by interruption of the integrative capacities of the hypothalamus, as he has found that anterior hypothalamic stimulation produces respiratory phase switching in QS, but not AS.

Frequent arousals may be important in protecting the organism from undesirable and potentially dangerous events which occur during sleep-events such as upper airway obstruction, gastro-oesophageal reflux and changes in

Table 11.1 Diagnostic Classification of Sleep and Arousal Disorders

DIMS: disorders of initiating & maintaining sleep (insomnias)

- Psychophysiological
  - Transient and situational
  - Persistent
- Associated with psychiatric disorders
  - Symptoms and personality disorders
  - Affective disorders
  - Other functional psychoses
- Associated with use of drugs and alcohol
  - Tolerance to or withdrawal from CNS depressants
  - Sustained use of CNS stimulants
  - Sustained use of or withdrawal from other drugs
  - Chronic alcoholism
- Associated with sleep-induced respiratory impairment
  - Sleep apnea DIMS syndrome
  - Alveolar hypoventilation DIMS syndrome
- Associated with sleep-related (nocturnal) myoclonus and 'restless legs'
  - Sleep-related (nocturnal) myoclonus DIMS syndrome
  - 'Restless legs' DIMS syndrome
- Associated with other medical, toxic and environmental conditions
- Childhood-onset DIMS
- Associated with other DIMS conditions
  - Repeated REM sleep interruptions
  - Atypical polysomnographic features
  - Not otherwise specified

DOES: disorders of excessive somnolence

- Psychophysiological
  - Transient and situational
  - Persistent
- Associated with psychiatric disorders
  - Affective disorders
  - Other functional disorders
- Associated with use of drugs and alcohol
  - Tolerance to or withdrawal from CNS stimulants
  - Sustained use of CNS depressants
- Associated with sleep-induced respiratory impairment
  - Sleep apnea DOES syndrome
  - Alveolar hypoventilation DOES syndrome
- Associated with sleep-related (nocturnal) myoclonus and 'restless legs'
  - Sleep-related (nocturnal) myoclonus DOES syndrome
  - 'Restless legs' DOES syndrome
- Narcolepsy
- Idiopathic CNS hypersomnolence

DOES: disorders of excessive somnolence (continued)

- Associated with other medical, toxic, and environmental conditions
- Associated with other DOES conditions
  - Intermittent DOES (periodic) syndromes
    - Kleine–Levin syndrome
    - Menstrual-associated syndrome
  - Insufficient sleep
  - Sleep drunkenness
  - Not otherwise specified
- No DOES abnormality
  - Longer sleeper
  - Subjective DOES complaint without objective findings
  - Not otherwise specified

Disorders of the sleep–wake schedule

- Transient
  - Rapid time zone change ('jet lag') syndrome
  - 'Work shift' change in conventional sleep–wake schedule
- Persistent
  - Frequently changing sleep–wake schedule
  - Delayed sleep phase syndrome
  - Advanced sleep phase syndrome
  - Non-24-hour sleep–wake syndrome
  - Irregular sleep–wake pattern
  - Not otherwise specified

Dysfunctions associated with sleep, sleep stages, or partial arousals (parasomnias)

- Sleepwalking (somnambulism)
- Sleep terror (pavor nocturnus, incubus)
- Sleep-related enuresis (bed-wetting)
- Other dysfunctions
  - Dream anxiety attacks (nightmares)
  - Sleep-related epileptic seizures
  - Sleep-related bruxism
  - Sleep-related headbanging (jactatio capitis nocturnus)
  - Familial sleep paralysis
  - Impaired sleep-related penile tumescence
  - Sleep-related painful erections
  - Sleep-related cluster headaches and chronic paroxysmal hemicrania
  - Sleep-related abnormal swallowing syndrome
  - Sleep-related asthma
  - Sleep-related cardiovascular symptoms
  - Sleep-related gastroesophageal reflux
  - Sleep-related hemolysis (paroxysmal nocturnal hemoglobinuria)
  - Asymptomatic polysomnographic finding
  - Not otherwise specified

ambient temperature (see Orr, 1982). Indeed, an arousal disorder has been suggested as one of the underlying abnormalities in the sudden infant death syndrome (Harper *et al.*, 1981). On the other hand, as sleep apneas can be benign, or associated with complaints of insomnia or hypersomnia, it is unclear what the relationship between the respiratory disorder and sleep–wakefulness actually is. Although apneas may lead to arousal it may be that, in some cases, a neurological defect triggers both the apneas and the additional sleep disorders.

The psychoses have been associated with abnormal sleep patterns although the detailed evidence is often conflicting and confusing (see Mendelson *et al.*, 1977; Weitzman, 1981). There is evidence that actively ill schizophrenics do not show a normal compensatory rebound in response to AS deprivation, and even that this treatment may produce clinical improvement (see Mendelson *et al.*, 1977). The depressive disorders have been researched with somewhat clearer results (see Weitzman, 1981, and chapters by Hume and Borbély). Depressives frequently complain of insomnia and daytime sleepiness. Monopolar depressives have a sleep pattern with repeated awakenings and premature early morning arousal, reduced amounts of slow wave sleep, and a shortened latency to AS. These last two features are also characteristic of bipolar depressives, who also show extended night sleep and excessive daytime napping. Depression has been found to respond to total sleep deprivation (Rudolf *et al.*, 1977), prolonged AS deprivation (Vogel *et al.*, 1980), and phase advancing the sleep time of patients (Wehr *et al.*, 1979). The second manipulation relieves depression in endogenous, but not reactive cases, and the third has been reported only with bipolar depressives.

Vogel *et al.*, (1980) have claimed that patients who respond to AS deprivation also respond to tricyclic drugs, such as imipramine. The efficacy of these drugs can be predicted by their success in suppressing AS. Contrastingly, ECT was effective with patients who did not respond to deprivation or tricyclics. These findings may indicate that a catecholaminergic disorder underlies both depression and the AS anomaly. As catecholamine systems often interact antagonistically with cholinergic ones, it is therefore interesting to note that Sitaram *et al.* (1980) have reported that infusions of the cholinergic agonist arecoline advance the next AS episode to a greater extent in remitted endogenous depressives than controls, although the patients did not show reduced AS latencies on placebo nights. The success in reversing the symptoms of bipolar depressives by advancing their sleep time by 6 h suggests that there may also be a disorder in the circadian control of AS. Borbély has, however, suggested a deficiency in process S may underlie both depression and the sleep abnormality (see Chapter 8). The relationship between abnormalities in circadian timing of active sleep, neurotransmitter function and the affective psychoses remains to be unravelled.

If bipolar depressives suffer from a phase advance in the triggering of active sleep and possible 'sleepiness' as well, they constitute only one kind of disorder of sleep scheduling. The significance of these disorders has only recently been appreciated. For example, a severe form of insomnia has on careful examination been revealed as a delayed sleep phase syndrome (DSPS). Patients with DSPS cannot fall asleep at the desired clock time and may remain insomniac up to as late as 06.00. If not forced into a strict time schedule, they do fall asleep, sleep normally and awake refreshed. They may not, however, go to sleep until 03.00 or 04.00. They cannot phase advance their sleeping times to a socially acceptable hour. Standard drug treatments and home remedies are also ineffective. These patients can be successfully treated by progressively phase delaying their normal sleeping time (see Weitzman *et al.*, 1981, for a discussion). Over a period of about a week they are allowed to sleep 3 h later each day until their sleeping time is reset at the desired point.

Weitzman (1981) argues that DSPS patients have a reduced ability to phase advance their sleep time. This ability is an essential one for entraining the sleep–wakefulness cycle to the biological day as the approximate non-entrained length of this cycle is 25 h in humans. It enables normal individuals to remain entrained despite minor fluctuations in their bedtimes and arousal times. DSPS patients seem less capable of accommodating to such fluctuations — they cannot readjust after a late night. Several patients have now been reported who are unable to entrain to a 24-h day at all. These hypernychthermal patients develop 25 to 27-h biological days despite all attempts to entrain them. Weizman (1981) argues that this syndrome differs only in degree from the DSPS. Both syndromes are characterized by a reduction or loss in phase advance capability.

Normal individuals also have a greater ability to phase delay than to phase retard, a fact which explains why jet lag is usually more prolonged after west –east flights compared to east–west ones. Czeisler *et al.* (1982) have applied this knowledge in improving a system of rotating shift schedules. Their study involved a factory in which workers operated 8-h shifts. Every week these were begun 8 h earlier. The experimenters kept workers on a shift for longer to allow time for the phase shift to stabilize and phase delayed rather than advanced. This manipulation was accompanied by improvements in subjective satisfaction and health, less personnel turnover and greater worker productivity. The possibility of a Hawthorne effect should not, however, be excluded.

Just as disorders of sleep scheduling may illuminate and be illuminated by studies of normal circadian and ultradian control of sleep, so in the long run may study of hypersomnias throw light on the mechanisms of sleep control. One such disorder is narcolepsy which occurs in 40 per 10,000 of people (Dement *et al.*, 1979). It is characterized by inappropriate attacks of sleep to which may be added three additional symptoms: cateplexy (sudden loss of tone in striated muscles), sleep paralysis (in which the victim may be fully conscious and terrified) and hypnagogic hallucinations. As Weitzman (1979) describes, the major advance in understanding narcolepsy has been the realization that these auxiliary symptoms constitute fragments of the AS state. AS periods at sleep onset, whether this is at night or during afternoon naps, are typical in narcoleptics. The development of a model of the narcolepsy-cataplexy complex in dogs (Mitler & Derment, 1977) has helped establish that the idiopathic form of the disorder is genetically transmitted as an autosomal recessive trait-relatives of narcoleptics have a 60-fold greater risk of having the condition.

Narcolepsy is controlled by stimulant drugs with catecholaminergic actions, such as amphetamines or the tricyclics, which have the general effect of reducing AS. CNS diseases, which cause narcoleptic symptoms, have been shown to involve damage to the pontomesencephalic reticular formation (Hobson, 1975). Further, monosynaptic reflex activity is lost during AS, cataplexy and sleep paralysis in both humans and dogs (see Weitzman, 1981). Idiopathic narcolepsy is therefore probably an inherited reticular formation dysfunction which affects the control of AS in a fairly selective manner. The disorder may affect the threshold for triggering AS in a general way or alter its circadian timing so as to cause sleep-onset AS episodes. Different forms of the disorder suggest that the components of AS are controlled by separate neural structures, the coherent activity of which can break down. These possibilities may be testable using canine models.

The fourth category of sleep disorders — dysfunctions associated with sleep or partial arousals — also support the view that QS and AS are basically different forms of sleep. The dysfunctions tend to be non-uniformly distributed across sleep stages. For example, somnambulism, sleep terror and sleep-related enuresis are mainly confined to Stages 3 and 4 of QS. Similarly, abnormalities associated with generalized epileptic seizures are more likely to occur in QS than in AS (Broughton, 1978). Conversely, penile tumescence is more common in AS than QS, so that its absence from AS is regarded as pathognomonic of organic impotence (Karacan *et al.*, 1982). Similarly, sleep-related cluster headaches and chronic paroxysmal hemicrania are closely linked to the occurrence of AS episodes (see Weitzman, 1981). Although some events such as gastro-oesophageal reflux have not yet been related to specific sleep stages (Orr, 1982), it is clear that many dysfunctional events are so related.

In summary then, study of sleep disorders is valuable apart from its clinical significance because of the light it can throw on normal sleep control systems. It may also increase understanding of sleep's relationship to other basic drives. For example, the Kleine–Levin syndrome, a rare periodic hypersomnia, usually emerging in young males, is also associated with several other motivational abnormalities. Patients may periodically develop enormous and bizarre appetites, disturbed social interactions, sexual hyperactivity and exhibitionism, mood changes, hallucinations and amnesia (see Weitzman, 1981). It is uncertain whether the lesions underlying this condition, which are probably in hypothanlamic and limbic system structures, are of neural systems which integrate behaviour across these different systems or whether a number of independent systems are usually disturbed.

11.3 New Techniques and the Mechanisms of Sleep

A recent application of techniques for measuring regional cerebral hemodynamics, during daytime naps and wakefulness, has shown that blood flow changes within the hemispheres and particularly in brainstem-cerebellar areas of narcoleptics are opposite those seen in sleep apnea patients and normal subjects (Sakai *et al.*, 1980). This finding corroborates ideas derived from other sources, but the use of new techniques has not always done this as was indicated in this chapter's introduction. Techniques for recording and analysing both single unit and EEG activity have developed in the past decade. The ability to record from identified neurons in freely moving animals has altered conceptions about sleep mechanisms. Spectral analysis of EEG may also turn out to be essential for understanding the mechanisms underlying, and the possible functions of different components of sleep.

In his chapter, Borbély shows that all-night spectral analysis of EEG is a more sensitive gauge of the after-effects of hypnotics than is a standard analysis of the sleep stage pattern. He also found that recovery from sleep deprivation was associated with a rise in low frequency across sleep stages, including Stage 2 and AS — a change that could not be fully reflected in a sleep stage analysis. Feinberg *et al.* (1982) have also shown that the after-effects of excessive sleep involved reduced delta activity in the first and third QS periods. In comparison with these computer-detected changes, visual analysis showed changes only in the first period. Feinberg *et al.* used period analysis and reported that in period one the reduction was mainly in delta amplitude, whereas in period three it was mainly in delta duration. Although the potential significance of delta amplitude and duration remain to be discovered, Borbély argues plausibly that it is slow wave activity which represents his sleep-dependent process S, in whatever sleep stage the activity occurs. Horne's obligatory sleep may be identified with such slow wave activity, which could explain why not only deep QS, but also the early AS episodes are obligatory. If slow wave activity is not confined to Stages 3 and 4 it is likely to be fairly prominent in AS early in the night when Borbély's process S is dominant.

The appearance of slow wave activity in sleep seems to require a reduction of tonic activity in midbrain reticular formation (MRF) neurons. Steriade's unit recordings show that these neurons have decreased activity before the onset of EEG sleep signs. The MRF neurons monosynaptically excite thalamic targets in the medial-intralaminar nuclei. The second group of neurons produce cortical activation, characteristic of wakefulness and AS, by sending projections to sensory, motor and association cortex as well as caudate. The projections are, however, to discrete sites, as the neurons show little bifurcation. Not all MRF neurons are involved in this activating system as Steriade reported that more dorsally placed units have often got different discharge characteristics and may project downstream to the paramedian pontine reticular formation. This heterogeneity among MRF neurons probably explains earlier conflicting results.

It is less certain why MRF activity reduces to initiate QS. In the 1970s it was generally believed that other structures, particularly in the brainstem, actively inhibited the MRF. Popular structures for serving this role were the nucleus of the solitary tract, the preoptic area of the basal forebrain and the raphe system. Carlton (1981) summarizes the evidence, mainly drawn from lesion and stimulation studies, that these structures are active hypnogenic systems. These studies are not unequivocal as, for example, the raphe is itself a heterogeneous set of nuclei, and also, effects may arise from disturbance of fibres of passage. There is no direct evidence that any structures increase their activity to trigger sleep. Although few single unit recording studies have been done on the relevant systems it is well established that most raphe neurons decrease activity during the waking–sleeping transition (see McGinty, 1973) and Nakamura *et al.*'s (1981) study of cerebral glucose utilization in 74 structures gave no support to the notion of active hynogenic structures.

Whether sleep is initiated by reduction in MRF neuron activity, arising from an active inhibition or a decline in the number of excitatory inputs, remains then an open issue. If the suprachiasmatic nucleus (SCN) is the circadian clock in mammals of the rest–activity cycle, then further research may well find a relationship between SCN and MRF activity prior to sleep. Similar work on the endogenous sleep factors, such as substance S, discussed in Borbély's chapter, may well prove to be rewarding. Although sleep is made more likely with sensory deafferentation, the major triggers are endogenous factors associated with the circadian clock and length of preceding wakefulness. How these act has not yet been determined.

As Steriade and Siegel discuss, many neurons in the raphe nuclei and the locus coeruleus show decreased acitivity at sleep onset, and may virtually cease to fire altogether during active sleep. These changes are consistent with the popular view, that the dorsal raphe in particular, inhibits phasic signs of active sleep such as PGO spikes. As these neurons are serotonergic, and PCPA depletes serotonin levels, Borbély's claim that the drug reduces sleep by raising the threshold for the C-process, rather than affecting the self-regulatory sleep process S, makes sense. The occurrence of disturbing phasic components of active sleep in all states of consciousness would be expected to raise the threshold for sleep. The generality of these results is, however, an open issue. They are based on studies with cats, and recent observations of rats have failed to find a PCPA-related change in the distribution of PGO spikes across states. Although PCPA did not affect the frequency or distribution of PGO spikes (which remained confined to active sleep periods), the rats showed a reduction of up to 70–80% in total sleep time, a complete elimination of active sleep, and 305-fold increase in locomotor activity (Kaufman & Morrison, 1981). Serotonergic raphe units or other serotonergic systems in the rats may therefore play a direct role in controlling sleep (Borbély's process S). It is a moot point whether cats are more representative of mammals in this respect. Although a popular model for sleep researchers they do not, for example, show the clear rest–activity cycle found in rats.

Siegel shows in his chapter that the pontomedullary brainstem systems are sufficient for generating AS although more anterior structures probably modulate the state. Separate brainstem systems control the various phasic and tonic components of AS as distinct lesions can produce PGO spikes without AS, AS without atonia, and ultradian rhythmicity without AS. Harper, Frostig and Taube's review of early ontogeny, in which there is progressive coalescence of physiological signs that in adults form coherent state clusters, draws a similar picture for both AS and QS. The systems responsible for such coordinations have not however, been identified.

Attempts to find brainstem neurons which increase their firing rate only at the transition to, and during AS have been largely unsuccessful. Sakai *et al.* (1982) have, however, claimed to find such neurons in parts of the locus coeruleus and medulla, which they believe form a system responsible for atonia in AS, as lesions to these regions prevent atonia occurring. The small proportion of neurons showing these effects may explain Siegel's failure to replicate their results although the problem needs more study. Even so, it is interesting to note that the locus coeruleus neurons involved, are not noradrenergic but probably cholinergic and that local cholinergic stimulation has several times been reported to produce atonia (see Sakai *et al.*, 1982).

AS probably does involve increased activity in MRF neurons and these may well be cholinergic. Systemic injections of acetylcholine cause EEG arousal and the same effect is achieved when cholinomimetics are applied directly to the ascending tegmental cholinergic pathways. Injections of atropine have the opposite effect, producing EEG slow waves and reducing behavioural alertness. Acetylcholine is also differentially released at the cortex during wakefulness and AS (see Koella, 1981, for a review). It is also known that cholinomimetic drugs increase the probability of AS, as well as PGO spikes. Koella argues that serotonergic neurons inhibit such cholinergic mechanisms and that this inhibition declines at the onset of AS. He also makes the more controversial claim (see above) that the critical level of serotonergic activity is necessary for the initiation and maintenance of sleep. He rests this claim partly on an interpretation of PCPA effects, but also on evidence showing that increasing serotonin levels, locally or generally, enhances slow wave sleep while inhibiting active sleep. He also cites evidence that brain and pineal gland serotonin levels show a circadian rhythm, which corresponds to changes in sleep density. The status of this evidence needs to be clarified as there are conflicting data. For example, as already mentioned, McGinty (1973) found that serotonergic raphe neurons decrease their activity at sleep onset.

If Koella's (1981) claim that some serotonergic system (possibly in the area postrema rather than the raphe nuclei) initiates and maintains QS when its activity increases, is polemical, so is his claim that noradrenergic and dopaminergic neurons play a key role in maintaining high levels of cerebral vigilance. Equally controversial is his view that a certain level of activity in noradrenergic neurons (probably in the locus coeruleus) is necessary for the initiation and maintenance of AS. Although drugs which increase noradrenergic activity may increase waking arousal and improve mood, their other predominant effect is the suppression of AS. In their recent review, Vanderwolf and Robinson (1981) argued that cholinergic systems maintained one aspect of aroused wakefulness and initiated AS, but that no direct evidence supports the view that catecholamine systems initiate waking arousal or AS. Instead, they proposed that a putative kind of EEG arousal, associated *inter alia* with voluntary movements, is mediated by a different system perhaps using an amino acid neurotransmitter.

There is then conflicting evidence about the relation of serotonergic activity to waking and sleep states. There is uncertainty about the role of the noradrenergic neurons of the locus coeruleus. Only in the case of cholinergic systems (which may include Steriade's MRF arousal neurons) does some confidence exist that a system (or systems) have been identified which are involved in initiating waking arousal and AS. Finally, other work weakly suggests that certain endogenous polypeptides and proteins may selectively play roles in initiating and maintaining QS and AS. The conflicts occur not only between results using different techniques (e.g. lesion vs. recording), but also between results using similar techniques. Technical improvements should therefore clarify many issues in the near future. Important clues are already available. For example, the serotonergic neurons of the dorsal raphe and the noradrenergic neurons of the locus coeruleus are known mutually to inhibit each other, as well as showing progressively decreasing activity as an animal moves from waking to QS to AS. Furthermore, both systems exert a widespread non-specific inhibitory effect on forebrain neurons. Many observers believe that the resulting reduced spontaneous activity leads to an increased signal-to-noise ratio in affected neurons. The relationship of this change to arousal warrants investigation.

11.4 Some Comments on the Possible Functions of Sleep

The traditional method of determining the function of a process by preventing its occurrence has not proved successful with sleep. It has, however, supported the view that sleep comprises an obligatory component, the amount of which depends on preceding wakefulness and a facultative component, the amount of which is determined by factors such as boredom and time of day. How does this dichotomy relate to the view that sleep is a behavioural adaptation which serves no restorative functions? This view may be addressed as it applies to mammals, by examining how sleep components vary as a function of a species' constitutional features and ecological arrangements. If QS time is regarded as a rough index of the obligatory sleep component and AS sleep is regarded as an index of the facultative sleep component, then the analysis in Meddis's chapter can be seen to illuminate possible sleep functions.

The analysis shows that AS time is reduced in species exposed to more predatory danger, which is consistent with this state being one of high vulnerability. Amounts of AS are also greater in species in which the major period of growth for nervous tissue is postnatal. Meddis interprets this as an instance of neoteny. In neoteny, foetal and infant characteristics develop more slowly and persist into adulthood — a process which may confer an adaptive advantage as a general strategy. It may be therefore that the specific increase in AS time is a neotenous epiphenomenon of no functional significance. These conclusions are compatible with Meddis's finding that the length of AS episodes was reduced in species exposed to danger (confirming the state's vulnerability) and also, in species of small size. The brains of such animals would be very vulnerable to the loss of thermoregulatory control which characterizes AS (but see Horne's Chapter 9 for an alternative view to the one that AS is a poikilothermic state).

Although initial inspection suggested that body weight and exposure to danger were both negatively related to the amount of QS shown by a species, Meddis argues that these relationships are artefactual. Grazing showed a stronger relationship to QS — grazers showed less QS than non-grazers — and an analysis confined to non-grazing species showed no relationship between QS and either body weight or exposure to danger. The grazing variable was treated as dichotomous. It could relate to a species' manner of foraging in which case the use of a non-dichotomous foraging variable might suggest a different pattern of relationships. Alternatively, it might relate to constitutional differences between grazers and non-grazers, in which case a foraging analysis would be irrelevant. The inclusion of further species in future analyses may, in any case, alter the pattern of correlations. At present however, QS (and perhaps then obligatory sleep) has not been clearly linked in cross-species comparisons to either constitutional or ecological factors.

The issues are controversial as Zepelin in Chapter 5 questions Meddis's conclusions and methods with respect to cross-species comparisons. Further, he argues that analysis of sleep changes across life span suggest that the need for sleep and its intensity decrease as metabolic rate decreases. Analysis also suggested that the same relationship to metabolic rate held for declining AS time, but not, however, for declining delta wave activity. As Zepelin has argued that mammals with high metabolic rates tend to be long sleepers (Zepelin & Rechtschaffen, 1974), he believes these two sources of evidence support a relationship between metabolic rate and need for sleep. If the age-related decline in delta activity is related to a sleep need (which is unproved), this kind of sleep, which corresponds to Horne's obligatory sleep, may then serve functions unconnected with metabolic rate.

Although Meddis's evidence is neutral with respect to a restorational function for QS, Horne cites evidence which makes such a restorative function seem plausible. Even in species for which sleep constitutes a severe ecological risk (as in the giraffe, blind Indus and bottlenose dolphin), the state persists — indeed, special adaptations occur to ensure its continuity. The problem is that, although Horne argues that obligatory sleep is unlikely to be primarily concerned with restoring bodily processes in advanced mammals, no-one has identified convincing candidates for cerebral restoration. Some cerebral process(es) must change as a function of wakefulness in a way that leads to maladaptive results, and this process must be reversed by the processes of obligatory sleep.

Resolution of these uncertainties by future research involves several issues. First, there needs to be careful examination of the putative distinction between obligatory and facultative sleep. Several contributors suggest a distinction along these lines, but in Horne's view obligatory sleep involves both QS and AS from early in the sleep period. Are the restorative functions then heterogeneous or will spectral analysis identify one sleep process common to these stages (but most intense in deep QS)? Such a process would be non-circadian and sensitive to prior wakefulness. If the process involves slow wave, i.e. delta, activity, it still needs to be determined whether parameters like amplitude, number of waves, patterning of waves, etc. are significant. Second, there needs to be a careful analysis of neuronal activity and metabolism during this state, particularly in the neocortex. The relationship of EEG measures to underlying neuronal firing patterns and metabolism is still only vaguely understood. If there are restorative changes, certain metabolic and activity measures should change as the process continues. During wakefulness the identified change should proceed in the opposite direction with results which should eventually be maladaptive.

The main problem with this programme is separating the operation of sleep mechanisms from sleep functions. Both a restorative process and a sleep-controlling process would perhaps show the same kinds of changes during waking and sleep, but only if changes are associated with the latter process will their effects be maladaptive during prolonged wakefulness. Such effects are difficult to ascertain — deprivation studies have provided little help. The problem of interpreting exercise effects on slow wave sleep makes a similar general point. Recent evidence suggests that intense exercise increases subsequent slow wave sleep only because it raises core temperature, as passive heating has the same effect (Horne, submitted for publication.) Is the raising of core temperature increasing the rate of change of some process which must be restored by slow wave sleep, for normal functioning to continue, or is it directly activating a sleep-triggering system, inducing a kind of hyperthermic torpor? The same question must be asked of any other variables which increase the 'need' for slow wave sleep.

Sleep, like wakefulness, is a highly complex state which probably serves many functions. Leaving no fossil record, its evolutionary origins remain obscure. The ubiquity of a sleep-like state, however, suggests that it may be coeval with life itself, a reflection of the circadian rhythm imposed on the inchoate biological 'soups'. If there is a primitive circadian rest–activity cycle it is likely to have been adapted and modified many times in the course of evolution. The structure of sleep (like wakefulness) will differ radically across animal groups and so may its functions. Indeed, the same point applies within a group such as the mammals. As Horne argues, less advanced mammals may need sleep for energy conservation, a function partially served in humans by relaxed wakefulness. Differences between mammalian sleep and that of both contemporary reptiles and the reptilean ancestors of mammals will be more dramatic. Attempts to find precursors of QS and AS in reptiles, although theoretically important, are perhaps simplistic (see discussions by Horne and Meddis). Reptilian sleep may seem to share features with both kinds of mammalian sleep but serve different adaptive ends. For example, the EEG spikes seen in reptilian sleep (see discussions by Meddis and Horne) may not be homologous with either the PGO spikes or the limbic spike of slow wave sleep, but a functionally separate phenomenon.

In humans, although there is an ineluctable drive to sleep, much of the process may be facultative in Horne's sense. The restorative function(s) of obligatory sleep remain to be identified. Such a function is probably not associated with AS. Historically, this seems peculiar for, if Foulkes is correct, dreaming, which is closely related to AS, is unique to humans, and many theorists have and do believe that dreams perform some kind of cognitive maintenance function. A popular version of this position is that dreaming (or AS) is important for the stablization of memories (see Fishbein, 1981, for a discussion of the recent evidence). Although disturbances of AS affect memory in animals and humans, these effects are probably caused by indirect actions such as those on arousal level (see Chapter 9). The time-scale of the sleep effects make a stimulation of consolidation processes seem unlikely (see Mayes, 1981). The firing rate of association cortex interneurons increases selectively in AS however (see Chapter 6), and it may that this activity is conducive to the modification of both new and established memories.

If dreaming and AS influence memory, they are more likely to do so through a rehearsal of new and old experience, i.e. by reorganizing memory. Obviously this process can be performed on waking. In AS, however, external distractions are minimized and processing of information may be somewhat different from that of ordinary waking. It may be more visuo-spatial as there is evidence of greater right hemisphere activity in this state (see Gordon *et al.*, 1982). This is hardly a vital restorative function, but even so human dreaming may play a distinctive role in processing and reorganizing significant experiences so that later retrieval is facilitated. In support of this notion, Fiss *et al.* (1977) reported that dreaming about pre-sleep stimuli aided their recall, although recall accuracy was unrelated to waking rehearsal or REM density.

References

ASSOCIATION OF SLEEP DISORDERS CENTERS (1979). Diagnostic classification of sleep and arousal disorders, 1st edn, Sleep Disorders Classification Committee, H. P. Roffwarg (Chairman). *Sleep*, **2**, 1–137.

BROUGHTON, R. J. (1978). Sleep and epilepsy. In: *Epilepsy*, Berkshire, England: British Epilepsy Association.

CARLSON, N. R. (1981). *Physiology of Behavior*, 2nd edn, Boston, Mass: Allyn and Bacon.

CZEISLER, C. A., MORRE-EDE, M. C. and COLEMAN, R. M. (1982). Rotating shift work schedules that disrupt sleep are improved by applying circadian principles. *Science*, **217**, 460–463.

DEMENT, W. C., CARSKADON, M. and LEY, R. (1973). The prevalence of narcolepsy II. *Sleep Research*, **2**, 147.

FEINBERG, I. FEIN, G. and FLOYD, T. C. (1982). Computer-detected patterns of

electroencephalographic delta activity during and after extended sleep. *Science*, **215**, 1131–1133.
FISHBEIN, W. (1981). *Sleep, Dreams and Memory*, Lancaster, England: MTP Press.
FISS, H., KREMER, E. and LITCHMAN, J. (1977). The mnemonic function of dreaming. Presented to the Association for the Psychophysiological Study of Sleep.
GORDON, H. W., FROOMAN, B. and LAVIE, P. (1982). Shift in cognitive asymmetries between wakings from REM and NREM sleep. *Neuropsychologia*, **20**, 99–104.
HARPER, R. M., LEAKE, B., HOFFMAN, H., WALTER, D. O., HOPPENBROUWERS, T., HODGMAN, J. and STERMAN, M. B. (1981). Periodicity of sleep states is altered in infants at risk for the sudden infant death syndrome. *Science*, **213**, 1030–1032.
HOBSON, J. A. (1975). Dreaming sleep attacks and desynchronised sleep enhancement: report of a case of brain stem signs. *Archives of General Psychiatry*, **32**, 1421–1424.
HOBSON, J. A., MCCARLEY, R. W. and WYZINSKI, P. W. (1975). Sleep cycle oscillation: reciprocal discharge by two brainstem neuronal groups. *Science*, **189**, 55–58.
HORNE, J. A. and STAFFE, L. H. E. (submitted for publication). Exercise and sleep: mediation by body heating.
KARACAN, I., WILLIAMS, R. L., DERMAN, S. and ASLAN, C. (1982). Impaired sleep-related penile tumescence in the diagnosis of impotence. In: M. R. ZALES (Ed.), *Eating, Sleeping and Sexuality*, pp. 186–199. New York: Brunner/Mazel.
KAUFMAN, L. S. and MORRISON, A. R. (1982). The effect of acute administration of PCPA on selected parameters of sleep and waking in albino rats. Paper given at the 27th Oholo Biological Conference on Behavioural Models and the Analysis of Drug Action. Israel Institute for Biological Research.
KOELLA, W. P. (1981). Neurotransmitters and sleep. In: D. WHEATLEY (Ed.), *Psychopharmacology of Sleep*, New York: Raven Press, pp. 19–52.
MCGINTY, D. J. (1973). Neurochemically defined neurons: behavioural correlates of unit activity of serotonin- containing cells. In: M. T. PHILLIPS (Ed.), *Brain Unit Activity During Behaviour*, Springfield. Ill: Thomas, pp. 244–267.
MAYES, A. (1981). The physiology of memory. In: G. UNDERWOOD and R. STEVENS, (Eds.), *Aspects of Consciousness*. Vol. 2, *Structural Issues*, New York: Academic Press, pp. 1–38.
MENDELSON, W. B., GILLIN, J. C. and WYATT, R. J. (1977). *Human Sleep and its Disorders*, New York: Plenum Press.
MITLER, M. M. and DEMENT, W. C. (1977). Sleep studies on canine narcolepsy: pattern and cycle comparisons between affected and normal dogs. *Electroencephalography and Clinical Neurophysiology*, **43**, 691–699.
NAKAMURA, R. K. KENNEDY, C., GILLIN, J. C., SUDA, S., ITO, M., STORCH, F., MENDELSON, W., MISHKIN, M. and SOKOLOFF, L. (1981). Hypnogenic center theory of sleep: no support from 2-deoxyglucose studies in monkeys. *Abstracts of the Society for Neurosciences*, **7**, 234.
ORR, W. C. (1982). The biology of sleep: recent developments and clinical applications. In: M. R. ZALES (Ed.), *Eating, Sleeping, and Sexuality*, New York: Brunner/Marzel, pp. 105–128.
PARMEGGIANI, P. (1979). Integrative aspects of hypothalamic influences on respiratory brain stem mechanisms during wakefulness and sleep. In: C. VON EULER and H. LAGERCRANTZ (Eds.) *Central Nervous Control Mechanisms in Breathing*, New York: Pergamon Press, pp. 53–69.
RUDOLF, G. A. E., SCHILGEN, B. and TOLLE, R. (1977). Anti-depressive behandlung mittels schlafentzug. *Nervenarzt*, **48**, 1–11.
SAKAI, F., MEYER, J. S., KARACAN, I., DERMAN, S. and YAMAMOTO, M. (1980). Normal human sleep: regional cerebral hemodynamics. *Annals of Neurology*, **7**, 471–478.
SAKAI, K., SASTRE, J. P., KANAMORI, N. and JOWET, M. (1981). State-specific neurons in the pontomedullary reticular formation with special reference to postural atonia during paradoxical sleep in the cat. In: O. POMPEIANO and C. AJMONE

MARSAN (Eds.), *Brain Mechanisms and Conscious Awareness*, pp. 405–429.
SITARAM, N., NURNBERGER, J. I. jun., GERSHON, E. S. and GILLIN, J. C. (1980). Faster cholinergic REM sleep induction in euthymic patients with primary affective illness. *Science*, **208**, 200–202.
VANDERWOLF, C. H. and ROBINSON, T. E. (1981). Reticulo-cortical activity and behaviour: a critique of the arousal theory and a new synthesis (with commentaries). *Behavioral and Brain Sciences*, **4**, 459–514.
VOGEL, G. W., VOGEL, F., MCABEE, R. S. and THURMOND, A. J. (1980). Improvement of depression by REM sleep deprivation. *Archives of General Psychiatry*, **37**, 247–253.
WEHR, T., WIRZ-JUSTICE, A., GOODWIN, F. K., DUNCAN, W. and GILLIN, J. C. (1979). Phase advance of the circadian sleep-wake cycle as an antidepressant. *Science*, **206**, 710–711.
WEIZMAN, E. D. (1981). Sleep and its disorders. *Annual Review of Neuroscience*, **4**, 381–417.
WEITZMAN, E. D., CZEISLER, C. A., COLEMAN, R. M. SPIELMAN, A. J., ZIMMERMAN, J. C., DEMENT, W., RICHARDSON, G. and POLLAK, C. P. (1981). Delayed sleep phase syndrome. *Archives of General Psychiatry*, **38**, 737–746.
ZEPELIN, H. and RECHTSCHAFFEN, A. (1974). Mammalian sleep, longevity and energy metabolism. *Brain, Behavior and Evolution*, **10**, 425–470.

Author Index

Subject Index